GENE THERAPY APPLICATIONS

Edited by **Chunsheng Kang**

Gene Therapy Applications
Edited by Chunsheng Kang

Published by InTech
Janeza Trdine 9, 51000 Rijeka, Croatia

Publishing Process Manager Romina Krebel

Technical Editor Teodora Smiljanic

Cover Designer InTech Design Team

Additional hard copies can be obtained from orders@intechopen.com

Gene Therapy Applications, Edited by Chunsheng Kang
p. cm.
ISBN 978-953-307-541-9

For EU product safety concerns:
IN TECH d.o.o., Prolaz Marije Krucifikse Kozulić 3, 51000 Rijeka, Croatia,
info@intechopen.com or visit our website at intechopen.com.

Meet the editor

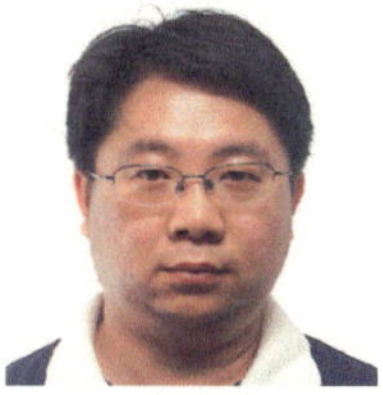

Dr. Chunsheng Kang is Professor and Vice-director at Lab of Neuro-oncology, Tianjin Neurological Institute, Department of neurosurgery, Tianjin Medical University General Hospital, P. R. China. He is a member of many professional societies, including American Association for Cancer Research and Chinese Neurosurgical Society. He is also a vice board chairman of Tianjin Genetics Society. Dr. Kang received his bachelor degree in medicine from Tianjin Medical University, P. R. China in 1993 and his Ph.D. in neurosurgery from Tianjin Medical University General Hospital, Tianjin, P. R. China in 2003. He specializes in RNAi in cancer, microRNA and signaling pathway in cancer, high-throughput analysis in cancer, nonviral gene delivery system. His research has received sustained funding from the Chinese Natural Science Foundation, "Program for New Century Excellent Talents in University" of Ministry of Education, Natural Science Foundation of Tianjin Municipal Science and Technology Commission and other foundations. Dr. Kang has supervised the research efforts of over 30 postdoctoral associates, doctoral candidates and master's level graduate students in the past 8 years.

Contents

Preface

In the face of extraordinary advances in the prevention, diagnosis, and treatment of human diseases, devastating illnesses such as heart disease, and cancer continue to deprive people of health. Recently, techniques have been developed for gene therapy, providing unprecedented opportunities for further studying and understanding human diseases. Although it is impossible to cure all human diseases, scientists and the public will gain immense new knowledge in the development of gene therapy that will likely hold remarkable potential for therapies.

This book aims to cover key aspects of the potential and existing problems in the emerging field of gene therapy application. With the contribution of leading pioneers in various disciplines of gene therapy, the book brings together major approaches of gene therapy application in one text. Given that a great deal of data has been gathered and insights have been provided by researchers around the world, we believe that it will provide detailed clinical experiences and facilitate research in gene therapy.

Dr. Chunsheng Kang
Professor at Lab of Neuro-oncology
Tianjin Neurological Institute
China

Part 1

Gene Therapy in Blood and Vascular System

1

Gene Therapy with Non-Viral Vectors For Critical Limb Ischemia: From Bench to Bedside

Erich Vinicius De Paula
Hematology and Hemotherapy Center, University of Campinas, Campinas, SP Brazil

1. Introduction

As knowledge about the cellular and molecular mechanisms that control vessel growth grew during the last two decades, therapeutic manipulation of angiogenesis was increasingly regarded as one of the most promising areas of translational research. Based on its potential to target key steps in the pathogenesis of disease groups with great impact on public health, therapeutic blockage and stimulation of angiogenesis emerged years ago, as the holy grail of research on new strategies to treat cancer and arterial occlusive diseases respectively. However, the result of these two related development processes were quite different. Anti-angiogenic therapy is today a reality in the treatment of cancer and diseases associated with pathological vessel growth such in the retina. In contrast, no strategy based on the concept of stimulating angiogenesis (usually referred as "therapeutic angiogenesis") has so far reached widespread clinical use.

1.1 The clinical problem: critical limb ischemia

Arterial occlusive disease (AOD) is the leading cause of morbidity and mortality in industrialized countries, and represents a problem of growing dimensions for developing countries (Beaglehole et al., 2003). Clinically, AOD includes acute myocardial infarction, stroke and peripheral arterial disease (PAD). PAD is defined as the obstruction of arterial blood flow, in areas other than the brain and heart (Garcia, 2006). When it affects the lower limbs, the clinical picture is silent in its early stages, progressing to intermittent claudication when the obstruction of blood flow reaches 50% of normal. Out of patients with intermitent claudication, between 15 and 20% are estimated to progress to critical limb ischemia (CLI) (Dormandy et al., 1989; Second European Consensus Document, 1991). The term critical limb ischemia (CLI) refers to the final stages of PAD, when chronic lack of blood supply sets off a cascade of pathophysiologic events that lead to rest pain, trophic lesions of the leg or both (Varu et al., 2010). The international consensus definition of CLI is the following: any patient with chronic ischemic rest pain, ulcers, or gangrene attributable to objectively proven arterial occlusive disease (Norgren et al., 2007). CLI patients represent approximately 1% of patients with PAD. The prognosis of these patients can be compared to some other malignancies, showing overall survival rates below 50% in 5 years (DormandyThomas, 1988).

The diagnosis of established CLI is straightforward, and based on the physical examination, the ankle:brachial index (ABI), and on several imaging methods. Despite progresses in medical care, the grim significance of CLI diagnosis does not seem to have changed significantly during the last decade, remaining a predictor of poor survival and poor outcomes (Varu et al., 2010). Observational studies of patients with CLI roughly agree on a 50% amputation-free rate after 1 year (with part of these patients still presenting symptoms), 25% of patients undergoing a major amputation and 25% will have died. In areas with poorer medical care, these numbers maybe even worse.

Current treatment of CLI is complex, involving both surgical and non-surgical approaches. The goal of treatment is to restore adequate blood supply. Ultimately, success should include relief of ischemic pain, healing of ischemic ulcers, prevention of limb loss, improvement of patient function and quality of life, while also prolonging survival. Revascularization, either surgical or endovascular, is the most straightforward and intuitive strategy to reach these goal. Unfortunately, revascularization is not always feasible for several reasons. First, CLI is not only a disease of large vessels, and widespread microvascular and/or surrounding tissues involvement at the time of diagnosis (resulting in poor outflow vessels in the limb) may hamper its success. Second, medical comorbidities, invariably present in CLI patients, may also limit surgery as a viable option. Last, even in patients referred to surgical revascularization, an extremely high immediate post-operative mortality rate that reaches 11.6% according to a recent meta-analysis (Albers et al., 2006) demonstrates the need for a thorough assessment of risks and benefits, underscoring the challenge of treating CLI. For patients for whom revascularization is not feasible for one of these reasons, limb loss rates after 6 months are near 50% (Brass et al., 2006), and amputation remains as the only option to treat CLI.

In conclusion, CLI represents a condition characterized by considerable morbidity and mortality, a high impact on quality of life, and suboptimal treatment options. These characteristics highlight the importance of devising new strategies to treat CLI.

1.2 Understanding the problem: pathophysiology of CLI

From a pathophysiological stand-point, CLI affects both macrovascular and microvascular systems, and is characterized by chronic deprivation of blood supply to limb tissues. With time, several changes in the structure and function of the vascular tree occur, including diminished sensitivity to vasodilatory stimuli, decreased wall to lumen ratio, lower nitric oxide production, and capillary microthrombi formation due to impaired anticoagulant function of the endothelium (Varu et al., 2010).

The natural response to tissue ischemia is the activation of several molecular and cellular pathways that result in the formation of new blood vessels, involving processes such as angiogenesis and arteriogenesis. However, in CLI patients, as in other forms of AOD, this response is not sufficient to provide the adequate amount of blood to ischemic tissues.

2. Therapeutic angiogenesis

Thirty years ago, Folkman observed that the development and maintenance of an adequate microvascular supply is as an essential condition for growth of neoplastic tissue (Folkman, 1971), laying the ground for the development of anti-angiogenic therapies and also for therapeutic angiogenesis. Later, the idea of boosting the formation of collateral vessels as a way to treat CLI, a strategy known as "therapeutic angiogenesis", was stimulated by angiographic and clinical observation that spontaneous development of collateral vessels was sufficient to preserve ventricular function in patients with ischemic heart disease (Habib et al., 1991). Therefore, it was not very long after the identification of the first angiogenic growth factors that the first experiments using Vascular endothelial growth factor (VEGF-A) were initiated, aiming to improve blood flow to ischemic tissues (Takeshita et al., 1994).

2.1 The rationale for therapeutic angiogenesis

For therapeutic angiogenesis to be justified from a theoretical standpoint, at least one of the following two conditions must be true: (1) the presence of decreased levels of angiogenic growth factors in ischemic tissues, or (2) the possibility of optimizing the endogenous response to ischemia through the use of supra-physiological doses of these factors. Regarding the first hypothesis, Schultz and colleagues demonstrated a positive correlation between the expression of VEGF-A stimulated by hypoxia in monocytes and the number of collaterals in the myocardium of patients with chronic coronary ischemia (Schultz et al., 1999). Furthermore, senile rabbits and mice exhibit subnormal angiogenic response, attributed to decreased levels of VEGF-A in ischemic tissues, and supplementation with exogenous VEGF-A reversed this subnormal angiogenic response (Rivard et al., 1999). A single study that evaluated the concentrations of these factors in muscle and skin of patients with PAD found normal levels of VEGF-A, and high levels of other angiogenic growth factor FGF-2, suggesting a relative deficiency of VEGF-A in these tissues (Palmer-Kazen et al., 2004). Regarding the second hypothesis, several studies have shown that supraphysiological doses of VEGF optimize the angiogenic response (Post et al., 2001), and this was indeed the rationale for most of the initial protocols for therapeutic angiogenesis. It should be noted however, that supraphysiological doses of VEGF-A and FGF-2 have also been shown to induce the formation of aberrant vessels (Sola et al., 1997; Ozawa et al., 2004), suggesting that the therapeutic window for this strategy may be narrow. For this reason, a detailed comprehension of the molecular and cellular events that govern the formation of new blood vessels is of paramount importance for the development of a successful therapeutic angiogenesis strategy.

2.2 The "how-to" of new blood vessels formation

In the human embryo, development of the vascular system begins with the formation of the blood islands, where hematopoietic and endothelial cell (EC) precursors (angioblasts) coexist (Choi et al., 1998). The differentiation of angioblasts in EC is called vasculogenesis, and is the process by which primitive tubes of EC are formed. Several additional steps are needed until a functional and mature vascular system is formed. During these processes, vascular sprouts emerge from pre-existing tubes, a process known as angiogenesis, and mural cells (pericytes and smooth muscle cells - SMC) are incorporated, a process termed arteriogenesis (Conway et al., 2001). The regulation of these steps is made through a complex network of vascular growth factors. To mention some, VEGF plays a critical role from early to later stages, which was demonstrated in knockout mice for the VEGF gene, which do not develop a vascular system (Carmeliet et al., 1997). Moreover, in an unusual observation, heterozygosity for the VEGF gene (+/-) determined the mortality of all animals, indicating the need for optimal concentrations of VEGF for vascular formation. The expression of VEGF occurs, among other stimuli, in response to hypoxia (Shweiki et al., 1992). It is now recognized that hypoxia induces expression of HIF-1α, which binds to a

promoter region of VEGF gene, driving its expression in ischemic areas (Kimura et al., 2000). FGF is another growth factor that promotes the proliferation and migration of EC. PDGF is essential for the recruitment of components of the vascular wall such as SMC, that stabilize EC by preventing their unregulated proliferation (Benjamin et al., 1998). Angiopoietin 1 is involved in the maintenance of vascular integrity (Thurston et al., 1999) and recruitment of smooth muscle cells (Suri et al., 1996). In conclusion, the formation of a mature arterial system starts with the proliferation of EC (vasculogenesis), followed by the sprouting of new capillaries (angiogenesis), and the maturation of the newly formed vessel by pericytes, smooth muscle cells and extracelular matrix (arteriogenesis).
Angiogenesis also occurs in post-embryonic life, in physiological situations such as the ovulatory cycle, wound healing, and in response to tissue ischemia, as in CLI. In addition, several pathological conditions are associated with increased angiogenesis, such as inflammation, proliferative retinopathy and growth and spread of tumors (Carmeliet, 2003). In general terms, it is acknowledged that post-natal angiogenesis recapitulates the mechanisms described in the embryo.

2.3 Gene therapy as the preferred platform for therapeutic angiogenesis

One of the most attractive aspects of therapeutic angiogenesis is that by increasing the formation of collateral vessels, one would be only intensifying what happens spontaneously in ischemic tissue. The simplicity of this idea, associated with the huge unmet needs of patients with CLI, resulted in a relatively rapid transition from preclinical to phase I and II trials, which were initiated with a level of expectation that was probably too unrealistic considering the amount of basic and translational research on post-natal angiogenesis available at that time.
Gene transfer was rapidly considered the preferred method for therapeutic angiogenesis. Using gene therapy (GT), genes of vascular growth factors could be directly injected into ischemic muscle, which would function both as the major therapeutic target, as well as a production site for these proteins. Several reasons make CLI an attractive target for GT. These include not only the limitations of available treatments for CLI, but also a series of very specific characteristics of CLI treatment that will be discussed next.

2.3.1 Requirement of lower levels of expression

A major obstacle to the success of GT in some hereditary diseases is the need to obtain high and sustained expression of the therapeutic gene. Initial observations suggested that therapeutic angiogenesis required minimal and only transient expression of angiogenic growth factors (Dor et al., 2002). This was interpreted as a possibility to obtain therapeutic effects with less and more simple vectors, resulting in higher safety, and lower costs.

2.3.2 Availability of animal models

The existence of animal models that reproduce the clinical outcome of CLI allowed the completion of preclinical studies and accelerated the development of clinical trials. In this model, hindlimb ischemia is generated by excision of the femoral artery of the animal (usually rabbit or rat) leg (Pu et al., 1993).

2.3.3 Expression of naked DNA by skeletal muscle

Perhaps the most important factor to boosted studies in GT-based therapeutic angiogenesis from the 90's on was an intriguing observation in 1990 by Wolff and colleagues, that pure

DNA or RNA could be absorbed and expressed by skeletal muscle cells of mice without the participation of any particular system of gene transfer (Wolff et al., 1990). Although the mechanism of DNA capture by the target cell remains unknown (Wolff et al., 2005), the confirmation of this observation opened the way for the use of non-viral vector (usually in the form of pure plasmid DNA) in CLI studies.

2.3.4 Lower complexity of strategies based on non-viral vectors

The major advantage of non-viral vectors is their safety profile. These vectors do not integrate into the host genome (no risk of insertional mutagenesis), do not trigger severe inflammatory reactions (absence of innate immune response to the vector), which would be a huge limitation in an already inflamed tissue, and their effectiveness is not limited by previous immunity of the host. In addition, non-viral vectors are simple to produce, at lower costs when compared to viral vectors.

3. Preclinical data

Using variations of the model of hind limb ischemia (Pu et al., 1993), the effectiveness of therapeutic angiogenesis in small animal models was demonstrated by intra-arterial, intravenous and intramuscular administration of recombinant proteins or by gene transfer of several vascular growth factors (Takeshita et al., 1994; Takeshita et al., 1994; Bauters et al., 1995; Tsurumi et al., 1996; Garcia-Martinez et al., 1999; Shimpo et al., 2002). However, as discussed in the next section, these studies should be regarded more a proof of concept tool than as an indicator of efficacy in clinical studies.

In order to have a more critical view of these studies, it is important to briefly review general characteristics of the hindlimb ischemia model and of tools to evaluate efficacy in these studies.

3.1 The hindlimb ischemia model

In the classic hindlimb ischemia model, ligation and excision of the iliac or femoral artery reduces blood flow to levels between 30%, inducing a series of events that trigger angiogenesis and arteriogenesis over 3-4 weeks, after which resting blood flow is restored to about 60-70% of baseline (Scholz et al., 2002). In order to more accurately reproduce the progressive clinical course of CLI, a minority of studies used stepwise ligation of vessels, as well as constricting devices (Tang et al., 2005). Angiographic study of these animals show that collaterals emerging from the side branches of internal iliac artery and reaching the distal portions of the foot, as well as an extensive network of capillaries throughout the ischemic muscle are responsible for the partial restoration of blood flow (Takeshita et al., 1997). Because revascularization in this model has been shown to involve the basic mechanisms of angiogenesis and arteriogenesis (Asahara et al., 1997; Scholz et al., 2002), the model has been widely used in preclinical studies of GT-based therapeutic angiogenesis. However, one should acknowledge that the model does not exactly mimic the slow progression of atherosclerosis observed in patients with PAD. In addition, revascularization that occurs in this model is associated with intense capillary proliferation, whose real significance for perfusion has been challenged.

As in other areas of medical research, the translation of results from small animal models to humans is problematic. This is even more relevant for studies using gene transfer by direct injection of non-viral vectors. Uptake and expression of non-viral vectors by skeletal muscle occurs mostly in the vicinity of the needle (Wolff et al., 1990). Therefore, the exposure of muscle fibers to vector is much higher in rats and rabbits, than in humans, even if multiple injections are used in humans. In addition, animals used in these studies are usually healthy and young, as opposed to patients with CLI. This is even more relevant because it has been shown that age impairs the angiogenic response (Zhuo et al., 2010).

3.2 Methods used to evaluate efficacy

Although the preclinical studies have unequivocally demonstrated that GT-based therapeutic angiogenesis increase capillary proliferation in ischemic tissues, the real significance of this increase to the effective perfusion remains uncertain. Thus, the use of functional methods to assess the clinical relevance of newly formed vessels is of utmost importance in preclinical studies. Usually, efficacy is measured by a combination of anatomic (usually counting of newly formed vessels in histological sections or angiographic studies) and functional methods. Perfusion studies with microspheres that are trapped in capillaries are considered the gold-standard, bur are time-consuming. Therefore, doppler tissue imaging, which measures the skin blood flow in the ischemic limb, is one of the most frequently used functional method. The method is based on the assumption that skin perfusion reflects whole limb perfusion. Alternative methods such as measurements of oxygen tension, sestamibi scintigrapy and heat detecting cameras have also been used, along with clinical scores that evaluate the presence of ulcer healing, necrosis, etc. Whichever the method used, one should bear in mind potential pros and cons to avoid over-interpretation of preclinical data.

4. Data from clinical trials

In humans, GT-based therapeutic angiogenesis was first used in 1994 in a patient with CLI, who received an intra-arterial (distal to the obstruction) injection of plasmid DNA containing the cDNA of VEGF-A (Isner et al., 1996). The authors reported angiographic improvement after 12 weeks, associated with the development of angiomas and unilateral edema, two characteristics that enforced the biological effect of the treatment. The first phase I study also used plasmid DNA of the VEGF-A cDNA, delivered by multiple intramuscular injections in 9 CLI patients for whom revascularization was not feasible. Treatment was considered safe, and transient edema was the only adverse event. In addition, the authors reported increased levels of VEGF-A in serum, and improvements in ABI and in skin lesions, which could avoid amputation in 3 patients (Baumgartner et al., 1998). Two years later similar results were reported by the same group in 50 patients (Baumgartner et al., 2000). Subsequently, additional phase I studies confirmed the safety of these strategies (Comerota et al., 2002), paving the way for phase II studies.

4.1 Phase II studies

The first randomized double-blind study involved 54 patients with PAD amenable to angioplasty. In this study, VEGF-A gene transfer (n=35) or placebo (n = 19) were delivered intra-arterially by catheter after angioplasty. Gene transfer was performed using adenovirus (n=18) or non-viral vectors (liposome/plasmid-DNA) (n=17). Treatment proved to be safe. However, despite s significant increase in the number of collaterals in the two treated groups compared to placebo, other efficacy parameters were not modified (Makinen et al.,

2002). In the second randomized doubleblind study, 54 patients with CLI and diabetes were randomized to intramuscular injections of placebo or plasmid DNA with the VEGF-A cDNA. The primary efficacy endpoint (amputation at 100th day) was not significantly modified by treatment, but authors reported significant improvements in ABI, and in ulcer healing in treated patients compared to placebo (Kusumanto et al., 2006). Though not using non-viral vectors, the RAVE (Regional Angiogenesis with Vascular Endothelial Growth Factor) trial deserves to be discussed. In this trial, 105 patients with unilateral, exercise-limiting claudication were randomized to directi intramuscular injections of low or high doses of adenoviral $VEGF_{121}$ (Kusumanto et al., 2006). Despite the observation of dose-dependnent peripheral edema, which suggests that bioactive VEGF was indeed produced, the authors observed no significant change in primary or secondary endpoints. These results raised several important questions: First, it could be possible that the use of an isoform of VEGF that could have a shorter tissue half-life (as is the case of $VEGF_{121}$ compared to $VEGF_{165}$) could have limited treatment efficacy. Alternatively, the lack of validated endpoints, privileging physician-oriented as opposed to patient-oriented outcomes could also explain the negative results. Finally, failure could simply mean that use a VEGF isolated is not an effective strategy to obtain clinicaly-relevant therapeutic angiogenesis in CLI (Gupta et al., 2009).

After the first phase I trial with gene transfer of FGF-1 reported improvements in wound healing, pain and transcutaneous oxygen pressure after intramuscular injection of naked plasmid FGF-1 (Comerota et al., 2002), results from a phase II trial were reported. In this trial (TALISMAN 201 phase II trial in patients with CLI), patients were randomized to intramuscular injections of NV1FGF (n=59) or placebo (n=66) (Nikol et al., 2008). After 25 weeks, the proportion of patients that reached the primary endpoint (ulcer healing) did not differ significantly between treatment and control groups. However, amputation rate was significantly lower in NV1FGF-treated patients compared to placebo (37.3 vs 55.4%) and the strategy moved on to a phase III trial.

Because of its properties to regulate the expression of multiple downstream mediators of the angiogenesis cascade, including VEGF, thus acting as a "master-switch" agent, the transcription factor hypoxia-inducible factor (HIF) 1-α has been intesively studied as a candidate therapeutic gene for therapeutic angiogenesis (Gupta et al., 2009).

The most extensively studied growth factor that is currently under clinical development for GT-based therapeutic angiogenesis is hepatocyte growth factor, a potent mitogen for several cell types (Bussolino et al., 1992). It has been shown that serum levels of HGF are elevated in patients with coronary artery disease, and that higher levels correlate with better prognosis (Lenihan et al., 2003). In the STAT phase II trial, 104 patients with CLI were randomized to treatment with placebo or HGF (Powell et al., 2008). No safety concerns were raised related to the therapeutic agent. On an intention-to-treat analysis, no significant differences in transcutaneous oxygen tension ($TcPO_2$) were observed among patients treated with HGF (in increasing dose levels) or placebo. However, when patients that presented increases in $TcPO_2$ before treatment were excluded, patients that received the highest dose level of HGF presented significant improvements in $TcPO_2$ compared to the remaining groups. Again, these observations demonstrate the impact of endpoint selection in trial results and highlight the importance of identifying the most relevant endpoint to be used in therapeutic angiogenesis trials.

Following this study, the same group recently reported the results of the HGF-0205 trial. Patients received three sets of eight intramuscular injections of HGF plasmid every 2 weeks

(Powell et al., 2010). Injection sites were selected on an individual basis based on arteriographically defined vascular anatomy. In total, 21 patients were randomized to HGF treatment and 6 to placebo. No safety concerns were raised. HGF-treated patients presented significant improvements in toe-brachial index and rest pain compared to patients that received placebo. Complete ulcer healing at 12 months occurred in 31% of patients compared to 0% of placebo, though this difference was not statistically significant. Amputation rates (HGF 29 % vs. placebo 33%) and mortality were similar between groups. These results suggest that tailoring treatment to patient indivual characteristics might improve treatment outcomes. If confirmed, it is possible that the classical strategy to inject naked DNA into predefined sites of ischemic tissue with poor knowledge of the pharmacological and geographic distribution of the actual treatment agent could justify several negative results reported in previous human trials. One should bear in mind that when using a delivery strategy that is characterized mostly by local transfection, the proportion of ischemic tissue actually treated in a mouse or rat is very unlikely to be reached even by multiple injections in humans.

Additional studies have been recently reported using HGF plasmid-based therapeutic angiogenesis. In a multicenter, randomized, double-blind, placebo-controlled trial, 40 patients also received injections in sites selected by angiographic evaluation, on days 0 and 28 (Shigematsu et al., 2010). The overall primary improvement rate of the primary endpoint (improvement of rest pain or reduction of ulcer size) was significantly higher in HGF-treated patients (70.4%) compared to the placebo group (30.8%). An evaluation of quality of life also showed benefits of HGF treatment. Very recently, HGF plasmid intramuscular injections was also shown to improve several efficacy endpoints such as ABI, ulcer size, pain, in another phase I/IIa trial that treated 22 patients with CLI with of 2 or 4 mg of HGF plasmid, 2 times (Morishita et al., 2011).

Finally, a phase II trial was also conducted using gene transfer of an extracellular matrix protein that induces angiogenesis indirectly by interaction with integrins, Developmentally regulated endothelial locus (Del-1). In the DELTA trial, 105 patients with PAD were randomized to intramuscular injections of Del-1 plasmid in association with poloxamer 188, an agent that enhances transfection (Grossman et al., 2007). The control group received poloxamer 188 alone. No safety concerns were raised, but neither primary nor secondary endpoints were modified. Notably, improvement in these endpoints occurred in both treated and control groups, highlighting the importance of placebo effect in studies using new strategies such as gene therapy.

4.2 Safety concerns

To date, more than 1000 subjects have been treated for gene therapy for therapeutic angiogenesis in phase I and II trials, with adverse event rates that are similar to those in control groups (Varu et al., 2010). Still, there are important long-term safety concerns, stemming from theoretical but rather intuitive and important considerations, that still need to be addressed and weighted against the benefits of gene therapy-based therapeutic angiogenesis. These include the risk of accelerating pathologic angiogenesis in tumors, retina and atherosclerotic plaques. So far no evidence of these effects has been reported. Dose-dependent hypotension or proteinuria (> 1g/24h) have been reported in studies using VEGF-A (Henry, Rocha-Singh et al., 2001) and FGF-2 (Laham et al., 2000; Unger et al., 2000; Cooper et al., 2001) in the form of recombinant proteins, but in studies with gene therapy, where lower levels of proteins are expected to be expressed, these were not observed.

Studies with hepatocyte growth factor have not raised significant safety concerns. Of note, in one recent study, circulating levels of HGF were not detected, suggesting a restricted distribution of the therapeutic agent (Morishita et al., 2011).

5. Next steps

Preclinical and clinical trials have demonstrated the safety and potential efficacy of this strategy. Currently, the area is going through a phase in which new strategies and conceptual changes, developed after reevaluation of early clinical results and after a return from bedside to bench, are being tested in clinical trials. After almost 2 decades since the first human trial of GT for CLI, it is clear that several factors can be optimized in order to maximize the effectiveness of therapeutic angiogenesis. These include:

- *Animals x humans:* differences between animal models and the progression of CLI in humans, should be acknowledged, thus avoiding over-interpretation of results from animal studies.
- *Efficacy outcomes (animals):* more relevant efficacy outcomes should be identified in preclinical models allowing more realistic translation of results from bench to bedside.
- *Efficacy outcomes (humans)*: CLI is diagnosed and monitored with the help of objective methods that include ABI determination, toe systolic pressures or transcutaneous partial pressure of oxygen ($TcPO_2$) (Varu et al., 2010). However, an important unanswered question that makes evaluation of treatment even more complex is the very definition of a salvageable versus a non-salvageable limb (Connelly et al., 2001; Rowe et al., 2009). As in other areas of medical research, treatment outcome measures are mostly physician- rather than patient oriented. In the context of CLI, outcomes such as ABI improvement, limb salvage and survival have always been considered the most significant outcomes that any new treatment should be able to improve. However, patient-oriented outcome research in the last years suggests that in selected populations these outcomes are not necessarily associated with improvements in quality of life (Varu et al., 2010). Whether classical outcomes such as ABI index, or more patient-oriented outcomes should be used as primary endpoint for efficacy assessment of therapeutic angiogenesis is an important and challenging question.
- *Basic science:* Continuing research efforts on the mechanisms of blood vessel formation are extremely important to allow more rational selection of therapeutic genes to treat CLI. These could include the use of "cocktails" of growth factor genes, or master-switch genes, that could induce an angiogenic response that is closer to that spontaneously observed during "physiologic" collateral formation.
- *Delivery strategies and vectors:* Better delivery strategies and/or more efficient non-viral vectors for GT-based therapeutic angiogenesis should be developed, allowing more widespread expression of the therapeutic gene in human skeletal muscle.
- *Towards a pharmacological approach to therapy:* Better understanding of variables that govern the pharmacokinetics of non-viral vector delivery to skeletal muscle, thus enabling a less empiric design of clinical trials are of paramount importance so that trial design with non-viral vectors delivered to skeletal muscle start to move towards a more pharmacological paradigm, that allow a more rational interpretation of data and planning of treatment. So far, actual "dosing" of the therapeutic proteins has not been possible. In fact, this could severely affect the possibility to to reproduce even very positive results in larger scale phase III trials.

6. Conclusions

Therapeutic manipulation of angiogenesis is increasingly regarded as a promising treatment alternative for patients with CLI, as results from a new generation of clinical trials are revealed. The rationale for the use of vascular growth factors to stimulate vessel growth in ischemic tissues is mainly the demonstration that ischemic tissues present a relative deficiency of these growth factors, and that their administration can boost vessel growth. In addition, several characteristics render CLI a very interesting target for gene therapy-based therapeutic angiogenesis. In this chapter we reviewed the molecular and cellular rationale of therapeutic angiogenesis, results from pre-clinical studies, and finally results from clinical trials that used gene therapy as a platform for therapeutic angiogenesis. In addition, we tried to provide a critical appraisal of limitations of small animal models (and of the translation of endpoints from these studies to clinical practice), as well as a discussion on the steps that still need to be taken in order to render gene therapy with non-viral vectors as a more predictable and controllable strategy.

7. Acknowledgment

This work was financially supported by FAPESP and CNPq, Brazil. The Hematology and Hemotherapy Center forms part of the National Institute of Science and Technology of Blood, Brazil (INCT do Sangue-CNPq/MCT/FAPESP).

8. References

Albers, M., M. Romiti, et al. (2006). Meta-analysis of popliteal-to-distal vein bypass grafts for critical ischemia. *J Vasc Surg*, Vol.43, No.3,(Mar), pp.498-503.

Asahara, T., T. Murohara, et al. (1997). Isolation of putative progenitor endothelial cells for angiogenesis. *Science*, Vol.275, No.5302,(Feb 14), pp.964-967.

Baumgartner, I., A. Pieczek, et al. (1998). Constitutive expression of phVEGF165 after intramuscular gene transfer promotes collateral vessel development in patients with critical limb ischemia. *Circulation*, Vol.97, No.12,(Mar 31), pp.1114-1123.

Baumgartner, I., G. Rauh, et al. (2000). Lower-extremity edema associated with gene transfer of naked DNA encoding vascular endothelial growth factor. *Ann Intern Med*, Vol.132, No.11,(Jun 6), pp.880-884.

Bauters, C., T. Asahara, et al. (1995). Site-specific therapeutic angiogenesis after systemic administration of vascular endothelial growth factor. *J Vasc Surg*, Vol.21, No.2,(Feb), pp.314-324; discussion 324-315.

Beaglehole, R., A. Irwin, et al. (2003). The World Health Report - Shaping the future. Geneva, World Health Organization: 204.

Benjamin, L. E., I. Hemo, et al. (1998). A plasticity window for blood vessel remodelling is defined by pericyte coverage of the preformed endothelial network and is regulated by PDGF-B and VEGF. *Development*, Vol.125, No.9,(May), pp.1591-1598.

Brass, E. P., R. Anthony, et al. (2006). Parenteral therapy with lipo-ecraprost, a lipid-based formulation of a PGE1 analog, does not alter six-month outcomes in patients with critical leg ischemia. *J Vasc Surg*, Vol.43, No.4,(Apr), pp.752-759.

Bussolino, F., M. F. Di Renzo, et al. (1992). Hepatocyte growth factor is a potent angiogenic factor which stimulates endothelial cell motility and growth. *J Cell Biol*, Vol.119, No.3,(Nov), pp.629-641.

Carmeliet, P. (2003). Angiogenesis in health and disease. *Nat Med*, Vol.9, No.6,(Jun), pp.653-660.

Carmeliet, P., L. Moons, et al. (1997). Insights in vessel development and vascular disorders using targeted inactivation and transfer of vascular endothelial growth factor, the tissue factor receptor, and the plasminogen system. *Ann N Y Acad Sci*, Vol.811,(Apr 15), pp.191-206.

Choi, K., M. Kennedy, et al. (1998). A common precursor for hematopoietic and endothelial cells. *Development*, Vol.125, No.4,(Feb), pp.725-732.

Comerota, A. J., R. C. Throm, et al. (2002). Naked plasmid DNA encoding fibroblast growth factor type 1 for the treatment of end-stage unreconstructible lower extremity ischemia: preliminary results of a phase I trial. *J Vasc Surg*, Vol.35, No.5,(May), pp.930-936.

Connelly, J., M. Airey, et al. (2001). Variation in clinical decision making is a partial explanation for geographical variation in lower extremity amputation rates. *Br J Surg*, Vol.88, No.4,(Apr), pp.529-535.

Conway, E. M., D. Collen, et al. (2001). Molecular mechanisms of blood vessel growth. *Cardiovasc Res*, Vol.49, No.3,(Feb 16), pp.507-521.

Cooper, L. T., Jr., W. R. Hiatt, et al. (2001). Proteinuria in a placebo-controlled study of basic fibroblast growth factor for intermittent claudication. *Vasc Med*, Vol.6, No.4,(Nov), pp.235-239.

Dor, Y., V. Djonov, et al. (2002). Conditional switching of VEGF provides new insights into adult neovascularization and pro-angiogenic therapy. *Embo J*, Vol.21, No.8,(Apr 15), pp.1939-1947.

Dormandy, J., M. Mahir, et al. (1989). Fate of the patient with chronic leg ischaemia. A review article. *J Cardiovasc Surg (Torino)*, Vol.30, No.1,(Jan-Feb), pp.50-57.

Dormandy, J. A. and P. R. Thomas (1988). What is the natural history of critically ischemic patient with and without his leg? Limb Salvage and Amputation for Vascular Disease. R. M. Greenhalgh and C. W. Jamieson. Philadelphia, WB Saunders: 11-26.

Folkman, J. (1971). Tumor angiogenesis: therapeutic implications. *N Engl J Med*, Vol.285, No.21,(Nov 18), pp.1182-1186.

Garcia-Martinez, C., P. Opolon, et al. (1999). Angiogenesis induced in muscle by a recombinant adenovirus expressing functional isoforms of basic fibroblast growth factor. *Gene Ther*, Vol.6, No.7,(Jul), pp.1210-1221.

Garcia, L. A. (2006). Epidemiology and pathophysiology of lower extremity peripheral arterial disease. *J Endovasc Ther*, Vol.13 Suppl 2,(Feb), pp.II3-9.

Grossman, P. M., F. Mendelsohn, et al. (2007). Results from a phase II multicenter, double-blind placebo-controlled study of Del-1 (VLTS-589) for intermittent claudication in subjects with peripheral arterial disease. *Am Heart J*, Vol.153, No.5,(May), pp.874-880.

Gupta, R., J. Tongers, et al. (2009). Human studies of angiogenic gene therapy. *Circ Res*, Vol.105, No.8,(Oct 9), pp.724-736.

Habib, G. B., J. Heibig, et al. (1991). Influence of coronary collateral vessels on myocardial infarct size in humans. Results of phase I thrombolysis in myocardial infarction (TIMI) trial. The TIMI Investigators. *Circulation*, Vol.83, No.3,(Mar), pp.739-746.

Isner, J. M., A. Pieczek, et al. (1996). Clinical evidence of angiogenesis after arterial gene transfer of phVEGF165 in patient with ischaemic limb. *Lancet*, Vol.348, No.9024,(Aug 10), pp.370-374.

Kimura, H., A. Weisz, et al. (2000). Hypoxia response element of the human vascular endothelial growth factor gene mediates transcriptional regulation by nitric oxide: control of hypoxia-inducible factor-1 activity by nitric oxide. *Blood*, Vol.95, No.1,(Jan 1), pp.189-197.

Kusumanto, Y. H., V. V. Weel, et al. (2006). Treatment with Intramuscular Vascular Endothelial Growth Factor Gene Compared with Placebo for Patients with Diabetes Mellitus and Critical Limb Ischemia: A Double-Blind Randomized Trial. *Hum Gene Ther*,(May 2),

Laham, R. J., N. A. Chronos, et al. (2000). Intracoronary basic fibroblast growth factor (FGF-2) in patients with severe ischemic heart disease: results of a phase I open-label dose escalation study. *J Am Coll Cardiol*, Vol.36, No.7,(Dec), pp.2132-2139.

Lenihan, D. J., A. Osman, et al. (2003). Evidence for association of coronary sinus levels of hepatocyte growth factor and collateralization in human coronary disease. *Am J Physiol Heart Circ Physiol*, Vol.284, No.5,(May), pp.H1507-1512.

Makinen, K., H. Manninen, et al. (2002). Increased vascularity detected by digital subtraction angiography after VEGF gene transfer to human lower limb artery: a randomized, placebo-controlled, double-blinded phase II study. *Mol Ther*, Vol.6, No.1,(Jul), pp.127-133.

Morishita, R., H. Makino, et al. (2011). Phase I/IIa clinical trial of therapeutic angiogenesis using hepatocyte growth factor gene transfer to treat critical limb ischemia. *Arterioscler Thromb Vasc Biol*, Vol.31, No.3,(Mar), pp.713-720.

Nikol, S., I. Baumgartner, et al. (2008). Therapeutic angiogenesis with intramuscular NV1FGF improves amputation-free survival in patients with critical limb ischemia. *Mol Ther*, Vol.16, No.5,(May), pp.972-978.

Norgren, L., W. R. Hiatt, et al. (2007). Inter-Society Consensus for the Management of Peripheral Arterial Disease (TASC II). *J Vasc Surg*, Vol.45 Suppl S,(Jan), pp.S5-67.

Ozawa, C. R., A. Banfi, et al. (2004). Microenvironmental VEGF concentration, not total dose, determines a threshold between normal and aberrant angiogenesis. *J Clin Invest*, Vol.113, No.4,(Feb), pp.516-527.

Palmer-Kazen, U., D. Wariaro, et al. (2004). Vascular endothelial cell growth factor and fibroblast growth factor 2 expression in patients with critical limb ischemia. *J Vasc Surg*, Vol.39, No.3,(Mar), pp.621-628.

Post, M. J., R. Laham, et al. (2001). Therapeutic angiogenesis in cardiology using protein formulations. *Cardiovasc Res*, Vol.49, No.3,(Feb 16), pp.522-531.

Powell, R. J., P. Goodney, et al. (2010). Safety and efficacy of patient specific intramuscular injection of HGF plasmid gene therapy on limb perfusion and wound healing in patients with ischemic lower extremity ulceration: results of the HGF-0205 trial. *J Vasc Surg*, Vol.52, No.6,(Dec), pp.1525-1530.

Powell, R. J., M. Simons, et al. (2008). Results of a double-blind, placebo-controlled study to assess the safety of intramuscular injection of hepatocyte growth factor plasmid to improve limb perfusion in patients with critical limb ischemia. *Circulation*, Vol.118, No.1,(Jul 1), pp.58-65.

Pu, L. Q., A. D. Sniderman, et al. (1993). Enhanced revascularization of the ischemic limb by angiogenic therapy. *Circulation*, Vol.88, No.1,(Jul), pp.208-215.

Rivard, A., J. E. Fabre, et al. (1999). Age-dependent impairment of angiogenesis. *Circulation*, Vol.99, No.1,(Jan 5-12), pp.111-120.

Rowe, V. L., W. Lee, et al. (2009). Patterns of treatment for peripheral arterial disease in the United States: 1996-2005. *J Vasc Surg*, Vol.49, No.4,(Apr), pp.910-917.

Scholz, D., T. Ziegelhoeffer, et al. (2002). Contribution of arteriogenesis and angiogenesis to postocclusive hindlimb perfusion in mice. *J Mol Cell Cardiol*, Vol.34, No.7,(Jul), pp.775-787.

Schultz, A., L. Lavie, et al. (1999). Interindividual heterogeneity in the hypoxic regulation of VEGF: significance for the development of the coronary artery collateral circulation. *Circulation*, Vol.100, No.5,(Aug 3), pp.547-552.

Second European Consensus Document (1991). Second European Consensus Document on chronic critical leg ischemia. *Circulation*, Vol.84, No.4 Suppl,(Nov), pp.IV1-26.

Shigematsu, H., K. Yasuda, et al. (2010). Randomized, double-blind, placebo-controlled clinical trial of hepatocyte growth factor plasmid for critical limb ischemia. *Gene Ther*, Vol.17, No.9,(Sep), pp.1152-1161.

Shimpo, M., U. Ikeda, et al. (2002). AAV-mediated VEGF gene transfer into skeletal muscle stimulates angiogenesis and improves blood flow in a rat hindlimb ischemia model. *Cardiovasc Res*, Vol.53, No.4,(Mar), pp.993-1001.

Shweiki, D., A. Itin, et al. (1992). Vascular endothelial growth factor induced by hypoxia may mediate hypoxia-initiated angiogenesis. *Nature*, Vol.359, No.6398,(Oct 29), pp.843-845.

Sola, F., A. Gualandris, et al. (1997). Endothelial cells overexpressing basic fibroblast growth factor (FGF-2) induce vascular tumors in immunodeficient mice. *Angiogenesis*, Vol.1, No.1pp.102-116.

Suri, C., P. F. Jones, et al. (1996). Requisite role of angiopoietin-1, a ligand for the TIE2 receptor, during embryonic angiogenesis. *Cell*, Vol.87, No.7,(Dec 27), pp.1171-1180.

Takeshita, S., T. Isshiki, et al. (1997). Microangiographic assessment of collateral vessel formation following direct gene transfer of vascular endothelial growth factor in rats. *Cardiovasc Res*, Vol.35, No.3,(Sep), pp.547-552.

Takeshita, S., L. Q. Pu, et al. (1994). Intramuscular administration of vascular endothelial growth factor induces dose-dependent collateral artery augmentation in a rabbit model of chronic limb ischemia. *Circulation*, Vol.90, No.5 Pt 2,(Nov), pp.II228-234.

Takeshita, S., L. P. Zheng, et al. (1994). Therapeutic angiogenesis. A single intraarterial bolus of vascular endothelial growth factor augments revascularization in a rabbit ischemic hind limb model. *J Clin Invest*, Vol.93, No.2,(Feb), pp.662-670.

Tang, G. L., D. S. Chang, et al. (2005). The effect of gradual or acute arterial occlusion on skeletal muscle blood flow, arteriogenesis, and inflammation in rat hindlimb ischemia. *J Vasc Surg*, Vol.41, No.2,(Feb), pp.312-320.

Thurston, G., C. Suri, et al. (1999). Leakage-resistant blood vessels in mice transgenically overexpressing angiopoietin-1. *Science*, Vol.286, No.5449,(Dec 24), pp.2511-2514.

Tsurumi, Y., S. Takeshita, et al. (1996). Direct intramuscular gene transfer of naked DNA encoding vascular endothelial growth factor augments collateral development and tissue perfusion. *Circulation*, Vol.94, No.12,(Dec 15), pp.3281-3290.

Unger, E. F., L. Goncalves, et al. (2000). Effects of a single intracoronary injection of basic fibroblast growth factor in stable angina pectoris. *Am J Cardiol*, Vol.85, No.12,(Jun 15), pp.1414-1419.

Varu, V. N., M. E. Hogg, et al. (2010). Critical limb ischemia. *J Vasc Surg*, Vol.51, No.1,(Jan), pp.230-241.

Wolff, J., D. L. Lewis, et al. (2005). Non-viral approaches for gene transfer. *Acta Myol*, Vol.24, No.3,(Dec), pp.202-208.

Wolff, J. A., R. W. Malone, et al. (1990). Direct gene transfer into mouse muscle in vivo. *Science*, Vol.247, No.4949 Pt 1,(Mar 23), pp.1465-1468.

Zhuo, Y., S. H. Li, et al. (2010). Aging impairs the angiogenic response to ischemic injury and the activity of implanted cells: combined consequences for cell therapy in older recipients. *J Thorac Cardiovasc Surg*, Vol.139, No.5,(May), pp.1286-1294, 1294 e1281-1282.

2

Cell-Based Gene Therapies and Stem Cells for Regeneration of Ischemic Tissues

Rosalinda Madonna[1,2] and Raffaele De Caterina[2,3]
[1]*Texas Heart Institute and University of Texas Medical School, Houston,*
[2]*Institute of Cardiology, "G. d'Annunzio" University – Chieti,*
[3]*Fondazione "G. Monasterio" – Pisa,*
[1]*Texas*
[2,3]*Italy*

1. Introduction

Coronary (CAD) and peripheral (PAD) artery disease are major causes of morbidity and mortality, requiring bypass surgery or angioplasty in approximately one million patients/year in the world (MERIT-HF Study Group, 1999). While collateral vessel formation as an alternative pathway for blood supply occurs in some of these patients, many do not form vascular networks adequate to compensate for the loss of the original blood supply (Hirsch et al., 2006). These patients might therefore benefit from stem cell transplantation therapies that would accelerate natural processes of postnatal collateral vessel formation, an approach referred to as therapeutic angiogenesis. On the other hand, recent seminal reports have indicated that the adult heart is self-healing and self-renewing. Specifically, these studies have demonstrated that there is a pool of resident cardiac stem cells (CSCs) that are clonogenic and multipotent and are capable of differentiating into new blood vessels or into new myocytes, and of cardiac progenitor cells (CPCs) (Marban, 2007). This suggests the possibility of using a therapeutic angiogenesis approach to complement other treatments (e.g., stem cell therapy) that facilitate myocardial repair. Such combined modalities may facilitate myocardial regeneration by inducing endogenous cardiac cells to migrate, differentiate, and proliferate *in situ*, replacing lost endothelial cells and cardiomyocytes (Urbaneket al., 2005). However, despite recent progress in applying the approaches of regenerative medicine to the treatment of such diseases, valid strategies aimed at repairing the infarcted heart and, in general, at treating end-organ ischemia continue to be elusive. Major obstacles are the difficulty in isolating and delivering stem cells that are specifically effective in myocardial repair, and in stimulating recruitment of endogenous stem cells to the ischemic tissue. To address these issues, there has been increasing focus on novel biotechnologies or pharmacological strategies to enhance the implantation of exogenous stem cells or to boost endogenous regeneration of myocardial tissue. By employing three fundamental "tools", namely stem cells, biomaterials and growth factors (GFs) (Lavik & Langer, 2004; Mikos et al., 2006), such tissue engineering strategies may enhance the efficacy of stem cell therapy in several ways: by mobilizing endogenous stem/progenitor cells *in vivo*; by promoting cell proliferation and differentiation; and by augmenting cell engraftment and survival in the injured myocardium. In general, because of the short half-lives of GFs in the body and the necessity to deliver them to specific target sites, GF injections themselves do not always produce the anticipated therapeutic effect. At present, GF delivery in regenerative medicine basically relies upon two strategies: 1) delivery of the GF genes; 2) direct delivery of GFs by incorporating them into a vehicle. In the gene delivery approach, delivery of the GF gene may result in higher and more constant levels of protein produced, since the gene - rather than a degradable protein - is being delivered (Haastert & Grothe, 2007). Two major problems are associated however with this approach: 1) the complexity of cloning and integrating the gene into the target cells; 2) safety and efficiency of transduction. At present, there are insufficient well-controlled long-term studies in the preclinical area to make any conclusive statements about the clinical suitability/efficacy of gene delivery in humans. If resolved, cell-mediated synthesis of GFs should be associated with more efficient targeting of receptors and, consequently, a more robust and predictable approach in ischemic tissue regeneration.

2. Stem cell basics and selection

Stem cells are a population of immature tissue precursor cells capable of self-renewal as well as of differentiation into a spectrum of different cell types in appropriate conditions. In general, they share the following characteristics: (1) a high capacity for self-renewal; (2) the potential for differentiation in multiple cell types; (3) the ability to be cultured *ex vivo* and used for tissue engineering; and (4) plasticity (transdifferentiation ability) (Vats et al., 2005). On the basis of their differentiating potential, stem cells can currently be classified into four categories: (1) totipotent, (2) pluripotent, (3) multipotent, and (4) oligopotent or monopotent. Totipotent stem cells have the potential to differentiate into cells of all three main germinal layers (the ectodermal, endodermal, and mesodermal) and embryo-derived tissues. Pluripotent stem cells have the ability to differentiate only into tissues derived from the ectoderm, endoderm and mesoderm. Multipotent stem cells can differentiate into tissue-specific progenitor cells within a given organ. For example, multipotent blood stem cell or hematopoietic stem cells can develop into red blood cells, white blood cells, or platelets. Oligopotent or monopotent stem cells can only give rise to one or few types of specialized cells. On the basis of their origin and biological properties, stem cells can also be classified as either (1) embryonic stem cells or (2) adult stem cells. Embryonic stem cells are derived from the inner layer mass of the blastocyst and can be harvested from three sources: aborted fetuses (cadaveric stem cells), embryos left over from *in vitro* fertilization (discarded embryos), and embryos created in the laboratory solely for the purpose of producing stem cells (research embryos). *In vitro* differentiation of human embryonic stem cells into cardiomyocytes has been demonstrated by Kehat et al. (Kehat et al., 2001). However, ethical issues have been raised against harvesting human embryonic stem cells, especially if this process requires destruction of an embryo. Other potential obstacles to using embryonic stem cells are that recipients often need to receive immunosuppressants, because embryonic stem cells are potentially allogenic and strongly immunogenic. Uncontrolled differentiation of embryonic stem cells may cause other problems, such as the development of cardiac or vascular neoplasm. Transplanted embryonic stem cells may form teratomas if some undifferentiated totipotent cells are still present. The formation of teratomas -i.e., tumors containing a mix of differentiated human cell types, including cells characteristic of the ectoderm, mesoderm, and endoderm-in severe combined immunodeficiency (SCID) mice after injection with human embryonic stem cells has been observed (Thomson et al., 1998).

Adult stem cells are the undifferentiated cells that exist in a differentiated tissue or organ and that are capable of specializing into cells of the tissue or organ from which they originated. Their capacity for self-renewal allows tissues and organs to maintain functional stability. Sources of adult stem cells include not only regenerating tissues, such as the heart, adipose tissue, bone marrow, blood, liver and epidermis, but also non-divisive tissues, such as the brain. Compared with embryonic stem cells, autologous adult stem cells are not faced with any major ethical or immunological controversies surrounding their use in the same individual from whom they were obtained. However, their ability to proliferate and differentiate is less powerful than that of embryonic stem cells; they are often difficult to identify, isolate, and purify; and they are not numerous enough for use in transplantation without being expanded *in vitro* substantially. For example, there is only one hematopoietic cell for every 1000-5000 bone marrow stromal cells (BMSCs). Adult stem cells do not replicate indefinitely in culture (Jiang et al., 2002), and they are referred to as multipotent or oligopotent stem cells. The partially differentiated cells are precursor or progenitor cells, which are characterized by the ability to proliferate. For instance, circulating endothelial progenitor cells (EPCs) can promptly differentiate into mature endothelial cells that replace dead or dying cells when the endothelium of arteries is injured by atherosclerosis (Urbich & Dimmeler, 2004).

Selection of a suitable type of stem cells is a key issue for the success of stem cell therapy. Stem/progenitor cells used for transplantation should have the following characteristics: (1) high rates of survival and proliferation; (2) high capability of differentiation; and (3) the potential for engraftment and integration with native or host cardiac cells. Currently, both embryonic and adult stem cells are used in experimental cardiac cell transplantation studies, while only adult stem cells (e.g., bone marrow-derived mesenchymal cells, skeletal myoblasts, endothelial progenitor cells) are used in clinical trials. Each stem cell type has unique biological properties that offer both advantages and limitations to their use. Therefore, selection of the most suitable stem cells for use in ischemic patients is still a major focus of current research. The skeletal myoblasts or satellite cells are precursor cells of human skeletal muscle that originate from muscle stem cells (Angelis et al., 1999). They normally lie in a quiescent state under the basal membrane of muscular fibers, and have the potential for reentry into the cell cycle in response to injury, where they can divide and differentiate into functional muscle cells. Skeletal myoblasts can be obtained from individual patients themselves. Other theoretical advantages of using autologous skeletal myoblast are their rapid expansion in culture and their lower likelihood of tumor formation after transplantation. In addition, these cells have a chance of engrafting with native cardiomyocytes and surviving in infarcted regions of the heart since they are relatively resistant to ischemia. Animal studies have demonstrated that skeletal myoblasts can successfully accommodate themselves in the infarcted region of the heart, forming striated muscle fibers with intercalated discs in the host myocardium under the influence of factors in the cardiac environment (Murry et al., 1996). Improvement in systolic function has been noted after skeletal myoblast transplantation in ischemic and non-ischemic heart failure models (Atkins et al., 1999; Hagegeet al., 2001; Siminiak & Kurpisz, 2003). Controversy still exists regarding the capability of stem cells to engraft and connect with native cardiomyocytes, despite promising results from preclinical studies (Suzuki et al., 2001; Menasche et al., 2003; Pagani et al., 2003; Smits et al., 2003). Bone marrow-derived stem cells are currently the most commonly used cells in cell transplantation therapy. The ideal stem cells from bone marrow for cardiac regeneration remain to be identified and many details remain to be elucidated. Yet, the clinical results from recent trials show the capability of these cells to ameliorate systo-diastolic heart function and decrease the size of the infarct region after intracoronary injection (Assmus et al., 2002; Strauer et al., 2002; Britten et al., 2003). Other studies (Perin et al., 2002; Perin et al., 2003) have demonstrated the safety and efficacy of transendocardial injection of autologous bone marrow mononuclear cells in patients with end-stage ischemic heart disease. Fetal cardiomyocytes still can enter the cell cycle and be expanded in culture. Successful cell transplantation using fetal cardiomyocytes was initially demonstrated in mice (Soonpaa et al., 1994; Li et al., 1995; Li et al., 1996), with findings in improvement of heart function and formation of new blood vessels in and around the cell graft area (Watanabe et al., 1998). These experiments show that fetal cardiomyocyte transplantation is feasible and potentially clinically relevant. Besides the ethical questions concerning the use of human fetal tissue, however, one limitation of using fetal cardiomyocytes is that lifelong immunosuppressive therapy may be necessary to prevent rejection. The optimal regimen and dose of immunosuppressive agents for cell transplantation would be here still unknown. A large number of studies have examined the differentiation of embryonic stem cells into cardiomyocytes, aiming at clarifying the mechanism of differentiation, identifying cell markers, and developing techniques for purifying embryonic stem cell-derived cardiomyocytes. The pluripotency of embryonic stem cells gives rise to their differentiation into more than 200 hundred kinds of cell lines. Protocols for the *in vitro* differentiation of embryonic stem cells into cardiomyocytes representing all specialized cell types of the heart, such as atrial-like, ventricular-like, sinus nodal-like, and Purkinje-like cells, have been established. Only 5-10% of these cells have been identified as cardiomyocytes. It may be ideal to separate cardiomyocytes from the undifferentiated ES cells before transplantation because of their potential to generate tumor-like tissue if implanted (Odorico et al., 2001). However, how to direct the differentiation of embryonic stem cells only into functional cardiomyocytes *in vivo* is still unclear. As stated above, another technical limitation is here the need for immunosuppressant therapy after transplantation. Endothelial progenitor cells can be identified in adult peripheral blood, bone marrow, and human umbilical cord blood.

Current experiments suggest that EPCs play an important role in vasculogenesis by differentiating into vascular endothelial cells, inhibiting ventricular remodeling through improvement in myocardial blood supply (Kamihata et al., 2001). Adipose tissue-derived stem cells may overcome major limitations in the use of adult stem cells harvested from essential organs such as muscle, skin, brain. liver and bone marrow. It has been shown that these cells can be induced to differentiate into multiple cell lineages, including adipose, cartilage and bone, muscle cells, neurons and endothelial cells (Zuk et al., 2001; Madonna et al., 2009). Injection of adipose tissue-derived stromal cells (ADSCs) has been recently shown to improve neovascularisation in the ischemic hind limb and the infarcted heart (see Madonna et al., 2009 for a general review of preclinical studies in the heart and hind limb ischemia models). Furthermore, recent studies (Puissant et al., 2005) have reported on the *in vivo* and *in vitro* immunosuppressive properties of ADSCs and their capability of escaping the immune surveillance. Therefore, major advantages of the adipose tissue as an alternative source of regenerative cells, include: 1. yield: a therapeutic dose of regenerative cells can be isolated in approximately one hour without cell culture; 2. safety: patients receive their own cells (autologous-use), with no risk of immune rejection or transmission; 3. versatility: stem cells from the adipose tissue benefit from multiple mechanisms of action. Recently it has been documented that the adult heart contains a pool of small cells expressing stem cell markers [c-kit, multi drug resistance 1 (MDR-1), and stem cell antigen 1 (Sca-1)]. Such cells also harbor telomerase activity, which is only present in replicating cells. These cardiac stem-progenitor cells (CSCs) not only can replenish the cardiomyocyte population, but are also able to regenerate coronary vessels (Beltrami et al., 2001). The actual number of CSCs remains controversial. Quantitative data in mouse, rat, dog, and human hearts have demonstrated that there is 1 CSC per approximately 30,000 to 40,000 myocardial cells: approximately 65% of all CSCs possess the 3 above-referred antigens (c-kit, MDR-1, and Sca-1-like); approximately 20% possess 2, and approximately 15% possess only 1. Approximately 5% each of all CSCs exclusively express c-kit, MDR-1, or Sca-1. Furthermore, more premature resident CSCs, such as cardiospheres and $isl1^+$ cardioblasts, have been recently identified (Messina et al., 2004). This variability in the number and type of CSCs reflects cells with distinct functional capacity and different stage of differentiation. *In vivo* experiments have shown that injected cardiospheres can produce functional improvement of the heart, with 37% improvement in fractional shortening in the injected group (Messina et al., 2004; Smith et al., 2007; Chimenti et al., 2010). Main advantages of CSCs are the following: 1. CSCs are autologous, and thus unlikely to trigger infectious or immunological complications; 2. CSCs are more cardiogenic than other adult stem cells; 3. CSCs trigger robust angiogenic responses after myocardial transplantation.

3. Growth factor selection and vehicle-based delivery approach

Vehicle-based delivery systems for growth factors, derived from diverse biomaterials, are used to increase their retention at treatment sites for a sufficient period of time to allow tissue regenerating cells to migrate into the area of injury, to proliferate and to differentiate, as well as to reduce the loss of bioactivity. They are also used to control toxicity induced by high concentrations of growth factors (Vasita & Katti, 2006; Chou & Leong, 2007). A major challenge inherent in these strategies is to identify growth factors and signaling pathways that selectively promote proliferation, migration, engraftment, and differentiation of resident CSCs or exogenous multipotent stem cells. This challenge relates also to the understanding of cellular uptake mechanisms, cell response to the mechanochemical microenvironment, the potential therapeutic utility of delivered biomolecules, and the exact requirements for multiple signals to drive the ischemic cardiovascular tissue regeneration process to completion. Current knowledge suggests that "cocktails" of biomolecules, or even cocktails of different types of stem cells, should be delivered locally, with specific and distinct pharmacokinetics/pharmacodynamics (e.g., the capacity of each single component of the cocktail to act distinctly in differentiating or in homing different endogenous stem cell/progenitor population), in order to mimic, as far as possible, the different requirements of the ischemic tissue during the various regeneration phases. Engineering natural and/or synthetic scaffolds to release several growth factors (or growth factor-encoding genes) in a sequential manner might affect more than one phase of the ischemic tissue healing process, for example, neovascularization and myogenesis, ultimately leading to cardiovascular tissue regeneration rather than repair. The growth factors that have been most intensively investigated in the regeneration of ischemic cardiovascular tissues include vascular endothelial growth factor (VEGF), transforming growth factor (TGF)-β, platelet-derived growth factors (PDGF, including PDGF-BB and PDGF-AA), insulin-like growth factor (IGF)-

1, basic fibroblast growth factor (b-FGF) (Beohar et al., 2010). Overall, results indicate that these growth factors elicit significant proliferative and angiogenic effects. It is now well established that the utilization of multiple growth factors, rather than one, capable to act in a concentration- and time-dependent manner, is essential in the processes involved in the regeneration of ischemic cardiovascular tissues (Chen et al., 2010). An example is given by the need of having VEGF and PDGF together in order to promote angiogenesis. Indeed, VEGF is an initiator of angiogenesis, while PDGF promotes blood vessel maturation. As an example for this, a polymer scaffold constructed from Poly (Lactide-co Glycolide) (PLG), capable of delivering VEGF and PDGF together, with better results in terms of formation of mature vessels compared with the delivery of VEGF or PDGF singularly, has been produced (Richardson et al., 2001). In the selection of growth factors potentially capable to boost the regeneration of ischemic cardiovascular tissue, we and others have investigated on hepatocyte growth factor (HGF) and its receptor receptor mesenchymal-epithelial transition factor (Met). Ligand-receptor systems such HGF and its receptor, the tyrosine kinase Met, are potential candidates for therapeutic angiogenesis and for boosting migration, engraftment and commitment of CSCs because they promote the translocation of CSCs into the injured area, activate their growth and differentiation, and stimulate endothelial cell migration (Rappolee et al., 1996; Forte et al., 2006; Madonna et al., 2010). The strategy of combining stem cells, either native or gene-engineered to overexpress growth factors, with biopolymers that are functionalized with growth factors such as HGF, would facilitate myocardial regeneration: a) by supplying exogenous stem cells or GFs that stimulate resident CSC migration, engraftment and commitment to cardiomyocytes, and that induce and modulate arterial responses to ischemia; b) by supporting the maintenance of GFs and transplanted stem cells in the damaged tissues through the use of biocompatible and biodegradable polymers for a period of time sufficient to allow histological and anatomical restoration of the damaged tissue. These polymers can provide vehicles to deliver bioactive factors and stem cells into the infarcted heart or ischemic cardiovascular tissues. Finally, this approach would promote the ability of resident CSCs or of exogenous multipotent stem cells, such as adipose tissue-derived mesenchymal stem cells (AT-MSCs), to induce the healing of damaged tissue, by recruiting and directing these cells into the damaged area, by improving angiogenesis and, finally, by promoting the reperfusion of ischemic tissues.

4. Growth factor-delivery systems and devices in the treatment of tissue ischemia

Many limitations of stem cell therapies could be resolved by stimulating specific cellular functions for cell populations that normally are quiescent in the adult heart or that are not capable of replacing the dying cells. Compounds (cytokines and growth factors) that are simply injected into the lesions quickly disappear from the site of injection because they are removed by the blood flow and degraded by specific enzymes located in the extracellular microenvironment. To overcome this drawback, a possible strategy is to install a polymer functionalized with growth factors and stem cells into the damaged heart to stimulate the natural process of cardiac repair. Polymers tested in the past for their ability to support transplanted cells, without any conjugation with functional molecules, have been marginally effective. More novel polymers are conjugated with functional molecules (growth factors, chemotactic factors, cytokines), and are capable of stimulating specific normally quiescent cellular functions (Tatard et al., 2005). They are known as "smart" polymers because they "persuade" and guide the regenerative process, and are "biomimetics" because they use strategies occurring during the physiological regenerative process. Unlike the previous ones, novel polymers are "smart", in that they can acquire several biological functions depending on the bioactive factor or stem cell type to which they are conjugated. These polymers can prolong and amplify specific stem cell functions. They can stimulate the recruitment of circulating and resident stem cells and subsequently promote their adhesion to the damaged area, and can enhance survival, proliferation, and differentiation of stem cells into cardiac and vascular cells (Madonna & De Caterina, 2009). Several of these features are critical to tissue regeneration, including restoration of the delivery of factors, nutrients, oxygen, and blood to necrotic tissues. To accomplish this, polymers must be functionalized by conjugation with bioactive factors. To date, delivery systems of growth factors are basically classified as: 1) reservoir systems; 2) environmentally responsive systems. Reservoir systems are one of the oldest methods used successfully to deliver drugs. The primary drug release mechanism from reservoir systems is diffusion-controlled release, characterized by an initial "burst release" phase followed by a phase of slower drug release from the carrier (Langer, 1983). Examples are hydrophilic matrices, that degrade when water enters and in this way release the drug (Franssen et al., 1999). Several reservoir systems have been developed to more closely control the release kinetics and avoid "burst type" release of the encapsulated factor(s). For example, the *in vitro* release of TGF-β from novel, injectable hydrogels based on the polymer oligo(poly(ethylene glycol) fumarate) (OPF) has been investigated (Holland et al., 2003). This system has been extended to enable the dual delivery of IGF-1 and TGF-β by loading the two growth factors into either the OPF hydrogel phase or the gelatin microparticle phase of composites. Release profiles were successfully manipulated by altering the phase of growth factor loading and the extent of microparticle cross linking (Holland et al., 2005).

Environmentally responsive systems are able to match a patient's physiological needs at the appropriate time and/or the correct site. They are able to deliver a certain amount of growth factor(s) in response to a biological state (Qiu & Park, 2001). They are constituted by sensitive hydrogels that can control the release of drugs by changing the gel structure according to environmental stimulation, such as temperature, pH, and/or ion concentration. Temperature-sensitive hydrogels are able to swell or shrink as the temperature of the surrounding fluid varies (Ramanan et al., 2006). The poly-N-isopropylacrylamide (PNIPAAm) hydrogel is a typical example of temperature-sensitive hydrogel, featuring sol-to-gel transition at a critical solution temperature of about 35 °C. This polymer releases the drug with the transition from gel to sol (Zhang et al., 2004), and is of particular interest in those clinical situations, such as tissue ischemia, characterized by low tissue temperature. Similarly, pH-sensitive polymers contain pendant acidic (e.g., carboxylic and sulphonic acids) or basic (e.g., ammonium salts) groups that either accept or release protons in response to changes in environmental pH (Qiu & Park, 2001). Such polymers can release a drug when the environmental pH decrease. These acidic pH-sensitive polymers may be useful for the treatment of tissue ischemia and inflammation (Matsusaki & Akashi, 2005). A very recent work has also shown the capability of new magnetic particles embedded in polymer gels, termed ferrogels, to release drugs in response to magnetic fields (Zhao et al., 2011). Here the authors created alginate-based porous scaffolds containing the arginine-glycine-aspartic acid amino acid sequence, covalently coupled with the alginate and embedded with 10 nm iron oxide particles. Under applied magnetic fields this superparamagnetic gel undergoes prompt deformation, causing water flow through the interconnected pores, thus triggering the release of biological agents. The authors here showed the capability of these ferrogels to promptly release several drugs, including mitoxantrone, plasmid DNA, chemokines, as well as cells under the control of external magnetic fields *in vitro* and *in vivo* (Zhao et al., 2011). In our laboratory, we have been working on a novel and still poorly investigated strategy using polymeric pharmacologically active microspheres (PAM), 50-100 μm in diameter, with an *in vivo* half-life of 1 month, that encapsulate bioactive factors gradually released into the injection area (Tatard et al., 2005; Madonna & De Caterina, 2009), and providing a vehicle for stem cell, drug, growth factors and gene delivery (Fig. 1). The chemical composition of these polymers is based on FDA-approved compounds, namely, polylactic acid (PLA), poly-D,L-lactic-co-glycolic (PLGA), and polycaprolactone (PCL) (Mudargi et al., 2008). PAM also satisfy the need for resistance to accelerated degradation that may happen in the harsh microenvironment of tissue ischemia. In addition, compared with other polymers, PLGA has more hydrophilic domains, which favors cell attachment, and therefore constitute a good support material for bioactive molecules that mobilize and home circulating progenitor/stem cells to the injured area (Tatard et al., 2005).

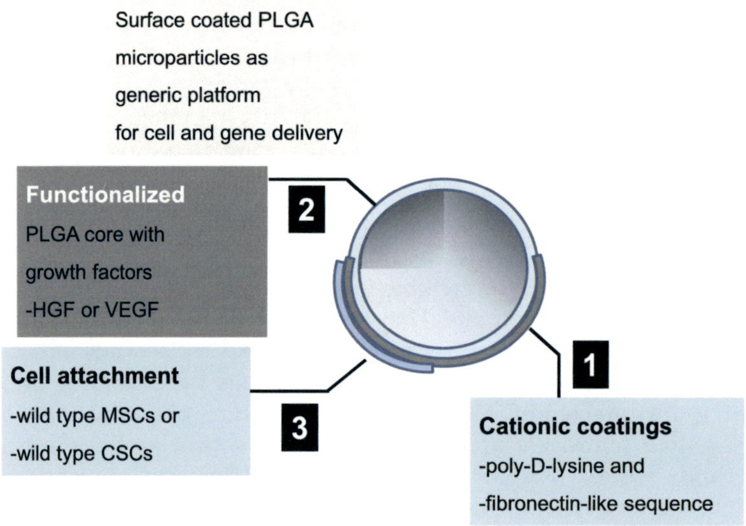

Fig. 1. The concept of multifunctional pharmacologically active microspheres (PAM). Surface-coated PLGA microparticles form a generic platform that can be functionalized with drugs, growth factors or genes and externally coated with stem cells. Abbreviations: PLGA, poly-D,L-lactic-co-glycolic; HGF, hepatocyte growth factor; VEGF, vascular endothelial growth factors; MSCs, mesenchymal stem cells; CSCs, cardiac stem cells.

5. The gene delivery approach

Beside the incorporation into a carrier vehicle, different approaches and strategies for direct delivery of growth factors have been employed, including the delivery of growth factor genes. In order to mimic the natural healing process of the tissue successfully, this strategy mostly requires a localized application of multiple, rather than one, genes that encode for and activate the synthesis of sequential multiple growth factors with synergistic effects on tissue regeneration (De Laporte et al., 2009; Donofrio et al., 2010; Fujii et al., 2011; Liu et al., 2011). However, low transfection efficiencies, inefficient gene targeting, low gene expression levels, and undesired gene integration into host DNA are all challenges that may undermine growth factor gene delivery as a better approach instead of the growth factor protein delivery (Juillerat-Jeanneret & Schmitt, 2007). Gene delivery can be performed either by directly introducing the delivery vector into the anatomical site (*in vivo*) or by harvesting cells from the patient, transferring the gene(s) to the cells in tissue culture and then transferring the genetically modified cells back into the patient (*ex vivo*). In another recent review article we have specifically discussed cell-mediated HGF/Met gene transfer for myocardial regeneration (Madonna et al., 2010). A more general overview of preclinical studies using *in vivo* and *ex vivo* gene delivery strategies is provided here.

***In vivo* approaches**

An *in vivo* gene delivery approach can be accomplished either by direct injection of viral vectors or transfection reagents into the site, or by attaching the delivery vector to the scaffold (Bleiziffer et al., 2007). This latter approach is more straightforward, but is limited by inefficient gene delivery and nonspecific cellular targeting. An early evaluation of *in vivo* gene delivery for therapeutic angiogenesis involved the direct intramyocardial injection of VEGF DNA using an adenovirus vector in patients with otherwise inoperable coronary artery disease and intractable angina pectoris (Rosengart et al., 1999). Phase I clinical trials documented the safety and feasibility, but not clear-cut clinically relevant efficacy of gene transfer using plasmid DNA, most likely because of the low levels of growth factor achieved with single injections of plasmid DNA (Rosengart et al., 1999). As of today, most clinical trials have failed to show any benefit of VEGF *in vivo* gene therapy, even by using different routes of intramyocardial administration that can achieve the transfer of high doses of the specific DNA, such as with percutaneous guidance catheter systems. The double-blind, placebo-controlled *NOGA angiogenesis Revascularization Therapy: assessment by RadioNuclide Imaging (NORTHERN)* study showed no benefit of plasmid DNA-VEGF gene therapy at 3 and 6 months in terms of change in myocardial perfusion from baseline in patients with refractory Canadian Cardiovasculart Society (CCS) class 3 angina (Stewart et al., 2009).

***Ex vivo* approaches**

Although traditional delivery of cells associated with growth factors is still a candidate strategy in laboratory-based trials , the most frequently investigated cell transplantation in tissue engineering to date is cell-based gene therapy. This therapy typically relies on transplanting cells, such as stem cells, lymphocytes, fibroblasts, or - alternatively - the cells of interest, that are removed from the body and injected after therapeutic transgene modifications (Fischer et al., 2009; Cho & Marban, 2010; Madonna et al., 2010). This *ex vivo* approach allows for targeting of specific cells for gene delivery, supplies cells that may directly participate in the regenerative process, allows for both autocrine and paracrine effects from the expressed growth factor, and avoids the safety risks of directly injecting viral vectors or transfection reagents *in vivo*. This approach, however, involves an extra step to manipulate and expand cells in tissue culture, and has the risk of contamination. Additionally, the *ex vivo* approach does not eliminate the possibility of retroviral vectors causing insertional activation of other genes, the over-expression of which may cause cancer, as experienced when using *ex vivo* gene therapy for the treatment of children with X-linked severe combined immune deficiency (Gansbacher & European Society of Gene

Therapy, 2003). Progress in the field of gene therapy has been limited by safety concerns related to delivery vectors. Genetically modified cells are potentially able to provide a stable source of growth factors at a level that is sufficient to elicit a biological response. Autologous cells may also be used in this approach via the isolation of a small number of differentiated adult cells or stem cells, followed by *in vitro* expansion to produce an appropriate supply. The cells may naturally secrete or be genetically modified *in vitro* to overexpress the factor, either transiently or permanently. After their genetic modification, the cells are allowed to grow *in vitro* and increase in number, so as to synthesize and secrete the desired growth factors at the site where they have been transplanted. This approach may be particularly appropriate for delivery of growth factors that act by paracrine or juxtacrine mechanisms.

6. Lentiviral and non-lentiviral vectors for gene delivery into stem cells

The introduction of growth factor genes in stem cells can be performed by using viral or non-viral vectors. In the choice of using viral vectors, important experimental variables for a successful gene therapy include the multiplicity of infection (MOI), time length for viral incubation and medium used for viral incubation. An optimal combination of such experimental conditions would increase gene transfer efficiency and possibly obviate the need for selective antibiotic-based enrichment and long-term culture, which may contribute to senescence or compromise the long-term engraftment efficiency and/or multipotency of grafted cells (Rombouts & Ploemacher, 2003). In addition, by increasing gene transfer efficiency, fewer cells may be required to achieve a therapeutic effect. This justifies the use of lentiviral vectors for transducing adult stem cells, by virtue of their ability to transduce both dividing and non-dividing cells and their relative ease of use and comparable nature to adeno-associated viral (AAV) vectors, which are clinically preferred. For the transduction of adult stem cells, lentivirus-based systems are virtually ideal, since they overcome most problems, including the short duration of gene expression and the occurrence of significant inflammatory responses, which plague other types of gene vectors (such as adenoviruses). Lentiviruses are a subgroup of retroviruses that include the human type 1 immunodeficiency virus (HIV). While retroviral systems are inefficient in transducing non-dividing or slowly dividing cells, lentivirus-based vectors, after being pseudotyped with vesicular stomatitis virus glycoprotein G (VSV-G) (i.e., using the glycoprotein envelope from the vesicular stomatitis virus to package recombinant retroviruses) (Emi et al., 1991), can mediate genome integration into both non-dividing and dividing cells (Fig. 2). There is evidence that lentiviral vectors can also transduce more primitive, quiescent progenitors with stable transgene integration (Case et al., 1999). In comparison with other retroviral vectors, lentiviral systems allow the immediate transduction without prior expansion, or with growth factor stimulation for only short exposure times. Compared with adenoviral vectors, lentiviral vectors also offer the major advantages of causing little or no disruption of the target cells and of not promoting any inflammatory response (Lever, 1996). AAV vectors represent an alternate type of vector that may also be used for long-term transgene expression in the heart through cell-based therapy (Svensson et al., 1999). Like lentiviruses, AAV can stably integrate into the host genome providing long-term transgene expression, with a minimum inflammatory response. However, AAV can cause insertional mutagenesis and can only carry genes which are less than 5 kb (Donsante et al., 2007). A possible drawback of the use of lentiviral and AAV vectors for delivering genes that encode for growth factors might be that they can cause a chronic overexpression of the protein, with an uncertain therapeutic effect. Short-term gene expression of the growth factor gene would be desirable if the goal is to deliver a secreted protein, such as insulin-like growth factor-1 (IGF-1), vascular endothelial growth factor (VEGF) and HGF, while long-term expression would be preferable if the goal is to express membrane proteins such as receptors for growth factors that require stable expression. Possible strategies to induce short-term gene expression of the transgene include plasmid transfection or the use of adenoviral vectors (Rabbany et al., 2009). Limitations of these strategies are the low transfection efficiency with plasmids and the immunogenic response of the host with adenoviruses.

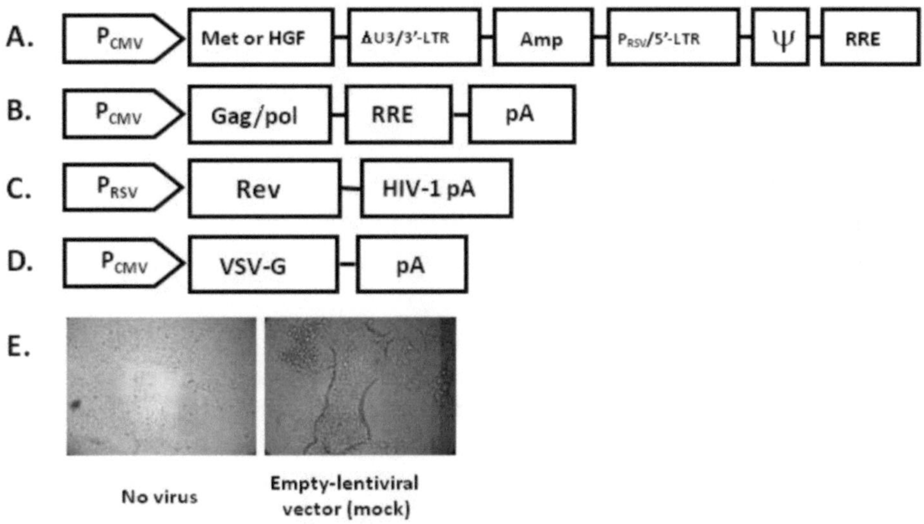

Fig. 2. Schematic representation of the transducing vector construct (a), packaging construct (b, c) and VSV-G Env-expressing construct (d). Abbreviations: Amp: ampicillin resistance gene; ΔU3: deleted region of the 3'LTR, which allows for biosafety of the vector; Gag, pol, env: genes codifying for envelope proteins; PCMV: cytomegalovirus promoter; 3'-LTR: 3'-long terminal repeats for viral packaging; PRSV: Rous Sarcoma Virus (RSV) enhancer/ promoter; 5'-LTR: 5'-long terminal repeats for viral packaging; w psi: packaging sequence for viral packaging; pA: polyadenylation signal; RRE: HIV-1 Rev response element; VSV-G: G glycoprotein gene from Vesicular Stomatitis Virus (VSV-G) as a pseudotyping envelope. (e) Photographs representing the experimental steps of production of the lentiviral stock (containing the packaged expression construct) by cotransfecting the packaging construct (b, c), the VSV-G Env-expressing construct (d) and transducing vector construct (a) into the 293FT virus-producing cell line. The expression of the VSV-G glycoprotein causes 293FT cells to fuse, resulting in the appearance of large, multinucleated cells known as syncytia.

7. Conclusions

Growth factor delivery and tissue engineering have emerged as new concepts that focus on tissue regeneration from cells with the support of biomaterials and growth factors

(Ikada, 2006). Various delivery methods are available to administer growth factors to ischemic tissues. Among these strategies, the cell-based delivery of growth factor genes is of great potential interest, since the *in situ* expression of the growth factor gene may result in higher and more constant levels of protein production. With respect to the delivery of growth factors, a major challenge is to identify growth factors and signaling pathways that selectively promote proliferation, migration, engraftment and differentiation of resident CSCs or exogenous multipotent stem cells. Current knowledge suggests that "cocktails" of biomolecules (growth factors or DNA), or even more cocktails of exogenous stem/committed progenitor cells (myogenic or angiogenic cells) with a wide spectrum of differentiation capabilities, should be delivered locally, in order to mimic, as far as possible, the different requirements of the ischemic tissue during the different regeneration phases. To deliver multiple growth factor genes and stem cells with distinct release and dynamic profiles, a greater understanding of the requirements for regenerating complex and functional tissues such as the myocardium is necessary. Challenges in this area revolve on controlling reciprocal interactions among those cells and signals. Winning these challenges would open a new era in stem cell and gene therapy research for both laboratory-based scientists and practicing physicians. From a bedside point of view, preclinical studies in large animals (such as porcine model) are required to carefully evaluate potential human therapies.

8. Acknowledgements

This work was supported by grants from the Italian Ministry of University and Scientific Research and from the Istituto Nazionale Ricerche Cardiovascolari (INRC).
The Authors declare no conflict of interest as related to the topics here discussed.

9. References

Angelis, D., L. Berghella, et al. (1999). "Skeletal myogenic progenitors originating from embryonic dorsal aorta coexpress endothelial and myogenic markers and contribute to postnatal muscle growth and regeneration." *J Cell Biol* 147: 869-77.

Assmus, B., V. Schachinger, et al. (2002). "Transplantation of progenitor cells and regeneration enhancement in acute myocardial infarction (TOPCARE-AMI)." *Circulation* 106: 3009-17.

Atkins, B. Z., M. T. Hueman, et al. (1999). "Myogenic cell transplantation improves in vivo regional performance in infracted rabbit myocardium." *J Heart Lung Transplant* 18: 1173-80.

Beltrami, A. P., K. Urbanek, et al. (2001). "Evidence that human cardiac myocytes divide after myocardial infarction." *N Engl J Med* 344: 1750-1757.

Beohar, N., J. Rapp, et al. (2010). "Rebuilding the damaged heart: the potential of cytokines and growth factors in the treatment of ischemic heart disease." *J Am Coll Cardiol* 56: 1287-1297.

Bleiziffer, O., E. Eriksson, et al. (2007). "Gene transfer strategies in tissue engineering." *J Cell Mol Med* 11: 206–223.

Britten, M. B., N. D. Abolmaali, et al. (2003). "Infarct remodelling after intracoronary progenitor cell treatment in patients with acute myocardial infarction (TOPCARE-AMI)." *Circulation* 108: 2212-8.

Camarata, P. J., R. Suryanarayanan, et al. (1992). "Sustained release of nerve growth factor from biodegradable polymer microspheres." *Neurosurgery* 30: 313–9.

Case, S. S., M. A. Price, et al. (1999). "Stable transduction of quiescent CD34(+)CD38(-) human hematopoietic cells by HIV-1-based lentiviral vectors." *Proc Natl Acad Sci U S A* 96(6): 2988-93.

Chen, F. M., M. Zhang, et al. (2010). "Toward delivery of multiple growth factors in tissue engineering." *Biomaterials* 31: 6279-6308.

Chimenti, I., R. R. Smith, et al. (2010). "Relative roles of direct regeneration versus paracrine effects of human cardiosphere-derived cells transplanted into infarcted mice." *Circ Res* 106(5): 971-80.

Cho, H. C. and E. Marban (2010). "Biological therapies for cardiac arrhythmias: can genes and cells replace drugs and devices?" *Circ Res* 106: 674-685.

Chou, C. and K. W. Leong (2007). "Biomaterials approach to expand and direct differentiation of stem cells." *Mol Therapy* 15: 467-480.

De Laporte, L., Y. Yang, et al. (2009). "Plasmid releasing multiple channel bridges for transgene expression after spinal cord." *Mol Therapy* 17: 318-326.

Donofrio, G., A. Capocefalo, et al. (2010). "Virally and physically transgenized equine adipose-derived stromal cells as a cargo for paracrine secreted factors." *BMC Cell Biol* 23: 11-73.

Donsante, A., D. G. Miller, et al. (2007). "AAV vector integration sites in mouse hepatocellular carcinoma." *Science* 317(5837): 477.

Emi, N., T. Friedmann, et al. (1991). "Pseudotype formation of murine leukemia virus with the G protein of vesicular stomatitis virus." *J Virol* 65: 1202–1207.

Fischer, K. M., C. T. Cottage, et al. (2009). "Enhancement of myocardial regeneration through genetic engineering of cardiac progenitor cells expressing Pim-1 kinase." *Circulation* 120: 2077-2087.

Forte, G., M. Minieri, et al. (2006). "Hepatocyte growth factor effects on mesenchymal stem cells: proliferation, migration, and differentiation." *Stem Cells* 24(1): 23-33.

Franssen, O., R. D. van Ooijen, et al. (1999). "Enzymatic degradation of cross-linked dextrans." *Macromolecules* 32: 2896-2902.

Fujii, H., S. H. Li, et al. (2011). "Repeated and targeted transfer of angiogenic plasmids into the infarcted rat heart via ultrasound targeted microbubble destruction enhances cardiac repair." *Eur Heart J* Jan 8.

Gansbacher, B. and European Society of Gene Therapy (2003). "Report of a second serious adverse event in a clinical trial of gene therapy for X-linked severe combined immune deficiency (X-SCID). Position of the European Society of Gene Therapy (ESGT)." *J Gene Med* 5: 261-262.

Haastert, K. and C. Grothe (2007). "Cardiovascular gene therapy: current status and therapeutic potential." *Br J Pharmacol* 152: 175-188.

Hagege, A. A., J. T. Vilquin, et al. (2001). "Regeneration of the myocardium: a new role in the treatment of ischemic heart disease? ." *Hypertension* 38: 1413-5.

Hirsch, A. T., Z. J. Haskal, et al. (2006). "ACC/AHA 2005 practice guidelines for the menagement of patients with peripheral arterial disease (lower extremity, renal, mesenteric, and abdominal aortic): a collaborative report from the American Association for Vascular Surgery/Society for Vacular Surgery, Society for Cardiovascular Abgiography and Interventions, Society for Vascular Medicine and Biology, Society of Interventional Radiology, and the ACC/AHA Task Force on Practice Guidelines (Writing Committee to Develop Guidelines for the Menagement of Patients with Peripheral Arterial Disease): endorsed by the American Association of Cardiovascular and Pulmonary Rehabilitation; National Heart, Lung, and Blood Institute; Society for Vascular Nursing; TransAtlantic Inter-Society Consensus; and Vascular Disease Foundation." *Circulation* 113: e463.

Holland, T. A., Y. Tabata, et al. (2003). " In vitro release of transforming growth factor-beta 1 from gelatin microparticles encapsulated in biodegradable, injectable oligo(poly(ethylene glycol) fumarate) hydrogels." *J Control Release* 91: 299–313.

Holland, T. A., Y. Tabata, et al. (2005). "Dual growth factor delivery from degradable oligo(poly(ethylene glycol) fumarate) hydrogel scaffolds for cartilage tissue engineering." *J Control Release* 101: 111–125.

Ikada, Y. (2006). "Challenges in tissue engineering." *J R Soc Interface* 3: 589–601.

Jiang, Y. H., B. N. Jahagirdar, et al. (2002). "Pluripotency of mesenchymal stem cells derived from adult marrow." *Nature* 418: 41-9.

Jollivet, C., A. Aubert-Pouessel, et al. (2004). "Striatal implantation of GDNF releasing biodegradable microspheres promotes recovery of motor function in a partial model of Parkinson's disease." *Biomaterials* 25: 933–42.

Juillerat-Jeanneret, L. and F. Schmitt (2007). "Chemical modification of therapeutic drugs or drug vector systems to achieve targeted therapy: looking for the grail." *Med Res Rev* 27: 574-590.

Kamihata, H., H. Matsubara, et al. (2001). " Implantation of bone marrow mononuclear cells into ischemic myocardium enhances collateral perfusion and regional function via side supply of angioblasts, angiogenic ligands, and cytokines." *Circulation* 104: 1046-52.

Kehat, I., D. Kenyagin-Karsenti, et al. (2001). "Human embryonic stem cells can differentiate into myocytes with structural and functional properties of cardiomyocytes." *J Clin Invest* 108: 407-414.

Krewson, C. E. and W. M. Saltzman (1996). "Transport and elimination of recombinant human NGF during long-term delivery to the brain." *Brain Res* 727: 169–81.

Langer, R. (1983). "Implantable controlled release systems." Pharmacol Ther 21: 35-51.

Lavik, E. and R. Langer (2004). "Tissue engineering: current state and perspectives." *Appl. Microbiol. Biotechnol* 65: 1-8.

Lever, A. M. (1996). "HIV and other lentivirus-based vectors." *Gene Ther* 3: 470–471.

Li, R. K., Z. Q. Jia, et al. (1995). "Cardiomyocyte transplantation improves heart function." *Ann Thorac Surg* 62: 654-661.

Li, R. K., D. A. Mickle, et al. (1996). " In vivo survival and function of transplanted rat cardiomyocytes." *Circ Res* 78: 283-288.

Liu, J., L. Xu, et al. (2011). "Temporally controlled multiple-gene delivery in scaffolds: a promising strategy to enhance bone regeneration." *Med Hypothesis* 76: 173-5.

Madonna, R. and R. De Caterina (2008). "In vitro neovasculogenic potential of resident adipose tissue precursors." *Am J Physiol - Cell Physiol* 295 (5): c1271-80.

Madonna, R. and R. De Caterina (2009). "Enhancement of the regenerative capacity of stem cells by the "Pharmacologically Active Microcarriers": a biomimetic support for cells and a growth factor delivery vector." *Acta* from the V workshop of the Italian Society of Cardiovascular Research I: 20-25.

Madonna, R., Y. J. Geng, et al. (2009). "Adipose Tissue-Derived Stem Cells. Characterization and Potential for Cardiovascular Repair." *Arterioscler Thromb Vasc Biol* 29: 1723-9

Madonna, R., R. Rokosh, et al. (2010). "Hepatocyte Growth Factor/Met Gene Transfer in Cardiac Stem Cells - Potential for Cardiac Repair." *Basic Card Res* 105: 443-52

Madonna, R., J. T. Willerson, et al. (2008). "Myocardin a enhances telomerase activities in adipose tissue mesenchymal cells and embryonic stem cells undergoing cardiovascular myogenic differentiation." *Stem Cells* 26(1): 202-11.

Marban, E. (2007). "Big cells, little cells, stem cells: agents of cardiac plasticity." *Circ Res* 100: 445–446.

Matsusaki, M. and M. Akashi (2005). "Novel fucntional biodegradable polymer IV: pH-sensitive controlled release of fibroblast growth factor-2 from a poly(gamma-glutamic acid)-sulfonate matrix for tissue engineering." *Biomacromolecules* 6(6): 3351-6.

Menasche, P., A. A. Hagege, et al. (2003). "Autologous skeletal myoblast transplantation for severe postinfarction left ventricular dysfunction." *J Am Coll Cardiol* 41: 1078-1083.

Menei, P., E. Jadaud, et al. (2004). "Stereotaxic implantation of 5- fluorouracil-releasing microspheres in malignant glioma." *Cancer* 100: 405–10.

Menei, P., J. M. Pean, et al. (2000). "Intracerebral implantation of NGF-releasing biodegradable microspheres protects striatum against excitotoxic damage." *Exp Neurol* 161: 259–72.

MERIT-HF Study Group (1999). "Effect of metoprolol CR/XL in chronic heart failure: Metoprolol CR/XL Randomised Intervention Trial in Congestive Heart Failure (MERIT-HF)." *Lancet* 353: 2001-2007.

Messina, E., L. De Angelis, et al. (2004). "Isolation and expansion of adult cardiac stem cells from human and murine heart." *Circ Res* 95: 911-921.

Mikos, A. G., S. W. Herring, et al. (2006). "Engineering complex tissues." *Tissue Eng* 12: 3307–3339.

Mittal, S., A. Cohen, et al. (1994). "In vitro effects of brain derived neurotrophic factor released from microspheres." *Neuroreport* 5: 2577–82.

Mudargi, R. C., V. R. Babu, et al. (2008). "Nano/micro technologies for delivering macromolecular therapeutics using poly(D,L-lactide-co-glycolide) and its derivatives." *J Control Release* 125(3): 193-209.

Murry, C. E., R. W. Wlseman, et al. (1996). "Skeletal myoblast transplantation for repair of myocardial necrosis." *J Clin Invest* 98: 2512-23.

Nakagami, H., K. Maeda, et al. (2005). "Novel autologous cell therapy in ischemic limb disease through growth factor secretion by cultured adipose tissue-derived stromal cells." *Arterioscler Thromb Vasc Biol* 25(12): 2542-7.

Odorico, J. S., D. S. Kaufman, et al. (2001). "Multilineage differentiation from human embryonic stem cell lines." *Stem Cells* 19: 193-204.

Pagani, F. D., H. DerSimonian, et al. (2003). "Autologous skeletal myoblasts transplantated to ischemia-damaged myocardium in humans. Histological analysis of cell survival and differentiation." *J Am Coll Cardiol* 41: 879-88.

Pean, J. M., P. Menei, et al. (2000). "Intraseptal implantation of NGF-releasing microspheres promote the survival of axotomized cholinergic neurons." *Biomaterials* 21: 2097–101.

Perin, E. C., H. F. R. Dohmann, et al. (2003). "Transendocardial, autologous bone marrow cell transplantation for severe, chronic ischemic heart failure." *Circulation* 107: 2294-2302.

Perin, E. C., G. V. Silva, et al. (2002). "Assessing myocardial viability and infarct transmurality with left ventricular electromechanical mapping in patients with stable coronary artery disease: validation by delayed-enhancement magnetic resonance imaging." *Circulation* 106: 957-61.

Puissant, B., C. Barreau, et al. (2005). "Immunomodulatory effect of human adipose tissue-derived adult stem cells: comparison with bone marrow mesenchymal stem cells." *Br J Haematol* 129: 118-129.

Qiu, Y. and K. Park (2001). "Environment-sensitive hydrogels for drug delivery." *Adv Drug Deliv Rev* 53: 321–339.

Rabbany, S. Y., J. Pastore, et al. (2009). "Continuous delivery of stromal cell-derived factor-1 from alginate scaffolds accelerates wound healing." *Cell Transpl.* doi:10.3727/096368909X481782.

Ramanan, R. M., P. Chellamuthu, et al. (2006). "Development of a temperature-sensitive composite hydrogel for drug delivery applications." *Biotechnol Prog* 22: 118-125.

Rappolee, D. A., A. Iyer, et al. (1996). "Hepatocyte growth factor and its receptor are expressed in cardiac myocytes during early cardiogenesis." *Circ Res* 78(6): 1028-36.

Rehman, J., D. Traktuev, et al. (2004). "Secretion of angiogenic and antiapoptotic factors by human adipose stromal cells." *Circulation* 109(10): 1292-8.

Richardson, T. P., M. C. Peters, et al. (2001). "Polymeric system for dual growth factor delivery." *Nature Biotechnology* 19: 1029-1034.

Rombouts, W. J. and R. E. Ploemacher (2003). "Primary murine MSC show highly efficient homing to the bone marrow but lose homing ability following culture." *Leukemia* 17: 160-170.

Rosengart, T. K., L. Y. Lee, et al. (1999). "Angiogensis gene therapy: phase I assessment of direct intramyocardial administration of an adenovirus vector expressing VEGF121 cDNA to individuals with clinically significant severe coronary artery disease." *Circulation* 100: 468-74.

Siminiak, T. and M. Kurpisz (2003). "Myocardial replacement therapy." *Circulation* 108: 1167-71.

Smith, R. R., L. Barile, et al. (2007). "Regenerative potential of cardiosphere-derived cells expanded from percutaneous endomyocardial biopsy specimens." *Circulation* 115(7): 896-908.

Smits, P. C., R. J. van Geuns, et al. (2003). "Catheter-based intramyocardial injection of autologous skeletal myoblasts as a primary treatment of ischemic heart failure: clinical experience with six-month follow-up." *J Am Coll Cardiol* 42: 2063-9.

Soonpaa, M. H., G. Y. Koh, et al. (1994). "Formation of nascent intercalated disks between grafted fetal cardiomyocytes and host myocardium." *Science* 264: 98-101.

Stewart, D. J., M. J. Kutryk, et al. (2009). "VEGF gene therapy fails to improve perfusion of ischemic myocardium in patients with advanced coronary disease: results of the NORTHERN trial." *Mol Therapy* 17: 1109-15.

Strauer, B. E., M. Brehm, et al. (2002). "Repair of infracted myocardium by autologous intracoronary mononuclear bone marrow cell transplantation in humans." *Circulation* 106: 1913-8.

Suzuki, K., B. Murtuza, et al. (2001). "Cell transplantation for the treatment of acute myocardial infarction using vascular endothelial growth factor-expressing skeletal myoblasts." *Circulation* 104: I107-212.

Svensson, E. C., D. J. Marshall, et al. (1999). "Efficient and stable transduction of cardiomyocytes after intramyocardial injection or intracoronary perfusion with recombinant adeno-associated virus vectors." *Circulation* 99: 201–205.

Tatard, V. M., M. C. Venier-Julienne, et al. (2005). "Pharmacologically active microcarriers: a tool for cell therapy." *Biomaterials* 26(17): 3727-37.

Thomson, J. A., J. Itskovitz-Eldor, et al. (1998). "Embryonic stem cell lines derived from human blastocysts." *Science* 282: 1145-7.

Urbanek, K., M. Rota, et al. (2005). "Cardiac stem cells possess growth factor-receptor systems that after activation regenerate the infarcted myocardium, improving ventricular function and long-term survival." *Circ Res* 97(7): 663-73.

Urbich, C. and S. Dimmeler (2004). "Endothelial progenitor cells, characterization and role in vascular biology." *Circ Res* 95: 343-353.

Vasita, R. and D. S. Katti (2006). "Growth factor-delivery systems for tissue engoneering: a materials perspective." *Expert Rev Med Devices* 3: 29-47.

Vats, A., R. C. Bielby, et al. (2005). "Stem cells." *Lancet* 366: 592-602.

Watanabe, E., D. M. Smith, et al. (1998). "Cardiomyocyte transplantation in a porcine myocardial infarction model." *Cell Transplant*: 239-46.

Zhang, X., D. Wu, et al. (2004). "Synthesis and characterization of partially biodegradable, temperature and pH sensitive Dex-MA/PNIPAAm hydrogels." *Biomaterials* 25: 4719-4730.

Zhao, X., J. Kimb, et al. (2011). "Active scaffolds for on-demand drug and cell delivery." *PNAS* 108: 67-72.

Zuk, P. A., M. Zhu, et al. (2001). "Multilineage cells from human adipose tissue: implications for cell-based therapies." *Tissue Eng* 7: 211-228.

3

Establishment of Conditional Transgenic Mice Model with Cavernous Hemangioma Using the Tet-On System

Jia Wei Zheng
College of Stomatolgy, Shanghai Jiao Tong University
China

1. Introduction

During the last two decades, fundamental insight into gene function has been efficiently provided through conventional knockout and transgenic experiments. Although genetically modified mice have provided important new information about the function of many genes, there are serious limitations to current animal models for a number of diseases. Introducing genetic changes to the germ line of a mouse may track down the effects of a particular gene but may also have severe developmental consequences, complicating or even precluding the desired experimental analysis. Good example illustrating these restrictions is embryonic lethality. In gene therapy, an ideal vector should include a regulatory system that is off in the resting state, exhibit tight regulation and allow for rapid and repeatable induction in response to a clinically approved inducer molecule. To overcome these undesired limitations and to precisely control gene expression, conditional mouse models are becoming increasingly popular. Although there are many kinds of inducible transgenic expression systems, tetracycline-controlled expression systems have been employed most frequently. The tet system developed by Gossen and co-workers includes two basic variants: one is the Tet-Off system (tTA system) and the other Tet-On system(rtTA system)(1.2). As a positive regulatory system, Tet-On system was used more widely in numerous transgenic animal models (3.4).

The original tet system contained two transcriptional units, transactivator and responder, on two plasmids. Currently available tetracycline-regulated transgenic methods require most of the generation of two transgenic strains, one carrying the transgene of interest under the control of the tet operator, and the other the reverse transactivator (rtTA). Crossing the lines generates progeny with both transgenes, allowing the regulation of the gene of interest through the administration of tetracycline. However, crossing and analysis of animals transgenic for the individual components of the system is costly and time consuming. Therefore, the generation of a vector containing the two units in a single plasmid may provide advantages for the simplified generation of conditional transgenic animals, as well as for gene therapy, and the successful use of a single construct containing the two elements has been reported (5.6.7). In addition, improvements of newly created tet-based systems should be focused on the elimination of background expression, increased sensitivity to tetracycline or its derivative doxycyline (Dox), and increased inducibility.

We designed and constructed two conditional transgenic vectors combining the two transcriptional units on a single plasmid. In addition, in order to eliminate the background expression of the gene of interest, the most powerful repressor domain containing a 'kruppel-associated box' (KRAB) of the zinc finger protein NK10 (8.9) was used and fused to tetR. The transactivator was placed under the control of CMV promoter, and the tet responsive element, driving the gene of interest, was inserted downstream into the same vector. To minimize any potential interference between the two elements, they were spaced by a 1.2Kb cHS4 insulator. To shield the transgene from the affection of chromosomal position effect and improve the transgene's expression efficiency, we inserted another cHS4 insulator into the upstream of the transgene cassette, and the two insulators were in the same orientation. One of the transgenes was introduced into the mouse genomic DNA through microinjection, and the transgenic mice developed venous malformation after the induction of transgene expression.

2. Plasmid construction

2.1 The construction of regulatory units

2.1.1 Cloning of cHS4 insulator, NK10 and teTR gene

The first step of the study was the cloning of cHS4 insulator from chicken genomic DNA. The primers used were: forward primer, 5′ AAAACGCCTCCAGGAAACCACTCT3′; and reverse primer, 5′CAGCAATATTCCCCCATCCTCACT3′. To ensure the sequence be in frame with the targeting sequence, pfu enzyme was used for the PCR experiments. PCR conditions were 95℃ for 5 minutes and then 34 cycles of 94℃ for 30s, 60.1℃for 40s, and 72℃ for 2m40s, followed by 72℃ for 10minutes.

NK10 gene was cloned from brain tissues cDNA. The primers used were: forward primer, 5′GAATTCGGAATGGCCCCGAGACCT3′; and reverse primer, 5′CTGCAGTCAATGCCCC TGGATAGCGACATT 3′. EcoR1 and Pst1 restriction site sequences were incorporated into the 5' end of the PCR primers, respectively. PCR conditions were 95℃ for 5 minutes and then 34 cycles of 94℃ for 30s, 61℃ for 40s, and 72℃ for 1minutes,followed by 72℃ for 10minutes.

TetR gene was cloned from the plasmid of ptet-off. The primers used were: forward primer, 5′AAACTCGAGCCCGGGATGGCTAGATTAGATAAAAG 3′; and reverse primer, 5′AAA GAATTCCTTTCTCTTCTTTTTGGCGACCCACTTTCACATTT 3′. The Xho1 and EcoR1 restriction sites sequences were introduced into the 5' end of the PCR primers, respectively. PCR conditions were 95°C for 5 minutes and then 34 cycles of 94°C for 30s, 61.5°C for 40s,and 72°C for 1minutes,followed by 72℃ for 10minutes.

2.1.2 Cloning the PCR products in pSK-

The 1.36Kb cHS4 insulator was digested by Sac II and Ssp II and the Sac II Ssp I fragment(1.2Kb) was subcloned into the Sac II-EcoRV fragment of plasmid pSK-,constructing the plasmid of pBShs4.The NK10 and tetR PCR products were subcloned into T-vector, respectively. The pMD-NK10 plasmid was digested by Pst I and EcoR1, and the pMD-tetR was digested by Xho I and EcoR I .The Pst I-EcoR1 fragment containing NK10 gene and the Xho I Eco I fragment containing tetR gene were subcloned into the Pst I-Xho I fragment of the pSK- plasmid, forming the plasmid of pBSNK10-tetR,in which the NK10-tetR gene will be translated into a fusion protein. The plasmid of pBSNK10-tetR was digested by Xho I. After the end blunted and purified, the fragment was then digested by

Not I. The plasmid of pIRES-EGFP was first digested by Bstx I and after the end blunted and purified the fragment was also digested by Not I, cutting off the EGFP gene. The Xho I-Not I insert fragment containing NK10-tetR gene and the Bstx I-Not I vector fragment were ligated together to generate the plasmid pIRES-NK10-tetR.To build the plasmid of pVP16-NK10-tetR, a EcoR I-Pst I digestion was carried out on the plasmid of pIRES- NK10-tetR, generating the 4Kb EcoR I-Pst I vector fragment, and a BamH1- Pst1 double digestion was also performed on the same plasmid to obtain the 1.6Kb BamH1- Pst1 insert fragment. The ptet-on plasmid was digested by EcoR1 and BamH I, isolating the 1.6Kb EcoR I- BamH I insert fragment rtTA. The three fragments, EcoR I-Pst I vector fragment, BamH I- Pst I insert fragment and EcoR I- BamH I insert fragment, which were all sticky ends were ligated in one ligation reaction, and the pVP16-NK10-tetR plasmid was constructed. pVP16-NK10-tetR plasmid was digested with BamH1 and Not1 cutting off the IRES- NK10-tetR fragment ,and then ligated itself after the end blunted, generating the plasmid of pVsp-teton.

2.2 The construction of responsive element

2.2.1 The cloning of MT gene

The plasmid pPyMT1 containing MT gene was digested by Bstx1 restriction enzyme. A 0.8% agarose gel electrophoresis that was loaded with all samples was used to isolate the 1.53Kb fragments. After the ends blunted and purified, the fragments were then digested by HindIII, and the Bstx I (blunting) - HindIII fragment(1.48Kb)containing ORF of MT gene was subcloned into the Sma I -HindⅢ fragment of pSK- ,forming the plasmid of PbsMT. A BamH I-HindIII digestion reaction was done on the plasmid of PbsMT, and the BamH I-HindIII fragment containing MT gene was cloned to the BamH I-HindIII vector fragment of the pTRE2 plasmid, forming the vector of pTREMT.

The pBSHS4 plasmid was first digested with Cla I, and then Sac I digestion was done on the same fragment after the Cla I ends were blunted. The 1.2Kb Cla I (blunt)-Sac I insert fragment containing Hs4 insulator was ligated with the Sac I -EcoR I vector fragment of pN2-EGFP plasmid that the EcoR I ends were also blunted, and this plasmid was labeled pHs4-N2EGFP. The Xho I-BamH I fragment of pTRE2 plasmid containing TRE gene was cloned to the Sal1-BamH1 vector fragment of pHs4-N2EGFP plasmid. As the Xho I is an isoschizomer of Sal I,this ligation reaction was sticky-ends, and the plasmid was named pHs4TRE-N2EGFP. The next step was to replace the EGFP gene of pHs4TRE-N2EGFP vector with MT. The experiments were as follows: pHs4TRE-N2EGFP was digested with BamH I and Not I, and the Not I ends were blunted. The vector fragment ligated with the BamH I-EcoRV insert fragment of pTRE-MT plasmid containing the MT gene, and this plasmid was designated as pN2-Hs4TRE-MT.

2.3 Ligation of the regulatory unit and the responsive element

The Ssp I -Vsp I insert fragment of pVP16-NK10-tetR plasmid(2.5Kb) and pVsp-teton(1.9Kb) were ligated with the Nhe I - Vsp I vector fragment of pN2-Hs4TRE-MT, respectively, whose Nhe I ends were blunted. Thus the plasmid of pVP16NK10-Hs4-TREMT and pVP16-Hs4-TREMT were constructed.

In order to insert another Hs4 insulator upstream of the transgene cassette, a plasmid was constructed. First, a pair of primers were designed: forward primer, 5' AAAATCG ATCATATGGCGGAGCGAGGAACTGAG3' having Cla I and Nde I restriction site sequences; and reverse primer, 5' AAACTCGAGGATATCCATATGCCGCCCTGGGAA3' having Xho I , EcoRV and Nde I restriction site sequences, and the template DNA was

1.5Kb MT gene originated from pBSMT plasmid. PCR was carried out to amplify a 500bp fragment. The product as a spacer was digested with Cla1 and Xho1 and cloned to the Cla1-Xho I vector fragment of pBS Hs4.Thus the pBSHs4-Nde plasmid was constructed, in the upstream of the spacer there was Nde I restriction site and the downstream were Nde I and EcoV. Therefore, the Vsp I -Ssp I insert fragments of pVP16NK10-hs4-TREMT(6.9Kb) and pVP16-Hs4-TREMT(5.4Kb) could be cloned to the pBSHs4-Nde' s Nde I -EcoRV vector fragment(4.2Kb).However, we tried many times and failed. So we changed the strategies: pBSHs4-Nde plasmid was first digested with Vsp1 and Nde1. The 1.4Kb fragment containing two kinds of DNAs was extracted and the Ssp1 digestion was done on it. Thus two kinds of DNAs were divided, and the 1.4Kb fragment which contained 1.2Kb insulator flanking Vsp I, Nde I sticky ends was cloned to the Vsp I site of plasmid of pVP16NK10-hs4-TREMT and pVP16-Hs4-TREMT, respectively, constructing the final plasmids, pHs4-VP16NK10-hs4-TREMT and pHs4-VP16-Hs4-TREMT, and the Bstx1 digestion was performed to determine the insert directions.

3. Experiments of the two plasmids *in vitro*

3.1 Transient transfection

To testify the function of the two plasmids, transient transfection was carried out. COS7 cells were cultivated in DMEM for 72 h and transfected by electroporation with the same amount of substance of the two plasmids. The electroporation conditions were: voltage, 220V; electrical capacity, 975uF; No. of pulse,1. After the electroporation and adding 1.5ml DMEM to the cuvette, the cells were carefully transfered into two culture dishes equally, respectively. Dox(15μg/ml DMEM) was added to one dish three hours after the electroporation, and the other was used as control.

3.2 Semi-quantitative RT-PCR experiment

A semi-quantitative RT-PCR(reverse transcription-polymerase chain reaction) method was applied to measure the marker genes expression of the two plasmids. Total RNA was isolated from the cells by TRIzol method, according to manufacturer's instructions (Invitrogen, Cergy-Pontoise, France), after 72 hours of incubation. In order to resolve the problem of genomic DNA contamination ,2μg RNA was digested with RNase Free Dnase I (New England BioLab, England). RT-PCR was carried out to 1μg DNase-digested RNA. The cDNA was generated using First-Strand Synthesis System for RT-PCR (TaKaRa, Dalian city, China), followed which was the PCR amplification of marker gene, and the expression of β-actin, a housekeeping gene which is assumed to be expressed at roughly equal levels in different cell types and under different conditions, was examined as an internal control. The primers and templates were the same amount of substances in different reactions. The primers used were: MT forward primer, 5′ AAAGAATTCCCATTTTTTGGCTGG GCAGATATCGCGGAGCGAGGAACTGAG3′; MT reverse primer, 5′ AAAAAGCTT CCATTTTTTGGATGGCGAGATATCCGCCCTGGGAATGATAG 3′. β-actin PCR primers were kindly provided by Dr Fei (IBCB, Shanghai Institutes for Biological Sciences, Chinese Academy of Sciences, Shanghai, China), which was designed spaning an intron of the genomic sequence , and this will result in a PCR product from genomic contamination that will be larger in size than the product generated from the cDNA. The PCR conditions were 95°C for 5 minutes and then 27 cycles of 94°C for 30s, 60°C for 1m30s, and 72°C for 1m, followed by 72°C for 10minutes. 0.8% agarose gel loaded with the same volume of PCR products was run to test the differences of the marker genes expression levels.

4. Transgenic mice

The 8.5 kb microinjection construction of the plasmid pHs4-VP16NK10-hs4-TREMT was excised from the vector by digestion with SSP I and VSP I, and separated by agarose gel electrophoresis, followed by purification. The purified fragment was microinjected at a concentration of 10 μ g/ml in phosphate-buffered saline into fertilized C57/BL6 mouse eggs. Transgenic animals were identified by PCR of tail-tip genomic DNA. The sense and antisense primers were 5′-GCGGAGCGAGGAACTGAG- 3′ and 5′-CCGCCCTGGGA ATGATAG-3′, respectively. Founder mouse mate with wild type C57/BL6 mouse was used to obtain the F1 generation. Dox (0.5 mg/ml) and Sucrose (1 %) were added to drinking water to induce the expression of MT in 6-week-old F1 mice. Skin and tumor samples were fixed in formaldehyde (10% in phosphate-buffered saline) and embedded in paraffin. Sections were cut at 5 μ m and stained with hematoxylin-eosin.

5. Results

In construction of the vectors the following plasmids were used: pTtet-On , pTet-Off , pTRE2, PBSsk-, pIRES2-EGFP and pEGFP-N2, and the vector backbone of the final plasmid was pEGFP-N2.The tet-off and tet-on systems have been developed to regulate transgene expression which provided negative and positive control of transgene expression, respectively. Although the tet-on system produces high basal expression in the absence of an inducer, as it is positive regulation, it is still applied widely. In order to eliminate the basal expression, in this study, we cloned the 'kruppel-associated box' (KRAB) silenceing domain of the zinc finger protein NK10 gene, a powerful transcriptional repressor, and ligated it with tet repressor to translate a fusion protein .The fusion protein binds to the tet operator sequences in the response element only in the absence of Dox and reduce leaked gene transcription. As dox added, the silencer dissociates from the tet operator, relieving the transcriptional inhibition, while the rtTA binds to the TRE and activate the gene's expression. To compare the efficiency and the effectiveness of diverse operating systems, two different Tet-On based inducible expression systems carried in a single cassette were constructed (Fig.1) .

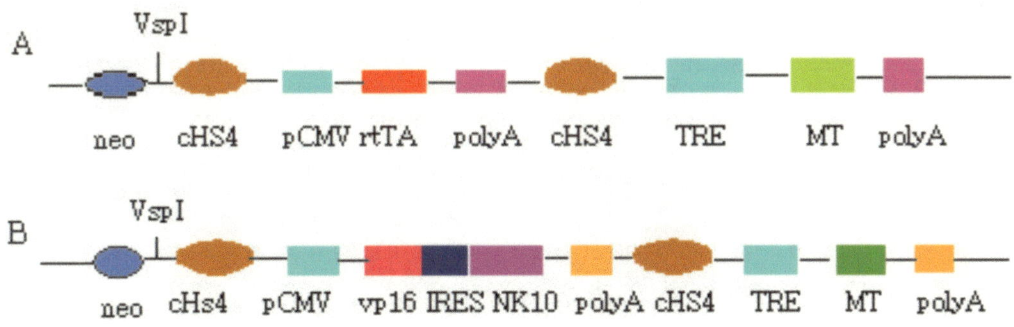

Fig. 1. The maps of the plasmids pHs4-VP16-Hs4-TREMT(A) and pHs4-VP16NK10-hs4-TREMT(B) after the SspI digestion.

In this study, three genes were successfully cloned by PCR method, and the sequences were right through the identification of sequencing and restriction enzyme digestion (Fig.2).

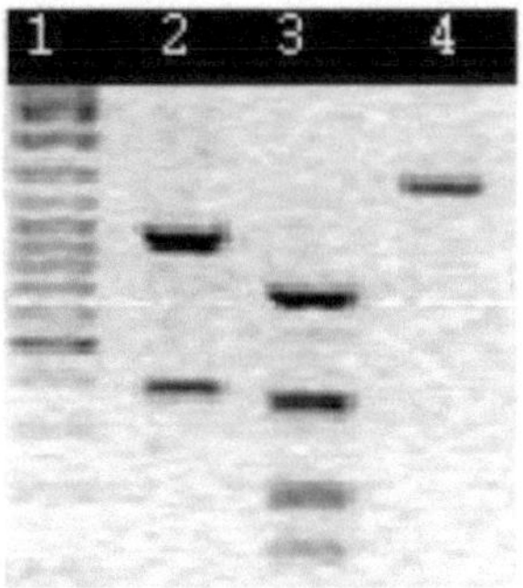

Fig. 2. CHS4 insulator restriction enzyme digestion. Lane 1: Marker, lane 2: Hind III, lane 3: Pst I, lane 4: cHS4 PCR product.

Restriction digestions were carried out to identify the final two transgene vectors, and analysis of the gel showed the two plasmids were constructed successfully (Fig.3).

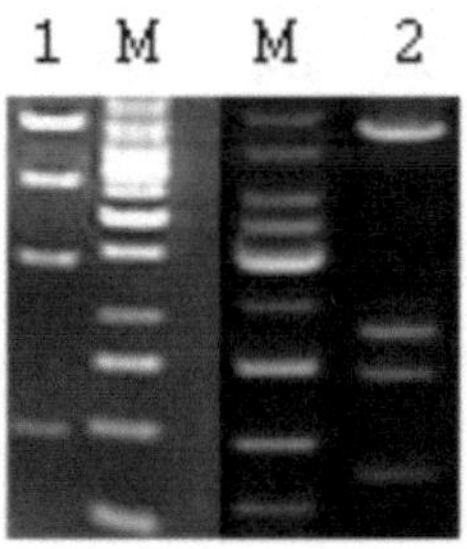

Fig. 3. The EcoRI digestion results of the two plasmids, pHs4-VP16-Hs4-TREMT(1) and pHs4-VP16NK10-hs4-TREMT(2).

The relative quantification of MT transcripts (target) was analyzed by semi-quantitative RT-PCR method in mRNA samples, by comparison with the mRNA abundance of β-actin (control), a housekeeping gene, which is assumed to be expressed at roughly equal levels in different cell types and under different conditions. The results showed that the two plasmids, pHs4-VP16NK10-hs4-TREMT and pHs4-VP16-Hs4-TREMT, had certain levels of transgene expression in the absence of tetracycline, and the inducibility of the latter was higher than that of the former (Fig.4).

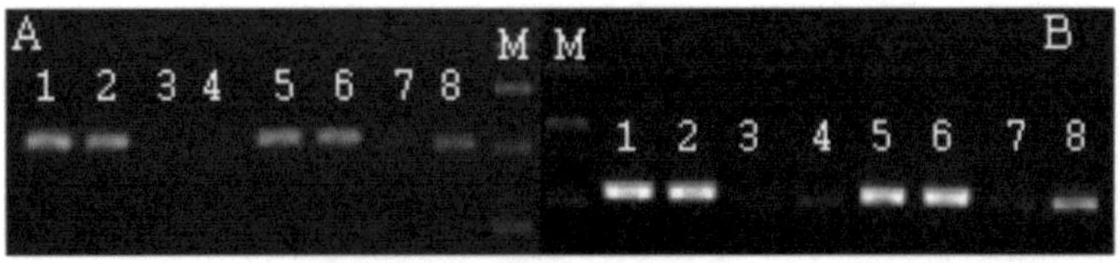

Fig. 4. The results of semi-quantitative RT-PCR of the two plasmids, pHs4-VP16NK10-hs4-TREMT(lane 1,2,3,4) and pHs4-VP16-Hs4-TREMT(lane 5,6,7,8) . The cycles were 22(A) and 24(B).There was no DOX added in the lanes 1,3,5 and 7, while dox added in lanes 2,4,6, and 8. There was no difference in the beta-actin expression before and after the DOX added (lane 1,2,5,6).

Five founders were identified by PCR analysis of DNA from tail biopsies. As expected from the inducible nature of transgene expression, no apparent phenotype was observed. After hybridization, three F1 mice were obtained, Dox (0.5mg/ml) and Sucrose (1%) were added to drinking water to induce the expression of MT in 6-week-old F1 mice .Two months later 2 mice developed vascular anomalies in brain and skin. The lesion was more venous malformation than hemangioma in histopathology (Fig.5., Fig.6.) .

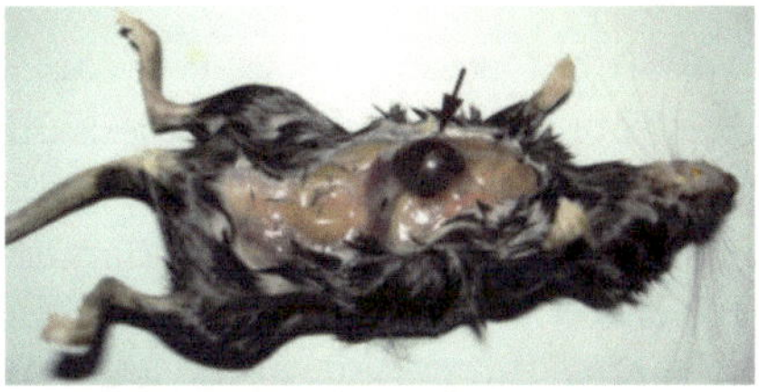

Fig. 5. Cystic tumor developed in the chest and skin of the mouse after 2 months of induction (arrow shows).

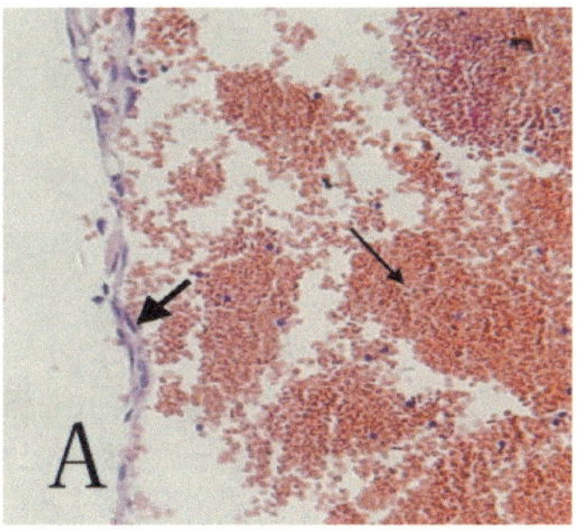

Fig. 6. Histological analysis of vascular anomalies induced in F1mice. The tumor was cystic and lined by endothelial cells(thick arrow shows). The cyst was full of red blood cells (thin arrow shows)

6. Discussion

The concept of gene therapy was originally introduced to treat inherited genetic disorders with the goal of replacing the defective gene with a normal one in diseased cells. This early concept has rapidly switched to a broader vision of gene therapy that uses genetic materials to alter the disease process. Currently, clinical trials are ongoing to examine the use of gene therapy in life-threatening diseases, such as malignant tumors and inherited genetic disorders. In gene therapy, the choice of gene delivery systems is most important.

Transgenic models have provided a wealth of information about the function of specific genes. However, the limitations of promoter-controlled transgene expression have become clear. The constitutive system has no control over the time of expression, which depends entirely on the properties of the promoters used. The promoters in this setting are active constitutively, many staring early in embryonic stages. The target gene is activated as soon as the promoter becomes active. If the transgene product happens to be toxic to the organism, especially during gestation, it can be detrimental to the developing embryo. This will results in a failure to generate live progeny carrying the transgene and that of the transgene cannot be studied past embryogenesis. If the gene product is not toxic to the embryos, the animals are viable and many demonstrated an interesting phenotype. However, there will still be questions remaining such as whether the phenotype is the results of transgene expression or is that of the mutation of endogenous genes. To deal with the limitations a number of investigators have established transgenic systems in which the expression of the transgene can be externally regulated. Although a variety of approaches have been utilized, tetracycline-controlled expression systems have been employed most frequently (10).

In the present study, we constructed a single plasmid containing both a tet-responsive transactivator together with the transgene responder successfully. This strategy circumvents the need to generate two independent transgenetic lines in the first place and greatly facilitates the mouse breeding strategy as effector and responder will not segregate.

Recent development of gene transfer approaches in plants and animals has revealed that transgene can undergo silencing after integration in the genome (11.12.13). Gene expression is influenced not only by the presence or absence of nearby transcription factors but also by the structure of surrounding chromatin. Variable repression of transcription often is associated with heterochromatin and frequently manifests itself as position effect variegation. In an extensive study of this phenomenon, Cerutti et al. (12) arrived at the conclusion that in C.reinhardtii the local heterochromatin structure rather than DNA methylation has a role in transgene inactivation. Insulators are DNA sequence elements that function as blocking the action of an enhancer and shielding a transgene from chromosomal position effect in transgenic animals and cell lines (14). Flanking a transgene with two copies of an insulator can shield it from chromosomal position effect following stable integration. In our preliminary study we attempted to insert two copies of 1.2Kb insulators in the flank of the transgene cassette, if that there will be three copies of direct repeat sequences in one plasmid and the plasmid will be unstable. We tried many times to construct it , but failed, though the STBL4 competent cells that are capable of stabilizing direct repeat sequences was used. As transgenes are usually found to be inserted into a single chromosomal location as multiple copies forming head-to-tail concatermers (10), so insulators can still be effective when placed on only one side of transgenes when in multi-copy arrays. This strategy has been employed successfully in this study and others (15.16.17).Theoretically only the end copy of the transgene would be susceptible to position effect after the concatemers integrated with germ lines genomic DNA. This not only can help save some cloning time and lower the plasmid size, but also can improve the transgene's expression efficiency.

Theoretically tetracycline inducible transgene expression systems should have negligible basal expression levels and high inducibility. Unfortunately, these goals are not achievable in our project. The results of this study showed that background expressions still existed in the two vectors, pVP16NK10-hs4-TREMT and pVP16-Hs4-TREMT, but the former's was much lower than that of the latter, and the inducibility of the later was much higher than that of the former. The reasons were as follows : first, in the two plasmids there was a enhancer/promoter of neo gene which could also act on the CMV minipromoter of TRE at a distance promoting the expression of the target gene. In *in vivo* experiment this factor will be excluded after the linearization of the plasmid with Vsp I and Ssp I digestions. Second, in the plasmid of pVP16NK10-hs4-TREMT the products of rtTA and tetR-NK10 can form heterodimers that do not function appropriately and compromise the overall inducibility of this system. On the other hands, competition existed between rtTA and tetR-NK10 for the DNA binding sites of TRE which could also lower the Dox-inducibility. This plasmid would be modified in our next project. Basal expression was also associated with the site(s) of integration of the transgenic constructs, and enhancer sequences near the target gene have been repeatedly demonstrated to increase basal target gene expression, thereby compromising the tight regulation that is desired (18.19). To eliminate the basal expression, insulator was used to block the effect of enhancer near the transgene integration sites on TRE in our study. Although the results in the test of transient transfections showed a degree of leakage expression, in some circumstances, the leak is acceptable and does not negate the ability of the experimental system to appropriately address the hypothesis that is being investigated. In the upstream of our transgene cassettes there was a neo gene, respectively. If the vectors were only digested with Ssp I this gene being a selective marker will be included in the transgene cassettes, and this will benefit stable transfection of the two vectors.

Vascular anomalies are classified into hemangiomas and vascular malformations. Hemangiomas are the most common cutaneous tumors of infancy, which demonstrated by rapid growth after birth followed by a slow spontaneous involution or regression within five to seven years. Unlike hemangiomas, vascular malformations enlarge proportionately with the growth of the child and do not undergo spontaneous involution (Mulliken JB and Glowacki J. 1982). Vascular malformations can be subdivided based on blood flow rate: "slow flow" (capillary, venous, lymphatic or mixed) vs "fast flow" (arterial, arteriovenous, fistulae or shunt) subtypes. Vascular anomalies occur mostly in the head and neck regions, and there is no useful animal model with this disease until now. In our study, we established conditional transgenic mice model with cavernous malformations base on tet-on system, and this animal model could be a useful tool to investigate the pathogenesis and intervention of venous malformation, as well as the function of PyMT gene.

In summary, in the present study we combined the two expression units of Tet-On system on a single plasmid constructing two conditional transgenic vectors, one of which contained Nk10 gene fused to TetR. CHS4 insulator elements were utilized in the construction of the vectors to eliminate the basal expression and transgene silencing. Our study *in vitro* demonstrated that the two "two-in-one" systems were functional. This would minimize the breeding and genotyping required for phenotypic characterization. Above all, If the vectors were only digested with Ssp I a neo gene as a selection marker will be included in the transgene cassettes. Therefore, the Tet-On system presented here may be easy to use and widely applicable to the study of gene function in transfected cells and gene therapy, as well as for the creation of conditional transgenic animal models to study disease and development *in vivo*. As the Dox-inducibility of pHs4-VP16NK10-hs4-TREMT was lower, modifications should be made on this plasmid in the future.

7. Reference

[1] Gossen M, Bujard H. Tight control of gene expression in mammalian cells by tetracycline-responsive promoters. Proc Natl Acad Sci U S A. 1992;89(12):5547-51.

[2] Gossen M, Freundlieb S, Bender G, Muller G, Hillen W, Bujard H. Transcriptional activation by tetracyclines in mammalian cells. Science. 1995;268(5218):1766-9.

[3] Vitale-Cross L, Amornphimoltham P, Fisher G, Molinolo AA, Gutkind JS. Conditional expression of K-ras in an epithelial compartment that includes the stem cells is sufficient to promote squamous cell carcinogenesis. Cancer Res. 2004;64(24):8804-7.

[4] Zabala M, Wang L, Hernandez-Alcoceba R, Hillen W, Qian C, Prieto J, Kramer MG. Optimization of the Tet-on system to regulate interleukin 12 expression in the liver for the treatment of hepatic tumors. Cancer Res. 2004;64(8):2799-804.
[5] Lottmann H, Vanselow J, Hessabi B, Walther R. The Tet-On system in transgenic mice: inhibition of the mouse pdx-1 gene activity by antisense RNA expression in pancreatic beta-cells. J Mol Med. 2001;79(5-6):321-8.
[6] Backman CM, Zhang Y, Hoffer BJ, Tomac AC. Tetracycline-inducible expression systems for the generation of transgenic animals: a comparison of various inducible systems carried in a single vector. J Neurosci Methods. 2004;139(2):257-62.
[7] Mizuguchi H, Xu ZL, Sakurai F, Mayumi T, Hayakawa T. Tight positive regulation of transgene expression by a single adenovirus vector containing the rtTA and tTS expression cassettes in separate genome regions. Hum Gene Ther. 2003;14(13):1265-77.
[8] Thiel G, Lietz M, Bach K, Guethlein L, Cibelli G. Biological activity of mammalian transcriptional repressors. Biol Chem. 2001;382(6):891-902.
[9] Lange R, Christoph A, Thiesen HJ, Vopper G, Johnson KR, Lemaire L, Plomann M, Cremer H, Barthels D, Heinlein UA.Developmentally regulated mouse gene NK10 encodes a zinc finger repressor protein with differential DNA-binding domains. DNA Cell Biol. 1995;14(11):971-81.
[10] Zhu Z, Ma B, Homer RJ, Zheng T, Elias JA. Use of the tetracycline-controlled transcriptional silencer (tTS) to eliminate transgene leak in inducible overexpression transgenic mice. J Biol Chem. 2001;276(27):25222-9.
[11] Ingelbrecht I, Van Houdt H, Van Montagu M and Depicker A. Posttranscriptional silencing of reporter transgenes in tobacco correlates with DNA methylation. Proc. Natl Acad. Sci. USA. 1994;91(22):10502–6.
[12] Cerutti H, Johnson AM, Gillham NW and Boynton JE. Epigenetic silencing of a foreign gene in nuclear transformants of Chlamydomonas. Plant Cell. 1997;9(6):925-45.
[13] Finnegan EJ, Genger RK, Peacock WJ and Dennis ES. DNA methylation in plants. Annu Rev Plant Physiol Plant Mol Biol. 1998;49:223-247.
[14] Burgess-Beusse B, Farrell C, Gaszner M, Litt M, Mutskov V, Recillas-Targa F, Simpson M, West A, Felsenfeld G. The insulation of genes from external enhancers and silencing chromatin. Proc Natl Acad Sci U S A. 2002;99 (Suppl 4):16433-7.
[15] Boeda B, Weil D and Petit C. A specific promoter of the sensory cells of the inner ear defined by transgenesis. Hum Mol Genet. 2001;10(15): 1581-9.
[16] Rivella S, Callegari JA, May C, Tan CW and Sadelain M. The cHS4 insulator increases the probability of retroviral expression at random chromosomal integration sites. J Virol. 2000;74:(10):4679-87.
[17] Taboit-Dameron F, Malassagne B, Viglietta C, Puissant C, Leroux-Coyau M, Chereau C, Attal J, Weill B and Houdebine LM. Association of the 5'HS4 sequence of the chicken beta-globin locus control region with human EF1 alpha gene promoter induces ubiquitous and high expression of human CD55 and CD59 cDNAs in transgenic rabbits. Transgenic Res. 19998;8(3): 223-35.
[18] Furth PA, St Onge L, Boger H, Gruss P, Gossen M, Kistner A, Bujard H, Hennighausen L. Temporal control of gene expression in transgenic mice by a tetracycline-responsive promoter. Proc Natl Acad Sci U S A. 1994;91(20):9302-6.
[19] Zheng T, Zhu Z, Wang Z, Homer RJ, Ma B .Inducible targeting of IL-13 to the adult lung causes matrix metalloproteinase- and cathepsin-dependent emphysema. J Clin Invest. 2000;106(9):1081-93.

4

Potential Gene Therapy: Intravenous Administration of Phagocytes Transfected Ex Vivo with FGF4 DNA/Biodegradable Gelatin Complex Promotes Angiogenesis in Animal Model of Myocardial Ischemia/Reperfusion Injury

Toru Shizuma, Chiharu Tanaka, Hidezo Mori and Naoto Fukuyama
Department of Physiology, School of Medicine, Tokai University, 143, Shimokasuya, Isehara, Kanagawa, Japan

1. Introduction

Conventional gene therapies still require improvement in various respects, such as transfection efficiency for targeting organs or tissues, safety (Li Q et al., 2001; Pfeifer A & Verma IM, 2001; Watson DJ et al., 2002), and so on. For example, transfection of naked plasmid DNA requires the use of a large quantity of DNA because of enzymatic degradation in the human body. Conventional non-viral vectors seem to be inferior to viral ones in efficiency, except for nucleofection (Nishikawa M & Hashida M, 2002; Schakowski F et al., 2004). On the other hand, gene therapy using viral vectors such as adenovirus, retrovirus etc., may induce tissue inflammation (Tomasoni S & Benigni A, 2004), though the efficiency of transfection is often relatively high. Also, the safety of viral transfection remains an issue, because of the risk of toxicity or mutation of viruses (Ferber D, 2001; Isner JM, 2002; Kay MA et al., 2001). Moreover, in vivo gene delivery to localized target tissues usually necessitates an invasive approach; for example, direct gene transfection to cardiomyocytes requires a surgical approach (Losordo DW et al.,1998) or catheterization (Kornowski R et al., 2000; Laitinen M et al., 2000). On the other hand, ex vivo gene transfection is less invasive. However, targeting of specific tissues by intravenous injection is usually inefficient.

Macrophages accumulate in ischemic tissues through chemotaxis (Ramsay SC et al., 1992). Therefore, we considered that intravenously administered macrophages might target ischemic tissue in vivo. Tabata, et al. reported that particles of gelatin are phagocytized by macrophages (Tabata Y & Ikada Y, 1987; Tabata Y & Ikada Y, 1988). Gelatin is a natural polymer derived from collagen, and is widely used in pharmaceutical or medical applications, i.e., it is safe and suitable for use in humans (Young S et al., 2005). Further, its isoelectric point (Ip) can be adjusted by modification of its residues, and positively charged gelatin can be impregnated with negatively charged substances (Ikada Y & Tabata Y, 1998), such as nucleic acid (Kasahara H et al., 2003). Therefore, gelatin may be suitable as a vector for transfecting phagocytes ex vivo.

Here, we describe a study aimed at examining the feasibility of a new concept for less-invasive, cell-based gene therapy by means of ex vivo gene transfection into isolated phagocytes (macrophages/monocytes) using a gelatin carrier, followed by intravenous injection of the transfected phagocytes. The present method has significant advantages over conventional cell-based gene delivery (Panetta CJ et al., 2002; Xie Y et al., 2001), in that the intravenously injected cells (phagocytes) not only produce protein from the transfected gene, but also have the potential for high tissue targeting ability. This method should be suitable for clinical gene therapy. Indeed, its clinical efficacy in patients with cardiovascular disease has recently been reported (Komeda M et al., 2009; Marui A et al., 2007; Tabata Y, 2009).

2. Main body

2.1 Methods

This study was performed in accordance with the Guideline of Tokai University School of Medicine on Animal Use, which conforms to the NIH Guide for the Care and Use of Laboratory Animals, (DHEW publication No. (NIH) 86-23, Revised 1985, Offices of Science and Health Reports, DRR/NIH, Bethesda, MD, 20205).

2.1.1 Animals

One hundred and twenty-one Fisher rats (male, 10 weeks old, Clea Japan Inc., Tokyo) and 61 nude SCID mice (male, 6 weeks old, Shizuoka Animal Center, Shizuoka, Japan) were used. Rats were anesthetized by inhalation of diethyl ether for harvesting of macrophages and with isofluran (1.5-3%) for thoracotomy, after which they were mechanically ventilated with a mixture of oxygen and nitrous oxide. Mice were anesthetized by intraperitoneal injection of sodium pentobarbital (40 mg/kg).

A model of myocardial ischemia-reperfusion injury was prepared in 41 rats. The remaining 80 rats were used for collecting activated macrophages. The heart was exposed via thoracotomy, and the proximal left anterior descending coronary artery was ligated (Gidh-Jain M et al.,1996) for 180 min, followed by reperfusion. A model of hindlimb ischemia was prepared in 61 mice. The left femoral artery was ligated and resected (Takeshita S et al., 1994).

2.1.2 Cells

Macrophages were obtained from 80 rats. Thioglycolate (4%, 8 ml) was injected into the peritoneal cavity, and after 4 days, peritoneal macrophages were collected (Ribeiro RA et al.,1991). Monocytes were obtained from peripheral blood of healthy volunteers. Leukocyte-rich plasma was obtained by dextran 500 sedimentation and layered onto Nycoprep 1.068 (Nycomed, Birmingham, UK). The monocyte-containing layer was aspirated, washed twice and allowed to adhere to the dish for 90 minutes. Fibroblasts (NIH 3T3, Invitrogen Corporation, Carlsbad, CA) were also used. The cells were resuspended in RPMI 1640 medium (Sigma) containing 5% heat-inactivated fetal calf serum and cultured for 7-14 days. The cell viability and type were determined by trypan blue exclusion and by immunostaining using anti-macrophage antibody, up to 14 days.

2.1.3 Genes and vector

Complementary DNA (cDNA) of green fluorescent protein (GFP), Renilla luciferase or human hst1/fibroblast growth factor 4 (FGF4) (Kasahara H et al., 2003) was inserted into the expression vector pRC/CMV (Invitrogen Corporation, Carlsbad, CA) and the constructs were designated as pRC/CMV-GFP, pRC/CMV-luciferase and pRC/CMV-HST1-10, respectively. Preparation and purification of the plasmid from cultures of pRC/CMV-GFP-, pRC/CMV-luciferase-, or pRC/CMV-HST1-10-transformed *Escherichia coli* were performed by equilibrium centrifugation in cesium chloride-ethidium bromide gradients.

Gelatin was prepared from porcine skin (Tabata Y & Ikada Y, 1987). After swelling in water the gelatin particles used in this study were spheroids with a diameter of approximately 5-30 μm, water content of 95%, and pI of 11. Gelatin (2 mg) was incubated with 50 μg of the plasmid for 7 days at 4 °C to make a gelatin-DNA complex (Tabata Y & Ikada Y, 1987).

2.1.4 *Ex vivo* gene transfection

Macrophages, monocytes, and fibroblasts (1 x 10^6) were cultured with the gelatin-DNA complex (2 mg of gelatin plus 50 μg of DNA) for 14 days on a culture dish (100 mm in diameter). Gene expression of GFP was evaluated by fluorescence microscopy and fluorescence-activated cell sorting. Luciferase activity in the cell lysate was evaluated with a photon counter system after cell lysis (Fukuyama N et al., 1996).

2.1.5 Organ distribution of phagocytes injected intravenously and directly into ischemic muscle

To examine tissue-targeting by intravenous injection of transfected phagocytes, the distribution of the cells into organs was evaluated by immunohistochemistry. In the rat model of myocardial ischemia-reperfusion injury, the GFP-gene-transfected macrophages (1.0 x 10^6 each) were injected into the superficial dorsal vein of the penis at the initiation of reperfusion (n=7 and 5, respectively). In the mouse model of hindlimb ischemia, the GFP-gene-transfected monocytes (1.0 x 10^6) were injected into the caudal vein 14 days after induction of ischemia (n=5). To examine the tissue targeting by direct local injection of transfected phagocytes, the distribution of the cells into organs was also evaluated. In the rat model of myocardial ischemia-reperfusion injury (n=7) and the mouse model of hindlimb ischemia (n=5), the same numbers of transfected macrophages and monocytes were directly injected into ischemic myocardium and ischemic skeletal muscle, respectively. Tissue samples were obtained 24 hours after cell administration. Each tissue was homogenized and the homogenate was cytospun. Immunohistochemical analysis was done with anti-GFP antibody (GFP monoclonal antibody; Clontech, USA). GFP-positive macrophages were counted in each tissue and expressed as a percentage of total GFP-positive cells.

2.1.6 Amelioration of ischemia by intravenous injection of angiogenic gene-transfected phagocytes

The angiogenic effect of intravenously injected FGF4-gene-transfected phagocytes on the ischemia models was evaluated. In the rat model of myocardial ischemia-reperfusion injury, FGF4-gene-transfected macrophages (n=5), non-transfected macrophages (1.0 x 10^6 each) (n=5), or saline (n=5) were injected into the superficial dorsal vein of the penis, or naked FGF4-DNA (50 μg) was injected directly into the ischemic myocardium (n=5), at the initiation of reperfusion. Fourteen days after the cell administration, blood flows in the ischemic and non-ischemic regions in the heart were evaluated with a noncontact laser

Doppler flowmeter (FLO-N1, Omegawave Corporation). Then, tissue samples were obtained and histological analysis was performed. In a mouse model of hindlimb ischemia, just after induction of ischemia, FGF4-gene-transfected monocytes (n=15), non-transfected monocytes (n=8) (1.0×10^6 each), or saline (n=10) were injected into the caudal vein, or naked FGF4-DNA (50 μg) was injected directly into the ischemic muscle (n=12). Fourteen days after induction of ischemia, blood flows in the limbs were evaluated with the noncontact laser Doppler flowmeter (FLO-N1, Omegawave Corporation).

2.1.7 Histology

Ten-micrometer sections were cut from formalin-fixed, paraffin-embedded tissue. Two sections were used for H.E. staining and Azan staining, and eight sections were used for immunohistochemical staining. Immunohistochemical staining was performed by an indirect immunoperoxidase method. Anti-GFP antibody, anti-Mac1 antibody (BMA Biomedicals Ag, Switzerland), and anti-CD31 antibody (Serotec, UK) were used as primary antibodies. Mac1-antigen is specific to macrophages/monocytes. Anti-Ig, peroxidase-linked species-specific F(ab')2 fragments (Amersham Pharmacia Biotech UK Ltd., UK), were used as a secondary antibody. Double staining was performed with alkaline staining and peroxidase staining. The density of vessels stained with von Willebrand factor-antibody was calculated by morphometric assessment in 16 randomly selected fields for each heart and expressed as number / mm^2.

2.1.8 Statistical analysis

Data are presented as mean values±SD. Differences were assessed by means of ANOVA (analysis of variance) with Scheffe's multiple comparisons test. A value of $P<0.05$ was considered statistically significant.

2.2 Results

2.2.1 *Ex vivo* gene transfection

We studied whether genes could be transfected into isolated rat macrophages, human monocytes, and mouse fibroblasts ex vivo by using gelatin. Transfection of the GFP gene into isolated rat macrophages (Figs. 1A and B) and human monocytes (Figs. 1C and D), but not into mouse fibroblasts (data not shown), was achieved by culture with gelatin-DNA complex for 14 days. The gene transfection efficiency into rat macrophages was 68±11% (30 experiments, Fig. 2A) and that into human monocytes was 78±8% (30 experiments) as determined with a fluorescence-activated cell sorter. Sequential analysis after luciferase-gene transfection into rat macrophages revealed high expression after 14 days of culture (Fig. 2B).

2.2.2 Organ distribution of phagocytes injected intravenously or directly into ischemic muscle

We studied quantitatively whether intravenously injected luciferase-gene-transfected phagocytes could target ischemic tissues (Table 1). In non-ischemic rats, the injected macrophages were found almost exclusively in the spleen (98±4%) (n=7, Table 1). In non-ischemic mice, similar results were observed (n=7, data not shown). In a rat with myocardial ischemia-reperfusion injury, some of the intravenously injected macrophages were incorporated into the heart (Table 1).

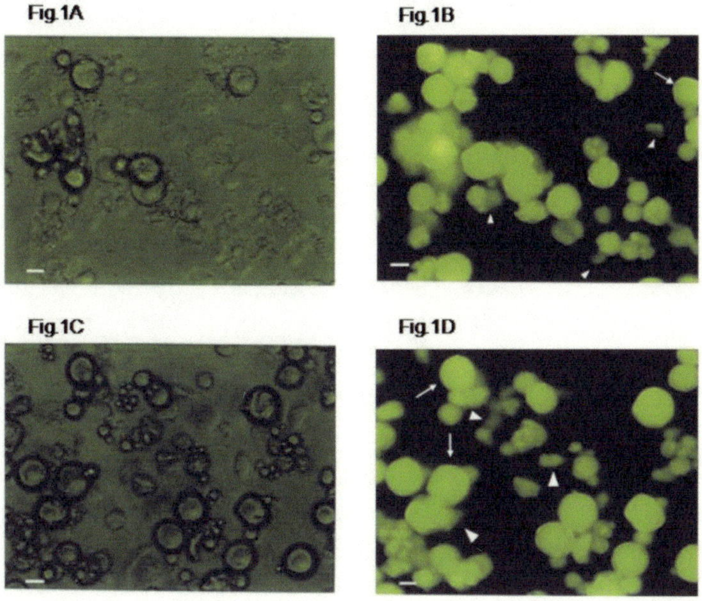

Fig. 1. Fluorescent presentation of ex vivo gene transfection with gelatin-DNA complex in macrophages/monocytes as well as fibroblasts. Rat macrophages (A and B) and human monocytes (C and D) were cultured with gelatin-GFP-gene complex for 14 days. Transmittance microscopic images (A and C) and fluorescence images (B and D) of the cells are shown. Macrophages (B) and monocytes (D) show fluorescence due to GFP. Arrowheads indicate GFP-expressing cells. Arrows indicate gelatin particles themselves. Bars=20 μm (Fukuyama N et al., 2007).

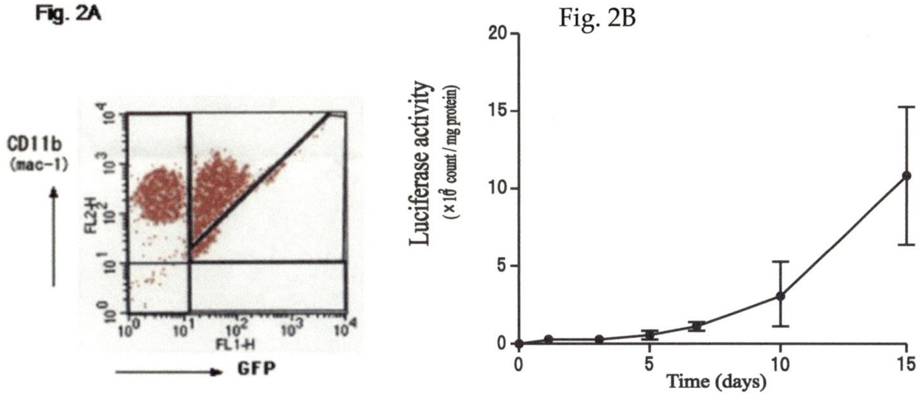

Fig. 2. Quantitative assessment of gene transfection into rat macrophages. A, Fluorescence-activated cell sorting analysis of transfected macrophages done on day 14 of culture with reference to GFP-positive and Mac1-positive cells. B, Sequential changes of luciferase activity in cultured macrophages in the presence of luciferase-gene-gelatin complex. Values are mean±SD. The number of experiments is shown in parentheses (Fukuyama N et al., 2007).

Organ	Normal i.v. (7 rats)	Myocardial injury i.v. (7 rats)	Myocardial injury i.m. (7 rats)	Hindlimb ischemia i.v. (7 mice)	Hindlimb ischemia i.m. (7 mice)
Heart	0±0	13±6	86±10	0±0	0±0
Hindlimb muscle	0±0	0±0	0±0	13±7	88±6
Spleen	98±4	84±6	13±10	84±6	11±6
Lung	1±2	1±1	1±2	1±2	1±1
Liver	1±2	1±1	1±1	1±2	1±1
Brain	0±0	0±0	0±0	0±0	0±0
Kidney	0±0	0±0	0±0	0±0	0±0
Intestine	0±0	0±0	0±0	0±0	0±0

Table 1. Organ-distribution of phagocytes injected into the vein and into local tissue. Each value shows a distribution ratio (%) into organs of transfected macrophages/monocytes (mean±SD). i.v., intravenous injection into the vein; i.m. direct injection into the jeopardized muscle (Fukuyama N et al., 2007).

Fig. 3A

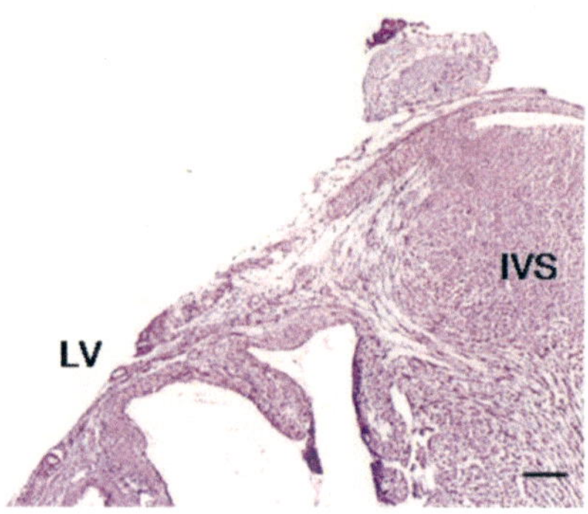

Fig. 3B

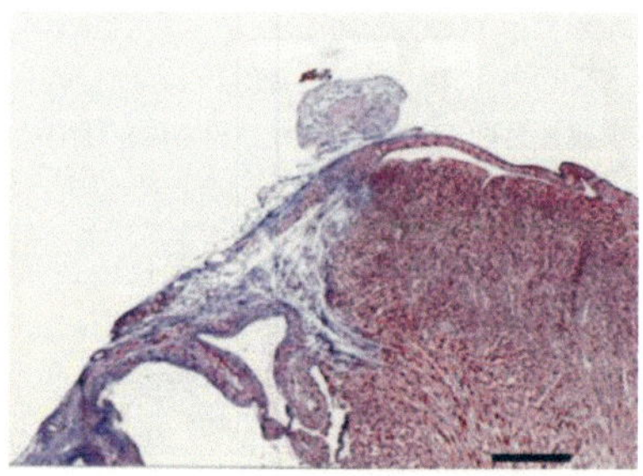

Fig. 3C

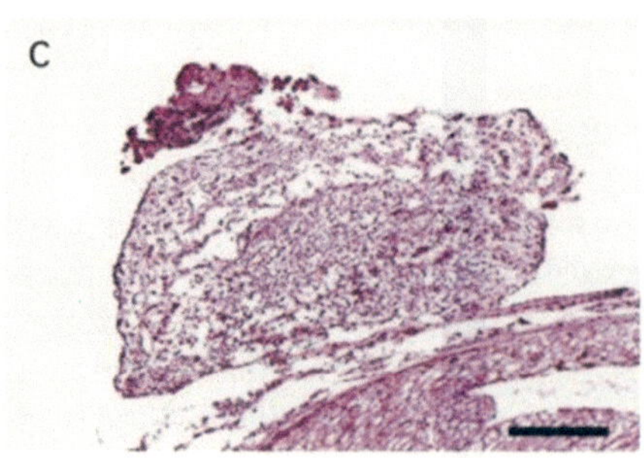

Fig. 3D

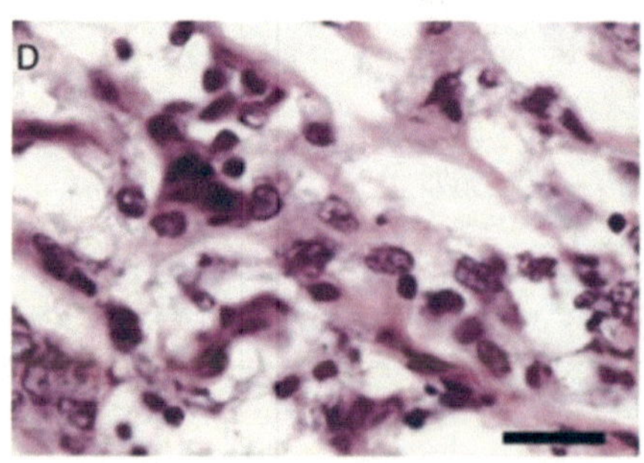

Fig. 3E

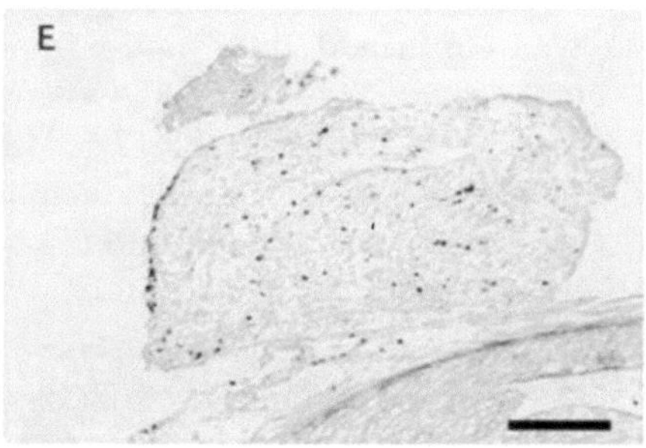

Fig. 3F

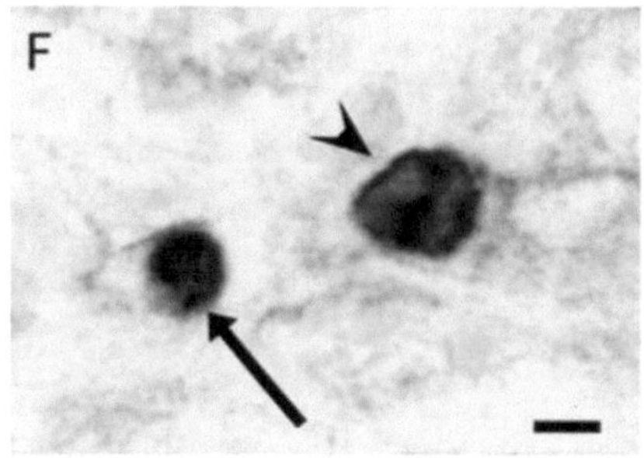

Fig. 3G

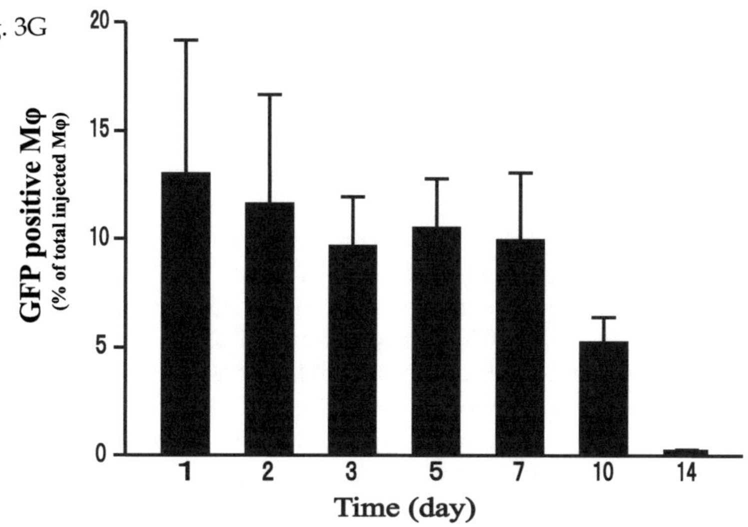

Fig. 3. Incorporation of injected macrophages into the heart. GFP-transfected macrophages were injected into the vein in a rat model of myocardial ischemia-reperfusion injury. A and B, Low-resolution images of ischemic myocardial tissue with hematoxylin-eosin staining and Azan staining, respectively. IVS, the interventricular septum; LV, the left ventricular free wall; RV, the right ventricular free wall. Original magnification x20. Bars=500 μm. C and D, Medium-and high-resolution images of ischemic myocardial tissue with hematoxylin-eosin staining; Original magnification x100 and x300; Bars=100 and 20 μm, respectively. E and F, Double immunohistochemical stainings of GFP- (red) and Mac1- (blue) antigens. Arrow indicates a GFP- and Mac1-antigen double-positive cell and arrowhead a Mac 1-antigen single-positive cell. Original magnification x100 and x400; Bars=100 and 10 μm, respectively. G, The time course of GFP-transfected macrophages (Mφ) accumulation into heart (Fukuyama N et al., 2007).

The incorporation into the post-ischemic pericardium amounted to 13±6% (n=7) (non-ischemic rats 0±0%, n=7, Table 1). The incorporated cells expressed GFP (Fig. 3). Fibrosis with inflammatory infiltrates was recognized in the anterior wall of the left ventricle, extending to the interventricular septum (Figs. 3A and B). These infiltrates were mainly polymorphonuclear leukocytes and macrophages (Figs. 3C and D). Approximately 20 % of the macrophages showed GFP-positivity in this area (Figs. 3E and F). Similar tissue-targeting by intravenously injected monocytes was confirmed in a mouse model with hindlimb ischemia (13±7%, n=7, Table 1). Furthermore, we studied whether local intramuscular injection increased the degree of tissue targeting (Table 1). After direct injection of phagocytes into ischemic muscle, 86±10% and 88±6% of the cells remained in the target tissue in the two models. Thirteen and 11% of phagocytes injected into the cardiac or hindlimb muscle migrated to the spleen. In the other organs, accumulation of phagocytes was negligible.

2.2.3 Amelioration of ischemia by intravenously injected angiogenic-gene-transfected phagocytes

In the rat model with myocardial ischemia-reperfusion injury, we studied the angiogenic effect of intravenously injected macrophages transfected with FGF4 gene by using gelatin. Intravenous injection of these macrophages (1.0 x 10^6) significantly increased the regional blood flow in the ischemic myocardium (78±7.1%, n=8, in terms of ischemic/non-ischemic myocardium flow ratio) compared with the other three treatments (P<0.05, ANOVA), that is, intravenous administration of saline (35±10%, n=8), intramuscular administration of naked DNA encoding FGF4 (50 µg, direct intramyocardial injection after thoracotomy) (58±5.3%, n=8), and intravenous administration of the same number of non-transfected macrophages (42±12%, n=8) (Fig. 4A). Histological analyses revealed angiogenesis in the ischemic tissue after the administration of transfected cells (Figs. 4B and C). Similar results were observed in the mouse model with hindlimb ischemia. Intravenous injection of FGF4-gene-transfected monocytes (1.0 x 10^6) enhanced regional blood flow in the ischemic leg (Fig. 4D). The increase of blood flow in the mice with transfected monocytes (93±22% in terms of flow ratio in the ischemic/non-ischemic leg) was significantly larger than those obtained with the other three treatments described above (38±12, 55±12, and 39±15%, P<0.05, ANOVA). Neither lymph node swelling in any part of the body nor pathologic change in the spleen or lung, such as angioma or abnormal immune response, was found in any of the animals.

Fig. 4A

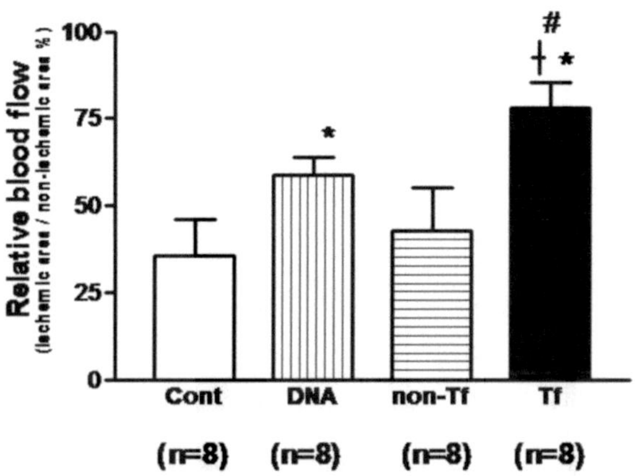

Fig. 4B

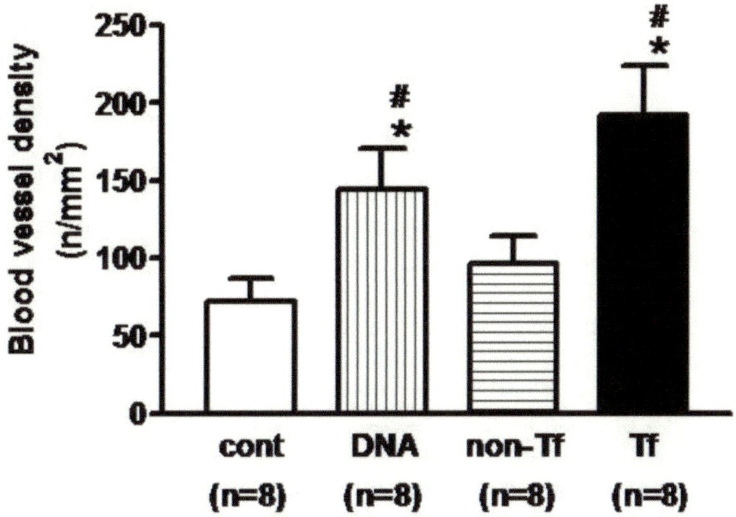
Blood vessel density
(n/mm²)
250
200
150
100
50
0
#
*
#
*
cont
(n=8)
DNA
(n=8)
non-Tf
(n=8)
Tf
(n=8)

Fig. 4C

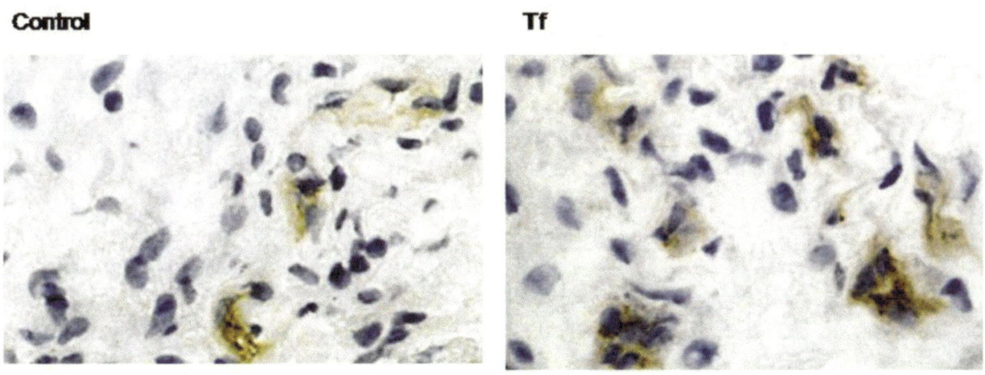
Control
Tf

Fig. 4D

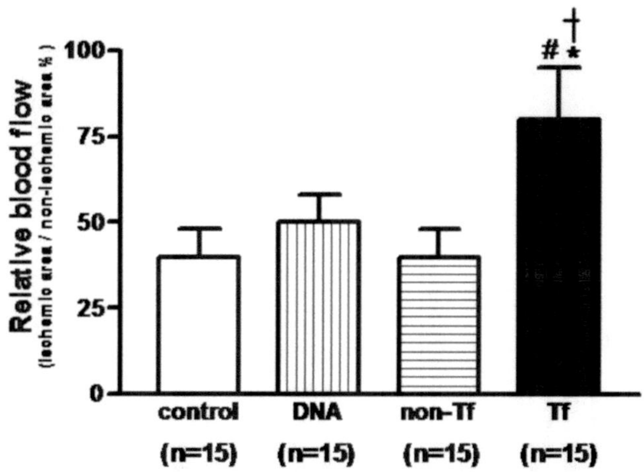

Fig. 4. Therapeutic effects of angiogenic-gene-transfected phagocytes on ischemia. FGF4-transfected macrophages were injected into the vein or naked DNA encoding FGF4 was injected directly into the myocardium in a rat model of myocardial ischemia-reperfusion injury (A-C). FGF4-transfected monocytes were injected into the vein or naked DNA encoding FGF4 was injected directly into the ischemic muscle in a mouse model of hindlimb ischemia (D). A, Relative blood flow in the ischemic myocardium. Each flow represents a relative value with respect to non-ischemic region. The number of animals is shown in parentheses. B, Quantification of vessel density in the ischemic myocardium. The number of observation fields is shown in parentheses. C, Immunohistochemical staining in the ischemic myocardium with anti-CD31 antibody. D, Relative blood flow in the ischemic leg. Each flow represents a relative value with respect to non-ischemic leg. The number of animals is shown in parentheses. Control represents animals injected with saline into the vein; DNA, naked DNA encoding FGF4 was injected directly into the ischemic muscle; non-Tf, non-transfected phagocytes were injected intravenously Tf, FGF4-gene-transfected phagocytes were injected intravenously. Values are mean±SD. $P<0.05$ vs *Cont, †DNA, and #non-Tf (ANOVA) (Fukuyama N et al., 2007).

2.3 Discussion

The advantages of the present method are as follows. First, genes can easily be transfected into phagocytes (macrophages/monocytes). In preliminary experiments, we found that genes can also be transfected into endothelial progenitor cells (Nagaya N et al., 2003). Compared with other transfection methods, the transfection efficiency was high (68±11%) and it is not necessary to use a potentially hazardous viral vector (Kobinger GP et al., 2004; Lei Y et al., 2004; Watson DJ et al., 2002). Second, the phagocytes can target pathologic tissues by chemotaxis even after intravenous injection, and targeting should be considerably improved if they are administered locally. Moreover, the injection is repeatable. We confirmed that the angiogenic gene-transfected phagocytes enhanced angiogenesis after ischemia-reperfusion injury in rat heart and ameliorated ischemia in a mouse hindlimb model. Gelatin prepared as described here is not rapidly degraded in the human body, and should be effective for prolonged transfection gene therapy, as well as for drug delivery

systems, etc.. This method appears to be suitable for safe and effective cell-based gene therapy.
The injected phagocytes migrated into pathologic tissues, presumably in response to the release of cytokines such as monocyte chemoattractant protein 1 by injured endothelial cells (Yoshimura T & Leonard EJ, 1990). Adhesion molecules such as P-selectin (Ikada Y et al., 2002) are probably involved in the recruitment of phagocytes to the vessel wall. The injected phagocytes also migrated to the spleen, but no pathologic change was found in the spleen.
The present method has several advantages over conventional methods of cell-based gene therapy, such as fibroblast-based and smooth muscle cell-based approaches (Koch K-C et al., 2006; Ott HC et al., 2005; Xie Y et al., 2001). For example, monocytes do not aggregate in vessels, whereas fibroblasts or smooth muscle cells cannot be injected intravenously because of aggregation. The transfected phagocytes not only synthesize protein from the transfected gene, but also are partially targeted to the impaired tissue. In addition, the transfection rate was better than those of methods such as lipofection, viral vectors and electroporation (Kobinger GP et al., 2004; Veit K et al., 1999). The newly developed technique of nucleofection has a transfection efficiency of 40-70% (Maasho K et al., 2004), which is similar to that of our method, but our procedure is easier to use (Maasho K et al., 2004; Mertz KD et al., 2002).

3. Conclusion

The therapeutic effect obtained here (intravenous administration of phagocytes transfected ex vivo with FGF4 DNA/biodegradable gelatin complex) was superior to that of conventional gene therapy, which we reported previously, i.e., intramuscular injection of naked DNA, in heart and leg ischemia models. The major disadvantage of our method is the cell preparation time of 2 weeks before therapy can be started, and further work is needed to speed up this process. However, our results suggest that this method may an effective therapeutic option from the viewpoint of regenerative medicine.

4. Ackowledgement

The authors wish to thank Jobu Itoh, Yoshiko Shinozaki, and Takayuki Hasegawa for their technical work.

5. References

Ferber, D. (2001). Gene therapy. Safer and virus-free? *Science*, vol.294:1638-1642

Fukuyama, N.; Ichimori, K.; Su, Z.; Ishida, H. & Nakazawa H. (1996). Peroxynitrite formation from activated human leukocytes. *Biochem Biophys Res Commun*, vol.224:414-419

Fukuyama, N.,Tanaka, E., Tabata, Y., Fujikura, H., Hagihara, M., Sakamoto, H., Ando, K., Nakazawa, H. & Mori, H.(2007). Intravenous injection of phagocytes transfected ex vivo with FGF4 DNA/biodegradable gelatin complex promotes angiogenesis in a rat myocardial ischemia/reperfusion injury model. Basic Res Cardiol, vol. 102:209-216

Gidh-Jain, M.; Huang, B.; Jain P. & el-Sherif N. (1996). Differential expression of voltage-gated K+ channel genes in left ventricular remodeled myocardium after experimental myocardial infarction. *Circ Res*, vol.79:669-675

Ikada, Y. & Tabata, Y. (1998). Protein release from gelatin matrices. *Adv Drug Deliv Rev*, vol.31:287-301

Ikada, Y.; Young, LH. & Lefer, AM. (2002). Attenuation of neutrophil-mediated myocardial ischemia-reperfusion injury by a calpain inhibitor. *Am J Physiol Heart Circ Physiol*, vol.282:H1421-H1426

Isner JM. (2002). Myocardial gene therapy. *Nature*, vol.415:234-239

Kasahara, H.; Tanaka, E.; Fukuyama, N.; Sato, E.; Sakamoto, H.; Tabata, Y.; Ando,K.; Iseki, H.;Shinozaki, Y.; Kimura, K.;Kuwabara, E.; Koide, S.; Nakazawa, H.& Mori, H. (2003). Biodegradable gelatin hydrogel potentiates the angiogenic effect of fibroblast growth factor 4 plasmid in rabbit hindlimb ischemia. *J Am Coll Cardiol*, vol.41:1056-1062

Kay, MA.;Glorioso, JC.& Naldini, L. (2001). Viral vectors for gene therapy: the art of turning infectious agents into vehicles of therapeutics. *Nat Med*, vol.7:33-40

Kobinger, GP.; Deng, S.; Louboutin, JP.; Vatamaniuk, M.; Matschinsky, F.; Markmann, JF.; Raper, SE. & Wilson JM. (2004). Transduction of human islets with pseudotyped lentiviral vectors. *Hum Gene Ther*, vol.15:211-219

Koch, K-C.; Schaefer, WM.; Liehn, EA.; Rammos, C.; Mueller, D.; Schroeder, J.; Dimassi, T.; Stopinski, T. & Weber, C. (2006). Effect of catheter-based transendocardial delivery of stromal cell-derived factor 1α on left ventricular function and perfusion in a porcine model of myocardial infarction. *Basic Res Cardiol*, vol.101:69-77

Komeda, M.; Marui, A.; Tambara, K.; Yamamoto, M.; Saji, Y.; Nishina, T. & Tabata, Y. (2009). Biologic anastomosis: the first case of biologic coronary bypass surgery. *J Thorac Cardiovasc Surg*, vol.138:775-777

Kornowski, R.; Leon, MB.; Fuchs, S.; Vodovotz, Y.; Flynn, MA.; Gordon, DA.; Pierre, A.; Kovesdi, I.;Keiser, JA. & Epstein, SE. (2000). Electromagnetic guidance for catheter-based transendocardial injection: a platform for intramyocardial angiogenesis therapy. Results in normal and ischemic porcine models. *J Am Coll Cardiol*, vol.35:1031-1039

Laitinen, M.; Hartikainen, J.; Hiltunen, MO.; Eränen, J.; Kiviniemi, M.; Närvänen, O.; Mäkinen, K.; Manninen, H.; Syvänne, M.; Martin, JF.; Laakso, M. & Ylä-Herttuala, S. (2000). Catheter-mediated vascular endothelial growth factor gene transfer to human coronary arteries after angioplasty. *Hum Gene Ther*, vol.11:263-270

Lei,Y.; Haider, HKh.; Shujia, J. & Sim, ES. (2004). Therapeutic angiogenesis; Devising new strategies based on past experiences. *Basic Res Cardiol*, vol.99:121-132

Li, Q.;Bolli, R.; Qiu, Y.; Tang, XL.; Guo Y. & French, BA. (2001). Gene therapy with extracellular superoxide dismutase protects conscious rabbits against myocardial infarction. *Circulation*, vol.103:1893-1898

Losordo, DW.; Vale, PR.; Symes, JF.; Dunnington, CH.; Esakof, DD.; Maysky, M.; Ashare, AB.; Lathi, K.& Isner, JM. (1998). Gene therapy for myocardia angiogenesis:initial clinical results with direct myocardial injection of phVEGF165 as sole therapy for myocardial ischemia. *Circulation*, vol.98:2800-2804

Maasho, K.; Marusina, A.; Reynolds, NM.; Coligan, JE. & Borrego, F.(2004). Efficient gene transfer into the human natural killer cell line, NKL, using the Amaxa nucleofection system. *J Immunol Methods*, vol.284 :133-140

Marui, A.; Tabata, Y.: Kojima, S.; Yamamoto, M.; Tambara, K.; Nishina, T.; Saji, Y.; Inui, K.; Hashida, T.; Yokoyama, S.; Onodera, R.; Ikada, T.; Fukushima, M. & Komeda, M. (2007). A novel approach to therapeutic angiogenesis for patients with critical limb ischemia by sustained release of basic fibroblast growth factor using biodegradable gelatin hydrogel: an initial report of the phaseI-IIa study. *Circ J*, vol.71:1181-1186

Mertz, KD.; Weisheit, G.; Schilling, K.& Lűers, GH. (2002). Electroporation of primary neural cultures: a simple method for directed gene transfer in vitro. *Histochem Cell Biol*, vol.118:501-506

Nagaya, N.; Kangawa, K.; Kanda, M.; Uematsu, M.; Horio, T.; Fukuyama, N.; Hino, J.; Harada-Shiba, M.; Okumura, H.; Tabata, Y.; Mochizuki, N.; Chiba, Y.; Nishioka, K.; Miyatake, K.; Asahara, T.; Hara, H.& Mori, H. (2003). Hybrid cell-gene therapy for pulmonary hypertension based on phagocytosing action of endothelial progenitor cells. *Circulation*, vol.108:889-895

Nishikawa, M. & Hashida, M. (2002). Nonviral approaches satisfying various requirements for effective in vivo gene therapy. *Biol Pharm Bull*, vol.25:275-283

Ott, HC.; McCue, J.& Taylor, DA. (2005). Cell-based cardiovascular repair: The hurdles and the opportunities. *Basic Res Cardiol*, vol.100:504-517

Panetta, CJ.; Miyauchi, K.; Berry, D.; Simari, RD.; Holmes, DR.; Schwartz, RS.& Caplice, NM. (2002). A tissue-engineered stent for cell-based vascular gene transfer. *Hum Gene Ther*, vol.13:433-441

Pfeifer, A. & Verma, IM. (2001). Gene therapy: promises and problems. *Annu Rev Genomics Hum Genet*, vol.2:177-211

Ramsay, SC.; Weiller, C.; Myers, R.; Cremer, JE.; Luthra,SK.; Lammertsma, AA. & Frackowiak, RS. (1992). Monitoring by PET of macrophage accumulation in brain after ischaemic stroke. *Lancet*, vol.339:1054-1055

Ribeiro, RA.; Flores CA.; Cunha, FQ.& Ferreira, SH. (1991). IL-8 causes in vivo neutrophil migration by a cell-dependent mechanism. *Immunology*, vol.73:472-477

Schakowski, F.; Buttgereit, P.; Mazur, M.; Märten, A.; Schőttker, B.; Gorschlűter M.& Schmidt-Wolf, IG. (2004). Novel non-viral method for transfection of primary leukemia cells and cell lines. *Genet Vaccines Ther*, vol.2:1

Tabata, Y. & Ikada, Y. (1987). Macrophage activation through phagocytosis of muramyl dipeptide encapsulated in gelatin microspheres. *J Pharm Pharmacol*, vol.39:698-704

Tabata, Y. & Ikada, Y. (1988). Macrophage phagocytosis of biodegradable microspheres composed of L-lactic acid/glycolic acid homo- and copolymers. *J Biomed Mater Res*, vol.22:837-858

Tabata, Y. (2009). Biomaterial technology for tissue engineering applications. *J R Soc Interface*, suppl.3:S311-S324

Takeshita, S.; Zheng, LP.; Brogi, E.; Kearney, M.; Pu, LQ.; Bunting, S.; Ferrara, N.; Symes, JF. & Isner, JM. (1994). Therapeutic angiogenesis. A single intraarterial bolus of vascular endothelial growth factor augments revascularization in a rabbit ischemic hind limb model. *J Clin Invest*, vol.93:662-670

Tomasoni, S. & Benigni, A. (2004). Gene therapy: how to target the kidney. Promises and pitfalls. *Curr Gene Ther*, vol.4:115-122

Veit. K.; Boissel, JP.; Buerke, M.; Grosser, T.; Meyer, J. & Darius H. (1999). Highly efficient liposome-mediated gene transfer of inducible nitric oxide synthase in vivo and in vitro in vascular smooth muscle cells. *Cardiovasc Res*, vol.43:808-822

Watson, DJ.; Kobinger, GP.; Passini, MA.; Wilson, JM. & Wolfe, JH. (2002). Targeted transduction patterns in the mouse brain by lentivirus vectors pseudotyped with VSV, Ebola, Mokola, LCMV, or MuLV envelope proteins. *Mol Ther*, vol.5:528-537

Xie, Y.; Yang, ST. & Kniss, DA. (2001). Three-dimensional cell-scaffold constructs promote efficient gene transfection: implications for cell-based gene therapy. *Tissue Eng*, vol.7:585-598

Yoshimura, T. & Leonard, EJ. (1990). Human monocyte chemoattractant protein-1 (MCP-1). Immunol Today, vol.11:97-101

Young, S.; Wong, M.; Tabata, Y. & Mikos, AG. (2005). Gelatin as a delivery vehicle for the controlled release of bioactive molecules. *J Control Release*, vol.109:256-274

5

Approaches in Gene Therapy of Cancer and Cardiovascular Diseases

Gardlik Roman[1], Dovinova Ima[2] and Chan Julie Y.H.[3]
[1]Institute of Molecular Biomedicine, Faculty of Medicine Comenius University, Bratislava,
[2]Institute of Normal and Pathological Physiology, Slovak Academy of Sciences, Bratislava,
[3]Center for Translational Research in Biomedical Science, Chang-Gung Memorial Hospital, Kaohsiung Medical Center, Kaohsiung,
[1,2]Slovakia
[3]Taiwan

1. Introduction

In this chapter we will focus on few topics. First, we summarize and discuss angiogenic gene therapy of cancer and cardiovascular diseases, with RNA interference in a separate section. Second, we briefly review delivering systems in gene therapy, their advatages and limitations and further focus on bacterial vectors. Last, we summarize antioxidant gene therapy of cardiovascular diseases and hypertension.

Considering the fact that the fundamental discoveries and new findings in medicine are being crystallized on genetic and genomic levels, gene therapy is one of the potential mechanisms for therapeutic intervention. Gene therapy in a broad sense, i.e. all the therapeutic strategies employing nucleic acids as carriers of genetic information, found its utilization in most areas of medicine, including angiogenesis research. Similarly to classical "non-gene" therapy, the research in gene therapy is happening on the preclinical level using appropriate animal models, with cancer and cardiovascular diseases being the most abundant indications. There are several different strategies known. Besides the delivery of therapeutic gene (replacement of the mutated gene by a functional one or delivery of the gene because of lack of the gene product), novel strategies are also being widely used based on blocking the function of a specific gene by application of RNA interference inducing sequences, antisense inhibition etc.

One of the key advantages of gene approaches is the endogenous production of the therapeutic molecule. Furthermore, targeted gene delivery specifically into the target tissue or only to a certain cell type can dramatically decrease the likelihood of adverse effects. Along with the development of new vectors and regulatory systems, the ability to control the expression of therapeutic gene in time and space is being improved. This is of great importance in affecting such complex and complicated processes as angiogenesis. Currently, almost three quarters of indications addressed by gene therapy clinical trials are represented by cancer and cardiovascular diseases

2. Angiogenic gene therapy

After birth, angiogenesis still contributes to organ growth. However, in adults, the majority of blood vessels remains in quiescence with the most active angiogenesis during menstruation cycle in the uterus and pregnancy in the placenta. In spite of this, endothelial cells do preserve the ability to quickly proliferate and react to physiological stimulus such as hypoxia and inflammation.

If the stimulus is too excessive, the fine balance between stimulants and inhibitors can be disrupted and thus lead to so-called "angiogenic switch". The best described pathological states with dysregulated angiogenesis include cancer, cardiovascular disorders, inflammatory eye disorders as well as many other processes such as obesity, metabolic diseases, asthma, diabetes mellitus, cirrhosis, sclerosis multiplex, rheumatoid arthritis, macular degeneration, psoriasis, atherosclerosis, restenosis, diabetic retinopathy, endometriosis, bacterial infections and autoimmune diseases (Cao, 2010; Webb & Vande Woude, 2000).

2.1 Gene therapy of cancer

Gene therapy-based angiogenesis inhibiting strategies have gained much attention thanks to their advantages over the conventional antiangiogenic treatments. Given that effective inhibition of pathological angiogenesis requires long term treatment, gene therapy may be of importance for selective gene transfer to the affected areas and prolonged expression of therapeutic genes. Apart from that, gene therapy provides a possibility to circumvent the issues associated with recombinant proteins production, stability and solubility. Gene transfer allows for appropriate folding and stability of encoded proteins *in vivo* in the natural environment. An interesting advantage is also the ability to selectively target the gene transfer into certain tissues enabling localized expression and high regional drug concentration without increasing systemic levels. One of the key justifications for using gene therapy is also an insufficient efficiency of "non-gene" therapies based on inhibition of VEGF and other growth factors signal pathways in humans (Gridelli et al., 2007). The most commonly used gene therapy approach in cancer is so called suicide cytotoxic therapy using thimidin kinase or other chemosensitizing genes that allow the conversion of inactive prodrug (ganciclovir) into a cytotoxic product (Both, 2009).

2.1.1 Preclinical studies

Antiangiogenic gene therapy of cancer has been tested on a preclinical level in various carcinogenesis models. Most of the studies performed so far have used viral vectors (adenoviruses, retroviruses, lentiviruses, adeno-associated viruses, herpes simplex viruses) encoding endogenous angiogenesis inhibitor genes such as cytokines/chemokines (IFN-α, IFN-β, IFN-γ, CXCL10, IL-12, IL-18, TNF-α), VEGF blockers (sFlt-1, Flk-1), proteolytic fragments (angiostatin, endostatin, vasostatin, tumstatin) and others (Persano et al., 2007). For example, in a colorectal cancer model an adenovirus-based therapy using genes encoding IFN-β (Tada et al., 2001) and endostatin (Oliner et al., 2004) as well as plasmids encoding Flk-1 (W.J. Kim et al., 2006) and tumstatin (Yao et al., 2005) have been successfully applied. In a model of malignant melanoma, retrovirus vectors carrying gene encoding CXCL10 (Feldman et al., 2002) and plasmids encoding vasostatin (Jazowiecka-Rakus et al., 2006) and MCP-1 (Koga et al., 2008) genes have been successfully used, all exerting a clear antiangiogenic effect. Recently, a systemically available antiangiogenic gene therapy using adenovirus bearing soluble VEGF receptor gene has been proven to be effective in suppressing tumor growth in various oral cancer cell line xenografts in mice (Okada et al., 2010).

Several studies have been performed using gene delivery of endogenous angiogenesis inhibitor endostatin. A liposome-encapsulated adenovirus encoding endostatin was applied in therapy of ovarian cancer (Yang et al., 2010). Systemic administration was well-tolerated and resulted in marked suppression of tumor growth, which was associated with a decreased number of micro-vessels and increased apoptosis of tumor cells. An interesting novel therapeutic approach for pancreatic cancer has been employed in a study using vaccinia virus encoding the endostatin-angiostatin fusion gene (Tysome et al., 2009). Besides high selectivity of the used vector, inhibition of angiogenesis and a clear antitumor potency has been observed. In another study, combined antiangiogenic and proapoptotic gene therapy involving endostatin and sTRIAL (soluble tumor necrosis factor-related apoptosis-inducing ligand) effectively suppressed hepatocellular carcinoma growth and angiogenesis in nude mice (Zhang et al., 2009). At last, adenovirus-mediated endostatin gene delivery combined with cisplatin treatment was effective in a lung cancer murine model (Ning et al., 2008). These studies represent a future direction in cancer research in which instead of targeting a single molecule, a combinatorial approach targeting multiple factors and/or an additional therapeutic approach is applied to cover multiple pathways of cancer progression.

2.1.2 Clinical studies

Despite a relatively high number of clinical studies using cancer gene therapy, specifically antiangiogenic gene therapy has only been exploited in a few studies. Intratumoral injection of adenovirus encoding immunostimulatory cytokine IL-12 has been tested in patients with advanced gastrointestinal cancer (liver, colorectal, pancreatic tumors) in phase I study (Sangro et al., 2004). Therapy was well tolerated, although only a moderate antitumor effect was observed. In another study, plasmid bearing IL-12 gene was applied to patients with malignant melanoma (Heinzerling et al., 2005). In two out of nine patients, the disease was stabilized for period of over three years and a complete remission was achieved in one patient. In these patients, a localized reduction in angiogenesis has been proven by immunohistochemistry. However, the rest of the patients showed only temporal response to the therapy. A recent phase I clinical trial of IL-12 plasmid/lipopolymer complexes has also shown a clinical benefit in treatment of recurrent ovarian cancer without adverse events (Anwer et al., 2010). In a different phase I study, adenovirus vector carrying IFN-β gene has been used in therapy of malignant pleural mesothelioma (Sterman et al., 2007). In all the above-mentioned studies, however, inhibition of angiogenesis was not the primary goal, yet a part of the antitumor effect.

2.2 Gene therapy of cardiovascular diseases

In view of the many advances in explaining the molecular mechanisms of angiogenesis high hopes were put in gene therapy. However, in the clinical studies with genes encoding for individual proangiogenic growth factors (similar to recombinant proteins) only moderate success has been observed so far, thus creating a space for development of new vectors and alternative approaches (Vincent et al., 2007).

Progress in the field of gene therapy for cardiovascular disease has been modest; one of the key reasons for this limited progress is the lack of gene delivery systems for localizing gene therapy to specific sites to optimize transgene expression and efficacy. However, progress toward the site-specific delivery of cardiovascular gene therapy is still ongoing and promising novel approaches are being tested (Fishbein et al., 2010).

2.2.1 Preclinical studies

A lot of studies have been performed on a preclinical level with very promising results. Angiogenic gene therapy using intramuscular injection of plasmids encoding VEGF and plasminogen activator has been applied in a mouse model of myocardial infarction (ligation of coronary artery) and hind limb ischemia (ligation of arteria femoralis) (Traktuev et al., 2007). Authors were able to detect functionally significant angiogenesis that clearly improved the pathological consequences of disease induction. The model of hind limb ischemia is actually a commonly used model to prove the efficiency of proangiogenic viral and non-viral gene delivery in ischemic disease (Schgoer et al., 2009). Bosch-Marce *et al.*, have used this model to test adenovirus vector carrying the gene encoding for constitutively active HIF-1α, resulting in a sufficient induction of reperfusion of the affected areas even in older animals (Bosch-Marce et al., 2007). These results suggest that the HIF-1α activity is necessary and sufficient for mobilization of angiogenic cells and that gene therapy using HIF-1α gene can compensate the pathological effects of ageing. Gene therapy using gene encoding VEGF has further shown a clear beneficial effect in a rat model of myocardial infarction (Tang et al., 2010). In a mouse model of myocardial infarction, the ultrasound-targeted gene delivery of VEGF or stem cell factor resulted in increased vascular density and improved myocardial perfusion and ventricular function (Fujii et al., 2009). Yockman *et al.*, used an ischemia-inducible plasmid construct expressing VEGF to treat myocardial ischemia and infarction (Yockman et al., 2009). Ischemia-inducible system was superior to constitutively expressed gene construct in reducing the infarct size. A different regulation system for VEGF gene delivery based on tetracycline-inducible AAV-based vector has been employed by Tafuro *et al.*, in a hind limb ischemia model (Tafuro et al., 2009). These results clearly indicate that the fine tuning of VEGF expression is required to achieve the formation of a stable vasculature able to sustain functional neovascularization. Hypothesizing that the transient nature of VEGF gene expression provokes instability of neovasculature, Olea *et al.*, compared single vs. repeated transfection in a rabbit model of hind limb ischemia by injecting a plasmid encoding human $VEGF_{165}$ (Olea et al., 2009). Repeated, but not single, VEGF gene transfection resulted in increased microvasculature, which in turn afforded effective protection against ischemic muscle damage. Pajusola *et al.*, have compared the virus vector-mediated delivery of genes encoding VEGF and HIF-1α into the muscle of mice (Pajusola et al., 2005). Results of this study show that HIF-1α gene therapy is able to ensure increased expression of numerous proangiogenic molecules and, thus, can circumvent the shortcomings associated with overexpression of a single growth factor. A rationale for combination proangiogenic therapy has been provided in two studies, in which a synergistic effect of concurrent application of plasmids encoding FGF-2 and PDGF-BB by intramuscular injection was observed in a rabbit/rodent hind limb ischemia model (Li et al., 2010).

2.2.2 Clinical studies

Results from several interesting clinical studies have been published recently. In a phase I study testing the safety of intramuscular injection of VEGF-encoding plasmid vector in 9 patients suffering from serious peripheral arterial disease of the lower extremities a significant improvement in most of the measured parameters has been observed regardless of the dose (Kim et al., 2004). However, the serum VEGF levels were not elevated and the control group was missing in that study. Interestingly, no significant improvement in primary and secondary endpoints between groups was achieved in two recent multicenter, double-blind, placebo-controlled phase II trials exploring intramuscular application of plasmid encoding angiogenic factors (Grossman et al., 2007; Rajagopalan et al., 2003). Authors of Euroinject One phase II trial analyzed the effect of gene transfer using plasmid encoding $VEGF_{165}$ gene on myocardial perfusion, left ventricle function and clinical symptoms in 80 patients suffering from stable severe ischemic heart disease (Kastrup et al., 2005). A direct intramyocardial injection of plasmid did not improve the study endpoints compared to placebo, although a regional improvement in ventricle wall movement was achieved. Results thus show the safety of direct intramyocardial injection, but not the efficiency. In the REVASC trial, a total of 67 patients with ischemic heart disease and severe angina pectoris were enrolled to the study (Stewart et al., 2006). Here, the intramyocardial injection of replication-deficient adenovirus vector bearing $VEGF_{121}$ gene significantly ameliorated the primary endpoint (exercise time needed for 1mm ST segment depression) as well as overall exercise time and exercise time to moderate angina after 26 weeks of therapy in patients with exercise-induced ischemia. On the other hand, in a recent double-blind, placebo-controlled study VEGF gene therapy failed to improve perfusion of ischemic myocardium in patients with advanced coronary artery disease (Stewart et al., 2009). Further, intramuscular injection of plasmid with VEGF gene was compared against placebo (saline) in 54 diabetic patients suffering from severe peripheral arterial disease (Kusumanto et al., 2006). Although a significant improvement of some of the parameters (hemodynamic status, skin ulcerations) has been achieved, the primary endpoint of this study - amputation of lower extremity after 100 days - stayed unchanged. Moreover, long-term safety of VEGF gene therapy has been proven in an eight-year safety follow-up of coronary artery disease patients after intracoronary VEGF gene transfer (Hedman et al., 2009). Local intracoronary VEGF gene delivery is, thus, considered safe and does not increase the risk of major adverse cardiovascular events, arrhythmias, cancer, diabetes or other disease.

So far the only clinical study testing the delivery of HIF-1α gene was a randomized, double-blind, placebo-controlled phase I trial enrolling 34 patients with peripheral arterial disease (Rajagopalan et al., 2007). Treatment based on direct intramuscular administration of adenovirus vector carrying the HIF-1α gene was well tolerated and provided relief of rest pain one year after the therapy, supporting the necessity for more clinical trials.

The second generation of angiogenic gene therapeutics is represented by constructs enabling the expression of two or more proangiogenic cytokines. Analogous to gene therapy using the master regulatory gene HIF-1α, these "multivalent" approaches may provide a benefit against the classical "monovalent" ones (Vincent et al., 2007).

Overall, we might conclude that only slight clinical benefit of gene therapy in cardiovascular diseases has been observed so far on the level of multicenter, randomized, placebo-controlled clinical trials. This finding, however, is in direct contrast to promising and convincing results from preclinical studies and, thus, further stimulates searching for new and alternative approaches in experimental as well as clinical settings. New viruses have been introduced and new results have been collected from preclinical and clinical studies. Recent results from preclinical developments and clinical trials have been reviewed (Karvinen & Yla-Herttuala, 2010).

2.3 RNA interference in therapeutic modulation of angiogenesis

Since the first discoveries of RNA interference mechanism (RNAi) 13 years ago, much new information has shown up and a new age of gene therapy, in broad sense, has actually begun. This molecular phenomenon found its usage, besides in functional genetic studies, also in therapy based on silencing the expression of disease-causing genes (so called gene knock-down).

One of the main obstacles in achieving *in vivo* gene silencing using RNAi is the means of delivery. The siRNA molecules are, if present outside the cell, unstable and are subject to rapid degradation. Therefore, they are being chemically modified or incorporated into vectors like in the case of classical gene delivery. Within such a vector siRNA are encoded as so called short hairpin RNA (shRNA) that are expressed inside the target cell.

One of the break-through experiments was based on intravenous administration of chemically modified siRNA against endogenous apolipoprotein B (apoB) in mice leading to apoB mRNA silencing in liver and jejunum as well as decrease in plasma levels of apoB and overall cholesterol (Soutschek et al., 2004). These siRNA even reduced the expression of human apoB in transgenic mice, and the results further extended the potential of RNAi-based therapy of not only cardiovascular diseases.

Several studies have been performed to test the efficiency of RNAi in therapy/prevention of cardiovascular diseases. It is known that activation of NFkappaB pathway can be associated with development of cardiac hypertrophy and its transition to heart failure. Intramyocardial delivery of shRNA against NFkappaB in lentiviral vector has led to regression of cardiac hypertrophy in transgenic mice, suggesting the potential role of NFkappaB as a therapeutic target in prevention of hypertrophy/heart failure (Gupta et al., 2008). Similar results have been observed in a model of pressure-induced hypertrophy using systemic administration of siRNA against focal adhesion kinase (FAK), which acts as one of the hypertrophy mediators (Clemente et al., 2007). In the work of Jiang *et al.*, it was even proven that RNAi against HIF-1α inhibits the formation of foam cells *in vitro,* indicating that induction of HIF-1α by atherogenic factors may be a key step in coordinating the cellular processes leading to atherosclerotic lesions (Jiang et al., 2007). An alternative approach was tested in a study of Natarajan *et al.,* that, instead of using constitutively active HIF-1α, reduced the activity of HIF-1α prolyl hydroxylases by RNA interference (Natarajan et al., 2006). Small interfering RNAs (siRNA) managed not only to activate HIF-1α signaling *in vitro,* but also rescued the endangered myocardium in a mouse model of overall ischemia. Thus, the authors proved that indirect activation of HIF-1α signaling is not only possible, but also efficient. In another study the systemic administration of siRNA against β1-adrenergic receptors has been proven to be specific for β1 receptors expression without influencing β2 receptors (Arnold et al., 2007). This therapy significantly reduced the hypertrophy and the blood pressure in spontaneously hypertensive rats. Moreover, preventive application of β1-specific siRNA 3 days before myocardial infarction improved the heart function and reduced cardiomyocyte apoptosis.

Antiangiogenic therapy using RNAi has found its broad experimental application (Hadj-Slimane et al., 2007). Silencing of HIF-1α by RNAi leads to transient stasis or regression of tumors *in vivo* and silencing in early stage tumors is more effective than in stable tumors (Li et al., 2005). In addition, siRNA against HIF-1α inhibit the expression of this transcription factor in cancer cells and in endothelial progenitor cells even in hypoxic conditions, when it is naturally activated. At the same time, differentiation, proliferation and migration of these cells are also inhibited. Effectiveness of anticancer therapy using siRNA against VEGF (naked or within a vector) has been proven to be effective *in vitro* and *in vivo* in a number of cancer models. Furthermore, a combination of oncolytic virus therapy and VEGF specific-siRNA has also been proven to be effective *in vitro* and *in vivo* (Yoo et al., 2007). Based on different physiological roles of VEGF family members, a combination therapy with siRNA vectors against VEGF-A and VEGF-C was used to suppress lymph node and metastasis in a mouse metastatic breast cancer model (Shibata et al., 2008). Another combined approach has been successfully used by Chen *et al.*, in therapy of laryngeal squamous cell carcinoma by concurrent application of plasmids encoding siRNA against VEGF, hTERT and Bcl-xl (Chen et al., 2008).

One of the most important papers in recent years was the study of Kleinman *et al.*, who have reported a sequence- and target-independent angiogenesis suppression by siRNA via toll-like receptor 3 (TLR3) (Kleinman et al., 2008). Here, the non-targeted siRNA suppressed dermal neovascularization in mice as effectively as VEGF siRNA. The effect was mediated through cell surface TLR3, its adaptor TRIF and induction of IFNgamma and IL-12. These results suggest that all siRNA-based RNAi strategies activating TLR3 have to face non-specificity, which, however, does not have to be considered a disadvantage. Even though a specific silencing is desired, a different approach/vector should be used to avoid activating of TLR3 pathway. Bacterial vectors are characterized by cellular entry into the host cell, where they can mediate their therapeutic effects. Thus, bacteria can represent an ideal system for delivery of RNAi.

Apart from RNAi, another big area of small RNA-related research that is gaining much more attention these days is the microRNA research. More importantly, microRNA have been found to play a key role in regulation of angiogenesis, both in cancer and ischemic diseases, indicating that the development of clinically relevant therapies can be expected in a short time period (Fasanaro et al., 2010).

3. Delivery systems

Vectors for transfer of therapeutic sequences into target cells can be divided into three basic groups: viral, non-viral (naked DNA) and bacterial. Each of these groups has different research and therapeutic indications, and features specific pros and cons (Gardlik et al., 2005 Chailertvanitkul and Pouton, 2010). Currently, the most frequently used vectors in gene therapy clinical trials include: adenoviruses (400 clinical trials; 23,8%), retroviruses (344 clinical trials; 20,5%), naked/plasmid DNA (304 clinical trials; 17,7%), adeno-associated viruses (75 clinical trials; 4,5%) and others (John Wiley & Sons, 2010).

Adenoviruses are the most commonly used gene-delivery vectors due to the efficiency of their *in vivo* gene transfer their ability to deliver double-stranded DNA to the nucleus efficiently. In addition, their large genome allows for extensive modification and incorporation of therapeutic genes. Since 1993, about 300 protocols using an adenoviral vector have been performed, although they have yet to be proven effective in clinical trials.

By 2009 over 350 protocols had been approved for clinical trials of gene therapy using attenuated adenoviral vectors, 210 of which were open, but only 5 of which were Phase III trials (for details see the Clinical Trials Worldwide Database at http://www.wiley.co.uk/genmed/clinical).

The adenovirus-based vector has been continuously improved by modification of the adenoviral genome and capsid, and novel adenovirus-delivery systems have been recently proposed (Shirakawa, 2008). Since their first clinical trial 20 years ago, retroviral vectors have now been used in more than 350 gene-therapy studies. Retroviral vectors are particularly suited for gene-correction of cells due to long-term and stable expression of the transferred transgene(s), and also because little effort is required for their cloning and production. Despite several unsuccessful attempts using retroviral therapeutics, a new generation of vectors with improved genome integration and safety characteristics are now available, making them a useful tool for several gene therapy applications (Maier et al., 2010). On contrary, adeno-associated vectors (AAV) are characterized by low frequency of random integration into the genome and moderate immune response. This makes AAV an attractive platform for vector design. Like in most other vector systems, the tropism of AAV vectors limits their utility for certain tissues especially upon systemic application. However, the tropism can be modified by targeted capsid modification and the use of different serotypes, thus making them a good cell-type specific delivery system (Michelfelder & Trepel, 2009).

Another group of delivery systems includes bacterial vectors (Gardlik et al., 2005). Owing to the specific ability of some bacterial strains to colonize hypoxic areas, bacteria found their primary application mainly in cancer therapy (Gardlik & Fruehauf, 2010). A number of experimental studies have been published to date and several clinical studies employing bacterial therapies are currently ongoing. Apart from live bacterial delivery systems, empty envelopes of Gram negative bacteria, so called bacterial ghosts are also being explored as a potential tool for gene delivery (Kudela et al., 2010). In the upcoming sections we specifically focus on modulation of angiogenesis-related events using bacterial vectors.

3.1 Bacteria – mediated gene therapy

The first attempts at using bacteria for therapeutic purposes were made more than 40 years ago. At this time, it was discovered that bacteria could predominantly replicate in solid tumors (Moese & Moese, 1964). However, the first indications of this phenomenon date back to 19th century. These findings remained largely unexplored until the turn of 20th century, when oncolytic bacteria capable of lysing host cells were first studied by various research groups (Theys et al., 2001; Yazawa et al., 2000).

Despite recent progress, only a few recent studies on bacterial tumor therapy have focused on antiangiogenic therapy. Although effects on the vasculature were observed in most of these studies, these changes seemed to be a consequence mainly of bacteria-mediated therapy. Bacteria-mediated antiangiogenesis tumor therapy, however, is a reasonable approach given that solid tumors are often characterized by increased vascularization. Herein we summarize latest research on cancer therapy using genetically modified bacteria with particular emphasis on the potential of blocking tumor angiogenesis.

3.2 Bacteria affecting angiogenesis

Pronounced angiogenesis is one of the hallmarks of solid tumors. Therefore, in order to search for more efficient anticancer drugs efforts are being made to block tumor angiogenesis. Despite notable successes achieved in studies using oncolytic bacteria for cancer treatment, bacteriolytic therapy in and of itself is often insufficient for complete eradication of experimental tumors (Agrawal et al., 2004). The idea of using combined therapy with bacteria and angiogenesis inhibition has therefore been suggested.

Below are reviewed four different approaches for using modified bacteria as anticancer therapeutics - bactofection, DNA vaccination, alternative gene therapy and bactoference - with a focus on angiogenesis suppression (Figure 1).

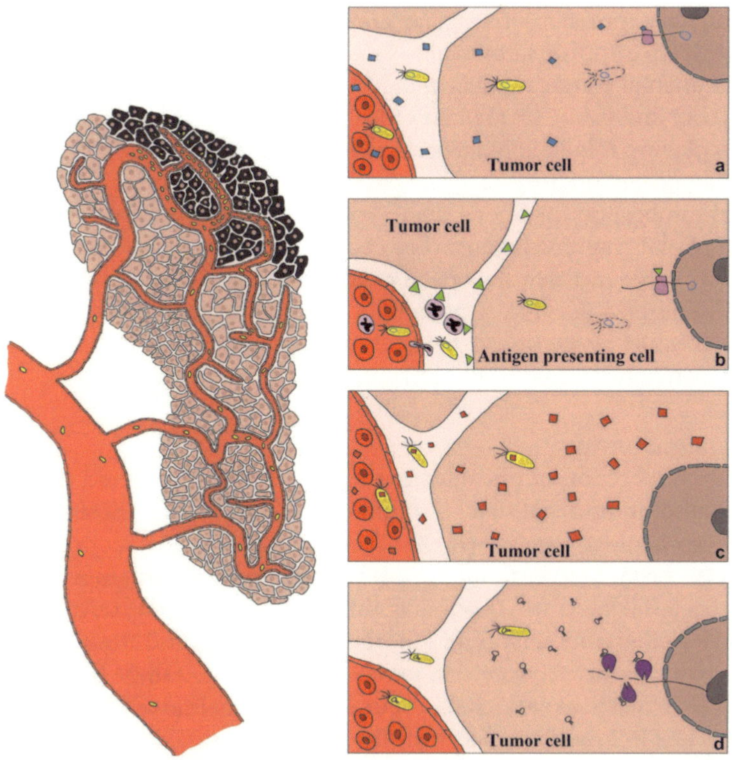

Fig. 1. Antitumor effect of bacteria colonizing tumor tissue. Auxotrophic bacteria specifically colonize tumors with necrotic and hypoxic areas (panel on the left). The anticancer effect of bacteria can be exerted in four different ways: (a) Bactofection - after escaping the vessel and entering the target cell, bacteria disrupt and release a plasmid vector encoding the therapeutic gene. The plasmid is transferred into the cell nucleus and the therapeutic protein is expressed by the host cell's expression system (blue square symbol). (b) DNA vaccination - bacteria deliver therapeutic plasmid into the host cell in a similar way as in bactofection. The host cell may in this case be an antigen presenting cell. The plasmid encodes a tumor cell-expressed antigen to help prime a T-cell response against the tumor antigen which is present on the surface of tumor cells leading to induction of humoral and cellular immune response against the tumor. (c) Bacterial protein delivery - bacteria, either in extracellular environment or inside tumor cells, express the therapeutic gene directly and serve as protein delivery vehicles (red square symbol). (d) Bacterial delivery of RNA interference - bacteria deliver plasmid encoding shRNAs or express the shRNAs to induce RNA interference against an oncogene or a tumor-expressed factor.

3.3 Bactofection

The use of bacteria as a vector for the delivery of therapeutic genes to target cells is known as bactofection, and several studies have used this approach to deliver genes encoding antiangiogenic molecules to tumor cells *in vivo*. A study was made using *Salmonella choleraesuis* strain bearing gene encoding endostatin on eukaryotic expression plasmid (Lee et al., 2004). The expression of endostatin was targeted exclusively to tumor tissues colonized by bacteria and significant inhibition of tumor growth (40-70%) with decreased intratumoral microvessel density and reduced expression of vascular endothelial growth factor (VEGF) was observed. Bactofection using auxotrophic salmonellae as vectors has also been effectively employed for therapy of experimental tumor models using expression plasmids carrying various cytokine genes such as IL-12 and GM-CSF (Yuhua et al., 2001), IL-4 and IL-18 (Agorio et al., 2007) or other molecules playing role in angiogenesis, such as Flt3 ligand (Yoon et al., 2007). Further, a dual tumoricidal and antiangiogenic effect of *S. choleraesuis* carrying an expression plasmid containing the thrombospondin-1 gene under control of eukaryotic promoter was observed in a murine model of malignant melanoma (Lee et al., 2005). A potential limitation of bactofection for cancer therapy is the fact that the effector molecule will likely be expressed exclusively in cells infected by bacteria, leaving a potentially large population of tumor cells untreated. However, if the product of the transgene is secreted outside the target cell, it may still have a therapeutic effect on non-infected tumor cells.

3.4 DNA vaccination

It is known that bactofection of plasmids encoding a tumor-expressed antigens can lead to induction of humoral and cellular immune response in the host thereby providing protective defense against tumors (R. Xiang et al., 2000). This approach, termed DNA vaccination, has been successfully implemented for antiangiogenic therapy. Oral antiangiogenic bacterial vaccines directed against VEGFR-2 were proven to be efficacious in animal models of malignant melanoma, colorectal carcinoma and lung cancer (Niethammer et al., 2002) as well as non-cancer diseases like stromal keratitis (Kim et al., 2006) and atherosclerosis (Petrovan et al., 2007). Furthermore, salmonella-mediated vaccination against murine VEGFR-2 has been successfully combined with classical gene therapy for the treatment of malignant melanoma (Lu et al., 2008). Bacterial vaccines directed against the apoptosis inhibitor survivin (Xiang et al., 2005) and the TGF-β1 co-receptor endoglin (Lee et al., 2006) also proved to be effective in inhibition of tumor angiogenesis. Taken together, these findings underscore the key role of angiogenesis in cancer as well as other diseases and, at the same time, highlight the complexity of this essential process.

3.5 Alternative gene therapy

Another means of using bacteria for gene therapy is the so-called alternative gene therapy (AGT) approach, which is also known as bacterial protein delivery (Palffy et al., 2006). It is based on transfer of bacterially expressed therapeutic proteins to the host organism using genetically modified (transformed) bacteria. As with bactofection, AGT is mostly used for treatment of tumors and employs primarily oncolytic and tumor-colonizing bacterial strains of *Clostridia, Bifidobacteria* or *Salmonellae* (Theys et al., 2001; Zheng et al., 2000). Li *et al.,* successfully used *Bifidobacterium adolescentis* as a vector for the expression of endostatin within tumors (Li et al., 2003). These authors showed a strong inhibition of angiogenesis was able to significantly to inhibit local tumor growth. In another study, *Bifidobacterium longum* was shown to efficiently deliver the antiangiogenic protein endostatin to murine liver tumors, and induce antitumor activity (Fu et al., 2005). Furthermore, the antitumor effect was enhanced by co-administration of the same bacterial strain expressing tumor necrosis factor-related apoptosis inducing ligand (TRAIL) (Hu et al., 2009). These findings emphasize the need for combination therapy, in which multiple antitumor pathways are inhibited. *In situ* production of cytokines by bacteria represents a cost-effective and safe alternative mainly to systemic administration which can be associated with unwanted side-effects. However, in recent study employing

Listeria monocytogenes as a vehicle for tumor specific gene and protein delivery, bactofection proved to be more efficient than AGT (Stritzker et al., 2008).

Interestingly, previously unknown antiangiogenic effects have recently been discovered for a variety of molecules involved in the immune response and cellular apoptosis mainly due to extensive ongoing research in the field of cancer therapy. Bacteria in gene therapy, differences between bactofection and AGT, advantages and disadvantages as well as specific application of both approaches are discussed in detail in our review article (Palffy et al., 2006).

In spite of great success in a preclinical setting, the application of bacteria for human tumor therapy has not been particularly efficacious, although this approach was well tolerated in most studies (Cunningham & Nemunaitis, 2001; Nemunaitis et al., 2003; Toso et al., 2002). In light of above-mentioned findings, however, we would suggest that angiogenesis would be a meaningful target for further experimental and clinical studies of bacteria-mediated anticancer therapy, particularly if used in conjunction with oncolytic strains of bacteria.

3.6 Bactoference – bacteria-mediated RNA interference

A promising new approach for bacteria-mediated anticancer therapy is the combination of two distinct methodologies: bacteriotherapy and RNA interference. Bacteria that have engineered to produce and deliver short interfering RNA (siRNA) represent a novel tool for the efficient induction of RNA interference (RNAi) in host cells. This concept herein termed "bactoference" was first tested at the *in vitro* level in 2005 by Zhao *et al.*, (Zhao et al., 2005). These authors showed that siRNAs produced by invasive *E. coli* strain could induce RNAi against in mammalian cell cultures. The first *in vivo* demonstration of bactoference was provided by Xiang *et al.*, who showed that invasive *E. coli* capable of producing beta-catenin shRNA could induce RNAi in colonic epithelial cells and colonic tumors xenografted into nude mice (Xiang et al., 2006). To date, however, bactoference has not been used to directly target angiogenesis, although some of the targets explored (beta-catenin, STAT3 and bcl-2) are known to augment angiogenesis via their effects on the expression of various proangiogenic factors. Thus, antitumor effects of knocking down these targets may, in part, be related to suppression of blood vessel formation. However, a number of studies using "non-bacterial" application of siRNA against VEGF (Jia et al., 2007), HIF-1α (Jiang et al., 2006) and other angiogenesis-related molecules indicates that inhibition of endothelial cell proliferation and new blood vessel formation is a viable target for RNAi-based treatment of cancer as well as other diseases.

4. Antioxidant gene therapy

Reactive oxygen and nitrogen species may remodel the extracellular matrix and blood vessels, cause endothelial dysfunction, induce apoptosis, exacerbate inflammatory reaction, regulate cell proliferation and key signal transduction pathways, and inhibit histone deacetylase activity involved in hypertension (Cohen and Tong, 2010; Fostermann, 2010).

Overproduction of reactive oxygen species plays an important role in a number of cardiovascular pathologies, including hypertension, atherosclerosis, myocardial infarction, ischemia/reperfusion injury, and restenosis after angioplasty.

In this section we focus on gene therapy research using experimental models of cardiovascular diseases and hypertension.

4.1 NO levels and the superoxide dismutases

There are at least two major strategies of modulation of nitric oxide (NO) levels in hypertension and cardiovascular diseases: (i) modulation of NO levels by NO synthase (NOS) stimulation, increase in NO bioavailability, administration of NO donors or precursors, and NOS gene incorporation; (ii) scavenging of superoxide and suppression of oxidative stress by activation of antioxidant gene expression or by suppression of selected genes via knock-out or RNA silencing (Dovinova, Gardlik et al., 2009).

NO reacts with superoxide at a rate three times faster than the dismutation of superoxide by superoxide dismutase (SOD). Because of the efficiency of the reaction, the local concentration of SOD is a key determinant of bioactivity (the biological half-life) of NO. Individual SOD isoform in different cell compartments (cytosol, mitochondria, extracellular space) protects against superoxide-mediated cytotoxicity and functioning as a signaling molecule (Mendez, 2005). SOD enzymes therefore play an important role in cardiovascular tissue by protecting NO against oxidative inactivation by superoxide and they are important in vasodilatation and in the protection of NO bioactivity in blood vessel walls (Gongora & Harrison, 2008).

Gene transduction of individual SOD genes (Chu et al., 2003; Zimmerman et al., 2004; Dovinova et al., 2008; Kamezaki et al., 2008) or combination of both SOD and NOS transgenes (Kung et al., 2008,) has positive influence on experimental hypertension. This protective effect is the end results of an increase in tissue level of NO and the decreases in oxidative stress (Chan et al., 2006) and peroxynitrite production (a cytotoxic molecule generated by reaction between superoxide and NO) (Kishi et al., 2004). The SOD genes are the first natural antioxidant defenses of an aerobic cellular system. The following subsection deals with gene therapies by individual SOD isoforms (alone or combined with other genes) and about their influence on the mechanisms of the cardiovascular disease.

4.2 Antioxidant gene therapy of the cardiovascular system with the SOD 1 gene

The connection between the influence of angiotensin II (Ang II) and the increased superoxide production by activation of NAPDH oxidase has been observed in animal studies (Paravicini and Touyz, 2004; Zimmerman et al., 2004, Chan et al., 2005) and patients with cardiovascular complications (Yokoyama et al., 2000). Peripheral angiotensin II exerts potent effects on blood pressure and cardiovascular function through its actions on neurons located in specialized brain regions called the circumventricular organs, in particular the subfornical organ (SFO). Zimmerman et al., (2004) reported that following peripheral infusion of Ang II at initially subpressor doses, there was a gradually developing hypertension paralleled by an increase in superoxide production in the SFO. Using the adenoviral vectors for *in vivo* gene delivery, they found that both the superoxide production and the hypertension were prevented by an overexpression of CuZnSOD (also known as SOD1) in the SFO, whereas ECSOD (also known as SOD3) was ineffective. Ang II receptors are also highly expressed in brain stem cardiovascular centers, including the rostral ventrolateral medulla (RVLM) and nucleus tractus solitarii (NTS). Activation of Ang II receptors in the RVLM (Gao et al., 2004; Kishi et al., 2004; Chan et al., 2005) or NTS (Hirooka, 2008) promotes neurogenic hypertension. This induced hypertension can also be prevented by protection against oxidative stress via treatment with *in situ* gene transduction of SOD1 (Chan et al., 2006). Using a gene therapy based on SOD1 gene transduction by a bacterial gene delivery system it was found that such application decreases the blood pressure, regulates SOD and NOS activities, and decreases oxidative stress response (Dovinova et al., 2008).

The overexpression of cytoplasm-targeted superoxide dismutase via an adenoviral vector (AdSOD1) efficiently scavenges angiotensin-II–induced increases in intracellular superoxide, markedly attenuates the increase in $[Ca^{2+}]_i$ and suggests a potential intracellular signaling mechanism involved in Ang II–mediated oxidant regulation of central neural control of blood pressure (Zimmerman et al., 2005).Genetically-altered mice and rats have been generated which overexpress SOD1. Compared with nontransgenic controls, mRNA for CuZn-SOD1 and SOD activity are increased several-fold in the vascular and non-vascular tissues, decreased vascular superoxide levels in atherosclerosis and diabetes to improve endothelial function and to protect in a model of fluid percussion injury that produces impairment of autoregulation (Faraci & Didion, 2004)

Downregulation of antioxidant gene expression and enzyme activity may underlie the augmented levels of superoxide and hydrogen peroxide in the RVLM, leading to oxidative stress and hypertension in the spontaneously hypertensive rats (SHR). A causative relationship between biochemical correlates of oxidative stress and neurological hypertension was established after a gene transfer by microinjection of adenovirus encoding SOD1 and MnSOD (also known as SOD2) or catalase (CAT) into brain (RVLM), which promoted a long-term reduction of blood pressure in SHR (Chan et al., 2006).

4.3 Antioxidant gene therapy of the mitochondrial dysfunction with the SOD 2 gene

Mitochondrial dysfunction is a prominent feature of most cardiovascular diseases and hypertension and is associated with the deterioration of mitochondrial energy production in several organs such as the liver, the heart and the brain (Chan et al., 2009a, b). In the myocardium of the SHR, the evidence that points to the occurrence of mitochondrial dysfunction includes the decrease of cytochrome oxidase activity, ATP production, and inorganic phosphate translocator activity (de Cavanagh et al., 2006). Attenuated intracellular ATP content, results in a long-term maintenance of elevated blood pressure by increasing in sympathetic outflow, whereas augmented ROS production following mitochondrial dysfunction lowers the capacity of the NO-dependent vascular relaxation. The stationary elevated blood pressure in chronic arterial hypertension should be regarded as a compensatory response to decreased mitochondrial ATP synthesis (Postnov et al., 2007). Depletion of p22*phox* subunit of NADPH oxidase with small interfering RNA inhibited Ang II–mediated mitochondrial ROS production. Ang II depletes mitochondrial glutathione, increases state 4 and decreased state 3 respirations, and diminishes the mitochondrial respiratory control ratio. It also prevents the Ang II–induced decrease in endothelial NO and mitochondrial membrane potential. Therefore, Ang II induces mitochondrial dysfunction via a protein kinase C–dependent pathway by activating the endothelial cell NADPH oxidase and formation of peroxynitrite. Furthermore, mitochondrial dysfunction in response to Ang II modulates endothelial NO and superoxide generation, which in turn has ramifications for the development of an endothelial dysfunction (Doughan et al., 2008). In the brain stem cardiovascular neurons in the RVLM, mitochondrial superoxide mediates the rebound hypertension induced by the eNOS transgene in SHR (Kung et al., 2008).

Mice lacking iNOS$^{(-/-)}$ exhibits extensive cytoplasmic swelling and degeneration of mitochondria, decrease in the resting indices of cardiac function as well as an impairment in the positive inotropic actions of isoproterenol following treatment with adriamycin compared to nTg mice. Cardiac troponin, creatine phosphokinase, and lactate dehydrogenase levels are significantly increased after adriamycin treatment in iNOS$^{(-/-)}$ mice However, when iNOS$^{(-/-)}$ mice are crossed with SOD2 overexpressing animals, mitochondrial injury is ameliorated to the level of the wild type (Cole, 2006). Mice completely deficient in Mn-SOD die within a few weeks after birth and exhibit a variety of phenotypes (depending on the genetic background) including neurodegeneration, cardiac abnormalities, and extensive mitochondrial damage (Faraci & Didion, 2004)

In Ang II-induced neurogenic hypertension or in SHR, mitochondrial electron transport capacity in the RVLM is reduced, accompanied by an increase in generation of mitochondrial superoxide and hydrogen peroxide (Chan et al., 2009a). Overexpression of SOD2 ameliorates mitochondrial oxidative stress and the induced antihypertension.

4.4 Antioxidant gene therapy of the cardiovascular system with the SOD 3 gene and RNA silencing

The degree of hypertrophy, ventricular dilatation, and myocardial fibrosis was markedly increased in mice lacking extracellular SOD (SOD3) and gene transfer of cDNA encoding membrane-bound SOD3 reduces vascular superoxide levels as well as arterial pressure in SHR (Chu et al., 2009). A deficiency in SOD3 does not alter the baseline blood pressure but increases the arterial pressure in models of hypertension that are greater in SOD3-deficient mice than in controls. Studies using overexpression strategies have revealed protective effects of SOD3 on blood vessels. Gene transfer of SOD3 reduced vascular superoxide levels during atherosclerosis in SHR. Effects of overexpression of SOD3 using this approach on endothelial function have varied (Faraci & Didion, 2004).

Depletion of NADPH oxidase subunits with small interfering RNAs - another approach in gene therapy - inhibits ROS production and, thus, has the potential to reduce blood pressure. Silencing of p22phox component of NADPH oxidase *in vivo* by RNAi resulted in reduced ROS and mean atrial pressure in angiotensin II-induced hypertension in rats (Modlinger et al., 2006). Knock-down of several molecular targets by silencing of matrix metalloproteinase-7 (Wang et al., 2009), angiotensin-converting enzyme (He et al., 2009) or $\beta 1$-adrenergic receptor (Arnold et al., 2007) using systemic RNAi results in attenuation of hypertension and stops the development of cardiac hypertrophy in SHR.

5. Conclusion

Modulation of angiogenesis is of great importance from experimental, pathophysiological and especially clinical point of view. However, further research is needed to fully delineate the most effective way to target angiogenesis for treatment of cancer and cardiovascular diseases. The application of new approaches using bacteria for the transfer of therapeutic genes or the production of therapeutic protein or small RNAs has the potential to significantly advance cancer gene therapy. Recent studies indicate that treatments targeting a single molecule/pathway, even if it has pleiotropic effects, are unlikely to be completely effective; however, if the natural anti-tumor activity inherent to some anaerobic bacteria strains can be successfully combined with their ability to deliver agents targeting tumor angiogenesis, apoptosis or the immune system, this will represent a significant step toward reaching this important goal.

This chapter summarizes the preclinical and clinical studies and the use of animal models to provide evidence for potential benefit from angiogenic and antioxidant gene therapy. Gene therapy with the use of antioxidant genes may offer a promising approach for treatment of cancer and cardiovascular diseases in patients not suitable for conventional therapies.

However, one must realize that in animal models before the experimental data can be translated to clinical trials, shortcomings of antioxidant gene therapy, for example the limited duration of transgene expression, low efficacy of the transgene expression in the target organs or tissues, and potential immune responses to the transgenes, must be resolved. Specifically related to the use of antioxidant enzymes in gene therapy is the fact that reactive oxygen species not only mediate pathological events but are also required for normal cell signaling. This double-edged sword nature of the reactive oxygen species in regulation of cellular phenotypes under physiological and pathological conditions poses challenges to the application of gene therapy for early treatment of disease condition.

6. Acknowledgment

This work is supported by grant SAS-NSC JRP 2010/1, Slovakia and NSC100-2923-B075B-001-MY3 (JYHC) from the National Science Council, Taiwan.

7. References

Agorio, C., Schreiber, F., Sheppard, M., Mastroeni, P., Fernandez, M., Martinez, M.A. & Chabalgoity, J.A. (2007). Live attenuated Salmonella as a vector for oral cytokine gene therapy in melanoma. *Journal of Gene Medicine,* Vol. 9, No. 5, pp. 416-423, 1099-498X

Agrawal, N., Bettegowda, C., Cheong, I., Geschwind, J.F., Drake, C.G., Hipkiss, E.L., Tatsumi, M., Dang, L.H., Diaz, L.A., Jr., Pomper, M., Abusedera, M., Wahl, R.L., Kinzler, K.W., Zhou, S., Huso, D.L. & Vogelstein, B. (2004). Bacteriolytic therapy can generate a potent immune response against experimental tumors. *Proceedings of the National Academy of Sciences of the United States of America,* Vol. 101, No. 42, pp. 15172-15177, 0027-8424

Anwer, K., Barnes, M.N., Fewell, J., Lewis, D.H. & Alvarez, R.D. (2010). Phase-I clinical trial of IL-12 plasmid/lipopolymer complexes for the treatment of recurrent ovarian cancer. *Gene Therapy,* Vol. 17, No. 3, pp. 360-369, 1476-5462

Arnold, A.S., Tang, Y.L., Qian, K., Shen, L., Valencia, V., Phillips, M.I. & Zhang, Y.C. (2007). Specific beta1-adrenergic receptor silencing with small interfering RNA lowers high blood pressure and improves cardiac function in myocardial ischemia. *Journal of Hypertension,* Vol. 25, No. 1, pp. 197-205, 0263-6352

Bosch-Marce, M., Okuyama, H., Wesley, J.B., Sarkar, K., Kimura, H., Liu, Y.V., Zhang, H., Strazza, M., Rey, S., Savino, L., Zhou, Y.F., McDonald, K.R., Na, Y., Vandiver, S., Rabi, A., Shaked, Y., Kerbel, R., Lavallee, T. & Semenza, G.L. (2007). Effects of aging and hypoxia-inducible factor-1 activity on angiogenic cell mobilization and recovery of perfusion after limb ischemia. *Circulation Research,* Vol. 101, No. 12, pp. 1310-1318, 1524-4571

Both, G.W. (2009). Recent progress in gene-directed enzyme prodrug therapy: an emerging cancer treatment. *Current Opinion in Molecular Therapeutics,* Vol. 11, No. 4, pp. 421-432, 2040-3445

Cao, Y. (2010). Adipose tissue angiogenesis as a therapeutic target for obesity and metabolic diseases. *Nature Reviews. Drug Discovery,* Vol. 9, No. 2, pp. 107-115, 1474-1784

Chailertvanitkul VA, Pouton CW. (2010). Adenovirus: a blueprint for non-viral gene delivery. Curr Opin Biotechnol. Vol.21, pp.627-632.

Chan SHH, Hsu KS, Huang CC, Wang LL, Ou CC, Chan JYH. (2005). NADPH oxidase-derived superoxide anion mediates angiotensin II-induced pressor effect via activation of p38 mitogen-activated protein kinase in the rostral ventrolateral medulla. Circ Res., Vol. 97, pp..772-780.

Chan SHH, Tai MH, Li CY, Chan JYH. (2006). Reduction in molecular synthesis and enzyme activity of superoxide dismutase and catalase contributes to oxidative stress and neurogenic hypertension in spontaneously hypertensive rats. Free Radic Biol Med. Vol.40, pp.2028-2039.

Chan SHH, Wu KLH, Chang AYW, Tai MH, Chan JYH. (2009a) Oxidative impairment of mitochondrial electron transport chain complexes in RVLM contributes to neurogenic hypertension. *Hypertension*, Vol. 53, pp. 217-227.

Chan SHH, Wu CA, Wu KLH, Ho YH, Chang AYW, Chan JYH (2009b). Transcriptional Upregulation of Mitochondrial Uncoupling Protein 2 Protects Against Oxidative Stress-associated Neurogenic Hypertension. *Circulation Research*, Vol. 105, pp. 886-896.

Chen, S.M., Wang, Y., Xiao, B.K. & Tao, Z.Z. (2008). Effect of blocking VEGF, hTERT and Bcl-xl by multiple shRNA expression vectors on the human laryngeal squamous carcinoma xenograft in nude mice. *Cancer Biology and Therapy,* Vol. 7, No. 5, pp. 734-739, 1555-8576

Chu Y, Iida S, Lund DD, Weiss RM, DiBona GF, Watanabe Y, Faraci FM, Heistad DD (2003).. Gene transfer of extracellular superoxide dismutase reduces arterial pressure in spontaneously hypertensive rats: role of heparin-binding domain. *Circ Res.*; Vol. 92, pp.461-468.

Clemente, C.F., Tornatore, T.F., Theizen, T.H., Deckmann, A.C., Pereira, T.C., Lopes-Cendes, I., Souza, J.R. & Franchini, K.G. (2007). Targeting focal adhesion kinase with small interfering RNA prevents and reverses load-induced cardiac hypertrophy in mice. *Circulation Research,* Vol. 101, No. 12, pp. 1339-1348, 1524-4571

Cohen RA, Tong X. (2010). Vascular oxidative stress: the common link in hypertensive and diabetic vascular disease. *J Cardiovasc Pharmacol.*; Vol. 55, pp. 308-316.

Cole MP, Chaiswing L, Oberley TD, Edelmann SE, Piascik MT, Lin SM, Kiningham KK, St Clair DK. (2006). The protective roles of nitric oxide and superoxide dismutase in adriamycin-induced cardiotoxicity.Cardiovasc Res.;69(1):186-97.

Cunningham, C. & Nemunaitis, J. (2001). A phase I trial of genetically modified Salmonella typhimurium expressing cytosine deaminase (TAPET-CD, VNP20029) administered by intratumoral injection in combination with 5-fluorocytosine for patients with advanced or metastatic cancer. Protocol no: CL-017. Version: April 9, 2001. *Human Gene Therapy,* Vol. 12, No. 12, pp. 1594-1596, 1043-0342

de Cavanagh E.M. V., Toblli J. E., Ferder L., Piotrkowski B., Stella . I. & Inserra F (2006). Renal mitochondrial dysfunction in spontaneously hypertensive rats is attenuated by losartan but not by amlodipine *Am J Physiol Regul Integr Comp Physiol* Vol. 290, R1616-R1625.

Dikalova AE, Bikineyeva AT, Budzyn K, Nazarewicz RR, McCann L, Lewis W, Harrison DG, Dikalov SI. (2010). Therapeutic targeting of mitochondrial superoxide in hypertension. *Circ Res;* Vol. 107, pp. 106-116.

Doughan A. K, Harrison D. G., Dikalov S.I. (2008). Molecular Mechanisms of Angiotensin II–Mediated Mitochondrial Dysfunction Linking Mitochondrial Oxidative Damage and Vascular Endothelial Dysfunction *Circ Res.*; Vol. 102, pp.488-496.

Dovinová I , Pálffy R, Gardlik, R, - Vranková, S, - Jendeková, L, Kristek, F, Sumbalová, Z, Paulíková, H. (2008). Antioxidant gene treatment of hypertension in spontaneously hypertensive rats. In Lifestyle-related diseases: cellular signaling and pathophysiology. Satellite symposium to the 22nd Scientific Meeting of International Society of Hypertension Bratislava: INPP, pp. 47-48.

Dovinova I, Gardlik R, Palffy R, Kristek F, Cacanyiova S. (2009). Modulation of antioxidative response in the therapy of hypertension and other cardiovascular diseases. *Neuro Endocrinol Lett.*, Vol.30, pp. 32-35.

Faraci Frank M., Didion Sean P. (2004). Vascular Protection Superoxide Dismutase Isoforms in the Vessel Wall *Arterioscler Thromb Vasc Biol.*; Vol.24, pp. 1367-1373.

Fasanaro, P., Greco, S., Ivan, M., Capogrossi, M.C. & Martelli, F. (2010). microRNA: emerging therapeutic targets in acute ischemic diseases. *Pharmacology and Therapeutics*, Vol. 125, No. 1, pp. 92-104, 1879-016X

Feldman, A.L., Friedl, J., Lans, T.E., Libutti, S.K., Lorang, D., Miller, M.S., Turner, E.M., Hewitt, S.M. & Alexander, H.R. (2002). Retroviral gene transfer of interferon-inducible protein 10 inhibits growth of human melanoma xenografts. *International Journal of Cancer*, Vol. 99, No. 1, (May 2002), pp. 149-153, 0020-7136

Fishbein, I., Chorny, M. & Levy, R.J. (2010). Site-specific gene therapy for cardiovascular disease. *Current Opinion in Drug Discovery and Development*, Vol. 13, No. 2, pp. 203-213, 2040-3437

Fostermann U. (2010). Nitric oxide and oxidative stress in vascular disease. *Pflugers Arch Eur J Physiol.* Vol.459, pp.923-939.

Fu, G.F., Li, X., Hou, Y.Y., Fan, Y.R., Liu, W.H. & Xu, G.X. (2005). Bifidobacterium longum as an oral delivery system of endostatin for gene therapy on solid liver cancer. *Cancer Gene Therapy*, Vol. 12, No. 2, pp. 133-140, 0929-1903

Fujii, H., Sun, Z., Li, S.H., Wu, J., Fazel, S., Weisel, R.D., Rakowski, H., Lindner, J. & Li, R.K. (2009). Ultrasound-targeted gene delivery induces angiogenesis after a myocardial infarction in mice. *JACC. Cardiovascular Imaging*, Vol. 2, No. 7, pp. 869-879, 1876-7591

Gardlik, R. & Fruehauf, J.H. (2010). Bacterial vectors and delivery systems in cancer therapy. *IDrugs*, Vol. 13, No. 10, pp. 701-706, 2040-3410

Gardlik, R., Palffy, R., Hodosy, J., Lukacs, J., Turna, J. & Celec, P. (2005). Vectors and delivery systems in gene therapy. *Med Sci Monit*, Vol. 11, No. 4, pp. RA110-121, 1234-1010

Gongora M.C., Harrison D.G. (2008). Sad heart from no SOD. Hypertension. Vol. 51(1), pp.28-30.

Gridelli, C., Maione, P., Del Gaizo, F., Colantuoni, G., Guerriero, C., Ferrara, C., Nicolella, D., Comunale, D., De Vita, A. & Rossi, A. (2007). Sorafenib and sunitinib in the treatment of advanced non-small cell lung cancer. *Oncologist*, Vol. 12, No. 2, pp. 191-200, 1083-7159

Grossman, P.M., Mendelsohn, F., Henry, T.D., Hermiller, J.B., Litt, M., Saucedo, J.F., Weiss, R.J., Kandzari, D.E., Kleiman, N., Anderson, R.D., Gottlieb, D., Karlsberg, R., Snell, J. & Rocha-Singh, K. (2007). Results from a phase II multicenter, double-blind placebo-controlled study of Del-1 (VLTS-589) for intermittent claudication in subjects with peripheral arterial disease. *American Heart Journal,* Vol. 153, No. 5, pp. 874-880, 1097-6744

Gupta, S., Young, D., Maitra, R.K., Gupta, A., Popovic, Z.B., Yong, S.L., Mahajan, A., Wang, Q. & Sen, S. (2008). Prevention of cardiac hypertrophy and heart failure by silencing of NF-kappaB. *Journal of Molecular Biology,* Vol. 375, No. 3, pp. 637-649, 1089-8638

Hadj-Slimane, R., Lepelletier, Y., Lopez, N., Garbay, C. & Raynaud, F. (2007). Short interfering RNA (siRNA), a novel therapeutic tool acting on angiogenesis. *Biochimie,* Vol. 89, No. 10, pp. 1234-1244, 0300-9084

He J, Bian Y, Gao F, Li M, Qiu L, Wu W et al., (2009). RNA interference targeting the ACE gene reduced blood pressure and improved myocardial remodelling in SHRs. *Clin Sci (Lond).* 116:249–255. In Blood Vessels Evidence for the Importance of ROS Compartmentalization

Hedman, M., Muona, K., Hedman, A., Kivela, A., Syvanne, M., Eranen, J., Rantala, A., Stjernvall, J., Nieminen, M.S., Hartikainen, J. & Yla-Herttuala, S. (2009). Eight-year safety follow-up of coronary artery disease patients after local intracoronary VEGF gene transfer. *Gene Therapy,* Vol. 16, No. 5, pp. 629-634, 1476-5462

Heinzerling, L., Burg, G., Dummer, R., Maier, T., Oberholzer, P.A., Schultz, J., Elzaouk, L., Pavlovic, J. & Moelling, K. (2005). Intratumoral injection of DNA encoding human interleukin 12 into patients with metastatic melanoma: clinical efficacy. *Human Gene Therapy,* Vol. 16, No. 1, pp. 35-48, 1043-0342

Hirooka Y. (2008). Role of reactive oxygen species in brainstem in neural mechanisms of hypertension. *Auton Neurosci.,* Vol. 142, pp.20-24.

Hu, B., Kou, L., Li, C., Zhu, L.P., Fan, Y.R., Wu, Z.W., Wang, J.J. & Xu, G.X. (2009). Bifidobacterium longum as a delivery system of TRAIL and endostatin cooperates with chemotherapeutic drugs to inhibit hypoxic tumor growth. *Cancer Gene Therapy,* Vol. 16, No. 8, pp. 655-663, 1476-5500

Jazowiecka-Rakus, J., Jarosz, M. & Szala, S. (2006). Combination of vasostatin gene therapy with cyclophosphamide inhibits growth of B16(F10) melanoma tumours. *Acta Biochimica Polonica,* Vol. 53, No. 1, pp. 199-202, 0001-527X

Jia, R.B., Zhang, P., Zhou, Y.X., Song, X., Liu, H.Y., Wang, L.Z., Luo, M., Lu, J., Ge, S.F. & Fan, X.Q. (2007). VEGF-targeted RNA interference suppresses angiogenesis and tumor growth of retinoblastoma. *Ophthalmic Research,* Vol. 39, No. 2, pp. 108-115, 0030-3747

Jiang, G., Li, T., Qiu, Y., Rui, Y., Chen, W. & Lou, Y. (2007). RNA interference for HIF-1alpha inhibits foam cells formation in vitro. *European Journal of Pharmacology,* Vol. 562, No. 3, pp. 183-190, 0014-2999

John Wiley & Sons, I. (2010). Gene therapy clinical trials worldwide, In: *The Journal of Gene Medicine,* March 17th 2011, Available from: <http://www.wiley.com/legacy/wileychi/genmed/clinical/>

Kamezaki F, Tasaki H, Yamashita K, Tsutsui M, Koide S, Nakata S, Tanimoto A, Okazaki M, Sasaguri Y, Adachi T, Otsuji Y. (2008). Gene transfer of extracellular superoxide dismutase ameliorates pulmonary hypertension in rats. *Am J Respir Crit Care Med.;* Vol.177, pp. 219-226.

Kao L, Wang W, Li YL, Schultz HD, Liu D, Comish KG, Zucker IH. (2004). Superoxide mediates sympathoexcitation in heart failure. Role of angiotensin II and NAD(P)H oxidase. *Circ Res.;* Vol. 95, pp. 937-944.

Karvinen, H. & Yla-Herttuala, S. (2010). New aspects in vascular gene therapy. *Current Opinion in Pharmacology,* Vol. 10, No. 2, pp. 208-211, 1471-4973

Kastrup, J., Jorgensen, E., Ruck, A., Tagil, K., Glogar, D., Ruzyllo, W., Botker, H.E., Dudek, D., Drvota, V., Hesse, B., Thuesen, L., Blomberg, P., Gyongyosi, M. & Sylven, C. (2005). Direct intramyocardial plasmid vascular endothelial growth factor-A165 gene therapy in patients with stable severe angina pectoris A randomized double-blind placebo-controlled study: the Euroinject One trial. *Journal of the American College of Cardiology,* Vol. 45, No. 7, pp. 982-988, 0735-1097

Kim, B., Suvas, S., Sarangi, P.P., Lee, S., Reisfeld, R.A. & Rouse, B.T. (2006). Vascular endothelial growth factor receptor 2-based DNA immunization delays development of herpetic stromal keratitis by antiangiogenic effects. *Journal of Immunology,* Vol. 177, No. 6, pp. 4122-4131, 0022-1767

Kim, H.J., Jang, S.Y., Park, J.I., Byun, J., Kim, D.I., Do, Y.S., Kim, J.M., Kim, S., Kim, B.M., Kim, W.B. & Kim, D.K. (2004). Vascular endothelial growth factor-induced angiogenic gene therapy in patients with peripheral artery disease. *Experimental and Molecular Medicine,* Vol. 36, No. 4, pp. 336-344, 1226-3613

Kim, W.J., Yockman, J.W., Jeong, J.H., Christensen, L.V., Lee, M., Kim, Y.H. & Kim, S.W. (2006). Anti-angiogenic inhibition of tumor growth by systemic delivery of PEI-g-PEG-RGD/pCMV-sFlt-1 complexes in tumor-bearing mice. *Journal of Controlled Release,* Vol. 114, No. 3, pp. 381-388, 0168-3659

Kishi T, Hirooka Y, Kimura Y, Ito K, Shimokawa H, Takeshita A. (2004). Increased reactive oxygen species in rostral ventrolateral medulla contribute to neural mechanisms of hypertension in stroke-prone spontaneously hypertensive rats. *Circulation;* Vol.109, pp.2357-2362.

Kleinman, M.E., Yamada, K., Takeda, A., Chandrasekaran, V., Nozaki, M., Baffi, J.Z., Albuquerque, R.J., Yamasaki, S., Itaya, M., Pan, Y., Appukuttan, B., Gibbs, D., Yang, Z., Kariko, K., Ambati, B.K., Wilgus, T.A., DiPietro, L.A., Sakurai, E., Zhang, K., Smith, J.R., Taylor, E.W. & Ambati, J. (2008). Sequence- and target-independent angiogenesis suppression by siRNA via TLR3. *Nature,* Vol. 452, No. 7187, pp. 591-597, 1476-4687

Koga, M., Kai, H., Egami, K., Murohara, T., Ikeda, A., Yasuoka, S., Egashira, K., Matsuishi, T., Kai, M., Kataoka, Y., Kuwano, M. & Imaizumi, T. (2008). Mutant MCP-1 therapy inhibits tumor angiogenesis and growth of malignant melanoma in mice. *Biochemical and Biophysical Research Communications,* Vol. 365, No. 2, pp. 279-284, 1090-2104

Kudela, P., Koller, V.J. & Lubitz, W. (2010). Bacterial ghosts (BGs)--advanced antigen and drug delivery system. *Vaccine,* Vol. 28, No. 36, pp. 5760-5767, 1873-2518

Kung, LC, Chan, SHH, Wu, KLH, Ou CC, Tai MH and Chan JYH. (2008). Mitochondrial respiratoryenzyme complexes in rostral ventrolateral medulla as cellular targets of nitric oxide and superoxide interaction in the antagonism of antihypertensive action of eNOS transgene. *Molecular Pharmacology*, Vol. 74, pp.1319-1332.

Kusumanto, Y.H., van Weel, V., Mulder, N.H., Smit, A.J., van den Dungen, J.J., Hooymans, J.M., Sluiter, W.J., Tio, R.A., Quax, P.H., Gans, R.O., Dullaart, R.P. & Hospers, G.A. (2006). Treatment with intramuscular vascular endothelial growth factor gene compared with placebo for patients with diabetes mellitus and critical limb ischemia: a double-blind randomized trial. *Human Gene Therapy*, Vol. 17, No. 6, pp. 683-691, 1043-0342

Lee, C.H., Wu, C.L. & Shiau, A.L. (2004). Endostatin gene therapy delivered by Salmonella choleraesuis in murine tumor models. *Journal of Gene Medicine*, Vol. 6, No. 12, pp. 1382-1393, 1099-498X

Lee, C.H., Wu, C.L. & Shiau, A.L. (2005). Systemic administration of attenuated Salmonella choleraesuis carrying thrombospondin-1 gene leads to tumor-specific transgene expression, delayed tumor growth and prolonged survival in the murine melanoma model. *Cancer Gene Therapy*, Vol. 12, No. 2, pp. 175-184, 0929-1903

Lee, S.H., Mizutani, N., Mizutani, M., Luo, Y., Zhou, H., Kaplan, C., Kim, S.W., Xiang, R. & Reisfeld, R.A. (2006). Endoglin (CD105) is a target for an oral DNA vaccine against breast cancer. *Cancer Immunology, Immunotherapy*, Vol. 55, No. 12, pp. 1565-1574, 0340-7004

Levonen AL, Vähäkangas E, Koponen JK, Ylä-Herttuala S. (2008). Antioxidant gene therapy for cardiovascular disease: current status and future perspectives. Circulation Vol. 117, pp.2142-2150.

Li, J., Yang, L., Liu, K., Yuan, C., Tang, Y., Quan, Q., Chen, P., Wang, W., Hu, H. & Wei, Y. (2010). Synergistic effects of FGF-2 and PDGF-BB on angiogenesis and muscle regeneration in rabbit hindlimb ischemia model. *Microvascular Research*, Vol. 80, No. 1, pp. 10-17, 1095-9319

Li, L., Lin, X., Staver, M., Shoemaker, A., Semizarov, D., Fesik, S.W. & Shen, Y. (2005). Evaluating hypoxia-inducible factor-1alpha as a cancer therapeutic target via inducible RNA interference in vivo. *Cancer Research*, Vol. 65, No. 16, pp. 7249-7258, 0008-5472

Li, X., Fu, G.F., Fan, Y.R., Liu, W.H., Liu, X.J., Wang, J.J. & Xu, G.X. (2003). Bifidobacterium adolescentis as a delivery system of endostatin for cancer gene therapy: selective inhibitor of angiogenesis and hypoxic tumor growth. *Cancer Gene Therapy*, Vol. 10, No. 2, pp. 105-111, 0929-1903

Lu, X.L., Jiang, X.B., Liu, R.E. & Zhang, S.M. (2008). The enhanced anti-angiogenic and antitumor effects of combining flk1-based DNA vaccine and IP-10. *Vaccine*, Vol. 26, No. 42, pp. 5352-5357, 0264-410X

Maier, P., von Kalle, C. & Laufs, S. (2010). Retroviral vectors for gene therapy. *Future Microbiology*, Vol. 5, No. 10, pp. 1507-1523, 1746-0921

Mendez J. Ignacio; Nicholson William J.; Taylor W. Robert (2005). SOD Isoforms and Signaling *Arteriosclerosis, Thrombosis, and Vascular Biology* , Vol.25, pp.887-888

Michelfelder, S. & Trepel, M. (2009). Adeno-associated viral vectors and their redirection to cell-type specific receptors. *Advances in Genetics,* Vol. 67, No., pp. 29-60, 0065-2660

Modlinger P, Chabrashvili T, Gill PS, Mendonca M, Harrison DG, Griendling KK et al., (2006). RNA silencing in vivo reveals role of p22phox in rat angiotensin slow pressor response. *Hypertension* , Vol. 47, pp. 238–244.

Moese, J.R. & Moese, G. (1964). Oncolysis by Clostridia. I. Activity of Clostridium Butyricum (M-55) and Other Nonpathogenic Clostridia against the Ehrlich Carcinoma. *Cancer Research,* Vol. 24, No. , pp. 212-216, 0008-5472

Natarajan, R., Salloum, F.N., Fisher, B.J., Kukreja, R.C. & Fowler, A.A., 3rd. (2006). Hypoxia inducible factor-1 activation by prolyl 4-hydroxylase-2 gene silencing attenuates myocardial ischemia reperfusion injury. *Circulation Research,* Vol. 98, No. 1, pp. 133-140, 1524-4571

Nemunaitis, J., Cunningham, C., Senzer, N., Kuhn, J., Cramm, J., Litz, C., Cavagnolo, R., Cahill, A., Clairmont, C. & Sznol, M. (2003). Pilot trial of genetically modified, attenuated Salmonella expressing the E. coli cytosine deaminase gene in refractory cancer patients. *Cancer Gene Therapy,* Vol. 10, No. 10, pp. 737-744, 0929-1903

Niethammer, A.G., Xiang, R., Becker, J.C., Wodrich, H., Pertl, U., Karsten, G., Eliceiri, B.P. & Reisfeld, R.A. (2002). A DNA vaccine against VEGF receptor 2 prevents effective angiogenesis and inhibits tumor growth. *Nature Medicine,* Vol. 8, No. 12, pp. 1369-1375, 1078-8956

Ning, T., Yan, X., Lu, Z.J., Wang, G.P., Zhang, N., Yang, J., Jiang, S., Wu, Y., Yang, L., Guan, Y.S. & Luo, F. (2008). Gene therapy with angiogenesis inhibitor endostatin in an orthotopic lung cancer murine model. *Human Gene Therapy,* Vol. 20, No. 2, pp. 103-111, 1557-7422

Okada, Y., Ueno, H., Katagiri, M., Oneyama, T., Shimomura, K., Sakurai, S., Mataga, I., Moride, M. & Hasegawa, H. (2010). Experimental study of antiangiogenic gene therapy targeting VEGF in oral cancer. *Odontology,* Vol. 98, No. 1, pp. 52-59, 1618-1255

Olea, F.D., Vera Janavel, G., Cuniberti, L., Yannarelli, G., Cabeza Meckert, P., Cors, J., Valdivieso, L., Lev, G., Mendiz, O., Bercovich, A., Criscuolo, M., Melo, C., Laguens, R. & Crottogini, A. (2009). Repeated, but not single, VEGF gene transfer affords protection against ischemic muscle lesions in rabbits with hindlimb ischemia. *Gene Therapy,* Vol. 16, No. 6, pp. 716-723, 1476-5462

Oliner, J., Min, H., Leal, J., Yu, D., Rao, S., You, E., Tang, X., Kim, H., Meyer, S., Han, S.J., Hawkins, N., Rosenfeld, R., Davy, E., Graham, K., Jacobsen, F., Stevenson, S., Ho, J., Chen, Q., Hartmann, T., Michaels, M., Kelley, M., Li, L., Sitney, K., Martin, F., Sun, J.R., Zhang, N., Lu, J., Estrada, J., Kumar, R., Coxon, A., Kaufman, S., Pretorius, J., Scully, S., Cattley, R., Payton, M., Coats, S., Nguyen, L., Desilva, B., Ndifor, A., Hayward, I., Radinsky, R., Boone, T. & Kendall, R. (2004). Suppression of angiogenesis and tumor growth by selective inhibition of angiopoietin-2. *Cancer Cell,* Vol. 6, No. 5, pp. 507-516, 1535-6108

Pajusola, K., Kunnapuu, J., Vuorikoski, S., Soronen, J., Andre, H., Pereira, T., Korpisalo, P., Yla-Herttuala, S., Poellinger, L. & Alitalo, K. (2005). Stabilized HIF-1alpha is superior to VEGF for angiogenesis in skeletal muscle via adeno-associated virus gene transfer. *FASEB Journal,* Vol. 19, No. 10, pp. 1365-1367, 1530-6860

Palffy, R., Gardlik, R., Hodosy, J., Behuliak, M., Resko, P., Radvansky, J. & Celec, P. (2006). Bacteria in gene therapy: bactofection versus alternative gene therapy. *Gene Therapy,* Vol. 13, No. 2, pp. 101-105, 0969-7128

Paravicini TM, Touyz RM. (2006). Redox signaling in hypertension. *Cardiovasc Res.*; Vol. 71, pp.247-258.

Persano, L., Crescenzi, M. & Indraccolo, S. (2007). Anti-angiogenic gene therapy of cancer: current status and future prospects. *Molecular Aspects of Medicine,* Vol. 28, No. 1, pp. 87-114, 0098-2997

Petrovan, R.J., Kaplan, C.D., Reisfeld, R.A. & Curtiss, L.K. (2007). DNA vaccination against VEGF receptor 2 reduces atherosclerosis in LDL receptor-deficient mice. *Arteriosclerosis, Thrombosis, and Vascular Biology,* Vol. 27, No. 5, pp. 1095-1100, 1524-4636

Piascik Michael T., Lin Shu-Mei ,. Kiningham Kinsley K, St. Clair Daret K. (2006). The protective roles of nitric oxide and superoxide dismutase in adriamycin-induced cardiotoxicity. *Cardiovascular Research,* Vol. 69, pp.186 - 197.

Postnov Y. V., Orlov S.N. Budnikov Y. Y., Doroschuk A. D., Postnov A. Y. (2007) Mitochondrial energy conversion disturbance with decrease in ATP production as a source of systemic arterial hypertension. *Pathophysiology,* Vol. 14, pp. 195–204.

Rajagopalan, S., Mohler, E.R., 3rd, Lederman, R.J., Mendelsohn, F.O., Saucedo, J.F., Goldman, C.K., Blebea, J., Macko, J., Kessler, P.D., Rasmussen, H.S. & Annex, B.H. (2003). Regional angiogenesis with vascular endothelial growth factor in peripheral arterial disease: a phase II randomized, double-blind, controlled study of adenoviral delivery of vascular endothelial growth factor 121 in patients with disabling intermittent claudication. *Circulation,* Vol. 108, No. 16, pp. 1933-1938, 1524-4539

Rajagopalan, S., Olin, J., Deitcher, S., Pieczek, A., Laird, J., Grossman, P.M., Goldman, C.K., McEllin, K., Kelly, R. & Chronos, N. (2007). Use of a constitutively active hypoxia-inducible factor-1alpha transgene as a therapeutic strategy in no-option critical limb ischemia patients: phase I dose-escalation experience. *Circulation,* Vol. 115, No. 10, pp. 1234-1243, 1524-4539

Sangro, B., Mazzolini, G., Ruiz, J., Herraiz, M., Quiroga, J., Herrero, I., Benito, A., Larrache, J., Pueyo, J., Subtil, J.C., Olague, C., Sola, J., Sadaba, B., Lacasa, C., Melero, I., Qian, C. & Prieto, J. (2004). Phase I trial of intratumoral injection of an adenovirus encoding interleukin-12 for advanced digestive tumors. *Journal of Clinical Oncology,* Vol. 22, No. 8, pp. 1389-1397, 0732-183X

Shibata, M.A., Morimoto, J., Shibata, E. & Otsuki, Y. (2008). Combination therapy with short interfering RNA vectors against VEGF-C and VEGF-A suppresses lymph node and lung metastasis in a mouse immunocompetent mammary cancer model. *Cancer Gene Therapy,* Vol. 15, No. 12, pp. 776-786, 1476-5500

Shirakawa, T. (2008). The current status of adenovirus-based cancer gene therapy. *Molecules and Cells,* Vol. 25, No. 4, pp. 462-466, 1016-8478

Schgoer, W., Theurl, M., Jeschke, J., Beer, A.G., Albrecht, K., Gander, R., Rong, S., Vasiljevic, D., Egger, M., Wolf, A.M., Frauscher, S., Koller, B., Tancevski, I., Patsch, J.R., Schratzberger, P., Piza-Katzer, H., Ritsch, A., Bahlmann, F.H., Fischer-Colbrie, R., Wolf, D. & Kirchmair, R. (2009). Gene therapy with the angiogenic cytokine secretoneurin induces therapeutic angiogenesis by a nitric oxide-dependent mechanism. *Circulation Research,* Vol. 105, No. 10, pp. 994-1002, 1524-4571

Soutschek, J., Akinc, A., Bramlage, B., Charisse, K., Constien, R., Donoghue, M., Elbashir, S., Geick, A., Hadwiger, P., Harborth, J., John, M., Kesavan, V., Lavine, G., Pandey, R.K., Racie, T., Rajeev, K.G., Rohl, I., Toudjarska, I., Wang, G., Wuschko, S., Bumcrot, D., Koteliansky, V., Limmer, S., Manoharan, M. & Vornlocher, H.P. (2004). Therapeutic silencing of an endogenous gene by systemic administration of modified siRNAs. *Nature,* Vol. 432, No. 7014, pp. 173-178, 1476-4687

Sterman, D.H., Recio, A., Carroll, R.G., Gillespie, C.T., Haas, A., Vachani, A., Kapoor, V., Sun, J., Hodinka, R., Brown, J.L., Corbley, M.J., Parr, M., Ho, M., Pastan, I., Machuzak, M., Benedict, W., Zhang, X.Q., Lord, E.M., Litzky, L.A., Heitjan, D.F., June, C.H., Kaiser, L.R., Vonderheide, R.H., Albelda, S.M. & Kanther, M. (2007). A phase I clinical trial of single-dose intrapleural IFN-beta gene transfer for malignant pleural mesothelioma and metastatic pleural effusions: high rate of antitumor immune responses. *Clinical Cancer Research,* Vol. 13, No. 15 Pt 1, pp. 4456-4466, 1078-0432

Stewart, D.J., Hilton, J.D., Arnold, J.M., Gregoire, J., Rivard, A., Archer, S.L., Charbonneau, F., Cohen, E., Curtis, M., Buller, C.E., Mendelsohn, F.O., Dib, N., Page, P., Ducas, J., Plante, S., Sullivan, J., Macko, J., Rasmussen, C., Kessler, P.D. & Rasmussen, H.S. (2006). Angiogenic gene therapy in patients with nonrevascularizable ischemic heart disease: a phase 2 randomized, controlled trial of AdVEGF(121) (AdVEGF121) versus maximum medical treatment. *Gene Therapy,* Vol. 13, No. 21, pp. 1503-1511, 0969-7128

Stewart, D.J., Kutryk, M.J., Fitchett, D., Freeman, M., Camack, N., Su, Y., Della Siega, A., Bilodeau, L., Burton, J.R., Proulx, G. & Radhakrishnan, S. (2009). VEGF gene therapy fails to improve perfusion of ischemic myocardium in patients with advanced coronary disease: results of the NORTHERN trial. *Molecular Therapy,* Vol. 17, No. 6, pp. 1109-1115, 1525-0024

Stritzker, J., Pilgrim, S., Szalay, A.A. & Goebel, W. (2008). Prodrug converting enzyme gene delivery by L. monocytogenes. *BMC Cancer,* Vol. 8, No. 94, pp. 1-10, 1471-2407

Tada, H., Maron, D.J., Choi, E.A., Barsoum, J., Lei, H., Xie, Q., Liu, W., Ellis, L., Moscioni, A.D., Tazelaar, J., Fawell, S., Qin, X., Propert, K.J., Davis, A., Fraker, D.L., Wilson, J.M. & Spitz, F.R. (2001). Systemic IFN-beta gene therapy results in long-term survival in mice with established colorectal liver metastases. *Journal of Clinical Investigation,* Vol. 108, No. 1, pp. 83-95, 0021-9738

Tafuro, S., Ayuso, E., Zacchigna, S., Zentilin, L., Moimas, S., Dore, F. & Giacca, M. (2009). Inducible adeno-associated virus vectors promote functional angiogenesis in adult organisms via regulated vascular endothelial growth factor expression. *Cardiovascular Research,* Vol. 83, No. 4, pp. 663-671, 1755-3245

Tang, J., Wang, J., Zheng, F., Kong, X., Guo, L., Yang, J., Zhang, L. & Huang, Y. (2010). Combination of chemokine and angiogenic factor genes and mesenchymal stem cells could enhance angiogenesis and improve cardiac function after acute myocardial infarction in rats. *Molecular and Cellular Biochemistry,* Vol. 339, No. 1-2, pp. 107-118, 1573-4919

Theys, J., Landuyt, A.W., Nuyts, S., Van Mellaert, L., Lambin, P. & Anne, J. (2001). Clostridium as a tumor-specific delivery system of therapeutic proteins. *Cancer Detection and Prevention,* Vol. 25, No. 6, pp. 548-557, 0361-090X

Toso, J.F., Gill, V.J., Hwu, P., Marincola, F.M., Restifo, N.P., Schwartzentruber, D.J., Sherry, R.M., Topalian, S.L., Yang, J.C., Stock, F., Freezer, L.J., Morton, K.E., Seipp, C., Haworth, L., Mavroukakis, S., White, D., MacDonald, S., Mao, J., Sznol, M. & Rosenberg, S.A. (2002). Phase I study of the intravenous administration of attenuated Salmonella typhimurium to patients with metastatic melanoma. *Journal of Clinical Oncology,* Vol. 20, No. 1, pp. 142-152, 0732-183X

Traktuev, D.O., Tsokolaeva, Z.I., Shevelev, A.A., Talitskiy, K.A., Stepanova, V.V., Johnstone, B.H., Rahmat-Zade, T.M., Kapustin, A.N., Tkachuk, V.A., March, K.L. & Parfyonova, Y.V. (2007). Urokinase gene transfer augments angiogenesis in ischemic skeletal and myocardial muscle. *Molecular Therapy,* Vol. 15, No. 11, pp. 1939-1946, 1525-0016

Tysome, J.R., Briat, A., Alusi, G., Cao, F., Gao, D., Yu, J., Wang, P., Yang, S., Dong, Z., Wang, S., Deng, L., Francis, J., Timiryasova, T., Fodor, I., Lemoine, N.R. & Wang, Y. (2009). Lister strain of vaccinia virus armed with endostatin-angiostatin fusion gene as a novel therapeutic agent for human pancreatic cancer. *Gene Therapy,* Vol. 16, No. 10, pp. 1223-1233, 1476-5462

Ulker S, McMaster D, McKeown PP, Bayraktutan U. (2003). Impaired activities of antioxidant enzymes elicit endothelial dysfunction in spontaneous hypertensive rats despite enhanced vascular nitric oxide generation. *Cardiovascular Res.*; Vol. 59, pp. 488–500.

Vincent, K.A., Jiang, C., Boltje, I. & Kelly, R.A. (2007). Gene therapy progress and prospects: therapeutic angiogenesis for ischemic cardiovascular disease. *Gene Therapy,* Vol. 14, No. 10, pp. 781-789, 0969-7128

Wang X, Chow FL, Oka T, Hao L, Lopez-Campistrous A, Kelly S et al., (2009). Matrix metalloproteinase-7 and ADAM-12 define a signaling axis in agonist-induced hypertension and cardiac hypertrophy. *Circulation,* Vol. 119, pp. 2480–2489.

Webb, C.P. & Vande Woude, G.F. (2000). Genes that regulate metastasis and angiogenesis. *Journal of Neuro-Oncology,* Vol. 50, No. 1-2, pp. 71-87, 0167-594X

Xiang, R., Lode, H.N., Chao, T.H., Ruehlmann, J.M., Dolman, C.S., Rodriguez, F., Whitton, J.L., Overwijk, W.W., Restifo, N.P. & Reisfeld, R.A. (2000). An autologous oral DNA vaccine protects against murine melanoma. *Proceedings of the National Academy of Sciences of the United States of America,* Vol. 97, No. 10, pp. 5492-5497, 0027-8424

Xiang, R., Mizutani, N., Luo, Y., Chiodoni, C., Zhou, H., Mizutani, M., Ba, Y., Becker, J.C. & Reisfeld, R.A. (2005). A DNA vaccine targeting survivin combines apoptosis with suppression of angiogenesis in lung tumor eradication. *Cancer Research,* Vol. 65, No. 2, pp. 553-561, 0008-5472

Xiang, S., Fruehauf, J. & Li, C.J. (2006). Short hairpin RNA-expressing bacteria elicit RNA interference in mammals. *Nature Biotechnology*, Vol. 24, No. 6, pp. 697-702, 1087-0156

Yang, L., Wang, L., Su, X.Q., Chen, X.C., Li, D., Luo, S.T., Shi, H.S., Chen, L.J. & Wang, Y.S. (2010). Suppression of ovarian cancer growth via systemic administration with liposome-encapsulated adenovirus-encoding endostatin. *Cancer Gene Therapy*, Vol. 17, No. 1, pp. 49-57, 1476-5500

Yao, B., He, Q.M., Tian, L., Xiao, F., Jiang, Y., Zhang, R., Li, G., Zhang, L., Hou, J.M., Wang, L., Cheng, X.C., Wen, Y.J., Kan, B., Li, J., Zhao, X., Hu, B., Zhou, Q. & Wei, Y.Q. (2005). Enhanced antitumor effect of the combination of tumstatin gene therapy and gemcitabine in murine models. *Human Gene Therapy*, Vol. 16, No. 9, pp. 1075-1086, 1043-0342

Yazawa, K., Fujimori, M., Amano, J., Kano, Y. & Taniguchi, S. (2000). Bifidobacterium longum as a delivery system for cancer gene therapy: selective localization and growth in hypoxic tumors. *Cancer Gene Therapy*, Vol. 7, No. 2, pp. 269-274, 0929-1903

Yockman, J.W., Choi, D., Whitten, M.G., Chang, C.W., Kastenmeier, A., Erickson, H., Albanil, A., Lee, M., Kim, S.W. & Bull, D.A. (2009). Polymeric gene delivery of ischemia-inducible VEGF significantly attenuates infarct size and apoptosis following myocardial infarct. *Gene Therapy*, Vol. 16, No. 1, pp. 127-135, 1476-5462

Yokoyama M, Inoue N, Kawashima S. (2000). Role of the vascular NADH/NADPH oxidase system in atherosclerosis. *Ann N Y Acad Sci.*; Vol. 902, pp.241-247.

Yoo, J.Y., Kim, J.H., Kwon, Y.G., Kim, E.C., Kim, N.K., Choi, H.J. & Yun, C.O. (2007). VEGF-specific short hairpin RNA-expressing oncolytic adenovirus elicits potent inhibition of angiogenesis and tumor growth. *Molecular Therapy*, Vol. 15, No. 2, pp. 295-302, 1525-0016

Yoon, W.S., Choi, W.C., Sin, J.I. & Park, Y.K. (2007). Antitumor therapeutic effects of Salmonella typhimurium containing Flt3 Ligand expression plasmids in melanoma-bearing mouse. *Biotechnol Lett*, Vol. 29, No. 4, pp. 511-516, 1573-6776

Yuhua, L., Kunyuan, G., Hui, C., Yongmei, X., Chaoyang, S., Xun, T. & Daming, R. (2001). Oral cytokine gene therapy against murine tumor using attenuated Salmonella typhimurium. *International Journal of Cancer*, Vol. 94, No. 3, pp. 438-443, 0020-7136

Zhang, Y., Qu, Z.H., Cui, M., Guo, C., Zhang, X.M., Ma, C.H. & Sun, W.S. (2009). Combined endostatin and TRAIL gene transfer suppresses human hepatocellular carcinoma growth and angiogenesis in nude mice. *Cancer Biology and Therapy*, Vol. 8, No. 5, pp. 466-473, 1555-8576

Zhao, H.F., L'Abbe, D., Jolicoeur, N., Wu, M., Li, Z., Yu, Z. & Shen, S.H. (2005). High-throughput screening of effective siRNAs from RNAi libraries delivered via bacterial invasion. *Nature Methods*, Vol. 2, No. 12, pp. 967-973, 1548-7091

Zheng, L.M., Luo, X., Feng, M., Li, Z., Le, T., Ittensohn, M., Trailsmith, M., Bermudes, D., Lin, S.L. & King, I.C. (2000). Tumor amplified protein expression therapy: Salmonella as a tumor-selective protein delivery vector. *Oncology Research*, Vol. 12, No. 3, (2000), pp. 127-135, 0965-0407

Zimmerman MC, Lazartigues E, Sharma RV, Davisson RL. (2004). Hypertension caused by angiotensin II infusion involves increased superoxide production in the central nervous system. *Circ Res.*; Vol.95, pp. 210-216.

Zimmerman M. C., Sharma R.V., Davisson R L.: (2005). Superoxide Mediates Angiotensin II–Induced Influx of Extracellular Calcium in Neural Cells *Hypertension*; Vol.45, pp. 717-723.

6

Rescue of Familial Hypertrophic Cardiomyopathy by Altering Sarcomeric Exposure and Response to Calcium

David F. Wieczorek[1] and Beata M. Wolska[2]
[1]*Department of Molecular Genetics, Biochemistry, & Microbiology University of Cincinnati Medical Center, Cincinnati,*
[2]*Department of Medicine, Section of Cardiology and Department of Physiology and Biophysics; University of Illinois at Chicago, USA*

1. Introduction

In 2006, the prevalence of total cardiovascular disease in the US was 81.1 million people, out of which 17.6 million people had coronary heart disease (1). Heart failure, the progressive loss of cardiac contractile performance, affects approximately 5 million Americans, with estimated medical costs of $21-50 billion dollars per year (2). Current pharmacologic therapies focus on symptomatic treatment and halting the progression of the disease (1). Interventional or surgical procedures in the treatment of cardiovascular disease are often restricted to a limited time frame, with heart transplantation patients reliant upon donor hearts that are in great demand.
In recent years, gene therapy studies have made significant progress in the successful treatment of numerous disease conditions using a variety of different approaches. Generally, gene therapy can be classified into two categories: germ line gene therapy where germ cells are modified by the introduction of functional genes which can subsequently be passed on to later generations, and somatic gene therapy where therapeutic genes are transferred into somatic cells of a patient. Another form of gene therapy known as cell-mediated gene therapy is where pluripotent stem cells or progenitor cells are delivered to the injured tissue/organ. The focus of this article will be the modification of disease phenotypes through genetic engineering and transgenic expression of contractile and calcium regulatory proteins.

2. Gene therapy and mouse models of disease

The diseases that were initially targeted for gene therapy were associated with blood disorders or cancers. For example, a decade ago, Pawlink et al demonstrated correction of sickle cell disease in a transgenic mouse model using a β globin gene variant being expressed in a lentiviral vector (3). Hemophilia A was successfully treated in mouse and dog models using adenoviral vectors expressing factor VIII (4). With the great promise of gene therapy in the treatment of disease, the field expanded rapidly with numerous mouse models having a wide variety of diseases being the target of various therapeutic approaches. For example, mouse models of cystic fibrosis, atherosclerosis, various cancers, and several retinal diseases using different methodological approaches showed great promise for successful treatment (5-10). Cardiovascular diseases have also been treated using gene therapy, targeting defined animal models of cardiac disease. Some of these models of cardiac disease were associated with ischemic heart disease, heart failure, and hypertrophic cardiomyopathy.

Currently, adeno-associated virus vectors are the most potent and promising vectors used for delivery of transgenes to the heart (11, 12). They exhibit efficient uptake, stable long-term expression of transferred genes, and tissue specificity dependent upon the viral serotype (13). Of the 11 identified serotypes of adeno-associated viruses, types 6, 8, and specifically 9, have tropism for the heart (14, 15). In addition to transgenes, these vectors can also deliver microRNAs to the heart which can regulate the simultaneous expression of multiple genes (11).

In this review, we discuss the current studies using *in vivo* models of hypertrophic cardiomyopathy. We describe various mouse models of hypertrophic cardiomyopathy and the different approaches that have been shown to be beneficial in improving cardiac pathology and function. In using these models and testing various therapeutic approaches, a determination of the most effective means for improving cardiomyopathic disease can be elucidated.

3. Familial hypertrophic cardiomyopathy

Familial Hypertrophic Cardiomyopathy (FHC) is a genetic disease caused by autosomal dominant mutations in genes encoding sarcomeric contractile proteins. Hundreds of disease causing mutations in any of 10 genes can result in FHC. These mutations occur in both thick and thin filament proteins, including myosin heavy and light chains, myosin binding protein C, actin, troponins I and T, and α-tropomyosin. Most of these mutations are missense mutations with single amino acid residue substitutions. The overall prevalence of hypertrophic cardiomyopathy is approximately 1 in 500 people; however, many of these individuals exhibit mild symptoms only with late onset in life. Pathologically, FHC is characterized by left and/or right ventricular hypertrophy that occurs in the absence of an increased external load, in addition to intraventricular septal hypertrophy (16). Left ventricular outflow tract obstruction, diastolic dysfunction, and myocyte hypertrophy and disarray are often found. Other common symptoms include myofibrillar disarray and fibrosis, increased calcium sensitivity of myofilaments, and cardiac arrhythmias that may lead to premature sudden death and/or heart failure. An interesting feature is that these symptoms are quite variable, ranging from mild cardiac hypertrophy and no symptoms to marked hypertrophy with diastolic heart failure and sudden death (17). These variable clinical phentoypes strongly suggest that a specific FHC mutation in a contractile protein seemingly can be modified by environmental factors and modifier genes. For example, pathological symptoms associated with FHC mutations in the troponin T gene appear to be minimal; however, most of these patients die of sudden cardiac arrest (18). Patients with FHC mutations in the α-tropomyosin (α-Tm) gene exhibit a wide phenotypic range of symptoms. In the United States, a small percentage (<5%) of FHC patients have mutations in α-Tm with relatively benign symptoms (19). In Japan, the incidence of FHC patients with mutations in α-Tm is still relatively low, but the symptoms are more pathological (20, 21).

Interestingly, in Finland, FHC mutations in the α-Tm gene have a very high incidence rate (11%) among contractile proteins and are a leading cause of FHC; this is most likely due to a "founder's effect" (22). The pathology of FHC with α-Tm mutations is quite severe in the Finnish population with a majority of the patients exhibiting a dramatic phenotype. This variability in incidence and phenotype associated with the Tm cases in different populations most likely reflects environmental factors and modifier genes in altering the onset and pathological symptoms of FHC.

There are 11 mutations in α-Tm that lead to FHC. These mutations are scattered throughout the α-Tm protein, with the majority of them occurring in one of the troponin T binding regions (amino acids 175-190). Since Tm is an α-helical coiled coil protein that dimerizes with itself, and binds to both actin and troponin T, the charge of each specific amino acid residue can play a critical role in both its own structure and in its interaction with its binding partners. In order to gain a greater understanding of the molecular and physiological mechanisms that lead to FHC, we developed 2 transgenic mouse models that incorporate FHC mutations in α-Tm (23-25). Since there is 100% amino acid conservation between mouse and human α-Tm sequence, the FHC mutant α-Tm protein in the transgenic mice is identical to the protein that is found in human patients. The first model entailed a substitution of an asparagine for aspartic acid at codon 175 (Asp175Asn). These mice develop a mild hypertrophic phenotype, coupled with systolic and diastolic dysfunction (23). The cardiac myofilaments demonstrate increased calcium sensitivity, which is in agreement with human studies (26). We also found a correlation between an increase in myofilament calcium sensitivity with a decrease in relaxation rate and a blunted response to β-adrenergic stimulation (27). The second transgenic mouse model was a substitution of glycine for glutamic acid at codon 180 (Glu180Gly) (24, 25). Pathological changes in the hearts of these mice are initially detected by 1 month and include ventricular concentric hypertrophy, fibrosis, and atrial enlargement. These disease-associated changes progressively increase and initially resulted in lethality by 6 months of age; more recently, some of these mice survive much longer probably due to modifying genes introduced when mating the FHC Tm 180 mice with commercial non-transgenic control mice. Physiological analyses show significant alterations in both contraction and relaxation of the heart, with increased sensitivity of the myofilaments to calcium. Isolated cardiomyocytes from the Glu180Gly FHC mice also exhibit an increase in calcium sensitivity of force production (28). Thus, FHC associated Tm proteins alter myofilament structure and properties in individual cardiomyocytes that collectively cause the aberrant function of the entire heart which leads to hypertrophic cardiomyopathy.

4. Rescue of cardiomyopathic mice by contractile proteins

To determine whether it is possible to rescue FHC mice from their lethality and cardiac hypertrophic phenotype, we and others have taken several approaches (29-32). The first approach was to target the myofilaments themselves through the incorporation of proteins that counteract the properties exhibited by the FHC mutant Tm 180 protein since myofilaments obtained from the hearts of FHC patients and animal models usually exhibit an increased sensitivity to calcium with respect to tension development. This is also true for the FHC Tm 180 myofilaments. To compensate for this increased calcium sensitivity, we generated a double-transgenic mouse expressing a chimeric Tm containing the α-Tm amino terminus and the carboxyl terminus of β-Tm, the fetal cardiac isoform (Chi 1) (30). Previous

work demonstrated that myofilaments from these Chi 1 mice have a decreased sensitivity to calcium (33, 34). The double-transgenic mice which were created by crossing the 2 lines displayed normalized myofilament calcium sensitivity. More importantly, the hearts of these mice exhibited a normal morphology with no pathological abnormalities and improved cardiac function (30). These mice also displayed a normal life span. These results demonstrate that alterations in calcium response by modifications in contractile proteins can prevent the pathological and physiological effects of FHC.
Restrictive cardiomyopathy (RCM) is a human condition that displays clinical features of biatrial dilation, a restricted left ventricle, and sudden cardiac death. Patients with this disease have mutations in cardiac z-line proteins, such as desmin and cardiac troponin I and T (35, 36). Recently, a transgenic mouse model was generated (cardiac TnI^{193His}) that displays many of the pathological changes that occur in human patients with RCM, including restrictive ventricles, biatrial enlargement, and sudden cardiac death (37, 38). These mice were crossed with another transgenic mouse line that expresses a cardiac TnI isoform that is truncated at the N-terminus (cTnI-ND) (31, 39); this is a naturally occurring TnI isoform that is found at low levels in normal hearts of all examined species. Transgenic mice expressing the cTnI-ND isoform exhibit a normal cardiac phenotype with no evidence of hypertrophy or histological abnormalites (31). Under hemodynamic stress and heart failure, the cTnI-ND isoform is increased in expression (40). The double transgenic mice (cardiac TnI^{193His} x cTnI-ND) rescued the lethal phenotype of the cardiac TnI^{193His} RCM mutant mice; cardiac function was significantly improved and the myofilaments' increased sensitivity to calcium was reversed (32). These results, which are similar to those found with the FHC Tm180 rescued mice, suggest that calcium desensitization in myofibrils is a therapeutic option for the treatment of diastolic dysfunction.

5. Rescue of cardiomyopathic mice through alterations in calcium handling

In addition to rescuing cardiomyopathic conditions through treatment with compensatory contractile proteins, recent studies have also addressed whether proteins involved with calcium handling can play a role in improving the pathological effects of heart disease. Reports suggest that Serca2a overexpression can modulate cardiac hypertrophy due to removal of calcium from the myofilament region (41-43). To test whether improvements in the hypertrophic phenotype can be achieved through increased Serca2 expression and/or activity, we recently treated the FHC Tm 180 mice with Serca2a, the protein involved in re-sequestering calcium from the cytoplasmic space into the sarcoplasmic reticulum of the cardiomyocyte (44). The approach that we implemented was gene transfer of Serca2a ligated to an adenoviral vector with injection into FHC Tm 180 neonatal hearts. Results demonstrated that a single dose of Serca2a in 1-day-old mice improved the heart morphology, altered hypertrophic gene expression, and improved cardiac function. Histological results showed there was a significant decrease in fibrosis, coupled with a decrease in the heart weight:body weight ratio. Molecular analysis shows that within the first 3 weeks, there is a significant decline in ANF and β-MHC expression in the Serca2a-treated FHC Tm 180 mice. *In situ* hemodynamic measurements show that by 3 months, the hearts from FHC Tm 180 mice treated with Serca2a have significantly improved their response to isoproterenol compared to control mouse hearts. These results demonstrate that gene transfer of a single dose of Serca2a can delay the hypertrophic phenotype and improve cardiac function in an FHC mouse model that is associated with increased myofilament calcium sensitivity. As such, the study strongly suggests that Serca2a expression should be considered as a potential therapeutic approach in the treatment of FHC.

The benefits for Serca2a overexpression on cardiac function has been demonstrated in both animal models and in human patients. The sodium-calcium exchanger (NCX), along with Serca2a, are the two principle pumps used to remove cytosolic Ca^{2+} in the heart. Both systolic and diastolic improvements occur with more efficient energy usage in removal of Ca^{2+} from the cytosol. Results show that Serca2a removes twice as much cytosolic Ca^{2+} as the NCX for each ATP that is hydrolyzed (12). During heart failure, there is decreased expression and function of Serca2a, which is compensated by increased NCX activity, which is a less efficient energy process. The ratio of Serca2a to NCX changes from approximately 75:25 in the healthy human heart to 50:50 in the failing human heart (45). Normalization of the Serca2a:NCX ratio in heart failure by transgenic or gene therapy approaches appears to hold great therapeutic promise. Studies show that delivery of Serca2a by gene transfer to experimental models of heart failure in sheep and swine can largely reverse cardiac dysfunction and improve systolic and diastolic performance of the heart (46, 47). Recently, percutaneous administration of Serca2a was conducted in phase 1 and 2 clinical studies in humans (48, 49). Heart failure patients were administered an adeno-associated virus expressing Serca2a. Results showed a majority of patients exhibited marked improvements within 6 months, which included improved ejection fraction and end-systolic volume measurements. Thus, the success of these human trials demonstrates that Serca2a may serve as a potential treatment modality for heart failure. Phase 3 clinical trials are expected to be initiated soon.

Another strategy that has been investigated in the treatment of hypertrophic mouse models has been to crossbreed these mice with phospholamban (PLB) knockout mice. PLB is a protein that normally inhibits Serca2a activity of calcium re-sequestration into the sarcoplasmic reticulum. Previous work demonstrated that when a heart failure mouse model due to overexpression of the β-adrenergic receptor was crossed with the PLB knockout mouse, systolic function was improved at 1 year; however, cardiac hypertrophy is still significant (50). In a FHC model of myosin binding protein C, cross-breeding with the PLB knockout mice failed to rescue the hypertrophy, fibrosis and functional parameters of the FHC mutant hearts (51). In a very recent study, we decided to cross the FHC Tm 180 mice with the PLB knockout mice (52). We hypothesized that since Tm is a thin filament protein in the sarcomere, which in FHC primarily affects diastolic function and calcium sensitivity, deletion of PLB may compensate for these altered physiological parameters by increasing the uptake of calcium into the sarcoplasmic reticulum and removing calcium from the myofilament space. Our results demonstrated that PLB ablation in the FHC Tm 180 mice rescued cardiac pathological changes and cardiac function for up to a year (52). The work with Serca2 overexpression and PLB knockout mice suggests that increased Ca^{2+} uptake by the sarcoplasmic reticulum may be a viable target for gene therapy in the treatment of FHC with thin filament contractile protein mutations.

Previous studies from the Metzger laboratory demonstrated that a calcium buffer, parvalbumin, could also play a role in ameliorating some of the FHC Tm180 physiological alterations (53). By crossing a parvalbumin transgenic mouse with the FHC Tm 180 mouse, they demonstrated that the decreased cardiac relaxation that occurs in the FHC mice was corrected. In addition, the relaxation performance was also corrected in cardiomyocytes that were isolated from double transgenic mouse hearts. Similarly, increased levels of parvalbumin expression were also able to rescue a slowed relaxation rate in FHC α-Tm cardiomyocytes that expressed parvalbumin and the FHC mutant Tm that substituted valine for alanine at codon 63 (53). Thus, these studies reinforce the concept that modification of calcium handling can rescue functional properties of FHC Tm myofilaments.

6. Conclusions

Familial hypertrophic cardiomyopathy is a common disease that is most often associated with mutations in the sarcomeric contractile proteins. Diagnosis and treatment of this condition is still in its infancy, although there have been significant advances in the understanding of the genetic causes of this disease and the molecular pathways that trigger cardiac hypertrophy. Recent studies implicate calcium itself, and the response to calcium by the sarcomere, as playing key roles in the development of hypertrophy. Various methods have been successfully used in animal models of FHC to treat and rescue mice from hypertrophy and heart failure. As such, they have demonstrated a "proof of principle" in the successful treatment of this disease. Some of these treatment methods revolve around re-supplying contractile proteins that counteract the physiological consequences caused by the mutant FHC proteins. For FHC mutations that occur in the thin filament and render the sarcomere most sensitive to calcium, the compensatory protein must exhibit properties associated with a decreased sensitivity to calcium. Other effective treatments focus on removing calcium from the region of the myofilament by enhanced uptake by the sarcoplasmic reticulum or the buffering of calcium. However, considering the large number of genes that activate different molecular pathways in contributing to the hypertrophic phenotype, it is unlikely that a single treatment strategy will be sufficient in addressing the various complexities of this disease. As such, a wide variety of experimental approaches should be pursued so as to design the most effective treatment strategies for the diverse hypertrophic phenotypes that are manifest in human patients.

7. Acknowledgements

The authors were like to acknowledge financial support by NIH NHLBI HL81680 (DFW) and HL79032 (BMW).

8. References

[1] Lavu M., S. Gundewar, and D. Lefer. Gene therapy for ischemic heart disease. J Mol Cell Cardiol. In press.

[2] Klein L, C. O'Connor, W. Gattis, M. Zampino, L. De Luca, A. Vitarelli, F. Fedele, and M. Gheorghiade. (2003) Pharmacologic therapy for patients with chronic heart failure and reduced systolic function: review of trials and practical considerations. Am J Cardiol 91 (suppl): 18F-40F.

[3] Pawliuk R, K. Westerman, M. Fabry, E. Payen, R. Tighe, E. Bouhassira, C. Eaves, R. Humphries, Y. Beuzard, R. Nagel, and P. Leboulch. (2001) Correction of sickle cell disease in transgenic mouse models by gene therapy. Science 294:2368-2371.

[4] Chuah M, G. Schiedner, L. Thorrez, B. Brown, M. Johnston, V. Gillijns, S. Hertel, N. Van Rooijen, D. Lillicrap, D. Collen, T. VanderDriessche, and S. Kochanek. (2003) Therapeutic factor VIII levels and negligible toxicity in mouse and dog models of

hemophilia A following gene therapy with high-capacity adenoviral vectors. Blood 101:1734-1743.
[5] Dorin J, R. Farley, S. Webb, S. Smith, E. Farini, S. Delaney, B. Wainwright, E. Alton, and D. Porteous. (1996) A demonstration using mouse models that successful gene therapy for cystic fibrosis requires only partial gene correction. Gene Ther. 3:797-801.
[6] Benoit P, F. Emmanuel, J Caillaud, L Bassinet, G. Castro, P. Galliz, J Fruchart, D. Branellec, P. Denefle, and N. Duverger. (1999) Somatic gene transfer of human apoA-I inhibits atherosclerosis progression in mouse models. Circulation 99:105-110.
[7] Collins S, A. Buhles, M. Scallan, P. Harrison, D. O'Hanlon, G. O'Sullivan, and M Tangney. (2010) AAV2-mediated in vivo immuno gene therapy of solid tumors. Genetic Vaccines and Therapy 8:8
[8] Allocca M, A. Manfredi, C. Lodice, U. Di Vicino and A. Auricchio. (2011) AAV-mediated gene replacement either alone or in combination with physical and pharmacological agents results in partial and transient protection from photoreceptor degeneration associated with beta PDE deficiency. Invest Ophthalmol Vis Sci. In press.
[9] Smith A., J. Bainbridge, and R. Ali. (2009) Prospects for retinal gene replacement therapy. Trends in Genetics 25:156-165.
[10] Ali R. (2004) Prospects for gene therapy. Novartis Found Symp. 255:165-172.
[11] Geisler A., A. Jungmann, J. Kurreck, W. Poller, H Katus, R. Vetter, H. Fechner, and O. Muller. (2011) microRNA122-regulated transgene expression increases specificity of cardiac gene transfer upon intravenous delivery of AAV9 vectors. Gene Therapy 18:199-209.
[12] Kawase Y. and R. Hajjar. (2008) The cardiac sarcoplasmic/endoplasmic reticulum calcium ATPase: a potent target for cardiovascular diseases. Nat Clin Pract Cardiovasc Med 5:554-565.
[13] Zincarelli C., S. Soltys, G. Rengo, W. Koch, and J. Rabinowitz. (2010) Comparative cardiac gene delivery of adeno-associated virus serotypes 1-9 reveals that AAV6 mediates the most efficient transduction in mouse heart. Clin Transl Sci 3:81-9.
[14] Njeim M. and R. Hajjar. (2010) Gene therapy for heart failure. Arch Cardiovasc Disease 103:477-485.
[15] Palomeque J., E. Chemaly, P. Colosi, J Wellman, S. Zhou, F. Del Monte, and R. Hajjar. (2007) Efficiency of eight different AAV serotypes in transducing rat myocardium in vivo. Gene Ther 14:989-997.
[16] Hughes SE. (2004) The pathology of hypertrophic cardiomyopathy. Histopathology 44:412-427.
[17] Maron BJ. (2002) Hypertrophic cardiomyhopathy: a systematic review. JAMA 287:1308-1320.
[18] Guinto P., R. Haim, C. Dowell-Martino, N. Sibinga, and J. Tardiff. (2009) Temporal and mutation-specific alterations in Ca2+ homeostasis differentially determine the progression of cTnT-related cardiomyopathies in murine models. Am J Physiol Heart Circ Physiol 297:H614-626.

[19] Tardiff J., (2005) Sarcomeric proteins and familial hypertrophic cardiomyopathy: linking mutations in structural proteins to complex cardiovascular phenotypes. Heart Fail Rev 10:237-248.
[20] Nakajima-Taniguichi C., H. Matsui, T. Kishimoto, and K. Yamauchi-Takinara. (1995) Novel missense mutation in α-tropomyosin gene found in Japanese patients with hypertrophic cardiomyopathy. J Mol Cell Cardiol 27:2053-2058.
[21] Yamauchi-Takihara, K. Nakajimataniguchi, H. Matsui, Y. Fujio, K. Kunisada, S. Nagata, and T. Kishimoto. (1996) Clinical implications of hypertrophic cardiomyopathy associated with mutations in the alpha-tropomyosin gene. Heart 63-65.
[22] Jaaskelainen, P., M. Soranta, R. Miettinen, L. Saarinen, J. Pihlajamaki, K. Silvennoinen, T. Tikanoja, M. Laakso, and J. Kuusisto. (1998) The cardiac β-myosin heavy chain gene is not the predominant gene for hypertrophic cardiomyopathy in the Finnish population. J. Am. Coll. Cardiol. 32:1709-1716.
[23] Muthuchamy, M., Pieples, K., Rethinasamy, P., Hoit, B., Grupp, I., Boivin, G., Wolska, B., Evans, C., Solaro, RJ., and Wieczorek, D. 1999. Mouse model of a familial hypertrophic cardiomyopathy mutation in α-tropomyosin manifests cardiac dysfunction. Circ Res. 85:47-56.
[24] Prabhakar, R., G. Boivin, I. Grupp, B. Hoit, G. Arteaga, R. J. Solaro, D. F. Wieczorek. (2001) A familial hypertrophic cardiomyopathy α-tropomyosin mutation causes severe cardiac hypertrophy and death in mice. J. Mol. Cell. Card. 33:1815-1828.
[25] Prabhakar R., N. Petrashevskaya, A. Schwartz, B. Aronow, G. Boivin, J. Molkentin, and D.F. Wieczorek. (2003) A mouse model of familial hypertrophic cardiomyopathy caused by a α-tropomyosin mutation. Mol Cell Biochem 251:33-42.
[26] Bottinelli R., D. Coviello, C. Redwood, M. Pellegrino, B. Maron, H. Watkinsw,and C. Reggiani. (1998) A mutant tropomyosin that causes hypertrophic cardiomyopathy is expressed in vivo and associated with an increased calcium sensitivity. Circ Res 82:106-115.
[27] Evans, C. J. Pena, R. Phillips, M. Muthuchamy, D. Wieczorek, R. Solaro, and B. Wolska. (2000) Altered hemodynamics in transgenic mice harboring a mutant tropomyosin (Asp175Asn) linked to hypertrophic cardiomyopathy. Amer. J. Physiol. Circ. Physiol. 279:H2414-2423.
[28] Michele D., F. Albayya, and J. Metzger. (1999) Direct, convergent hypersensitivity of calcium-activated force generation produced by hypertrophic cardiomyopathy mutant α-tropomyosins in adult cardiac myocytes. Nat Med 5:1413-1417.
[29] Alves M., R. Gaffin, and B. Wolska. (2010) Rescue of familial cardiomyopathies by modifications at the level of sarcomere and Ca2+ fluxes. J Mol Cell Cardiol. 48:834-842.
[30] Jagatheesan G., S. Rajan, N. Petrashevskaya, A. Schwartz, G. Boivin, G. Arteaga, R.J. Solaro, S. Liggett, and D.F.Wieczorek. (2007) Rescue of tropomyosin-induced familial hypertrophic cardiomyopathy mice by transgenesis. Am J Physiol Heart Circ Physiol 293:H949-958.
[31] Barbato J., Q. Huang, M. Hossain, M. Bond, and JP Jin. (2005) Proteolytic N-terminal truncation of cardiac troponin I enhances ventricular diastolic function. J Biol Chem 280:6602-6609.
[32] Li Y., P. Charles, C. Nan, J. Pinto, Y. Wang, J. Liang, G. Wu, J Tian, H. Feng, J. Potter, JP Jin, X. Huang. (2010) Correcting diastolic dysfunction by Ca^{2+} desensitizing

troponin in a transgenic mouse model of restrictive cardiomyopathy. J Mol. Cell Biol. 49:402-411.

[33] Jagatheesan G., S. Rajan, N. Petrashevskaya, A. Schwartz, G. Boivin, S. Vahebi P. de Tombe, R.J. Solaro, E. Labitzke, G. Hilliard, and D.F.Wieczorek. (2003) Functional importance of the carboxyl-terminal region of striated muscle tropomyosin. J Biol Chem. 278:23204-23211.

[34] Jagatheesan G., S. Rajan, and D.F. Wieczorek. (2010) Investigations into tropomyosin function using mouse models. J Mol Cell Cardiol. 48:893-898.

[35] Zhang J., A. Kumar, H. Stalker, G. Virdi, V. Ferrans, K. Horiba, F. Fricker, and M. Wallace. (2001) Clinical and molecular studies of a large family with desmin-associated restrictive cardiomyopathy. Clin Genet. 59:248-256.

[36] Mogensen J., T. Hubo, M. duque, W. Uribe, A. Shaw, R. Murphy, J Gimeno, P. Elliott, and W. McKenna. (2003) Idiopathic restrictive cardiomyopathy is part of the clinical expression of cardiac troponin I mutations. J Clin Invest 111:209-216.

[37] Du J., C. Zhang, J Liu, C. Sidky, and X. Huang. (2006) A point mutation (R192H) in the C terminus of human cardiac troponin I causes diastolic dysfunction in transgenic mice. Arch Biochem Biophys 456:143-150.

[38] Du J., J. Liu, H. Feng, M. Houssain, N. Gobara, C. Zhang, Y. Li, P. Jean-Charles, J Jin, and X Huang. (2008) Impaired relaxation is the main manifestation in transgenic mice expressing a restrictive cardiomyopathy mutation, R193H, in cardiac TnI. Am J Physiol Heart Circ Physiol 294:H2604-2613.

[39] Yu Z., L Zhang, and JP Jin. (2001) A proteolytic NH2-terminal truncation of cardiac troponin I that is up-regulated in simulated microgravity. J Biol Chem 276:15753-15760.

[40] Feng H., M. Chen, L. Weinstein, and JP Jin. (2008) Removal of the N-terminal extension of cardiac troponin I as a functional compensation for impaired myocardial β-adrenergic signaling. J Biol Chem. 283:33384-33393.

[41] Ito K., X. Yan, X Feng, W. Mannning, W. Dillmann, and B. Lorell. (2001) Transgenic expression of sarcoplasmic reticulum Ca^{2+}ATPase modifies the transition from hypertrophy to early heart failure. Circ Res 89:422-429.

[42] Sakata S., D. Lebeche, Y. Sakata, N. Sakata, E. Chemaly, L. Liang, C. Nakajima-Takenaka, T. Tsuji, N. Konishi, F. del Monte, R. Hajjar, and M. Takaki. (2007) Transcoronary gene transfer of SERCA2a increases coronary blood flow and decreases cardiomyocyte size in a type 2 diabetic rat model. Am J Physiol Heart Circ Physiol 292:H1204-H1207.

[43] Nakayama H., K. Otsu, O. Yamaguchi, K. Nishida, M. Date, K. Hongo, Y. Kusakari, T. Toyofuku, S. Hikoso, K. Kashiwase, T. Takeda, Y. Matsumura, S. Kurihada, M. Hori, and M. Tada. (2003) Cardiac-specific overexpression of a high Ca^{2+} affinity mutant of SERCA2a attenuates in vivo pressure overload cardiac hypertrophy. FASEB J 17:61-63.

[44] Pena J., A. Szkudlarek, C. Warren, L. Heinrich, R. Gaffin, G. Jagatheesan, F. del Monte, R. Hajjar, P. Goldspink R.J. Solaro, D.F. Wieczorek, and B. Wolska. (2010) J Mol Cell Cardiol. 49:993-1002.

[45] Hasenfuss G. (1988) Alterations of calcium-regulatory proteins in heart failure. Cardiovasc Res 37:279-293.

[46] Byrne M., J. Power, A. Preovolos, J Mariani, R. Hajjar, and D. Kaye. (2008) Recirculating cardiac delivery of AAV2/1SERCA2a improves myocardial function in an experimental model of heart failure in large animals. Gene Therapy 15:1550-1557.

[47] Kawase Y., H. Ly, F Prunier, D. Lebeche, Y. Shi, H. Jin, L. Hadri, R. Yoneyyama, K. Hoshino, Y. Takewa, S. Sakata, R. Peluso, K. Zsebo, J. Swathmey, J-C. Tardif, J Tanguay, and R. Hajjar. (2008) Reversal of cardiac dysfunction after long-term expression of SERCA2a by gene transfer in a pre-clinical model of heart failure. J Am Coll. Cardiol. 51:1112-1119.

[48] Jaski B., M. Jessup, D. Mancini, R. Cappola, D. Pauly, B. Gfrenberg, K. Borow, H. Dittrich, K. Zsebo, and R. Hajjar. (2009) Calcium upregulation by percutaneous administration of gene therapy in cardiac disease (CUPID trial), a first-in-human phase ½ clinical trial. J Card Fail. 15:171-181.

[49] Gwathmey J., A. Yerevanian, and R. Hajjar. (2011) Cardiac gene therapy with SERCA2a: from bench to bedside. J Mol Cell Cardiol. In press.

[50] Freeman K., I. Lerman, E. Kranias, T. Bohlmeyer, M. Bristow, R. Lefkowitz, G. Iaccarino, W. Koch, and L. Leinwand. (2001) Alterations in cardiac adrenergic signaling and calcium cycling differentially affect the progression of cardiomyopathy. J Clin Invest 107:967-974.

[51] Song Q., A. Schmidt, H. Hahn, A. Carr, B. Frank, L. Pater, M. Gerst, K. Young, B. Hoit, B. McConnell, K. Haghighi, C. Seidman, J. Seidman, G. Dorn, and E. Kranias. (2003) Rescue of cardiomyocytes dysfunction by phospholamban ablation does not prevent ventricular failure in genetic hypertrophy. J. Clin Invest. 111:859-867.

[52] Penia J., D. Urboniene, P. Goldspink, E. Kranias, D.F. Wieczorek, and B. Wolska. (2005) Phospholamban knockout prevents the development of hypertrophy and cardiac dysfunction in a FHC α-tropomyosin (Glu180Gly) mouse model. Keystone Symposium: molecular biology of cardiac diseases and regeneration. p. 61.

[53] Coutu P., C. Bennett, E. Favre, S. Day, and J. Metzger. (2004) Parvalbumin corrects slowed relaxation in adult cardiac myocytes expressing hypertrophic cardiomyopathy-linked α-tropomyosin mutations. Circ Res. 94:1235-1241.

7

Gene Therapy in Cardiovascular Disease

José Luis Reyes-Juárez[1] and Angel Zarain-Herzberg[2]
[1]*Department of Cardiac Surgery, Hospital Universitario Vall d'Hebron, Barcelona,*
[2]*Universidad Nacional Autónoma de México, Facultad de Medicina, Dept. Bioquímica,*
[1]*Spain*
[2]*México*

1. Introduction

Gene therapy is defined as the transference of nucleic acids to somatic cells of an individual resulting in a therapeutic effect (Yla-Herttuala & Martin, 2000). Among the advantages of gene therapy over the existent modalities of treatment are: the selective treatment of affected tissues, the possibility of using locally endogenous proteins in cases where its systemic application would incur in serious adverse secondary effects, and the possibility of therapeutic effects in the long term after a single application (Yla-Herttuala & Alitalo, 2003).
Despite medical advances in the last 30 years, cardiovascular diseases (CVD) constitute the main cause of death on the developed world. Ischemic Heart Disease (IHD) is one of the main morbidities in an ageing population. Over 5 million Americans are believed to have symptomatic Heart Failure (HF), and every year ~0.5 million patients are diagnosed, with a prevalence of 0.5-2% of the general population; the estimated direct and indirect costs of HF in the United States is ~$30 billion. HF is a disabling chronic disease and the most frequent discharge diagnosis for hospitalization among older adults. Despite the significant resources for its treatment, outcomes remain poor. The five-year survival for individuals diagnosed with HF is less than 50%, and in end-stage HF one-year survival may be as low as 25% regardless of medical therapy, which constitutes one of the dimmest prognosis compared with of any malignant disease, with the exception of lung and pancreatic carcinomas (Levy et al., 2002; Lloyd-Jones et al., 2002).
HF constitutes the end stage of most CVD, it has become one of the most researched fields in the last 10 years, with significant advances to understand its key mechanisms; and today presents a great challenge to modern medicine, because of its persistent high mortality and increasing incidence. This can be attributed partially, to the absence of therapies that are focused on the key molecular basis of the disease, although the therapeutic approach has improved in last the two decades, existing treatments are not ideal due to its broad scope and do not have a significant impact on the overall mortality, since they are not sufficient to support to the myocardium performance and to increase the global cardiac function. It is for this reason that new therapeutic approaches are required, focused to correct the molecular defects of HF.
Among the molecular defects observed during HF, that have been explored as therapeutic targets, are the alterations in Ca^{2+} handling during the excitation-contraction coupling (Hoshijima et al., 2002; Iwanaga et al., 2004; Kaprielian et al., 2002; Michele et al., 2004; Miyamoto et al., 2000; Most et al., 2004b; Most et al., 2007; Pleger et al., 2007; Pleger et al.,

2005; Szatkowski et al., 2001), alterations in the β-adrenergic receptors and their interaction with G proteins (Jones et al., 2004a; Koch, 2004; Maurice et al., 1999; Munch et al., 2005; Tevaearai et al., 2002), alterations of cellular signaling, including the members of the protein kinase C (PKC) family (Hambleton, 2006), and to the production of second messengers by the enzyme adenylyl cyclase (Lai et al., 2004). The apoptosis of cardiac myocytes also has been mentioned (Chatterjee et al., 2002; Tenhunen et al., 2006). Finally, the use of over-expressing angiogenic factors, also has been analyzed as alternatives in patients with HF secondary to ischemic cardiomyopathy.

As a therapeutic strategy for CVD, gene therapy is a field that during the last decade has experienced a substantial increase in research. Some diseases like hypertrophic cardiomyopathy, have a clear-cut genetic basis, arrhythmogenic right ventricular dysplasia, and as such constitute a theoretically obvious target. Nevertheless, gene therapy can also be used to normalize the expression of genes that undergo down regulation in pathological ventricular hypertrophy, where the cardiac myocyte responds to a physiological tension, such a pressure or volume overload, by means of the activation of a fetal genetic program, with a subsequent downgrade of performance, thus starting a deleterious cycle, with further deterioration of cardiac function, as observed in HF. The hypertrophic response is associated with a decrease of gene expression of several key proteins, such α– and β–myosin heavy chains, the Ca^{2+}-ATPase pump of the sarcoplasmic reticulum (SERCA2a) and its regulatory protein phospholamban (PLB), and the S100A1 regulatory protein.

There are diverse strategies used for the treatment of HF, mainly constituted by pharmacological therapy that it is mainly focused on a neurohormonal blockade; further treatment can be offered with more invasive therapies such as cardiac re-synchronization; mechanical unloading with different surgical strategies and the use of left ventricular assist devices, which can induce myocardial remodeling at the molecular level normalizing gene expression. Currently the only definitive strategy for treatment of end stage HF is cardiac transplantation. However, despite of the advances in the treatment of HF with the addition of new drugs and very effective devices, the number of patients with HF is increasing (Hamad et al., 2007). Without a great scale effective strategy, regenerative medicine including stem cells and gene therapy could provide with a solution to an increasing number of patients currently without a therapeutic option.

While most of the research of gene therapy in CVD has been for HF; it is not limited to normalize the expression of down regulated genes, it also offers the possibility of modulating inflammatory and angiogenic mediators, which have a key role in several other CVD. Ischemic heart disease continues to be one of the main causes of mortality in the developed world, and while the treatment by medical, interventional and surgical options, has greatly decreased the morbidity and mortality associated, there is still a subset of patients that cannot be successfully treated with the current therapeutic options. Thus therapeutic angiogenesis in ischemic myocardium, mediated by gene therapy may also be an option in a clinical setting. As mentioned the treatment by interventional cardiology (PTCA) and surgery (CABG), are highly effective strategies, both with some long term drawbacks, specifically intra-stent restenosis in the former, and vein graft disease in the later. In both cases gene therapy may provide a key role to enhance, already very successful therapies. For example, transient, nonintegrative gene expression has been shown to be sufficient to promote neovascularization in the case of angiogenesis. This may also apply to antiproliferative strategies for the prevention of neointima formation in patients that received PTCA, for the prevention of intra-stent restenosis, or for inhibition of atherosclerosis in venous and arterial grafts. Because cardiovascular diseases are diverse and as such have unique traits, they require precise tailoring of gene therapy strategies for particular disease. Those features, which may vary include mode of delivery, type of vector, length of gene expression, and target tissue. The angiogenic factors that have been object of a more exhaustive study are the vascular endothelial growth factor (VEGF) and the fibroblast growth factor (FGF). These cytokines can be administered in the form of recombinant protein or of the genes that they codify for these proteins. Each of these approaches presents a series of advantages and disadvantages that are being investigated in detail, in animal models and in clinical tests with humans; and may also become options in the clinical setting in a not so distant future.

Another exciting new target for gene therapy are the electrical and rhythm disturbances in the heart. While a number of tachy-arrhythmias have a clear genetic origin in channel protein mutations, or calcium modulating proteins, these monogenetic arrhythmias, may only benefit a small number of patients, but current research has shown encouraging results in the treatment of bradi- and tachy-arrhythmias of multifactorial origin, and also in atrial fibrillation.

In the last decade a significant number of molecular mechanisms have been identified as the molecular basis of HF (Yla-Herttuala & Alitalo, 2003). Likewise the possibility of perform transference of genomic material *in vivo*, has been made possible exploring this technique as an option to correct the defects present in CVD, under the premise of being a therapy able to correct the underlying defects present in the failing heart.

Although the treatment by transference of genetic material still presents many challenges, small clinical tests have already been performed, applying angiogenic factors in ischemic cardiomyopathy (Hedman et al., 2003; Kastrup et al., 2005; Stewart et al., 2006). In relation to other molecular mechanisms of the HF, as it is mentioned below, several of them are in clinical phases in different stages of proximity to a wider clinical setting. The potential that has this new therapeutic option, combined to the novelty of its mechanism of action, makes imperative that its advantages and disadvantages are known to be able to take advantage of this emergent therapeutic option.

During the late 1990s and early 2000s, gene therapy for CVD, experienced a significant expansion, searching for targets that could benefit a large number of patients; while the results where promising on experimental models, these were not translated to the clinical setting. This added to the rising of stem-cell research, resulted in an abandonment of the field, however with the increasing data identifying the molecular basis of HF, it has become clearer that a "silver bullet" is not feasible and a more combinatorial approach may be required. Thus the field of gene therapy has experienced a rebirth in the last years. Evidently an ideal gene therapy depends on the underlying cause of HF, and as such a multistep approach may be required. For example, when utilizing gene therapy for the most common cause of HF which is IHD, it may be needed to target endothelial cells to manage the atherosclerotic plaques and induce angiogenesis, providing means to inhibit apoptosis of hibernating myocardium, and long term inotropic support, reducing cardiac remodeling and reducing risk of arrhythmias. This approach clearly illustrates that a "one size fits all" approach is impossible, and that manipulation at several levels is needed, in most cases gene therapy would be needed to over-express target molecules, modifying of intracellular signaling, loss of function by the use of dominant negative molecule or introducing siRNA, correction of mutations in the genome; and also combine with cellular therapy by introducing genetically modified cells (Vinge et al., 2008). In 2010, the number of gene therapy clinical trials for CVD in the world was 144, representing 8.5% of the total, occupying the second place after gene therapy for cancer diseases that represented 64.5% of all ongoing gene therapy trials.

Therefore, it becomes clearer that the possibility that by gene therapy, we could improve the cardiovascular function through a normalization and/or modulation of gene expression in the near future is one of the most promising and active clinical investigation goals in the 21st century. The purpose of this chapter, is to review the current status of the literature in the basic and clinical settings, and analyze future perspectives for cardiovascular gene therapy.

2. Vectors used for cardiovascular gene therapy

The initial tests to transfer genetic material into the heart were done using plasmid DNA, chosen by its easy production and security. Although the first studies showed positive results (Fortuin et al., 2003; Tsurumi et al., 1996), in randomized larger tests, where genes coding for vascular endothelial growth factor (VEGF) as well other angiogenic factors were transferred, they showed that due to its very low efficiency was not a useful technique (Kastrup et al., 2005). The use of cationic liposomes in the transference of genetic material in cells in culture, does not increase the efficiency of transference *in vivo* (Laitinen et al., 1997; Wright et al., 2001). One of the main problems with the use of plasmid DNA, is the lack of response with an increasing dosage (Rutanen et al., 2004). The use of this vector, is considered relatively safe, but it has demonstrated in animal models that it can produce fever, inflammation and infarcts in the skeletal muscle and in the myocardium (Hedman et al., 2003). DNA and RNA oligonucleotides potential to be used as decoys, were mentioned over 10 year ago, but their minimum effectiveness in tissues, also discards them for some clinical application (Alexander et al., 2005). Due to above factors the viral vectors can be a better option for cardiovascular gene therapy (Table 1).

Small interference RNA (siRNA) is a useful tool to down-regulate the expression of genes *in vitro*, but as an isolated technique has proven to be inefficient in the preclinical and clinical setting; thus it was discarded over 10 years ago, as a viable option. However in the recent years its combination with viral vectors has reignited the interest on this strategy; and it may become a key tool for inhibiting the expression of genes with deleterious effects (Poller et al., 2010; Suckau et al., 2009; Yang et al., 2010).

Among the viral vectors, the retrovirus were the initial choice, because of the limited immune response generated and the possibility of a sustained expression (years), nevertheless, the retrovirus have several disadvantages for its use on CVD, including low efficiency of infection, limited cardiac tropism because they infect mainly dividing cells; and also concerns in their safety have been mentioned due to the oncogenic potential (Laitinen et al., 1997). Because of this reasons it is a vector in which the interest has decreased. Recently, lentivirus have been used mainly to transfer genetic material to cells of the vascular wall, they have demonstrated a high efficiency of infection in smooth muscle and elicit a minimum immune response, nevertheless, the tropism for myocardium is limited and its production in great amounts is difficult, thus currently is not a viable option and requires engineering of this vector to improve its utility on a large scale, facilitating its production (Kankkonen et al., 2004). Sendaivirus and herpesvirus, have been mentioned as possible useful vectors, but sufficient data to this date does not exist on their utility (Masaki et al., 2001). Currently the adenovirus (Ad), and the adeno associated virus (AAV), are the most studied vectors in the cardiovascular gene therapy, since both have demonstrated a great effectiveness in cardiac muscle, the vascular wall and the liver (Wright et al., 2001).

Vector	Advantages	Disadvantages
Naked plasmid DNA	Easy to produce. Safe.	Temporary expression. Low transfer rate.
Adenovirus	High transfer rate. Easy to produce substantial quantities. Transfer to quiescent cells. Big size transgene (7-30 kb). Multiple cell type tropisms.	Immune response, dose dependent. Temporary expression.
Adeno associated virus (AAV-1, 2, 5, 6, 8, 9)	Long-term expression. Moderate immune response. Transfer to quiescent cells. High tropism for skeletal muscle (AAV-1, -6) and cardiac (AAV-8, -9). Do not produce diseases in humans.	Limited transgene size (5 kb). High yield production difficulties.
Retrovirus	Long-term expression. Minimal immune response.	Low transfer rate. Non-controlled integration to genome. Limited tropism. Transfer only on dividing cells.
Antisense oligonucleotides, siRNA	Easy to produce.	Limited *in vivo* efficiency. Requires high transfer rate.

Table 1. Vectors used in Cardiovascular Gene Therapy.

The first generation Ad, have a very high initial expression, reaching their maximum effect in the first days after the material transference, but the expression is diminished after approximately 2 weeks (Poliakova et al., 1999; Rissanen et al., 2003; Rutanen et al., 2004). Therefore they seem to be useful when a high expression is required for a limited amount of time, like in therapeutic angiogenesis for wounds. The repeated administration of Ad for gene therapy is not useful in great mammals, since it evokes an important immune response. Small doses of Ad produce a minimum inflammatory response in the myocardium. The second and third generation Ad, produce a smaller immune response and seem to have a prolonged expression, but its utility in gene therapy trials in humans is not yet known (Wen et al., 2004). The security of the Ad has demonstrated to be very high in clinical trials, being the fever the most important complication.
The AAV have a number of characteristics that makes them potentially useful for cardiac gene therapy, they have a natural tropism towards vascular smooth muscle, skeletal muscle and myocardium (Gruchala et al., 2004). They are able to express genes in quiescent cells like Ad, and for a long period of time, although the maximum expression is reached in days

(Su et al., 2004). Because they do not produce diseases in the human, the inflammatory response that they generate is minimum; the native AAV are able to integrate themselves to the human genome, but modified AAV vectors cannot, and maintain their long term expression by means of episomal associations with the genomic DNA, thus reducing the risk of mutagenic and oncogenic insertions, a threat that at least theoretically is present with other vectors of long term expression like the retrovirus (Schnepp et al., 2003). In murine and rodent models single stranded (ss) AAV6, self-complementary (sc) AAV6 and ssAAV9 are capable of long term expression after transference of genetic material to the cardiomyocytes, however it has not been reproduced in large animals. Recently it has been proposed that the highest levels of expression in large animals, are obtained using scAAV6 vectors, delivered through surgical methods (White et al., 2011).

3. Routes of administration

The transference of genetic material to the heart can be obtained by three different routes, by intravascular transference, *ex-vivo* transference, and by intra-organ injection, in the following sections we describe in more detail these routes.

3.1 Intravascular transference

For the intravascular transference, different systems using catheters have been developed to improve penetration of the vectors through the intima vascular layer. Nevertheless the transference in vascular athrosclerotic injuries with calcifications, deposits of cholesterol, infiltrated and continuous inflammation are a significant obstacle to achieve satisfactory transfer (Laitinen et al., 1998). The use of porous stents, in which the vectors with therapeutic genes can be eluted, has been proposed as an option to improve the transference, but currently has not been sufficiently explored (Sharif et al., 2006; Walter et al., 2004). The ideal route of administration for gene therapy is an intravenous vector, but the required amount of virus to obtain an optimal expression in great mammals, is probably very high to consider it safe for humans.

3.2 *Ex vivo* transference

The *ex vivo* administration is a combination of the cellular therapy and gene therapy, it consists of the administration of the test-tube vector, to isolated stem cells from the bone marrow, or cultures of skeletal myoblasts, with the intent of later transferring these cells transformed with the transgenes into the patient (Assmus et al., 2006; Dib et al., 2005; Haider et al., 2008; Haider et al., 2007; Nasseri et al., 2007; Sim et al., 2007; Smits, 2004; Yau et al., 2005; Ye et al., 2005). This form of administration has been studied mainly in the expression of angiogenic factors, and cytokines (Assmus et al., 2006; Haider & Ashraf, 2008; Ye et al., 2005). Among the advantages of this form of administration it is the possibility of using efficient methods for the transference of genetic material, like cationic lipids or electroporation, that are not possible to use in the whole subject, and which in addition the location of the modified cells in the heart, has a localized, continuous expression and with constant levels, without systemic effects (Haider & Ashraf, 2008; Sim et al., 2007; Smits, 2004). The cardiomyocytes are by nature resistant to the transference of genetic material, and this form of administration avoids this complication. The *ex vivo* administration, has the potential to become a very useful tool, but at present it depends on stem cell research and their differentiation to the cardiac phenotype, so that it can be explored widely and to know its potentials and limitations. One of the major drawbacks with this route of administration is the location of the transferred cells to the patient. The intramuscular injection of *ex vivo* transformed cells to express the gene of interest has been mentioned, but the little distribution of the transferred cells has made difficult its use (Lee et al., 2000; Springer et al., 1998).

3.3 Intra-organ transference

The administration by intra-myocardial injection, at present it is considered the most efficient form to obtain the desired expression in the cardiac tissue, but it as has been reported the administration of a high volume of vector to obtain an expression, can be associated with a local injury and alterations in the structure of the myocardium wall (Kastrup et al., 2005; Rutanen et al., 2004; Vale et al., 2001). Different studies have demonstrated that the intra-arterial route is of little effectiveness unless the permeability of the endothelial lining is increased, or a high pressure gradient is used; in these cases a problem to consider is the increased tissue distribution and ectopic expression of the transferred gene (Lee et al., 2000; Rissanen et al., 2003; Wright et al., 2001). In animal models the most used techniques include the use of percutaneous devices, one is known as the antegrade epicardial coronary artery infusion, where the left main coronary artery is catheterized, simultaneously with the coronary sinus, isolating the coronary circulation by means of an oxigenator and a extracorporeal pump, where the solution with the vector is added and circulated through the coronary circulation continuously for the desired time (Kaye et al., 2007). This system is known as "V-Focus", and has shown satisfactory results in larger animal models. Another system which employs percutaneous devices, is the percutaneous antegrade myocardial gene transfer, in this system the left anterior coronary artery (LAD) and the circumflex artery are catheterized, while the great cardiac vein or the anterior descending vein are catheterized, when the vector is infused through the arterial catheters, a balloon is inflated in the venous catheter, thus creating a high pressure gradient for up to three minutes (Hayase et al., 2005). The system in which the greater effectiveness of transference has been observed, consist of perfusion of the myocardium by surgical methods, a technique known as Molecular Cardiac Surgery with Recirculating Delivery (MCARD); this consists in the establishment of conventional cardiopulmonary bypass, with isolation of the heart circulation and retrograde perfusion through the coronary sinus. MCARD allows performing surgical procedures in the heart while the transference of genetic material is occurring (Hayase et al., 2005; Katz et al., 2010; Raake et al., 2004; White et al., 2011). An option to avoid the ectopic expression of the transferred gene is to put the expression of the transferred gene under the control of a specific cardiac promoter, as is the case of the human cardiac calsequestrin gene (hCasq2) (Reyes-Juarez et al., 2007). At the moment, in our laboratory we are developing adenoviral vectors that contain the promoter of the gene hCasq2 and direct the expression of the calcium pump SERCA2a in specific form for the cardiac myocytes (unpublished results).

4. Heart failure: therapeutic targets

As it was mentioned briefly in the introduction, one of the main advantages of gene therapy as a therapeutic option is the possibility of modifying key molecular defects that are present in the failing heart. In the last years the knowledge of the molecular basis of HF has advanced significantly, and today multiple alterations that exist in the continuum of the natural history of HF are known. Although there is not an integrative model that is able to ensemble the multiple alterations described in HF (Braunwald & Bristow, 2000), due to multiple etiologies, the existing data allows us to identify targets for gene therapy. In the following sections we describe the different approaches that are being explored to treat cardiovascular diseases.

4.1 Alterations in calcium handling

Without doubt the area of greater interest in the molecular mechanisms of HF, are the alterations on the regulation of the concentrations of Ca^{2+} during the process of the excitation-contraction coupling, which have been demonstrated to play a critical role in the decreased contractile properties of the myocardium. Among the involved alterations are changes in the levels of the expression of regulatory proteins that act as sensors of the intracellular Ca^{2+} concentrations (Kaprielian et al., 2002).

These alterations include decreased levels of the sarcoplasmic reticulum Ca^{2+}-ATPase (SERCA2a), with a subsequent decrease of the recapture of Ca^{2+} to the sarcoplasmic reticulum (SR) during diastole, resulting in a smaller amount of Ca^{2+} available to be released in the following contraction cycle. The decrease of the functional levels of phosphorylated phospholamban (PLB), a regulator of the activity of SERCA2a, causes the activity of SERCA2a to be decreased during HF; this decrease is not only due to a smaller expression of the SERCA2a protein, but to alterations in the level of phosphorylation of PLB as a result of an increase in the levels of the members of the family of the protein kinase C (PKC), which phosphorylates the inhibitor of phophatase-1 (PP1), activating it, which causes a dephosphorylation of PLB. The Ca^{2+} release channel of the SR (Ryanodine Receptor, RyR), has been reported in an unstable state, dissociated of the protein calstabin, which results in a higher probability of opening of the channel, and spontaneous liberations of Ca^{2+} appear during diastole (diastolic leak) which are associated with ventricular arrhythmias and more importantly with a decrease of the reserve of Ca^{2+} available for contraction (Bers et al., 2003; Braunwald & Bristow, 2000; Yla-Herttuala & Alitalo, 2003).

The existing reports have focused to the correction of these defects; the therapeutic targets include the increase of the expression of SERCA2a, or blockade the expression of their regulator PLB, the regulatory protein S100A1, and parvalbumin in order to make more efficient the cardiac relaxation. In the following pages each of these strategies is detailed.

4.1.1 The sarcoplasmic reticulum Ca^{2+}-ATPase and phospholamban

The calcium pump SERCA2a has a fundamental role in the normal myocardium function during muscular relaxation, recapturing the majority (75%) of the released Ca^{2+} from the SR for contraction, and reloading the SR maintaining an amount of Ca^{2+} that is sufficient to achieve an optimal contraction. Due to this role it is a central point of the molecular basis of HF; where its expression is regulated in a negative manner, diminishing the capacity to reload the SR with Ca^{2+} after each contraction, resulting in a deficient contraction due to lack of Ca^{2+} inside the SR (Kaprielian et al., 2002). In the last years the expression of SERCA2a, became one of the most explored pharmacological targets in basic research, and to a lesser extent in clinical investigation and, although without conclusive positive results obtained (Zarain-Herzberg & Rupp, 2002; Zarain-Herzberg et al., 1996). The use of gene therapy, to over-express SERCA2a, has the advantage of eliminating the associated effects of drugs used to increase the expression of SERCA2a (Gianni et al., 2005).

In similar way that the induction of SERCA2a expression has been extensively explored by pharmacological means, the over-expression by transference of genetic material, also has been analyzed *in vitro* and *in vivo*. Over-expression of SERCA2a improves the contractile function and the energy consumption in animal models with HF, improving the thickness of the anterior wall, and reducing ventricular arrhythmias. Other studies have also shown a decrease of inflammatory mediators and pro-apoptotic markers after transference of viral vectors overexpressing SERCA2a in pressure overload induced HF inhibition of ventricular remodeling in ischemic and volume overload induced HF; (Beeri et al., 2010; Mariani et al., 2011; Miyamoto et al., 2000; Molina et al., 2010).

Recent studies suggest that the failing heart is not refractory to treatment as was previously believed. For example, the observation that a small percentage of subjects with left ventricular assist devices (LVADs) can be permanently weaned from the device, strongly suggests that damaged hearts are capable of recovering lost function (Baba & Wohlschlaeger, 2008; Entwistle, 2003; Kuhn et al., 2004).

Recently, in the United States a phase 2 clinical trial named CUPID (Calcium Up-Regulation by Percutaneous Administration of Gene Therapy in Cardiac Disease) of intracoronary delivery of AAV1/SERCA2a (MYDICAR®) to 39 patients with HF that started in 2007 was completed (Hajjar et al., 2008; Jaski et al., 2009). It was designed to evaluate the safety profile and biological effects of SERCA2a gene transfer; after 12 months follow-up, the patients showed an acceptable safety profile, and improvement of the functional class. There was no increase in adverse effects, disease-related events, laboratory abnormalities or arrhythmias. Currently, there are two other ongoing gene therapy clinical trials to express SERCA2a in the hearts of patients with HF using AAV6/SERCA2a; one in England and one in France. Therefore, the transfer of SERCA2a cDNA into cardiomyocytes is a promising approach to treat HF by gene therapy (Table 2).

In transgenic mice overexpressing SERCA2a subjected to ascending aortic constriction, the down-regulation of SERCA2a protein in hypertrophic hearts was prevented, however, the hearts showed no increase in inotropic response compared to the wild type mice hypertrophic hearts, suggesting that energy supply may be a limiting factor for the benefit of SERCA2a overexpression in hypertrophied hearts (Pinz et al., 2011). Therefore, it should be considered novel strategies combining energetic support with increasing SERCA2 activity might improve the therapeutic effectiveness for HF.

Closely related to SERCA2a is phospholamban (PLB), a peptide of 52 amino acids, that has a role as a regulator of the function of SERCA2a, inhibiting the pump in its native state, and dissociating from the pump when is phosphorylated by the protein kinase A (PKA), increasing the velocity of transport of Ca^{2+} by the enzyme. During HF, the SERCA2a/PLB ratio is diminished to a great extent by the diminution of SERCA2a, which causes that the amount of SERCA2a that is dissociated of PLB diminishes and with this its activity and capacity to recapture the Ca^{2+}, released during the contraction (Hoshijima et al., 2006).

The most used strategy of gene therapy that involves PLB, consists of the transference of a peptide that codifies for a pseudo-phosphorylated mutant of PLB, which imitates the conformational changes induced by phosphorylation, and competes with the native form of PLB, increasing the activity of SERCA2a (Hoshijima et al., 2002). The tests realized in animal models have used AAV vectors, and followed the evolution up to 6 months after the transference of genes. In animals with HF subjected to gene therapy with the PLB mutant, an improvement of cardiac function is observed, delaying the advance of HF, and approaching near normal levels, corroborated by hemodynamic values, besides this strategy prevents the remodeling of the cardiac wall and it even reverts the changes observed in HF, decreasing fibrosis (Iwanaga et al., 2004). Like in the case of S100A1 mentioned below, the

expressed fetal phenotype observed during HF reverts to the adult phenotype of the normal heart, thus improving its metabolism.
In the last few years, the use of siRNA molecules to down-regulate the expression of PLB, and improving the SERCA2 function has been explored with promising results in rat models in the short and medium term. As mentioned previously isolated siRNA is of little use in a clinical setting, thus it needs to be transferred with a viral vector, AAV9 was used in the experimental models with good results. PLB siRNA improves myocardial function by means of increasing the activity of SERCA2a in a pressure overload model in rats (Suckau et al., 2009; Tsuji et al., 2008). A cautionary note must be made when the choice is made to target PLB in HF, it is well documented that the knockout or continuous blocking expression of PLB results in cardiomyopathy and HF, thus the use of PLB as a target in gene therapy must be strictly controlled so that once the desired effect of restoring the heart to a correct function, the inhibition of PLB function and/or expression can be modulated, to avoid secondary effects (MacLennan & Kranias, 2003; Shanmugam et al., 2011).
Another strategy that involves PLB, is the inhibition of PP1, the enzyme responsible of dephosphorylate it, keeping SERCA2a in an activated state (Nicolaou et al., 2009). Overexpressing the inhibitor-2 gene in a dilated cardiomyopathy hamster model, significantly reduced the activity of PP1, increasing the activity of SERCA2a with an improvement in the handling of intracellular Ca^{2+} concentrations, and consequently with an improvement of the cardiac function, as well as a diminution of the ventricular remodeling diminishing fibrosis significantly (Yamada et al., 2006). The above studies indicate that gene therapy directed towards PLB or its regulation, is an area that can in the future be of importance, but requires further research with more studies in HF models, to be able to reach a phase of clinical investigation.

4.1.2 The S100A1 protein

The S100A1 protein is a member of the S100 family, binding Ca^{2+} and has an "EF-hand" domain. The members of this family are involved in several functions, among them signal transduction, control of the cellular cycle, interactions with the cytoskeleton, cellular differentiation. It has an important role in the function of the striated muscle; it is abundantly expressed in muscle tissue, particularly in cardiac muscle, where it co-localizes with SR and contractile filaments. Its expression is affected negatively during HF secondary to cardiomyopathies (Most et al., 2001; Most et al., 2004a). It has been demonstrated that S100A1 has a positive inotropic and lusitropic effect in the heart. The inotropic effects are due to the interaction with SR and its components, particularly SERCA2a, increasing its activity, thus promoting the recapture of Ca^{2+} during the relaxation of the myocardium, increasing the amount of Ca^{2+} available to release during the next contraction cycle, which is directly related to the contraction force. It also interacts with RyR, stabilizing it and diminishing the diastolic leak of Ca^{2+} (Most et al., 2001; Most et al., 2004a). These data indicate that S100A1 is involved in two of the key molecular processes of HF, added to the fact that its expression falls in HF, turns it into an objective of great value to explore.
In vitro tests have demonstrated that the over-expression of S100A1, improves the contractile function of the cardiomyocytes by means of the mechanisms before mentioned (Most et al., 2004b; Pleger et al., 2005). In animal models of HF, the S100A1 over-expression has been proven to be enough to preserve the myocardial function after an acute infarction, and to prevent the appearance of HF (Most et al., 2004b; Most et al., 2007). Recent reports using AAV have followed these models for prolonged periods (20 weeks), where it has been

observed that the S100A1 over-expression improves the myocardium function in sustained form, and in an independent and synergic effect to the treatment with β-blocker agents (Pleger et al., 2007), restoring the sensitivity of the myocardium to β-adrenergic agonists, that usually is very decreased in HF. In these models, over-expression of S100A1 is able to revert the phenotype of HF expressed by the myocardium, returning after two months to the normal pattern of the adult cardiac muscle, in similar form to that observed in patients with HF awaiting cardiac transplant, with devices of left ventricular assist, who can be weaned from the device after a prolonged period with a significant improvement of cardiac function (Entwistle, 2003; Kuhn et al., 2004). The available data, indicate that S100A1 is an important therapeutic target, but further research is needed before it can be used in a clinical or pre-clinical setting (Rohde et al., 2010).

4.1.3 Parvalbumin

Diastolic dysfunction is a component associated to HF, found mainly in patients older than 65 years; currently specific treatments for this type of dysfunction do not exist. In cardiac myocytes obtained of these patients it is observed that the required time to remove Ca^{2+} from the cytoplasm is increased; this slows down the relaxation of the heart and jeopardizes the filling of the cardiac chambers for the following beat. Parvalbumin is a soluble intracellular protein of low molecular weight, with capacity to bind Ca^{2+}, which is expressed importantly in fast-twitch skeletal muscle, but it is not expressed natively in the heart. Its main function is to accelerate the rate of decrease of the intracellular Ca^{2+} in an ATP-independent manner. The gene therapy interventions that involve parvalbumin, to this time have been limited to *in vitro* studies and to animal models followed by short terms of time (one week), these tests have demonstrated that the expression of parvalbumin in the heart, is associated with an increase of the speed of relaxation. The data can be used as the basis to express parvalbumin in the heart, by means of AAV vectors, to evaluate its effects in the long term. Although the effects that are obtained expressing parvalbumin in the heart are very similar to the observed ones with over-expression of SERCA2a, the ones obtained with parvalbumin do not require of ATP, avoiding compromising even more the energetic needs of the heart. Due to this, parvalbumin constitutes a therapeutic target that must be further explored in the future (Michele et al., 2004; Szatkowski et al., 2001).

4.2 β-Adrenergic system

Alterations of the β-adrenergic receptors during HF have been described extensively, including a decreased density of receptors in the myocardium, to desensitization to β-agonists. The desensitization of the receptors explains to a great extent the refractory response to the treatments directed to the adrenergic routes. The β-adrenergic receptors are coupled to G proteins that are regulated by protein kinases of receptors coupled to G proteins, known in the case the adrenergic receptors (Beta Receptor Adrenergic Kinase) βARK1 and βARK2, the expression of the two enzymes is up-regulated during HF and it plays a key role on the desensitization of the β-receptors (Koch, 2004). Transgenic mice with over-expression of the β1-receptors develop cardiomyopathy, whereas in animals that over-express β2-receptors contractility is increased without developing any pathology.

In animal models it has been demonstrated that the overexpression of β2-receptors directed to the cardiac tissue, is associated with an increased contractility and a greater response to isoproterenol (Jones et al., 2004a; Maurice et al., 1999; Tevaearai et al., 2002). In mice that over-express βARK1 a contractility-diminished response to isoproterenol is observed. An inhibitor of βARK1 has been developed, the transference of adenoviral vectors with βARK1ct in rabbits with acute infarct has been demonstrated to prevent the alterations in the β-adrenergic system, and improve the myocardial function and prevent the development of HF in short term basis (Koch, 2004). This same strategy was tested with AAV vectors to assess the long term effects, it improved the contractility, reversed ventricular remodeling and normalized the neuroendocrine axis, and intracellular adrenergic signaling, interestingly this work shows that addition of adrenergic antagonists, was not additive to the gene transfer, but treatment with pharmacological inhibitors yielded similar but less effective results (Rengo et al., 2009). These data suggest that manipulation of βARK1 function has an impact on cardiac function, and that is susceptible to be manipulated by gene therapy.

Another strategy used to modify the components of the β-adrenergic system by gene therapy, includes over-expression of the protein that re-uptakes norepinephrine in the heart (NE uptake-1). This protein is down-regulated during HF, which leads to an increase of extracellular catecholamine levels, resulting in a hyper-adrenergic state that it has a central role in the desensitization of the receptors. In rabbits with HF with an over-expression of the NE-uptake-1, the concentration of norepinephrine was kept near normal levels, and was associated with an improvement in cardiac function, and the cardiac hypertrophy was reverted, recovering the normal phenotype of the heart (Munch et al., 2005).

4.3 Intracellular signaling

In the pathogenesis of HF, the hyper-adrenergic state and the alterations in the intracellular concentrations of Ca^{2+} contribute to alter the activation of different intracellular signaling pathways, which turns them into potential targets for gene therapy. To this date, the adenylyl cyclase (AC), and the protein kinase C (PKC) have been explored as potential targets. The adenylyl cyclase is a key role molecule in the cardiac myocyte, particularly the type 6 (AC6) in animal models with HF is demonstrated that over-expression of the AC6 improves the cardiac function and increase the life span. In pigs with established HF (Gao et al., 1999) besides improving the hemodynamic values, the cardiac function, and the response to isoproterenol, the over-expression of the AC6 prevents the remodeling of the cardiac wall and the appearance of fibrosis (Lai et al., 2004). It is thought that in the treatment of the HF response to AC6 is not only elicited due to an increase of the levels of cAMP, but it also modifies expression of other genes favoring the expression of useful genes for the myocardial contraction (Phan et al., 2007). There is an ongoing clinical trial, in which AAV5 encoding human AC6 is being delivered by intracoronary injection to patients with congestive HF (Table 2).

There is evidence that damaged and inflamed tissues produce signals to attract stem cells to the injured tissue, and many of these signals have been identified including stromal-derived factor (SDF)-1. There has been growing evidence that the receptor of SDF-1 (CXCR4) participates in regulating myocardial repair after ischemic injury. SDF-1 has been shown to increase after myocardial ischemia, and several studies have shown that enhancing SDF-1 levels around the infarct improves myocardial remodeling after infarction. Currently, a clinical trial is exploring the effects of percutaneous injection of SDF-1 naked DNA directly into the myocardium of patients with ischemic heart disease (Agarwal et al., 2010) (Table 2).

The other target for gene therapy that has been explored in the intracellular signaling setting is the family of the PKC, which is a component of several routes of transduction associated to the cellular membrane. The PKCα isoform is the most abundant in the heart where it plays a central role regulating the cardiac contractility. The lost of the contractile function in HF goes accompanied of an increase in the levels of PKCα in the heart. On this basis, studies have been performed in animal models transferring a dominant negative of PKCα by means of an adenoviral vector to determine their viability as therapeutic option. In rats with post-infarction HF, the transference of a PKCα dominant negative improves myocardial contractility and improves the hemodynamic values (Hambleton, 2006; Palaniyandi et al., 2009). While most of the research on the role and susceptibility of PKC as a therapeutic target has been done with conventional pharmacological therapy, the data show that at the very least is an option to be explored for gene therapy.

4.4 Apoptosis

It is well described that during the dilation of heart cavities observed in HF exists a remodeling of the myocardial wall, it has been proposed as one of the mechanisms responsible for this processes, the apoptosis of the cardiac myocytes. Although the precise mechanisms by which the apoptosis contributes to the remodeling of the myocardial wall are not understood, several studies have been realized using gene therapy to block apoptotic pathways with positive results. The Bcl-2 factor is able to block apoptosis, and it has been administered by means of an adenoviral vector after a period of myocardial ischemia in rabbits and it was found to avoid deterioration in the short and long term cardiac function, and also being able to prevent the dilation of the heart cavities and the remodeling of the same (Chatterjee et al., 2002). It was also demonstrated that prevents apoptosis in the border of the injured area; although has not determined if the expression of Bcl-2 is required at the initial moment of the injury or if it is required in the long term expression (Weisleder et al., 2004).

The protein p38 is a member of mitogen-activated protein kinases (MAPK) that is a fundamental regulator of growth, life span and cellular death. It has been reported that after myocardial infarction the activity of p38 falls, contributing to the development of apoptosis in the heart, increasing the downgrading of the function and the remodeling of the myocardial wall. When post-infarcted rats are treated with an adenoviral vector to over-express p38, it prevents the deterioration of the myocardial function, has an anti-apoptotic effect, and avoids the fibrosis and remodeling of the ventricular wall (Bassi et al., 2008; Tenhunen et al., 2006).

5. Therapy for heart failure of genetic causes

Multiple causes of HF have been identified due to genetic mutations; nevertheless, it is known that these constitute a minimum percentage of the cases of HF. These causes involve several pathological mechanisms, mainly proteins of the sarcomere and the cytoskeleton (Bos et al., 2007; Chang et al., 2008; Karkkainen & Peuhkurinen, 2007; Lind et al., 2006; Ramaraj, 2008; van Spaendonck-Zwarts et al., 2008; Wiersma et al., 2007). Theoretically these causes of HF offer an immediate target for its treatment, since they are monogenic and have a direct pathological mechanism, and are isolated from the complicated networks involved in the regulation of other elements already mentioned. In this line of research, it has been demonstrated that when an exogenous sarcomeric protein is over-expressed it assembles to

Trial	Target Gene	Diseases	Route/Vector	Stage	Num. patients
CUPID	SERCA2a (cardiac sarcoplasmic reticulum Ca^{2+} ATPase)	HF, ischemic and nonischemic	Intracoronary/AAV1-SERCA2a (MYDICAR®)	Phase 2, completed	39
SERCA2a Gene Therapy in LVAD patients	SERCA2a	Advanced HF with LVAD, ischemic and nonischemic	Intracoronary/AAV6	Phase 2, enrolling	16
AGENT-HF	SERCA2a	HF, ischemic and nonischemic	Intracoronary/AAV6	Phase 2, enrolling	30
AC6 Gene transfer for CHF	AC6 (Adenylyl Cyclase-6)	HF, ischemic and nonischemic	IntracoronaryAdenovirus	Phase 1/2, enrolling	72
Study to evaluate the safety of a single dose of ACRX-100 in adults with ischemic HF	SDF-1 (Stromal-Derived Factor-1)	HF, ischemic only	Intramyocardial/naked DNA	Phase 1, enrolling	16

Table 2. Gene Therapy Clinical Trials for Heart Failure.

form organized and stoichiometric complexes in the cytoplasm. The idea of this type of therapy is to displace the endogenous protein that has the defect, when changing the stoichiometry inside the cell. This type of therapy has not been explored experimentally, although it is susceptible to be done with animal models that reproduce hereditary cardiomyopathies.

Mutations of larger proteins like dystrophin have also been identified as responsible in the genesis of muscular dystrophy of Duchenne, where several mutations have been described and it has even been proved to be caused by mutations that truncate the protein (Rodino-Klapac et al., 2007). In these cases the possibility of being treated by gene therapy presents major technical difficulties, although it has been demonstrated that the transference of a mini-gene of dystrophin can improve the symptoms of the disease (Goyenvalle et al., 2004; Townsend et al., 2007).

A phase 1 clinical trial of rAAV2.5-CMV-Mini-Dystrophin Gene Vector in Duchenne Muscular Dystrophy is in progress. This study investigates the safety and efficacy of the mini-dystrophin gene transferred to the biceps muscle for Duchenne muscular dystrophy patients, ages 5 to 12 years of age, using a recombinant AAV. The mini-dystrophin gene or a placebo agent (normal saline or empty viral capsids) is injected directly into both biceps muscles while under conscious sedation. Following the gene transfer, patients are admitted to the hospital for 48 hours of observation followed by weekly outpatient visits. A bilateral muscle biopsy is performed following 6 weeks with long-term follow up will consisting of bi-annual visits for the next 2 years.

6. Ischemic heart disease

Atherosclerotic cardiovascular diseases continue to be the main cause of morbidity and mortality in the world. According to the American Heart Association the direct and indirect costs of coronary heart disease (CHD) for the year 2010 add up to 177.1 billion dollars. Pharmacologic therapies for CHD and HF have multiple systemic side effects and are predisposed to several adverse drug interactions since polypharmacy is frequently involved in the treatment of such patients. Importantly, pharmacologic therapies aim to reduce symptoms and halt progression of disease but do not necessarily reverse the pathophysiology associated with CHD and HF. While revascularization procedures have a significant role in treating CHD, there are problems with this therapies further explained later, and frequently patients remain symptomatic despite maximal anti-anginal therapies and may require repeat revascularization procedures. While the obvious target for gene therapy in CHD is angiogenesis, one must keep in mind that there is a wide spectrum of mechanisms in its natural history, such as those of myocardial reperfusion injury during and after myocardial infarction (MI) and cell survival and apoptosis after MI, and during ventricular remodeling (Lavu et al., 2010).

A significant part of the research in CHD has been focused on the administration of angiogenic growth factors, in the form of recombinant protein or by gene transfer, to promote the development of additional collateral blood vessels that would act like endogenous conduits of bypass around the occluded native arteries; a strategy known as therapeutic angiogenesis. This strategy has demonstrated to increase the tissue perfusion by means of neovascularization in a considerable number of preclinical tests of ischemia. In patients with critical ischemia of the lower extremities or with coronary terminal arterial disease, the clinical tests have demonstrated a symptomatic improvement and have contributed new objective evidence of improvement in perfusion, suggesting that this strategy can constitute an alternative method for treatment in patients in whom the therapies available at the moment have failed or they are not viable. The next targets of the research in the field of angiogenesis are going to be to determine the optimal dose, the formulation, the route of administration and the combination of growth factors; to determine the needs of endothelial progenitor cells or the supplementation with stem cells; to provide an effective and safe therapeutic angiogenesis, as well as to adapt the angiogenesis to the individual needs of the patients.

Among the strategies to induce angiogenesis various growth factors have been used including the vascular endothelial growth factor (VEGF), the angiopoietines, the fibroblastic growth factor (FGF), the hypoxia-inducible factor-1α (HIF-1α), the monocyte chemotactic protein-1 of (MCP-1), the hepatic growth factor (HGF), and the stimulating factor of colonies of granulocytes and macrophages (GM-CSF). The strategy consists of transferring the genes that codify for some of the above proteins to the target tissue, favoring the development of neovascularization in the ischemic myocardium. In preclinical animal models this approach has demonstrated to be effective promoting the growth and generation of new capillaries, although the relevance for the myocardial tissue has not been evaluated (Shen & Vatner,

1995; Wijns et al., 1998). It has been shown that with an expression for more than 4 weeks the newly formed vessels undergo a tissue remodeling that allows them to remain even though the stimulus is no longer present.

There is increasing evidence that VEGF is the master regulator of angiogenesis and thus is the prototype of angiogenic growth factors for gene therapy (Yla-Herttuala & Alitalo, 2003; Yla-Herttuala et al., 2007). In animal models with HF secondary to myocardial ischemia, administration of gene therapy for angiogenesis using VEGF has been associated with an improvement of the myocardial perfusion after 3 weeks of administration, and the myocardial function was also improved. The angiogenesis induced by gene therapy, is one of the more explored strategies at present, to treat CVD in humans, up to date with more than 15 different clinical trials of phase 1 already completed and many clinical trials of phase 2/3 are ongoing using adenoviral gene therapy in patients with coronary artery disease, with different goals, including therapeutic angiogenesis to improve the myocardial perfusion, the prevention of re-stenosis of stents, the prevention of the fault of venous grafts in revascularization, however, the results obtained are difficult to interpret, mainly due to the variation among the used vectors, the therapeutic routes of administration and the targets (Zachary & Morgan, 2011). Besides, one of the problems to consider is that the efficiency of the transference of genes is reciprocal to the size of the guest, partly by the limited diffusion of the vector in a greater amount of tissue. For this reason although several studies are promising in animal models, the results could be difficult to reproduce in humans.

Most of the cardiovascular gene therapy trials have been designed to study therapeutic blood vessel growth. The use of therapies using recombinant VEGF, FGF-2 and granulocyte macrophage colony-stimulating factor proteins has been researched in peripheral and myocardial ischemia, but there were no clear improvements in the clinical outcome of the patients (Henry et al., 2003; Lederman et al., 2002; Lederman et al., 2001). Several VEGF gene therapies using naked DNA have been tested by intramyocardial injection or percutaneously into the ischemic myocardium with the NOGA catheter or via thoracotomy alleviated angina and reduced the area of ischemic myocardium (Reilly et al., 2005; Vale et al., 2001).

Some gene therapy clinical trials using FGF have been reported. In the phase 1/2 AGENT-1 trial, intracoronary administration of AdFGF-4 improved exercise time at 4 weeks in stable angina pectoris patients (Grines et al., 2002). Similarly, in the phase 2 AGENT-2 trial, was observed a reduction of the myocardial ischemic area (Grines et al., 2003). Nevertheless, the results obtained from the gene therapy clinical trials performed to date verify that gene therapy is a strategy with viability to treat patients who are not susceptible to be treated with more conventional alternatives.

Another potential target for gene therapy in CHD is the injury generated by oxidative stress, mainly observed in myocardial infarction and ischemia-reperfusion injury. The central point is the generation of reactive oxygen species, which produce lipid and protein oxidation, and also interact with several calcium handling proteins, leading to an augmented entry of calcium into the cell and a secondary elevation of intracellular concentration, which leads to cellular injury (Cantor et al., 2003; Dhalla et al., 2000; Maddika et al., 2009). Among the targets to prevent oxidative stress, is the over expression of the extracellular superoxide dismutase (Ec SOD), which has a central antioxidant role, has been tested pre-emptively in animals later subjected to myocardial infarction and it was observed that mimicking myocardial ischemic preconditioning, it leads to decreased infarct size (Agrawal et al., 2004;

Li et al., 2001). The Thioredoxins (Trx) are proteins that have a potent antioxidant role and protect against oxidative stress by decreasing the superoxide anion generation and interacting with intracellular signalling pathways as p38MAPK (Tao et al., 2006). In mice models of CHD and myocardial infarction, the over-expression of the Trx-1 gene has an angiogenic effect, decreases apoptosis and reduces the ventricular remodelling (Adluri et al., 2011; Samuel et al., 2010), thus the use of Trx as a potential target is exciting and guarantees further research. Finally, it has been demonstrated that nitric oxide has a protective role in myocardial infarction minimizing oxidative stress, in mice the transfer of adenoviral delivered nitric oxide synthase previous to the generation of an infarction, results in reduced infarct size, improved contractility and ventricular function. It also decreases the inflammation in the infracted area and decreases phosphorylation of the MAPK overall improving the outcome of the treated mice (Chen et al., 2010; Jones et al., 2004b).

As mentioned previously, cell survival and apoptosis plays a key role in the chronic evolution of CHD, after a myocardial infarction or chronic ischemia, some surviving cells will start apoptosis and lead to ventricular remodeling and deterioration of the function, we have previously mentioned the role and potential target of the MAPK pathway and Bcl-2. The use of heat shock proteins, specifically HSP72 over-expression, in rats subjected to ischemia-reperfusion injury, resulted in decreased levels of apoptosis, increased activity of intracellular antioxidant systems, increased levels of Bcl-2, thus showing a cardioprotective effect (Suzuki et al., 2002). Also the use of the troponin I type 3 interacting kinase (TNNI3K) a member of the MAP kinase family with angiogenic and myogenic roles, has been explored combined with cellular therapy, over expressing it on pluripotent progenitor cells, which are then transferred into infarcted mice hearts, the results show a decrease infarction injury, decreased remodeling, induction of myogenesis and inhibition of p38-JNK mediated apoptosis (Lai et al., 2008).

7. Arrhythmias

Cardiac arrhythmias constitute a significant cause of morbidity, and sudden cardiac death primary o secondary to other cardiac diseases constitutes the main cause of death in CVD. While most are susceptible to pharmacological treatment, these therapies have a global effect in the heart, meaning that while it has the desired effect on the affected region of the heart, it also modifies the behavior of other regions and may even have a pro-arrhythmic effect. It must also be mentioned that a number of cardiac arrhythmias are caused by genetic causes, and as previously mentioned these constitute the most obvious targets for gene therapy, but only a small number of arrhythmias have a monogenic origin.

While the vectors used in arrhythmia treatment follow the same principles as in other CVD, delivery constitutes a significant problem. Direct myocardial injection is limited due to the size, location and thickness of the atria. Intracoronary perfusion is suboptimal since the atria vasculature is not as well defined as that of the ventricles. At this time the most effective method of gene delivery in an experimental setting is known as epicardial gene panting, where a solution containing the vector, a polymerization compound and a diluted protease are applied over the surface of both atria, obtaining full wall thickness transfer (Kikuchi et al., 2005).

Atrial fibrillation (AF) is the most common arrhythmia encountered. In the United States only, AF affects 2-5 million people and it has an increasing incidence. AF may be of primary origin, or secondary to structural disease; while in the former case it is due to electrical imbalances, in the latter is mainly to atrial remodeling with fibrosis of the atria and remodeling (Benjamin et al., 1998). Thus it is mainly the primary AF which has been explored as a potential target for gene therapy. Therapeutic strategies in AF are to controlling cardiac rate or restoring sinus rhythm. Primary AF is an abbreviation of action potential duration and, therefore, refractory period. This provides the substrate for abbreviated reentrant wavelengths, which serve to stabilize the chaotic atrial electrical activity.

One approach that has been explored for restoring sinus rhythm is the use of a dominant negative mutant potassium channel KCNH2-G628S that blocks the ion channel pore region. The transfer of an adenoviral vector by epicardial painting in a pig model of AF, a significant prolongation of the monophasic action potential was observed, with a reversal of AF observed (Amit et al., 2010). These results constitute a significant pathway to be explored. A second approach researched mimics the rate control; a mutated constitutively active inhibitory G protein in a viral vector is transferred to pigs with induced AF, and a 20% decrease on the maximal ventricular rate is observed (Bauer et al., 2004; Donahue et al., 2000).

The ventricular arrhythmias (VT) constitute a significant cause of death in several CVD, they have been mainly attributed to the beat-to-beat variation of the action potential. The proposed mechanisms underlying these variations are alterations of ionic currents or of the calcium cycling, with a slop clearing of calcium during the relaxation. In hearts where a viral vector expressing SERCA2 is transferred, the susceptibility of mice hearts to ventricular arrhythmias after rapid pacing is decreased (Cutler et al., 2009). One of the most relevant groups in the VT spectrum are those secondary to myocardial ischemia and infarction. One of the probable mechanisms of this type of VT is the slow conduction due to altered gap junction expression and reduced velocity of the action potential. One of the proposed mechanisms for velocity is a more positive resting membrane potential in scar border myocytes, secondary to an inactivation of some of the sodium current carried by the Nav1.5 (SCN5A) channel. To correct these alterations, the transfer of a skeletal muscle sodium channel has been tested in a canine post-MI model, observing a significant reduction of induced VT (Lau et al., 2009). MicroRNAs have also been explored as targets for the treatment of VT, in post-MI hearts miR-1 is up-regulated, with a subsequent inhibition of the expression of ion channels, when antagomirs are transferred, a decrease of the arrhythmic potential is observed (Yang et al., 2007).

An increasing trend observed in an ageing population is the increasing incidence of bradi-arrhythmias. An abnormal generation of the electrical impulse in the atria (sinus node dysfunction) or its propagation to the ventricles (atrioventricular [AV] block) may result in the development of abnormally slow heart rate, and in most of the cases the only satisfactory option is the implantation of a definitive pacemaker. Pacemaker implantation lacks sufficient physiological feedback parameters to grant greater freedom to the recipient. Other disadvantages are the mechanical nature of the treatment and associated risks. The experimental approaches for bradi-arrhythmias are focused on altering the function of existing cardiomyocytes.

The basis of the treatment of bradi-arrhythmias, has been focused on reducing the diastolic repolarization currents by inhibiting diastolic currents, the approach described suppresses the diastolic entrance of potassium by transferring a mutant inactive channel of Kir2.1, afterwards a new ventricular activity is observed (Miake et al., 2002). Another alternative researched is the combination on gene and cell therapy, where mesenchymal stem cells were

electroporated with plasmid DNA of HCN2, and latter injected into the anterior wall of dogs who had previously been subjected to ablation of the AV node; after 10 days spontaneous ventricular activity was observed (Plotnikov et al., 2007).
Thus as we have briefly exposed, gene therapy for arrhythmias is an exciting field which has shown encouraging and promising results, but it is also true that is probably one of the fields in CVD, that is most distanced form a translational setting. With he current pace of research it is certainly a field to keep a close watch on the next years.

8. Vein graft disease

Myocardial revascularization either by coronary artery bypass graft surgery (CABG) or percutaneous transluminal coronary angioplasty (PTCA) has became the standard of care for ischemic heart disease; both techniques are highly successful and have significantly improved its prognosis. However both have significant long-term issues with their durability, in the case of CABG, it is due to the patency of graft used, while arterial grafts have an excellent long term patency, saphenous vein graft (SVG) are still widely used due to technical considerations. SVG are a useful and valid tool in CABG but their long term patency is impaired by what is known as vein graft disease (VGD), where a proliferation of smooth cells and endothelial cells lead to intimal hyperplasia, which gradually decreases the patent lumen of the graft. Conventional treatments can help to prevent VGD, but still constitutes a significant problem in surgically revascularized patients with coronary artery disease (Parang & Arora, 2009).
Thus VGD is another entity which may be susceptible to be treated by gene therapy, one of the main advantages when using gene therapy in this disease is the possibility of delivering the therapy ex vivo, after the graft has been harvested. The pathogenesis of it, results from the graft's adaptation to high pressure and the loss of inhibition of the endothelial layer, there is a proliferation and migration to the intima of smooth muscle cells. These cells release cytokines and degrade the surrounding matrix, creating an inflammatory environment, highly atherogenic. In the hyperplasia of the intima the E2F transcription factors have been identified as key in initiating it. A decoy oligonucleotide for E2F has been designed and tested successfully in animal models, a phase 3 clinical trial was designed to test its efficacy in preventing vein graft failure, denominated as the PREVENT IV trial. The results did not show a significant decrease in the rate of vein graft failure in the treated group; while this specific approach was not successful it has proven that gene therapy is a possible approach to VGD (Alexander et al., 2005).
Another potential target which has only been tested experimentally, is the transfer of the fibromodullin gene. As previously mentioned the remodelling of the extracellular matrix plays a key role in the genesis on intimal hyperplasia, here widely known proteins have been identified, one of them is TGF-β1, fibromodullin and decorin are leucine rich-proteoglycans, which possess TGF-β1 antagonist activity *in vitro* and *in vivo*. Adenoviral transfer of the fibromodullin gene to harvested human saphenous veins, revealed significantly reduced neointimal thickness (Ranjzad et al., 2009). This proves that while clinical trials have been unsuccessful in the past, there are still a number of target that can be researched in the future and may result in an effective gene therapy option for VGD.

8.1 Intra-stent restenosis

As mentioned PTCA is widely used in the treatment of coronary artery disease, briefly an atherosclerotic obstruction of the coronary vessel is identified and dilated with a high

pressure balloon, afterwards a metal stent is deployed to prevent new obstructions. As in CABG its main drawback it's the long-term patency of treated lesions, a similar phenomena is observed where a neointimal proliferation results in the restenosis of the stent. Currently the most used option to prevent this restenosis is the use of drug eluting stents, which are covered in different drugs that inhibit the neointimal proliferation. However there is still a high number of stents that will develop restenosis. This particular field presents another option for the delivery of gene therapy, by deploying gene-delivering stents.
Intrastent restenosis has been researched in animal models, one of the strategies involves the inhibition of cellular proliferation using the CREB binding protein, which is known as a regulator of cell proliferation and apoptosis in vascular endothelial and smooth muscle cells. Rats were subjected to endothelial injury and denudation of the carotid artery, afterwards the injured artery was treated with lentivirus expressing siRNA for CREB binding protein; after 4 weeks it significantly decreased the neointimal formation. Thus providing a new target to be researched in the future (Yang et al., 2010). Another researched strategy is the use of stents delivering the gene of the endothelial nitric oxide synthase (eNOS); it is well describe that NO is a critical molecule in the vessel wall as it is responsible for a variety functions including inhibition of platelet adhesion and aggregation, inhibition of leukocyte chemotaxis, inhibition of smooth muscle cell growth and migration, vasodilatation, and re-endothelialization, thus making it a very attractive target to prevent neointimal hyperplasia. In a rabbit model of intrastent restenosis gene-eluting stents which delivered eNOS had significantly less neointimal formation, also it is important to mention, that in this study the gene was delivered by a lipid based transfection instead of a viral vector.

9. Conclusions

Despite of the therapeutic advances CVD continue to be the main cause of morbidity and mortality in the world; gene therapy appears to be a promissory alternative, having the capacity to correct the observed fundamental defects in several CVD. Currently gene therapy is an area of basic and clinical research of great significance that should produce positive results for HF in the next few years. An increase in the knowledge of the underlying molecular mechanisms of HF, along with advances in gene therapy technology has led to important efforts in *in vitro* studies and pre-clinical testing of a number of gene targets and recently in the successful completion of the first phase 2 gene therapy trial for HF. Moreover, the safety of AAV vectors has been demonstrated for the treatment of HF combined with the efficacy of the use of SERCA2a in the treatment of HF, thus opening the field for testing new targets to modulate with more advanced vector systems for gene therapy. As we have briefly exposed, myocardial ischemia along with HF constitutes one of the most researched fields in the CVD spectrum, and probably is the area where gene therapy has advanced further, and it even has several pre-clinical and clinical studies, and while the results are still non conclusive and even in some cases discouraging, it only shows the many difficulties and the need for further research, before gene therapy can be established as an everyday available clinical tool. It must also be said that there is a need to diversify the efforts in research, since in the case of IHD most of it has focused on angiogenesis, while the other pathways as ischemia reperfusion injury and apoptosis have been only scratched in the basic setting, thus more research is needed in areas which can offer new and exciting promising targets for gene therapy. One of the majors obstacles that presents the basic research and clinical application of this and other therapeutic options, is the complexity of the underlying mechanisms, and as such it is required that these along with the indications are known and understood so that we can be able to explode to the maximum the new capacities that this therapeutic option offers, reason why is necessary to closely follow the advances in this field in the near future.

10. Acknowledgment

This work was supported by DGAPA-PAPIIT grant IN204410 and CONACYT 78750.

11. References

Adluri, R.S., Thirunavukkarasu, M., Zhan, L., Akita, Y., Samuel, S.M., Otani, H., Ho, Y.S., Maulik, G. & Maulik, N. (2011). Thioredoxin 1 enhances neovascularization and reduces ventricular remodeling during chronic myocardial infarction: a study using thioredoxin 1 transgenic mice. *J Mol Cell Cardiol*, Vol. 50, No. 1, (November 2010), pp. 239-247, ISSN 1095-8584

Agarwal, U., Ghalayini, W., Dong, F., Weber, K., Zou, Y.R., Rabbany, S.Y., Rafii, S. & Penn, M.S. (2010). Role of cardiac myocyte CXCR4 expression in development and left ventricular remodeling after acute myocardial infarction. *Circ Res*, Vol. 107, No. 5, (July 2010), pp. 667-676, ISSN 1524-4571

Agrawal, R.S., Muangman, S., Layne, M.D., Melo, L., Perrella, M.A., Lee, R.T., Zhang, L., Lopez-Ilasaca, M. & Dzau, V.J. (2004). Pre-emptive gene therapy using recombinant adeno-associated virus delivery of extracellular superoxide dismutase protects heart against ischemic reperfusion injury, improves ventricular function and prolongs survival. *Gene Ther*, Vol. 11, No. 12, (March 2004), pp. 962-969, ISSN 0969-7128

Alexander, J.H., Hafley, G., Harrington, R.A., Peterson, E.D., Ferguson, T.B., Jr., Lorenz, T.J., Goyal, A., Gibson, M., Mack, M.J., Gennevois, D., *et al.* (2005). Efficacy and safety of edifoligide, an E2F transcription factor decoy, for prevention of vein graft failure following coronary artery bypass graft surgery: PREVENT IV: a randomized controlled trial. *Jama*, Vol. 294, No. 19, pp. 2446-2454

Amit, G., Kikuchi, K., Greener, I.D., Yang, L., Novack, V. & Donahue, J.K. (2010). Selective molecular potassium channel blockade prevents atrial fibrillation. *Circulation*, Vol. 121, No. 21, (May 2010), pp. 2263-2270, ISSN 1524-4539

Assmus, B., Honold, J., Schachinger, V., Britten, M.B., Fischer-Rasokat, U., Lehmann, R., Teupe, C., Pistorius, K., Martin, H., Abolmaali, N.D., *et al.* (2006). Transcoronary transplantation of progenitor cells after myocardial infarction. *N Engl J Med*, Vol. 355, No. 12, (September 2006), pp. 1222-1232, ISSN 1533-4406

Baba, H.A. & Wohlschlaeger, J. (2008). Morphological and molecular changes of the myocardium after left ventricular mechanical support. *Curr Cardiol Rev*, Vol. 4, No. 3, (August 2008), pp. 157-169, ISSN 1875-6557

Bassi, R., Heads, R., Marber, M.S. & Clark, J.E. (2008). Targeting p38-MAPK in the ischaemic heart: kill or cure? *Curr Opin Pharmacol*, Vol. 8, No. 2, pp. 141-146

Bauer, A., McDonald, A.D., Nasir, K., Peller, L., Rade, J.J., Miller, J.M., Heldman, A.W. & Donahue, J.K. (2004). Inhibitory G protein overexpression provides physiologically relevant heart rate control in persistent atrial fibrillation. *Circulation*, Vol. 110, No. 19, (October 2004), pp. 3115-3120, ISSN 1524-4539

Beeri, R., Chaput, M., Guerrero, J.L., Kawase, Y., Yosefy, C., Abedat, S., Karakikes, I., Morel, C., Tisosky, A., Sullivan, S., *et al.* (2010). Gene Delivery of Sarcoplasmic Reticulum Calcium ATPase Inhibits Ventricular Remodeling in Ischemic Mitral Regurgitation. *Circulation: Heart Failure*, Vol. 3, No. 5, pp. 627-634

Benjamin, E.J., Wolf, P.A., D'Agostino, R.B., Silbershatz, H., Kannel, W.B. & Levy, D. (1998). Impact of atrial fibrillation on the risk of death: the Framingham Heart Study. *Circulation*, Vol. 98, No. 10, (September 1998), pp. 946-952, ISSN 0009-7322

Bers, D.M., Eisner, D.A. & Valdivia, H.H. (2003). Sarcoplasmic reticulum Ca2+ and heart failure: roles of diastolic leak and Ca2+ transport. *Circ Res*, Vol. 93, No. 6, (September 2003), pp. 487-490, ISSN 1524-4571

Bos, J.M., Ommen, S.R. & Ackerman, M.J. (2007). Genetics of hypertrophic cardiomyopathy: one, two, or more diseases? *Curr Opin Cardiol*, Vol. 22, No. 3, (April 2007), pp. 193-199, ISSN 0268-4705

Braunwald, E. & Bristow, M.R. (2000). Congestive heart failure: fifty years of progress. *Circulation*, Vol. 102, No. 20 Suppl 4, (November 2000), pp. IV14-23, ISSN 1524-4539

Cantor, E.J., Mancini, E.V., Seth, R., Yao, X.H. & Netticadan, T. (2003). Oxidative stress and heart disease: cardiac dysfunction, nutrition, and gene therapy. *Curr Hypertens Rep*, Vol. 5, No. 3, (May 2003), pp. 215-220, ISSN 1522-6417

Chang, A.N., Parvatiyar, M.S. & Potter, J.D. (2008). Troponin and cardiomyopathy. *Biochem Biophys Res Commun*, Vol. 369, No. 1, (December 2007), pp. 74-81, ISSN 1090-2104

Chatterjee, S., Stewart, A.S., Bish, L.T., Jayasankar, V., Kim, E.M., Pirolli, T., Burdick, J., Woo, Y.J., Gardner, T.J. & Sweeney, H.L. (2002). Viral gene transfer of the antiapoptotic factor Bcl-2 protects against chronic postischemic heart failure. *Circulation*, Vol. 106, No. 12 Suppl 1, pp. I212-217

Chen, L.L., Zhu, T.B., Yin, H., Huang, J., Wang, L.S., Cao, K.J. & Yang, Z.J. (2010). Inhibition of MAPK signaling by eNOS gene transfer improves ventricular remodeling after myocardial infarction through reduction of inflammation. *Mol Biol Rep*, Vol. 37, No. 7, (November 2009), pp. 3067-3072, ISSN 1573-4978

Cutler, M.J., Wan, X., Laurita, K.R., Hajjar, R.J. & Rosenbaum, D.S. (2009). Targeted SERCA2a gene expression identifies molecular mechanism and therapeutic target for arrhythmogenic cardiac alternans. *Circ Arrhythm Electrophysiol*, Vol. 2, No. 6, (December 2009), pp. 686-694, ISSN 1941-3084

Dhalla, N.S., Temsah, R.M. & Netticadan, T. (2000). Role of oxidative stress in cardiovascular diseases. *J Hypertens*, Vol. 18, No. 6, (JUne 2000), pp. 655-673, ISSN 0263-6352

Dib, N., Michler, R.E., Pagani, F.D., Wright, S., Kereiakes, D.J., Lengerich, R., Binkley, P., Buchele, D., Anand, I., Swingen, C., *et al.* (2005). Safety and feasibility of autologous myoblast transplantation in patients with ischemic cardiomyopathy: four-year follow-up. *Circulation*, Vol. 112, No. 12, (September 2005), pp. 1748-1755, ISSN 1524-4539

Donahue, J.K., Heldman, A.W., Fraser, H., McDonald, A.D., Miller, J.M., Rade, J.J., Eschenhagen, T. & Marban, E. (2000). Focal modification of electrical conduction in the heart by viral gene transfer. *Nat Med*, Vol. 6, No. 12, (December 2000), pp. 1395-1398, ISSN 1078-8956

Entwistle, J.W., 3rd (2003). Long-term mechanical ventricular assistance toward myocardial recovery. *Cardiol Clin*, Vol. 21, No. 1, pp. 75-82, ISSN 0733-8651

Fortuin, F.D., Vale, P., Losordo, D.W., Symes, J., DeLaria, G.A., Tyner, J.J., Schaer, G.L., March, R., Snell, R.J., Henry, T.D., *et al.* (2003). One-year follow-up of direct myocardial gene transfer of vascular endothelial growth factor-2 using naked plasmid deoxyribonucleic acid by way of thoracotomy in no-option patients. *Am J Cardiol*, Vol. 92, No. 4, pp. 436-439

Gao, M.H., Lai, N.C., Roth, D.M., Zhou, J., Zhu, J., Anzai, T., Dalton, N. & Hammond, H.K. (1999). Adenylylcyclase increases responsiveness to catecholamine stimulation in transgenic mice. *Circulation*, Vol. 99, No. 12, (March 1999), pp. 1618-1622, ISSN 0009-7322

Gianni, D., Chan, J., Gwathmey, J., del Monte, F. & Hajjar, R. (2005). SERCA2a in heart failure: role and therapeutic prospects. *J Bioenerg Biomembr*, Vol. 37, No. 6, pp. 375-380

Goyenvalle, A., Vulin, A., Fougerousse, F., Leturcq, F., Kaplan, J.C., Garcia, L. & Danos, O. (2004). Rescue of dystrophic muscle through U7 snRNA-mediated exon skipping. *Science*, Vol. 306, No. 5702, (November 2004), pp. ISSN 1796-1799

Grines, C.L., Watkins, M.W., Helmer, G., Penny, W., Brinker, J., Marmur, J.D., West, A., Rade, J.J., Marrott, P., Hammond, H.K., *et al.* (2002). Angiogenic Gene Therapy (AGENT) trial in patients with stable angina pectoris. *Circulation*, Vol. 105, No. 11, (March 2002), pp. 1291-1297, ISSN 1524-4539

Grines, C.L., Watkins, M.W., Mahmarian, J.J., Iskandrian, A.E., Rade, J.J., Marrott, P., Pratt, C. & Kleiman, N. (2003). A randomized, double-blind, placebo-controlled trial of Ad5FGF-4 gene therapy and its effect on myocardial perfusion in patients with stable angina. *J Am Coll Cardiol*, Vol. 42, No. 8, pp. 1339-1347

Gruchala, M., Bhardwaj, S., Pajusola, K., Roy, H., Rissanen, T.T., Kokina, I., Kholova, I., Markkanen, J.E., Rutanen, J., Heikura, T., *et al.* (2004). Gene transfer into rabbit arteries with adeno-associated virus and adenovirus vectors. *J Gene Med*, Vol. 6, No. 5, pp. 545-554

Haider, H. & Ashraf, M. (2008). Strategies to promote donor cell survival: combining preconditioning approach with stem cell transplantation. *J Mol Cell Cardiol*, Vol. 45, No. 4, (June 2008), pp. 554-566, ISSN 1095-8584

Haider, H.K., Elmadbouh, I., Jean-Baptiste, M. & Ashraf, M. (2008). Nonviral vector gene modification of stem cells for myocardial repair. *Mol Med*, Vol. 14, No. 1-2, (November 2007), pp. 79-86, ISSN 1076-1551

Haider, H.K., Ye, L. & Ashraf, M. (2007). Skeletal muscle derived stem cells for myocardial repair. *Recent Pat Cardiovasc Drug Discov*, Vol. 2, No. 3, (January 2008), pp. 205-213, ISSN 1574-8901

Hajjar, R.J., Zsebo, K., Deckelbaum, L., Thompson, C., Rudy, J., Yaroshinsky, A., Ly, H., Kawase, Y., Wagner, K., Borow, K., *et al.* (2008). Design of a phase 1/2 trial of intracoronary administration of AAV1/SERCA2a in patients with heart failure. *J Card Fail*, Vol. 14, No. 5, (June 2008), pp. 355-367, ISSN 1532-8414

Hamad, E., Mather, P.J., Srinivasan, S., Rubin, S., Whellan, D.J. & Feldman, A.M. (2007). Pharmacologic therapy of chronic heart failure. *Am J Cardiovasc Drugs*, Vol. 7, No. 4, (August 2007), pp. 235-248, ISSN 1175-3277

Hambleton, M. (2006). Pharmacological- and Gene Therapy-Based Inhibition of Protein Kinase C / Enhances Cardiac Contractility and Attenuates Heart Failure. *Circulation*, Vol. 114, No. 6, pp. 574-582

Hayase, M., Del Monte, F., Kawase, Y., Macneill, B.D., McGregor, J., Yoneyama, R., Hoshino, K., Tsuji, T., De Grand, A.M., Gwathmey, J.K., *et al.* (2005). Catheter-based antegrade intracoronary viral gene delivery with coronary venous blockade. *Am J Physiol Heart Circ Physiol*, Vol. 288, No. 6, (May 2005), pp. H2995-3000, ISSN 0363-6135

Hedman, M., Hartikainen, J., Syvanne, M., Stjernvall, J., Hedman, A., Kivela, A., Vanninen, E., Mussalo, H., Kauppila, E., Simula, S., *et al.* (2003). Safety and feasibility of catheter-based local intracoronary vascular endothelial growth factor gene transfer in the prevention of postangioplasty and in-stent restenosis and in the treatment of chronic myocardial ischemia: phase II results of the Kuopio Angiogenesis Trial (KAT). *Circulation*, Vol. 107, No. 21, pp. 2677-2683

Henry, T.D., Annex, B.H., McKendall, G.R., Azrin, M.A., Lopez, J.J., Giordano, F.J., Shah, P.K., Willerson, J.T., Benza, R.L., Berman, D.S., *et al.* (2003). The VIVA trial: Vascular endothelial growth factor in Ischemia for Vascular Angiogenesis. *Circulation*, Vol. 107, No. 10, (March 2003), pp. 1359-1365, ISSN 1524-4539

Hoshijima, M., Ikeda, Y., Iwanaga, Y., Minamisawa, S., Date, M.O., Gu, Y., Iwatate, M., Li, M., Wang, L., Wilson, J.M., *et al.*(2002).Chronic suppression of heart-failure progression by a pseudophosphorylated mutant of phospholamban via in vivo cardiac rAAV gene delivery. *Nat Med*, Vol. 8, No. 8, pp. 864-871

Hoshijima, M., Knoll, R., Pashmforoush, M. & Chien, K. (2006). Reversal of calcium cycling defects in advanced heart failure toward molecular therapy. *J Am Coll Cardiol*, Vol. 48, No. 9 Suppl 1, pp. A15-23

Iwanaga, Y., Hoshijima, M., Gu, Y., Iwatate, M., Dieterle, T., Ikeda, Y., Date, M.O., Chrast, J., Matsuzaki, M., Peterson, K.L., *et al.* (2004). Chronic phospholamban inhibition prevents progressive cardiac dysfunction and pathological remodeling after infarction in rats. *J Clin Invest*, Vol. 113, No. 5, pp. 727-736

Jaski, B.E., Jessup, M.L., Mancini, D.M., Cappola, T.P., Pauly, D.F., Greenberg, B., Borow, K., Dittrich, H., Zsebo, K.M., Hajjar, R.J., *et al.* (2009). Calcium upregulation by percutaneous administration of gene therapy in cardiac disease (CUPID Trial), a first-in-human phase 1/2 clinical trial. *J Card Fail*, Vol. 15, No. 3, (March 2009), pp. 171-181, ISSN 1532-8414

Jones, J., Wilson, K., Steenbergen, C., Koch, W. & Milano, C. (2004). Dose dependent effects of cardiac beta2 adrenoceptor gene therapy. *J Surg Res*, Vol. 122, No. 1, pp. 113-120

Kankkonen, H.M., Vahakangas, E., Marr, R.A., Pakkanen, T., Laurema, A., Leppanen, P., Jalkanen, J., Verma, I.M. & Yla-Herttuala, S. (2004). Long-term lowering of plasma cholesterol levels in LDL-receptor-deficient WHHL rabbits by gene therapy. *Mol Ther*, Vol. 9, No. 4, pp. 548-556

Kaprielian, R., del Monte, F. & Hajjar, R.J. (2002). Targeting Ca2+ cycling proteins and the action potential in heart failure by gene transfer. *Basic Res Cardiol*, Vol. 97 Suppl 1, No., pp. I136-145

Karkkainen, S. & Peuhkurinen, K. (2007). Genetics of dilated cardiomyopathy. *Ann Med*, Vol. 39, No. 2, (April 2007), pp. 91-107, ISSN 0785-3890

Kastrup, J., Jorgensen, E., Ruck, A., Tagil, K., Glogar, D., Ruzyllo, W., Botker, H.E., Dudek, D., Drvota, V., Hesse, B., *et al.* (2005). Direct intramyocardial plasmid vascular endothelial growth factor-A165 gene therapy in patients with stable severe angina pectoris A randomized double-blind placebo-controlled study: the Euroinject One trial. *J Am Coll Cardiol*, Vol. 45, No. 7, pp. 982-988

Katz, M.G., Swain, J.D., Fargnoli, A.S. & Bridges, C.R. (2010). Gene therapy during cardiac surgery: role of surgical technique to minimize collateral organ gene expression. *Interact Cardiovasc Thorac Surg*, Vol. 11, No. 6, pp. 727-731

Kaye, D.M., Preovolos, A., Marshall, T., Byrne, M., Hoshijima, M., Hajjar, R., Mariani, J.A., Pepe, S., Chien, K.R. & Power, J.M. (2007). Percutaneous cardiac recirculation-mediated gene transfer of an inhibitory phospholamban peptide reverses advanced heart failure in large animals. *J Am Coll Cardiol*, Vol. 50, No. 3, (July 2007), pp. 253-260, ISSN 1558-3597

Kikuchi, K., McDonald, A.D., Sasano, T. & Donahue, J.K. (2005). Targeted modification of atrial electrophysiology by homogeneous transmural atrial gene transfer. *Circulation*, Vol. 111, No. 3, (January 2005), pp. 264-270, ISSN 1524-4539

Koch, W.J. (2004). Genetic and phenotypic targeting of beta-adrenergic signaling in heart failure. *Mol Cell Biochem*, Vol. 263, No. 1-2, pp. 5-9

Kuhn, M., Voss, M., Mitko, D., Stypmann, J., Schmid, C., Kawaguchi, N., Grabellus, F. & Baba, H.A. (2004). Left ventricular assist device support reverses altered cardiac expression and function of natriuretic peptides and receptors in end-stage heart failure. *Cardiovasc Res*, Vol. 64, No. 2, pp. 308-314, ISSN 0008-6363

Lai, N.C., Roth, D.M., Gao, M.H., Tang, T., Dalton, N., Lai, Y.Y., Spellman, M., Clopton, P. & Hammond, H.K. (2004). Intracoronary adenovirus encoding adenylyl cyclase VI increases left ventricular function in heart failure. *Circulation*, Vol. 110, No. 3, pp. 330-336

Lai, Z.F., Chen, Y.Z., Feng, L.P., Meng, X.M., Ding, J.F., Wang, L.Y., Ye, J., Li, P., Cheng, X.S., Kitamoto, Y., *et al.* (2008). Overexpression of TNNI3K, a cardiac-specific MAP kinase, promotes P19CL6-derived cardiac myogenesis and prevents myocardial infarction-induced injury. *Am J Physiol Heart Circ Physiol*, Vol. 295, No. 2, (June 2008), pp. H708-716, ISSN 0363-6135

Laitinen, M., Makinen, K., Manninen, H., Matsi, P., Kossila, M., Agrawal, R.S., Pakkanen, T., Luoma, J.S., Viita, H., Hartikainen, J., *et al.* (1998). Adenovirus-mediated gene transfer to lower limb artery of patients with chronic critical leg ischemia. *Hum Gene Ther*, Vol. 9, No. 10, pp. 1481-1486, ISSN 1043-0342

Laitinen, M., Pakkanen, T., Donetti, E., Baetta, R., Luoma, J., Lehtolainen, P., Viita, H., Agrawal, R., Miyanohara, A., Friedmann, T., *et al.* (1997). Gene transfer into the carotid artery using an adventitial collar: comparison of the effectiveness of the plasmid-liposome complexes, retroviruses, pseudotyped retroviruses, and adenoviruses. *Hum Gene Ther*, Vol. 8, No. 14, pp. 1645-1650

Lau, D.H., Clausen, C., Sosunov, E.A., Shlapakova, I.N., Anyukhovsky, E.P., Danilo, P., Jr., Rosen, T.S., Kelly, C., Duffy, H.S., Szabolcs, M.J., *et al.* (2009). Epicardial border zone overexpression of skeletal muscle sodium channel SkM1 normalizes activation, preserves conduction, and suppresses ventricular arrhythmia: an in silico, in vivo, in vitro study. *Circulation*, Vol. 119, No. 1, (December 2008), pp. 19-27, ISSN 1524-4539

Lavu, M., Gundewar, S. & Lefer, D.J. (2010). Gene therapy for ischemic heart disease. *Journal of Molecular and Cellular Cardiology*, Vol., No., pp. 1-9

Lederman, R.J., Mendelsohn, F.O., Anderson, R.D., Saucedo, J.F., Tenaglia, A.N., Hermiller, J.B., Hillegass, W.B., Rocha-Singh, K., Moon, T.E., Whitehouse, M.J., *et al.* (2002). Therapeutic angiogenesis with recombinant fibroblast growth factor-2 for intermittent claudication (the TRAFFIC study): a randomised trial. *Lancet*, Vol. 359, No. 9323, (June 2002), pp. 2053-2058, ISSN 0140-6736

Lederman, R.J., Tenaglia, A.N., Anderson, R.D., Hermiller, J.B., Rocha-Singh, K., Mendelsohn, F.O., Hiatt, W.R., Moon, T., Whitehouse, M.J. & Annex, B.H. (2001). Design of the therapeutic angiogenesis with recombinant fibroblast growth factor-2 for intermittent claudication (TRAFFIC) trial. *Am J Cardiol*, Vol. 88, No. 2, (July 2001), pp. 192-195, A196-197, ISSN 0002-9149

Lee, R.J., Springer, M.L., Blanco-Bose, W.E., Shaw, R., Ursell, P.C. & Blau, H.M. (2000). VEGF gene delivery to myocardium: deleterious effects of unregulated expression. *Circulation*, Vol. 102, No. 8, pp. 898-901

Levy, D., Kenchaiah, S., Larson, M.G., Benjamin, E.J., Kupka, M.J., Ho, K.K., Murabito, J.M. & Vasan, R.S. (2002). Long-term trends in the incidence of and survival with heart failure. *N Engl J Med*, Vol. 347, No. 18, (November 2002), pp. 1397-1402, ISSN 1533-4406

Li, Q., Bolli, R., Qiu, Y., Tang, X.L., Guo, Y. & French, B.A. (2001). Gene therapy with extracellular superoxide dismutase protects conscious rabbits against myocardial infarction. *Circulation*, Vol. 103, No. 14, (April 2001), pp. 1893-1898, ISSN 1524-4539

Lind, J.M., Chiu, C. & Semsarian, C. (2006). Genetic basis of hypertrophic cardiomyopathy. *Expert Rev Cardiovasc Ther*, Vol. 4, No. 6, (December 2006), pp. 927-934, ISSN 1744-8344

Lloyd-Jones, D.M., Larson, M.G., Leip, E.P., Beiser, A., D'Agostino, R.B., Kannel, W.B., Murabito, J.M., Vasan, R.S., Benjamin, E.J. & Levy, D. (2002). Lifetime risk for developing congestive heart failure: the Framingham Heart Study. *Circulation*, Vol. 106, No. 24, (December 2002), pp. 3068-3072, ISSN 1524-4539

MacLennan, D.H. & Kranias, E.G. (2003). Phospholamban: a crucial regulator of cardiac contractility. *Nat Rev Mol Cell Biol*, Vol. 4, No. 7, (July 2003), pp. 566-577, ISSN 1471-0072

Maddika, S., Elimban, V., Chapman, D. & Dhalla, N.S. (2009). Role of oxidative stress in ischemia-reperfusion-induced alterations in myofibrillar ATPase activities and gene expression in the heart. *Can J Physiol Pharmacol*, Vol. 87, No. 2, (February 2009), pp. 120-129, ISSN 0008-4212

Mariani, J.A., Smolic, A., Preovolos, A., Byrne, M.J., Power, J.M. & Kaye, D.M. (2011). Augmentation of left ventricular mechanics by recirculation-mediated AAV2/1-SERCA2a gene delivery in experimental heart failure. *European Journal of Heart Failure*, Vol. 13, No. 3, pp. 247-253

Masaki, I., Yonemitsu, Y., Komori, K., Ueno, H., Nakashima, Y., Nakagawa, K., Fukumura, M., Kato, A., Hasan, M.K., Nagai, Y., *et al.* (2001). Recombinant Sendai virus-mediated gene transfer to vasculature: a new class of efficient gene transfer vector to the vascular system. *Faseb J*, Vol. 15, No. 7, pp. 1294-1296

Maurice, J.P., Hata, J.A., Shah, A.S., White, D.C., McDonald, P.H., Dolber, P.C., Wilson, K.H., Lefkowitz, R.J., Glower, D.D. & Koch, W.J. (1999). Enhancement of cardiac function after adenoviral-mediated in vivo intracoronary beta2-adrenergic receptor gene delivery. *J Clin Invest*, Vol. 104, No. 1, pp. 21-29

Miake, J., Marban, E. & Nuss, H.B. (2002). Biological pacemaker created by gene transfer. *Nature*, Vol. 419, No. 6903, (September 2002), pp. 132-133, ISSN 0028-0836

Michele, D.E., Szatkowski, M.L., Albayya, F.P. & Metzger, J.M. (2004). Parvalbumin gene delivery improves diastolic function in the aged myocardium in vivo. *Mol Ther*, Vol. 10, No. 2, pp. 399-403

Miyamoto, M.I., del Monte, F., Schmidt, U., DiSalvo, T.S., Kang, Z.B., Matsui, T., Guerrero, J.L., Gwathmey, J.K., Rosenzweig, A. & Hajjar, R.J. (2000). Adenoviral gene transfer of SERCA2a improves left-ventricular function in aortic-banded rats in transition to heart failure. *Proc Natl Acad Sci U S A*, Vol. 97, No. 2, pp. 793-798

Molina, E.J., Gupta, D., Palma, J., Gaughan, J.P. & Macha, M. (2010). Right ventricular beneficial effects of intracoronary SERCA2a gene transfer in an experimental model of heart failure. *Folia Biol (Praha)*, Vol. 56, No. 1, pp. 1-8

Most, P., Bernotat, J., Ehlermann, P., Pleger, S.T., Reppel, M., Borries, M., Niroomand, F., Pieske, B., Janssen, P.M., Eschenhagen, T., *et al.* (2001). S100A1: a regulator of myocardial contractility. *Proc Natl Acad Sci U S A*, Vol. 98, No. 24, pp. 13889-13894

Most, P., Eicher, C., Volkers, M., Pleger, S. & Katus, H. (2004a). Hope for a broken heart? *Trends Biotechnol*, Vol. 22, No. 10, pp. 487-489

Most, P., Pleger, S., Volkers, M., Heidt, B., Boerries, M., Weichenhan, D., Loffler, E., Janssen, P., Eckhart, A., Martini, J., *et al.* (2004b). Cardiac adenoviral S100A1 gene delivery rescues failing myocardium. *J Clin Invest*, Vol. 114, No. 11, pp. 1550-1563

Most, P., Remppis, A., Pleger, S., Katus, H. & Koch, W. (2007). S100A1: a novel inotropic regulator of cardiac performance. Transition from molecular physiology to pathophysiological relevance. *Am J Physiol Regul Integr Comp Physiol*, Vol. 293, No. 2, pp. R568-577

Munch, G., Rosport, K., Bultmann, A., Baumgartner, C., Li, Z., Laacke, L. & Ungerer, M. (2005). Cardiac overexpression of the norepinephrine transporter uptake-1 results in marked improvement of heart failure. *Circ Res*, Vol. 97, No. 9, pp. 928-936

Nasseri, B.A., Kukucka, M., Dandel, M., Knosalla, C., Potapov, E., Lehmkuhl, H.B., Meyer, R., Ebell, W., Stamm, C. & Hetzer, R. (2007). Intramyocardial delivery of bone marrow mononuclear cells and mechanical assist device implantation in patients with end-stage cardiomyopathy. *Cell Transplant*, Vol. 16, No. 9, (February 2008), pp. 941-949, ISSN 0963-6897

Nicolaou, P., Hajjar, R.J. & Kranias, E.G. (2009). Role of protein phosphatase-1 inhibitor-1 in cardiac physiology and pathophysiology. *J Mol Cell Cardiol*, Vol. 47, No. 3, (June 2009), pp. 365-371, ISSN 1095-8584

Palaniyandi, S.S., Sun, L., Ferreira, J.C. & Mochly-Rosen, D. (2009). Protein kinase C in heart failure: a therapeutic target? *Cardiovasc Res*, Vol. 82, No. 2, (January 2009), pp. 229-239, ISSN 1755-3245

Parang, P. & Arora, R. (2009). Coronary vein graft disease: pathogenesis and prevention. *Can J Cardiol*, Vol. 25, No. 2, (February 2009), pp. e57-62, ISSN 1916-7075

Phan, H.M., Gao, M.H., Lai, N.C., Tang, T. & Hammond, H.K. (2007). New signaling pathways associated with increased cardiac adenylyl cyclase 6 expression:

implications for possible congestive heart failure therapy. *Trends Cardiovasc Med*, Vol. 17, No. 7, (October 2007), pp. 215-221, ISSN 1050-1738

Pinz, I., Tian, R., Belke, D., Swanson, E., Dillmann, W. & Ingwall, J.S. (2011). Compromised myocardial energetics in hypertrophied mouse hearts diminish the beneficial effect of overexpressing SERCA2A. *J Biol Chem*, Vol., No., (February 2011), ISSN 1083-351X

Pleger, S., Most, P., Boucher, M., Soltys, S., Chuprun, J., Pleger, W., Gao, E., Dasgupta, A., Rengo, G., Remppis, A., *et al.* (2007). Stable myocardial-specific AAV6-S100A1 gene therapy results in chronic functional heart failure rescue. *Circulation*, Vol. 115, No. 19, pp. 2506-2515

Pleger, S., Remppis, A., Heidt, B., Volkers, M., Chuprun, J., Kuhn, M., Zhou, R., Gao, E., Szabo, G., Weichenhan, D., *et al.* (2005). S100A1 gene therapy preserves in vivo cardiac function after myocardial infarction. *Mol Ther*, Vol. 12, No. 6, pp. 1120-1129

Plotnikov, A.N., Shlapakova, I., Szabolcs, M.J., Danilo, P., Jr., Lorell, B.H., Potapova, I.A., Lu, Z., Rosen, A.B., Mathias, R.T., Brink, P.R., *et al.* (2007). Xenografted adult human mesenchymal stem cells provide a platform for sustained biological pacemaker function in canine heart. *Circulation*, Vol. 116, No. 7, (July 2007), pp. 706-713, ISSN 1524-4539

Poliakova, L., Kovesdi, I., Wang, X., Capogrossi, M.C. & Talan, M. (1999). Vascular permeability effect of adenovirus mediated vascular endothelial growth factor gene transfer to the rabbit and rat skeletal muscle. *J Thorac Cardiovasc Surg*, Vol. 118, No. 2, pp. 339-347

Poller, W., Hajjar, R., Schultheiss, H.P. & Fechner, H. (2010). Cardiac-targeted delivery of regulatory RNA molecules and genes for the treatment of heart failure. *Cardiovascular Research*, Vol. 86, No. 3, pp. 353-364

Raake, P., von Degenfeld, G., Hinkel, R., Vachenauer, R., Sandner, T., Beller, S., Andrees, M., Kupatt, C., Schuler, G. & Boekstegers, P. (2004). Myocardial gene transfer by selective pressure-regulated retroinfusion of coronary veins: comparison with surgical and percutaneous intramyocardial gene delivery. *J Am Coll Cardiol*, Vol. 44, No. 5, (September 2004), pp. 1124-1129, ISSN 1558-3597

Ramaraj, R. (2008). Hypertrophic cardiomyopathy: etiology, diagnosis, and treatment. *Cardiol Rev*, Vol. 16, No. 4, (June 2008), pp. 172-180, ISSN 1538-4683

Ranjzad, P., Salem, H.K. & Kingston, P.A. (2009). Adenovirus-mediated gene transfer of fibromodulin inhibits neointimal hyperplasia in an organ culture model of human saphenous vein graft disease. *Gene Ther*, Vol. 16, No. 9, (May 2009), pp. 1154-1162, ISSN 1476-5462

Reilly, J.P., Grise, M.A., Fortuin, F.D., Vale, P.R., Schaer, G.L., Lopez, J., JR, V.A.N.C., Henry, T., Richenbacher, W.E., Losordo, D.W., *et al.* (2005). Long-term (2-year) clinical events following transthoracic intramyocardial gene transfer of VEGF-2 in no-option patients. *J Interv Cardiol*, Vol. 18, No. 1, (March 2005), pp. 27-31, ISSN 0896-4327

Rengo, G., Lymperopoulos, A., Zincarelli, C., Donniacuo, M., Soltys, S., Rabinowitz, J.E. & Koch, W.J. (2009). Myocardial Adeno-Associated Virus Serotype 6- ARKct Gene Therapy Improves Cardiac Function and Normalizes the Neurohormonal Axis in Chronic Heart Failure. *Circulation*, Vol. 119, No. 1, pp. 89-98

Reyes-Juarez, J.L., Juarez-Rubi, R., Rodriguez, G. & Zarain-Herzberg, A. (2007). Transcriptional analysis of the human cardiac calsequestrin gene in cardiac and skeletal myocytes. *J Biol Chem*, Vol., No. 282, No. 49, (December, 2007) pp. 35554-35563, ISSN 0021-9258

Rissanen, T.T., Markkanen, J.E., Gruchala, M., Heikura, T., Puranen, A., Kettunen, M.I., Kholova, I., Kauppinen, R.A., Achen, M.G., Stacker, S.A., *et al.* (2003). VEGF-D is the strongest angiogenic and lymphangiogenic effector among VEGFs delivered into skeletal muscle via adenoviruses. *Circ Res*, Vol. 92, No. 10, pp. 1098-1106

Rodino-Klapac, L.R., Chicoine, L.G., Kaspar, B.K. & Mendell, J.R. (2007). Gene therapy for duchenne muscular dystrophy: expectations and challenges. *Arch Neurol*, Vol. 64, No. 9, (September 2007), pp. 1236-1241, ISSN 0003-9942

Rohde, D., Brinks, H., Ritterhoff, J., Qui, G., Ren, S. & Most, P. (2010). S100A1 gene therapy for heart failure: A novel strategy on the verge of clinical trials. *Journal of Molecular and Cellular Cardiology*, Vol., No., pp. 1-8

Rutanen, J., Rissanen, T.T., Markkanen, J.E., Gruchala, M., Silvennoinen, P., Kivela, A., Hedman, A., Hedman, M., Heikura, T., Orden, M.R., *et al.* (2004). Adenoviral catheter-mediated intramyocardial gene transfer using the mature form of vascular endothelial growth factor-D induces transmural angiogenesis in porcine heart. *Circulation*, Vol. 109, No. 8, pp. 1029-1035

Samuel, S.M., Thirunavukkarasu, M., Penumathsa, S.V., Koneru, S., Zhan, L., Maulik, G., Sudhakaran, P.R. & Maulik, N. (2010). Thioredoxin-1 gene therapy enhances angiogenic signaling and reduces ventricular remodeling in infarcted myocardium of diabetic rats. *Circulation*, Vol. 121, No. 10, (March 2010), pp. 1244-1255, ISSN 1524-4539

Schnepp, B.C., Clark, K.R., Klemanski, D.L., Pacak, C.A. & Johnson, P.R. (2003). Genetic fate of recombinant adeno-associated virus vector genomes in muscle. *J Virol*, Vol. 77, No. 6, pp. 3495-3504

Shanmugam, M., Gao, S., Hong, C., Fefelova, N., Nowycky, M.C., Xie, L.H., Periasamy, M. & Babu, G.J. (2011). Ablation of phospholamban and sarcolipin results in cardiac hypertrophy and decreased cardiac contractility. *Cardiovasc Res*, Vol. 89, No. 2, (September 2010), pp. 353-361, ISSN 1755-3245

Sharif, F., Hynes, S.O., McMahon, J., Cooney, R., Conroy, S., Dockery, P., Duffy, G., Daly, K., Crowley, J., Bartlett, J.S., *et al.* (2006). Gene-eluting stents: comparison of adenoviral and adeno- associated viral gene delivery to the blood vessel wall in vivo. *Hum Gene Ther*, Vol. 17, No. 7, pp. 741-750, ISSN 1043-0342

Shen, Y.T. & Vatner, S.F. (1995). Mechanism of impaired myocardial function during progressive coronary stenosis in conscious pigs. Hibernation versus stunning? *Circ Res*, Vol. 76, No. 3, (March 1995), pp. 479-488,
ISSN 0009-7330

Sim, E.K., Ye, L. & Haider, H. (2007). New strategy for cardiac repair: genetically modified skeletal myoblasts. *Asian Cardiovasc Thorac Ann*, Vol. 15, No. 3, (June 2007), pp. 183-184, ISSN 1816-5370

Smits, P.C. (2004). Myocardial repair with autologous skeletal myoblasts: a review of the clinical studies and problems. *Minerva Cardioangiol*, Vol. 52, No. 6, (February 2005), pp. 525-535, ISSN 0026-4725

Springer, M.L., Chen, A.S., Kraft, P.E., Bednarski, M. & Blau, H.M. (1998). VEGF gene delivery to muscle: potential role for vasculogenesis in adults. *Mol Cell*, Vol. 2, No. 5, pp. 549-558

Stewart, D.J., Hilton, J.D., Arnold, J.M., Gregoire, J., Rivard, A., Archer, S.L., Charbonneau, F., Cohen, E., Curtis, M., Buller, C.E., *et al.* (2006). Angiogenic gene therapy in patients with nonrevascularizable ischemic heart disease: a phase 2 randomized, controlled trial of AdVEGF(121) (AdVEGF121) versus maximum medical treatment. *Gene Ther*, Vol. 13, No. 21, pp. 1503-1511

Su, H., Joho, S., Huang, Y., Barcena, A., Arakawa-Hoyt, J., Grossman, W. & Kan, Y. (2004). Adeno-associated viral vector delivers cardiac-specific and hypoxia-inducible VEGF expression in ischemic mouse hearts. *Proc Natl Acad Sci U S A*, Vol. 101, No. 46, pp. 16280-16285

Suckau, L., Fechner, H., Chemaly, E., Krohn, S., Hadri, L., Kockskamper, J., Westermann, D., Bisping, E., Ly, H., Wang, X., *et al.* (2009). Long-Term Cardiac-Targeted RNA Interference for the Treatment of Heart Failure Restores Cardiac Function and Reduces Pathological Hypertrophy. *Circulation*, Vol. 119, No. 9, pp. 1241-1252

Suzuki, K., Murtuza, B., Sammut, I.A., Latif, N., Jayakumar, J., Smolenski, R.T., Kaneda, Y., Sawa, Y., Matsuda, H. & Yacoub, M.H. (2002). Heat shock protein 72 enhances manganese superoxide dismutase activity during myocardial ischemia-reperfusion injury, associated with mitochondrial protection and apoptosis reduction. *Circulation*, Vol. 106, No. 12 Suppl 1, (October 2002), pp. I270-276, ISSN 1524-4539

Szatkowski, M.L., Westfall, M.V., Gomez, C.A., Wahr, P.A., Michele, D.E., DelloRusso, C., Turner, II, Hong, K.E., Albayya, F.P. & Metzger, J.M. (2001). In vivo acceleration of heart relaxation performance by parvalbumin gene delivery. *J Clin Invest*, Vol. 107, No. 2, pp. 191-198

Tao, L., Gao, E., Hu, A., Coletti, C., Wang, Y., Christopher, T.A., Lopez, B.L., Koch, W. & Ma, X.L. (2006). Thioredoxin reduces post-ischemic myocardial apoptosis by reducing oxidative/nitrative stress. *Br J Pharmacol*, Vol. 149, No. 3, (August 2006), pp. 311-318, ISSN 0007-1188

Tenhunen, O., Soini, Y., Ilves, M., Rysa, J., Tuukkanen, J., Serpi, R., Pennanen, H., Ruskoaho, H. & Leskinen, H. (2006). p38 Kinase rescues failing myocardium after myocardial infarction: evidence for angiogenic and anti-apoptotic mechanisms. *Faseb J*, Vol. 20, No. 11, pp. 1907-1909

Tevaearai, H.T., Eckhart, A.D., Walton, G.B., Keys, J.R., Wilson, K. & Koch, W.J. (2002). Myocardial gene transfer and overexpression of beta2-adrenergic receptors potentiates the functional recovery of unloaded failing hearts. *Circulation*, Vol. 106, No. 1, pp. 124-129

Townsend, D., Blankinship, M.J., Allen, J.M., Gregorevic, P., Chamberlain, J.S. & Metzger, J.M. (2007). Systemic administration of micro-dystrophin restores cardiac geometry and prevents dobutamine-induced cardiac pump failure. *Mol Ther*, Vol. 15, No. 6, (April 2007), pp. 1086-1092, ISSN 1525-0016

Tsuji, T., Del Monte, F., Yoshikawa, Y., Abe, T., Shimizu, J., Nakajima-Takenaka, C., Taniguchi, S., Hajjar, R.J. & Takaki, M. (2008). Rescue of Ca2+ overload-induced left ventriclur dysfunction by targeted ablation of phospholamban. *AJP: Heart and Circulatory Physiology*, Vol. 296, No. 2, pp. H310-H317

Tsurumi, Y., Takeshita, S., Chen, D., Kearney, M., Rossow, S.T., Passeri, J., Horowitz, J.R., Symes, J.F. & Isner, J.M. (1996). Direct intramuscular gene transfer of naked DNA encoding vascular endothelial growth factor augments collateral development and tissue perfusion. *Circulation*, Vol. 94, No. 12, pp. 3281-3290

Vale, P.R., Losordo, D.W., Milliken, C.E., McDonald, M.C., Gravelin, L.M., Curry, C.M., Esakof, D.D., Maysky, M., Symes, J.F. & Isner, J.M. (2001). Randomized, single-blind, placebo-controlled pilot study of catheter-based myocardial gene transfer for therapeutic angiogenesis using left ventricular electromechanical mapping in patients with chronic myocardial ischemia. *Circulation*, Vol. 103, No. 17, (May 2001), pp. 2138-2143, ISSN 1524-4539

van Spaendonck-Zwarts, K.Y., van den Berg, M.P. & van Tintelen, J.P. (2008). DNA analysis in inherited cardiomyopathies: current status and clinical relevance. *Pacing Clin Electrophysiol*, Vol. 31 Suppl 1, No., (March 2008), pp. S46-49, ISSN 1540-8159

Vinge, L.E., Raake, P.W. & Koch, W.J. (2008). Gene therapy in heart failure. *Circ Res*, Vol. 102, No. 12, (June 2008), pp. 1458-1470, 1524-4571

Walter, D.H., Cejna, M., Diaz-Sandoval, L., Willis, S., Kirkwood, L., Stratford, P.W., Tietz, A.B., Kirchmair, R., Silver, M., Curry, C., *et al.* (2004). Local gene transfer of phVEGF-2 plasmid by gene-eluting stents: an alternative strategy for inhibition of restenosis. *Circulation*, Vol. 110, No. 1, pp. 36-45, ISSN 1524-4539

Weisleder, N., Taffet, G.E. & Capetanaki, Y. (2004). Bcl-2 overexpression corrects mitochondrial defects and ameliorates inherited desmin null cardiomyopathy. *Proc Natl Acad Sci U S A*, Vol. 101, No. 3, (January 2004), pp. 769-774, ISSN 0027-8424

Wen, S., Graf, S., Massey, P.G. & Dichek, D.A. (2004). Improved vascular gene transfer with a helper-dependent adenoviral vector. *Circulation*, Vol. 110, No. 11, pp. 1484-1491

White, J.D., Thesier, D.M., Swain, J.B.D., Katz, M.G., Tomasulo, C., Henderson, A., Wang, L., Yarnall, C., Fargnoli, A., Sumaroka, M., *et al.* (2011). Myocardial gene delivery using molecular cardiac surgery with recombinant adeno-associated virus vectors in vivo. *Gene Therapy*, Vol., No., pp. 1-7

Wiersma, A.C., Leegwater, P.A., van Oost, B.A., Ollier, W.E. & Dukes-McEwan, J. (2007). Canine candidate genes for dilated cardiomyopathy: annotation of and polymorphic markers for 14 genes. *BMC Vet Res*, Vol. 3, No., (October 2007), pp. 28, ISSN 1746-6148

Wijns, W., Vatner, S.F. & Camici, P.G. (1998). Hibernating myocardium. *N Engl J Med*, Vol. 339, No. 3, (July 1998), pp. 173-181, ISSN 0028-4793

Wright, M.J., Wightman, L.M., Latchman, D.S. & Marber, M.S. (2001). In vivo myocardial gene transfer: optimization and evaluation of intracoronary gene delivery in vivo. *Gene Ther*, Vol. 8, No. 24, pp. 1833-1839

Yamada, M., Ikeda, Y., Yano, M., Yoshimura, K., Nishino, S., Aoyama, H., Wang, L., Aoki, H. & Matsuzaki, M. (2006). Inhibition of protein phosphatase 1 by inhibitor-2 gene delivery ameliorates heart failure progression in genetic cardiomyopathy. *Faseb J*, Vol. 20, No. 8, pp. 1197-1199

Yang, B., Lin, H., Xiao, J., Lu, Y., Luo, X., Li, B., Zhang, Y., Xu, C., Bai, Y., Wang, H., *et al.* (2007). The muscle-specific microRNA miR-1 regulates cardiac arrhythmogenic potential by targeting GJA1 and KCNJ2. *Nat Med*, Vol. 13, No. 4, (April 2007), pp. 486-491, ISSN 1078-8956

Yang, J., Jiang, H., Chen, S.-S., Chen, J., Li, W.-Q., Xu, S.-K. & Wang, J.-C. (2010). Lentivirus-mediated RNAi targeting CREB binding protein attenuates neointimal formation and promotes re-endothelialization in balloon injured rat carotid artery. *Cell Physiol Biochem*, Vol. 26, No. 3, pp. 441-448

Yau, T.M., Kim, C., Ng, D., Li, G., Zhang, Y., Weisel, R.D. & Li, R.K. (2005). Increasing transplanted cell survival with cell-based angiogenic gene therapy. *Ann Thorac Surg*, Vol. 80, No. 5, (October 2005), pp. 1779-1786, ISSN 1552-6259

Ye, L., Haider, H., Jiang, S., Ling, L.H., Ge, R., Law, P.K. & Sim, E.K. (2005). Reversal of myocardial injury using genetically modulated human skeletal myoblasts in a rodent cryoinjured heart model. *Eur J Heart Fail*, Vol. 7, No. 6, (October 2005), pp. 945-952, ISSN 1388-9842

Yla-Herttuala, S. & Alitalo, K. (2003). Gene transfer as a tool to induce therapeutic vascular growth. *Nat Med*, Vol. 9, No. 6, pp. 694-701

Yla-Herttuala, S. & Martin, J.F. (2000). Cardiovascular gene therapy. *Lancet*, Vol. 355, No. 9199, pp. 213-222

Yla-Herttuala, S., Rissanen, T.T., Vajanto, I. & Hartikainen, J. (2007). Vascular endothelial growth factors: biology and current status of clinical applications in cardiovascular medicine. *J Am Coll Cardiol*, Vol. 49, No. 10, (March 2007), pp. 1015-1026, ISSN 1558-3597

Zachary, I. & Morgan, R.D. (2011). Therapeutic angiogenesis for cardiovascular disease: biological context, challenges, prospects. *Heart*, Vol. 97, No. 3, (October 2010), pp. 181-189, ISSN 1468-201X

Zarain-Herzberg, A. & Rupp, H. (2002). Therapeutic potential of CPT I inhibitors: cardiac gene transcription as a target. *Expert Opin Investig Drugs*, Vol. 11, No. 3, pp. 345-356, ISSN 1354-3784

Zarain-Herzberg, A., Rupp, H., Elimban, V. & Dhalla, N.S. (1996). Modification of sarcoplasmic reticulum gene expression in pressure overload cardiac hypertrophy by etomoxir. *Faseb J*, Vol. 10, No. 11, pp. 1303-1309, ISSN 0892-6638

Part 2

Gene Therapy in Orthopedics

8

Potential Gene Therapy for Intervertebral Disc Degeneration

Kotaro Nishida, Koichiro Maeno, Kakutani Kenichiro,
Takashi Yurube, and Masahiro Kurosaka
Department of Orthopaedic Surgery,
Kobe University Graduate School of Medicine
Kobe,
Japan

1. Introduction

Degenerative spinal disorders including low back pain are one of the most common and costly problems for modern society. It has been recognized that these disorders are directly or indirectly associated with intervertebral disc degeneration. The disc is a cartilaginous connective tissue, composed of the nucleus pulposus(NP), annulus fibrosus and endplates, which connects adjacent vertebrae (the functional spinal unit) and plays major roles in promoting the flexibility and stability of the lumbar spine. The NP is comprised of chondrocytic cells (nucleus pulposus cells) in an extensive extra-cellular matrix such as proteoglycan or collagen. Large molecules of proteoglycan exist in collagen networks and the high osmotic pressure produced by proteoglycan can result in inbibing water into the encapsulated NP, leading to high positive pressure inside the disc (Nachemson et al., 1970). The maintainance of this high positive presure inside of the disc is important in ensuring the biomechanical strength of the disc (Figure 1).

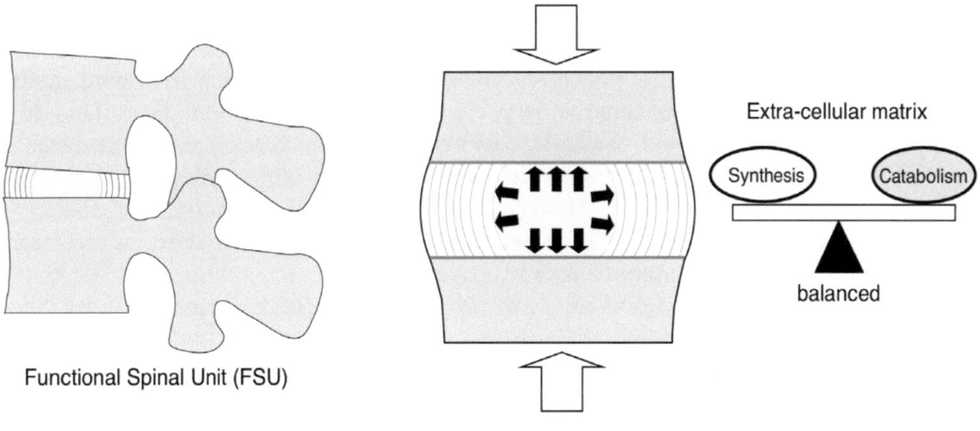

Fig. 1. Functional spinal unit and the biomechanical stability of the normal disc.

In the process of disc degeneration, the loss of an important extra-cellular matrix such as proteoglycan leading to loss of water from the nucleus pulposus, results in loss of the biomechenical stability of the disc. In this process, since the capability for regeneration of the degenerated disc is very limited, clinical treatment of degenerative disc disorders, especially if there is mechanical instability in this segment, often necessitates removal of the degenerated disc and fusion of this segment (spinal fusion) with or without metal instruments (Figure 2). Spinal fusion has been one of the main surgical treatments for degenerative disc disorders with acceptable clinical results. However, there are several problems associated with spinal fusion surgery, such as accerelated degeneration in the disc adjacent to the fused segnment (Lee, 1988), breakage of instruments and damage to the nerve tissue during the instumentation procedure (West et al., 1991). In addition, the procedure is highly invasive, costly, and the risc of infection is comparatively high.

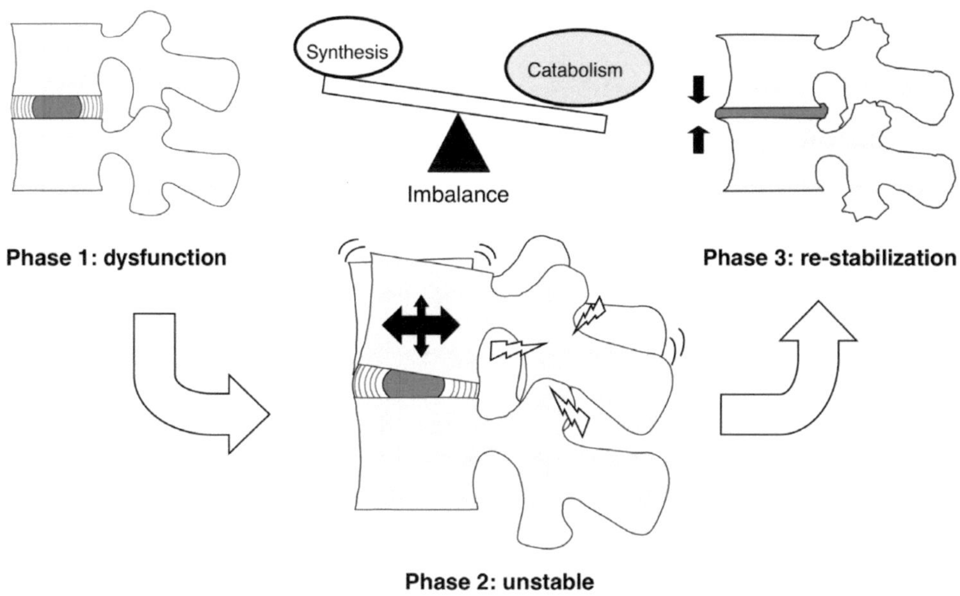

Fig. 2. Theoretical disc degeneration process (Kirkaldy & Farfan, 1982).

To overcome these problems attention has recently turned to biological treatment methods in an effort to stimulate the regeneration process of the degenerated discs. Due to the relatively well encapsulated and avascular enviroment of the disc, it seems preferable to deliver bioactive materials into the disc to obtain positive biological effects which can maintain or regenearate disc tissue. Biological treatment for the degenerated disc can be divided into three major categories: 1) growth factor injection with or without a carrier, 2) cell transplantation including stem cells, and 3) gene therapy. However, it is clear that the disc has unique anatomical and physiological properties, which challenge many traditional biological approaches. Therefore, we discuss the possiblity of biological treatment approaches especially from the view point of delivery of molecular materials to the disc. One of the most significant advantages of gene therapy may be the sustained biological effect making it potentially suitable in the treatment of chronic diseases such as spinal disorders, particularly those disorders associated with disc degeneration.

2. Intradiscal gene therapy

2.1 Previously reported intradiscal gene therapy

In vitro gene therapy approaches for the disc were first reported in 1997 and *in vivo* approaches in 1998. Attempts at intradiscal gene therapy using viral vectors have been made; however, due to the potential risks associated with viral gene therapy, the non-virus mediated intradiscal gene transfer method has been developed (see later discussion).

2.1.1 Virus vector-mediated intradiscal gene therapy

In 1997, Wehling et al. reported gene transfer to the chondrocytic cells from bovine intervertebral endplates using retrovirus vector *in vitro* (Wehling et al., 1997). This was the first report of gene therapy targeting the disc *in vitro*, and the authors indicated the potential use of indirect, ex vivo gene therapy for the degenerated disc by re-injecting genetically modified chondrocytic end-plate cells into the disc or surrounding tissue.

In 1998, Nishida and Kang et al. reported intradiscal direct gene transfer to the disc using an adenoviral vector *in vivo* with a rabbit model. This report was recognised as the first gene therapy approach targeting nucleus pulposus cells *in vitro* and *in vivo*. In their report, reporter gene expression continued *in vivo* at a seemingly undiminished level for at least 12 weeks. Later, their follow-up report using two different reporter genes showed the longevity of the transgene expression extended over 1 year. The results of these reports suggested that the adenoviral vector might be suitable for delivery of therapeutic genes to the disc, using an *in vivo*, direct gene therapy approach for the treatment of spinal disorders.

In their next study, Nishida and Kang et al. reported an *in vivo* study using the rabbit model once again to determine the feasibility of the adenovirus-mediated transfer of a therapeutic gene to the intervertebral disc. They used an adenovirus construct containing a human transforming growth factor-beta1 (TGF-beta1) encoding gene (Ad/CMV-TGF beta1). In vivo injection of Ad/CMV-TGF beta 1 into the normal nucleus pulposus was revealed to result in an approximately six-fold increase in total (i.e., active + latent) TGF- beta 1 production over that of the intact control discs. The discs of the therapeutic gene group exhibited a statistically significant two-fold increase in proteoglycan synthesis compared to the intact control discs. This study demonstrated the efficacy of adenovirus-mediated transfer of a therapeutic gene to the intervertebral disc *in vivo*. The observation of a significant increase in proteoglycan synthesis secondary to gene transfer suggested that gene therapy might have potential applications in changing the time-course of degenerative disc disease.

Recently, Liang et al. reported the successful curative effects of gene therapy for the treatment of the degenerated disc in a novel mice model by adenoviral mediation of the human growth and differentiation factor-5 (GDF-5) gene (Liang et al., 2010). Their study confirmed the long-term expression of the target protein in the disc *in vivo* and also demonstrated the physiological improvements occurring in the disc.

Meanwhile, Lattermann et al. reported adeno-associated virus (AAV) vector-mediated gene transfer to intervertebral disc *in vivo* (Lattermann et al., 2005). AAV vectors are understood to be less immunogenic than adenoviral vectors and as yet have not been linked with any disease in humans or mammals. The overall transgene expression was approximately half of that seen with the adenovirus, and the *in vivo* gene expression was associated with a 4–6 week latency period. They concluded that due to safety concerns over the use of adenoviral vectors for human gene therapy, the AAV vector might offer a valuable alternative to the adenovirus as a delivery vehicle for therapeutic gene transfer into the intervertebral disc.

Liu et al. reported the usefulness of baculovirus for the disc (Liu et al., 2006). Baculovirus is an insect virus able to deliver exogenous genes to mammalian cells including nondividing cells with no cell toxicity in vitro or in vivo. They concluded that baculovirus could transfer exogenous genes into rabbit nucleus pulposus cells safely and with high efficiency both *in vitro* and *in vivo*.

2.1.1 Nonvirus vector-mediated intradiscal gene therapy

Although the development of more sophisticated viral vectors such as non-toxic and safer vectors is still being investigated, progress in intradiscal gene therapy has been delayed by worries over the safety and potential costs of using recombinant viral vectors. Therefore, a number of non-virus mediated gene transfer techniques have been developed. However, the lower transfection efficiency compared with viral vector-mediated methods has been a major limitations of the non-virus mediated method, making the *in vivo*, direct gene transfer approach infeasible.

In 2006, Nishida et al. reported the efficacy of so-called "microbubble-enhanced ultrasound gene therapy" to the disc. More recent evidence suggested an appropriate intensity of ultrasound exposure could make a small transient hole on the cell membrane in a phenomenon called sonoporation, without causing cell toxicity. Additionally, it was reported that a kind of ultrasonography contrast agent called "micro-bubble" makes a cavitation with the exposure of ultrasound and this results in the bursting of the microbubbles leading to a distribution of material over a specific area of interest. Both these phenomenon, sonoporation and cavitation, are thought to have synergistic effects for increased transfection efficiency (Lawrie et al., 1999, 2000).

They demonstrated this micro-bubble enhanced ultrasound gene therapy in the intervertebral disc *in vivo* using a rat model. In their study, two different reporter plasmid DNA were used. They discovered that the ultrasound group demonstrated approximately an 11-fold increase in transgene expression over the plasmid DNA-only group. Moreover, transgene expression mediated by this method was seen, at least up to 24 weeks. These results demonstrate that ultrasound-mediated destruction of microbubbles loaded with plasmid-DNA is a feasible and efficient technique for local gene delivery within the intervertebral disc.

2.2 New strategy for intradiscal gene therapy

Despite much research effort, the successful biological treatment of degenerated discs is still limited to the injury induced disc degeneration (stub injury) model using relatively small animals. There are considerable limitations arising from the unique anatomy and physiology of the disc.

2.2.1 Limitations of biological approaches for degenerated disc

The lumbar intervertebral disc is known to be the largest avascular organ in the human body and the main path of nutrition or oxygen supply is passive diffusion via the endplates, resulting in poor nutrition and low oxygen tension, especially near the center of the disc (Grunhagen et al., 2006). Therefore, the metabolism in this area has to be relatively anaerobic, leading to the production of lactate, which in turn produces low pH inside of the disc (Nachemson, 1969). Low nutrition and oxygen tension, low pH, and high positive pressure make the interior of the intervertebral disc a harsh biological environment.

Therefore, NP cells existing in this environment must be highly differentiated to survive, which results in relative stability in terms of cell proliferation. Moreover, probably due to the low nutrition supply, the NP has a very low cell number compared with the rich extra-cellular matrix and a significantly low cellular metabolism.

Up to now, the main focus of intradiscal gene therapy and growth factor injection or cell therapy approaches has been to stimulate matrix synthesis. However, when taking the disc environment into consideration, methods requiring more resources or energy to up-regulate or stimulate matrix synthesis as well as cell proliferation seem less likely to result in successful disc regeneration. For successful biological treatment, taking into consideration of the characteristics of the target organ/tissue, and careful selection of the treatment strategy is necessary. As such, a different approach requiring less energy or fewer resources may have a better chance of promoting disc regeneration.

One of these approaches is the down-regulation of gene expressions that are potentially harmful for the physiological condition of the disc, and thus may induce degenerative change in the disc. This kind of approach focuses more on prophylactic treatment of disc degeneration. However, theoretically, it could become a regenerative treatment over an extended period (Figure 3). RNA interference (RNAi) is known to be a powerful means of sequence-specific gene silencing and would thus be a good candidate for this new strategy.

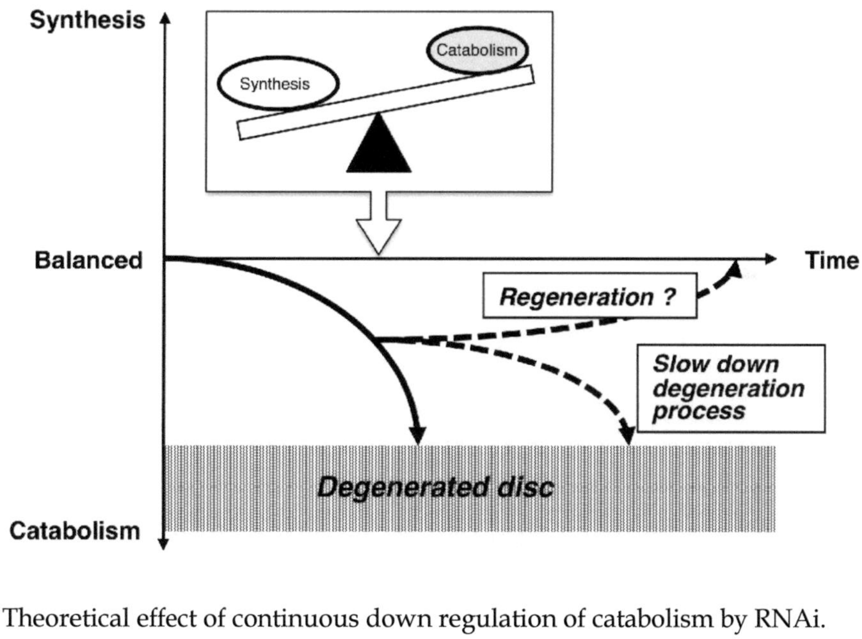

Fig. 3. Theoretical effect of continuous down regulation of catabolism by RNAi.

2.1.2 Potential application of RNA interference for treatment degenerated disc associated disorders

RNAi was first reported in 1998 by Fire et al. who demonstrated that double-stranded RNA induced sequence-specific silencing of gene expression in nematode cells (Fire et al., 1998). Elbashir et al. demonstrated that RNAi can be achieved in mammalian cells using oligoribonucleotide duplex 21 or 22 bases in length (small interfering RNA; siRNA)

(Elbashir et al., 2001). Since then, a numbers of RNAi applications for a variety of organs/diseases have been intensively investigated.

In 2006, Kakutani and Nishida et al. reported for the first time that RNAi targeting exogenous reporter gene is effective in silencing transgene expression in nucleus pulposus cells in humans and rats *in vitro*. In their study, two reporter luciferase plasmids (Firefly and Renilla) were used. These plasmids were co-transfected with siRNA targeting Firefly luciferase to the nucleus pulposus cells extracted from rats and scoliosis patients. The inhibitory effects were evaluated by dual luciferase assay for 3 weeks. The results showed the expression of Firefly Luciferase was drastically inhibited both in rats (94.7%) and in humans (93.7%). These inhibitory effects continued for 3 weeks. The study thus demonstrated that siRNA-mediated gene silencing in rat and human disc cells *in vitro* is feasible and effective in down regulating specific gene expression.

In their follow-up study, Suzuki and Nishida et al. reported the effectiveness of the DNA vector-based RNAi technique *in vitro* for a prolonged RNAi effect. Furthermore, they demonstrated the simple unmodified siRNA-mediated RNAi effect in intervertebral discs *in vivo* (rat coccygeal discs) resulted in a prolonged period of up to 24 weeks (168 days). Additionally, this study demonstrated long-term down-regulation is possible not only for the exogenous reporter gene, but also for the endogenous gene (Fas ligand) expression in rat discs in vivo. As a result of the prolonged silencing effect after a single intradiscal transduction of unmodified siRNA, this gene delivery method is suitable as a local therapy for disc degeneration and associated disorders by down-regulating some harmful genes for the normal physiology of the disc, which may cause disc degeneration. (Figure 4)

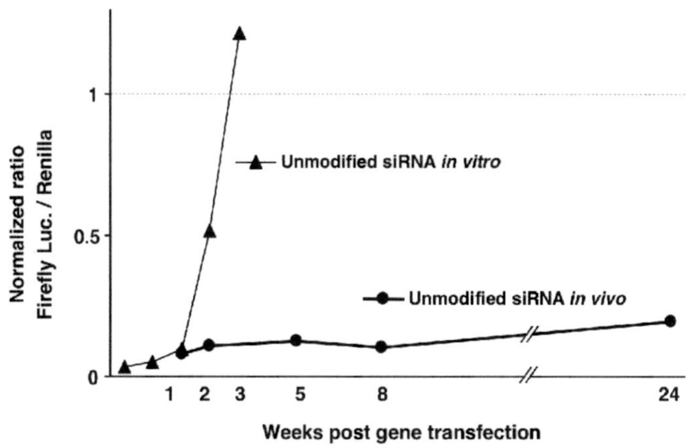

Fig. 4. Long-term RNAi effect mediated by unmodified siRNA in the nucleus pulposus *in vivo* (Modified from Suzuki et al., 2009).

More recently, Sudo and Minami reported successful RNAi in the degenerative process of the disc by down regulating Apotosis related factor caspase 3 (Sudo & Minami, 2011). In their report, they investigated the effects of siRNA targeting caspase 3 on rabbit nucleus pulposus (NP) cells *in vitro*. The researchers concluded that these findings indicated caspase 3 knockdown in intervertebral disc cells is effective in preventing apoptotic cell death, and thus could regulate intervertebral disc degeneration.

3. Conclusion

The gene therapy approach for the degenerated disc initially used a viral vector to transfer genes to stimulate important matrix synthesis for the disc such as proteoglycan. However, due to problems associated with a virus vector, a non-virus mediated gene transfer technique has been explored while the development of more sophisticated virus vectors remain a subject of investigation.

The difficulties of disc regeneration using a biological approach originate from the unique anatomical and physiological character of the disc. However, if we disregard these specific properties and the associated limitations of the disc, there may be little chance for successful regeneration. The successful treatment strategy for osteoporosis patients suggests us that the down-regulation of catabolic factors may be a more suitable strategy especially for organs/tissues with low cell metabolism and extensive extra-cellular matrix including bone or interverteral disc. As such, RNAi has been applied to the disc to down-regulate catabolic factors in the disc and correct imbalance between anabolic and catabolic factors with minimal nutrition requirements. This kind of approach would focus more on prophylactic treatment of disc degeneration. However, the potential exists for it to become a regenerative treatment over an extended period.

There are many issues to be overcome before the clinical use of RNAi can be permitted in patients suffering from degenerated discs and associated diseases. However, the demonstration that siRNA transfected by a nonvirus-mediated method can effectively inhibit specific gene expression in nucleus pulposus cells *in vivo* for an extended period lead the way for the exploration of siRNA as a novel strategy in gene therapy for the treatment of disc degeneration and associated diseases.

4. Acknowledgment

The authors thank Mrs. Tubby for their help in preparing the manuscript. Partial of this work was supported by Grant-in-Aid for Scientific Research (B) (19300184 and 21300189) from the Ministry of Education, Culture, Sports, Science and Technology of Japan.

5. References

Elbashir, SM., Harborth, J., Lendeckel, W., Yalcin, A., Weber, K., & Tuschl, T. (2001). Duplexes of 21-nucleotide RNAs mediate RNA interference in cultured mammalian cells. *Nature,* Vol. 411, pp. 494–8

Fire, A., Xu, S., Montgomery, MK., Kostas, SA., Driver, SE., & Mello, CC. (1998). Potent and specific genetic interference by double-stranded RNA in Caenorhabditis elegans. *Nature,* Vol. 391, pp.806–11

Grunhagen, T., Wilde, G., Soukane, DM., Shirazi-Adl, SA., & Urban, JP. (2006). Nutrient supply and intervertebral disc metabolism. *J Bone Joint Surg,* Vol. 88-A, pp. 30–35

Kirkaldy-Willis, W. & Farfan, H. (1982). Instability of the lumbar spine. *Clin Orthop Relat Res,* Vol. 165, pp. 110-23

Lattermann, C., Oxner, WM., Xiao, X., Li, J., Gilbertson, LG., Robbins, PD., & Kang JD. (2005). The adeno associated viral vector as a strategy for intradiscal gene transfer in immune competent and pre-exposed rabbits. *Spine,* Vol. 30, pp. 497–504

Lawrie, A., Brisken, AF., Francis, SE., Tayler, DI., Chamberlain, J., Crossman, DC., Cumberland, DC., & Newman, CM. (1999). Ultrasound enhances reporter gene expression after transfection of vascular cells in vitro. *Circulation*, Vol. 99, pp. 2617–20

Lawrie, A., Brisken, AF., Francis, SE., Cumberland, DC., Crossman, DC., & Newman, CM. (2000). Microbubble-enhanced ultrasound for vascular gene delivery. *Gene Ther*, Vol. 7, pp. 2023–27

Lee, CK. (1988). Accelerated degeneration of the segment adjacent to a lumbar fusion. *Spine*, Vol. 13, pp. 375-7

Liang, H., Ma, SH., Feng, G., Shen FH., & Li, XJ. (2010). Therapeutic effects of adenovirus-mediated growth and differentiation factor-5 in a mice disc degeneration model induced by annulus needle puncture. *Spine J*, Vol. 10, pp. 32-41

Liu, X., Li, K., Song, J., Liang, C., Wang, X., & Chen, X. (2006). Efficient and stable gene expression in rabbit intervertebral disc cells transduced with a recombinant baculovirus vector. *Spine*, Vol. 31, pp. 732–35

Nachemson, A. & Elfstrom, G. (1970). Intravital dynamic pressure measurements in lumbar discs: a study of common movements, maneuvers and exercises. *Scand J Rehabil Med Suppl*, Vol. 1, pp. 1- 40

Nachemson, A. (1969). Intradiscal measurements of pH in patients with lumbar rhizopathies. *Acta Orthop Scand*, Vol. 40, pp. 23–42

Sudo, H. & Minami, A. Caspase 3 as a thrapeutic target for regulation of intervertebral disc degeneration. (2011). *Arthritis Rheum*, Jan 21, doi:10.1002/art.30251. [Epub ahead of print]

Wehling, P., Schulitz, KP., Robbins, PD., Evans, CH., & Reinecke, JA. (1997). Transfer of genes to chondrocytic cells of the lumbar spine. Proposal for a treatment strategy of spinal disorders by local gene therapy. *Spine*, Vol. 22, pp.1092–97

West, JL., Ogilvie, JW., Bradford, DS. (1991). Complications of variable screw plate pedicle screw fixation. *Spine*, Vol. 16, pp. 576-9

9

Conditioning and Scaffolding of Chondrocytes: Smart Steps Towards Osteoarthritis Gene Therapy

Muhammad Farooq Rai[2], Annemarie Lang[1], Matthias Sieber[1] and Michael F.G. Schmidt[1]
[1]*Institute of Immunology and Molecular Biology, Department of Veterinary Medicine, Freie Universität Berlin, Berlin,*
[2]*Department of Orthopaedic Surgery, Washington University School of Medicine at Barnes-Jewish Hospital, St. Louis, MO*
[1]*Germany*
[2]*United States*

1. Introduction

Osteoarthritis (OA), the most common form of arthritis, is a chronic degenerative joint disease that remains a leading cause of chronic disability in the aged population and a financial burden on healthcare resources. It affects approximately 15% of the world's human population over 60 years of age (Wolf & Pfleger, 2003) and has even higher prevalence in dogs (Johnston, 1997), cats (Godfrey, 2005) and horses (Trumble et al., 2001). It is established that OA in dogs and horses has a model character for the human disease since it parallels the human form of OA in all aspects (Innes & Clegg, 2010).

The pathogenesis of OA is characterized by an imbalance in the network of anabolic and catabolic processes through complex interactions of mechanical and biochemical forces (M.B. Goldring, 2001; Sandell & Aigner, 2001). This imbalance leads, inevitably, to progressive articular cartilage destruction, osteophyte formation, subchondral bone remodelling and chronic inflammation (M.B. Goldring & S.R. Goldring, 2007; Martel-Pelletier & Pelletier, 2007). These events are further manifested by a loss of both tissue architecture and joint functionality, painful limited movement, disability and an inferior quality of life (Abramson & Yazici, 2006; Buckwalter et al., 2006; Pelletier et al., 2001). Despite major progress over the last few years, we still have a lot more to understand about the aetiology, pathogenesis and progression of OA.

A complete therapy for OA still remains elusive as manifold efforts made in this direction failed to provide a successful long-term remedy. The therapeutic strategies for OA have been predominantly directed to (i) alleviate symptomatic pain by suppressing the inflammatory process, (ii) reducing the cartilage degenerative process or (iii) enhancing cartilage regeneration. However, none has so far been applied to achieve all the three objectives.

Non-pharmacologic and pharmacologic treatments have been employed for early OA while surgical interventions for partial or total joint replacement are often indicated in advanced

OA when the symptoms cannot be controlled by non-invasive means. The long-term use of pharmacologics is commonly concomitant with side-effects while surgery contributes little to reduce the process of joint destruction and inflammation (Katz et al., 2010; Wei et al., 1998).

Articular cartilage destruction is a key pathological characteristic of OA and rheumatoid arthritis (RA). Therefore, attempts have been made to repair the OA-related cartilage defects. In this context, autologous chondrocyte transplantation (ACT) offers a practical solution (Brittberg et al., 1994). Evidence suggests that damaged cartilage plays a pivotal role in disease progression and severity (Buckwalter et al., 2006). ACT attempts to build hyaline repair tissue, delays total or partial joint replacement, helps to temporarily relieve pain and improves the joint function (Minas et al., 2010; Peterson et al., 2002). A further developed alternative technique is the matrix associated ACT, where the cultivated cells are seeded on a tissue-engineered (biomaterial) scaffold and the cell–scaffold complex is then implanted into the defect. The ACT/scaffold coupling paved the way for the use of functional tissue substitutes in the treatment of cartilage defects (Tuli et al., 2003). However, inflammatory mediators in the arthritic joint could negatively affect the implanted cells, potentiating the need to suppress inflammation (Hennerbichler et al., 2008).

Gene therapy represents another promising approach for OA treatment (Bandara et al., 1992; Evans et al., 2004; Evans et al., 2009). This concept utilizes viral or non-viral vectors to deliver genetic information encoding biological agents into the target tissue for their local expression. It appears that viral strategies provide high transfection efficiency and many additional assets for a clinical development (Mease et al., 2010) but immunogenicity and possible mutagenicity are their main drawbacks. Non-viral strategies, on the other hand, have a fascinating preclinical development in arthritis. They are safer but less efficient. Of major concern is the regulated expression of the therapeutic genes. Ideally, gene therapy outperforms the systemic intake of medicines by only affecting the transfected joint. Normally, drugs can be applied in a controlled dosage, while transgene expression is switched by intrinsic, normally immutable, regulatory elements. In other words, the expression of the therapeutic candidate gene should be limited to the site of OA occurrence and only applied in the presence of inflammation or other significant markers of OA arising in the affected joint. Moreover, the gene expression should ideally be self-limiting (=conditioned) and not constitutive (Geurts et al., 2007; Rachakonda et al., 2008a).

The information presented above provides evidence for a limited success of several efforts towards achieving effective therapeutic strategies for OA. This is mainly because they are associated with one or the other limitation. Nonetheless, it is tempting to speculate that gene therapy (coupled with tissue-engineering) has great potential for improvement. It is therefore very likely that it becomes a leading force for future OA treatment if suitably improved. This chapter will provide extended information on this topic and discuss as well as suggest some novel ways to improve the current gene therapy procedures for their safe application.

2. Non-pharmacological and pharmacological therapies

Pain is the presenting symptom in OA. Thus, the therapeutic efforts for OA specifically aim at the pain relief through the combination of non-pharmacological and pharmacological interventions. Non-pharmacological approaches include exercise therapy, weight loss, social support, self-management and awareness of patients to OA (Clouet et al., 2009). These

approaches help partially prevent the disease, reduce pain and may delay the degenerative process in early-stage OA but do not offer a long-term remedy. Pharmacological therapy improves the quality of life of OA patients also through alleviating pain. Acetaminophen treatment followed by non-steroidal anti-inflammatory drugs (NSAIDs) inhibits the activation of immune cells while NSAIDs suppress the inflammatory process by intervening with the prostaglandin synthesis. Long-term usage of NSAIDs is often accompanied by adverse side-effects such as gastrointestinal, renal or cardiovascular disorders, as most of these compounds inhibit cyclooxygenases (COX)-1 and -2 indiscriminatorily (Hotz-Behofsits et al., 2003; Scarpignato & Hunt, 2010; Wolfe et al., 1999).
Selective COX-2 inhibitors reduce pain through prostaglandin blockade, but owing to their harmful effects on cardiovascular events they were recalled from the market (Park et al., 2006). Later on, the application of some disease-modifying OA drugs (DMOADs) was being enhanced by advances in imaging and biomarkers that serve as validated surrogate endpoints for key clinical outcomes (Abramson & Yazici, 2006). However, the clinical development program for DMOADs is complicated due to the slowly progressive nature of OA.
Intra-articular injections of corticosteroids (Habib et al., 2010) or hyaluronic acid (Liao et al., 2005) exert pain reducing effects that last for a couple of weeks but do not significantly improve the physical function of the joint. Nutritional supplements such as chondrotin sulphate and glucosamine are asymptomatic slow-acting safe drugs for the management of OA, but their efficacy in OA is questionable (Dougados, 2006) just like avocado, soybean, unsaponifiables and Vitamin E (Clouet et al., 2009).

3. Surgical treatment

Surgical intervention offers another option for OA therapy after medications have failed to restore joint function. Arthroscopic lavage and debridement of the arthritic joint is only indicated in cases of superimposed structural lesions in the affected joint such as meniscal tear (Katz et al., 2010). Osteotomy is performed by trimming the joint resulting in a spread of the mechanical load which relieves the defect area (Parker et al., 2011). Partial or total joint replacements are the last resorts in orthopaedic surgery for OA. But these procedures are more prone to fail in young and middle-aged patients (Wei et al., 1998). In addition, the evidence supporting the use of various surgical approaches is limited mainly by the poor study design and relatively small sample size (Katz et al., 2010).

4. Concept of gene therapy in OA

The term gene therapy is commonly understood to mean the use of molecular methods to replace defective or absent genes or to counteract those that are over-expressed. The key technologies needed for gene therapy are the methods by which genes are isolated (cloned), manipulated (engineered), and transferred (delivered) into host cells. Since its inception, the field of gene therapy in medicine has received much attention, but still remains a great challenge for routine clinical applications to treat diseases including OA and RA (Gibbons & Hyrich, 2009).

4.1 *In vivo* gene delivery in the arthritic joint

OA is well-suited for local, intra-articular gene delivery because it affects a limited number of joints and lacks obvious extra-articular manifestations (Bandara et al., 1992). Thus, the delivery of locally expressed gene products may have therapeutic benefits for localized areas of cartilage damage with minimal systemic side-effects. In this approach genes encoding biological agents are introduced directly into the intra-articular tissues through viral and non-viral vectors. Despite its simplicity, the *in vivo* route has a number of disadvantages that limit its application. For example, targeting the appropriate cells may be difficult (Evans et al., 2004). In spite of that there are many published reports in which *in vivo* gene delivery has been the main subject (see Table 1).

Vector	Transgene	Animal model	Reference
Adenovirus	IL-1Ra	Dog ACLT	Pelletier et al., 1997
Plasmid	IL-1Ra	Rabbit meniscectomy	Fernandes et al., 1999
Adenovirus	IL-1Ra	Horse osteochondral defects	Frisbie et al., 2002
rAAV	bFGF	Rabbit osteochondral defects	Cucchiarini & Madry, 2005
Plasmid	BMP-2	Rabbit cartilage defects	Di Cesare et al., 2006
Plasmid	HSP-70	Rat MIA injection	Grossin et al., 2006
Adenovirus	TSP-1	Rat ACLT	Hsieh et al., 2010

Table 1. *In vivo* gene delivery in experimentally induced OA in animal models. Abbreviations: IL-1Ra=interleukin-1 receptor antagonist; ACLT=anterior cruciate ligament transection; rAAV=recombinant adeno-associated virus; bFGF=basic fibroblast growth factor; BMP-2= bone morphogenic protein-2; HSP-70=heat shock protein-70; MIA=mono-iodoacetate; TSP-1=thrombospondin-1.

4.2 *Ex vivo* gene delivery in arthritic joint

An efficient targeting of specific types of cells *in vivo* by using vectors is presently not possible. Therefore, most applications requiring selective cell transduction involve the removal of cells from the body and their genetic manipulation *in vitro* before re-implantation. This is known as *ex vivo* gene delivery. The logic behind such an approach is mainly to augment the expression of a therapeutic gene of interest or an inhibition of the expression of disease-associated genes (Jorgensen & Apparailly, 2010). Through *ex vivo* gene transfer the amount of genetic material introduced in a target cell can be controlled and expression levels monitored before application. A selection of transfection methods used in routine lab and clinical studies is listed in Table 2 and a comparison of *in vivo* and *ex vivo* gene transfer methods is presented in Figure 1.

4.3 Selective anti-catabolic gene products

The pro-inflammatory cytokines interleukin-1 beta (IL-1β) and tumour necrosis factor alpha (TNFα) secreted by chondrocytes, synovial cells and invading immune cells, are important mediators of matrix degeneration and cell apoptosis in OA (M.B. Goldring, 2001). Therefore, inhibitors of these cytokines may counteract inflammatory destruction of cartilage. Besides cytokines, matrix metalloproteinases (MMPs) and aggrecanases such as ADAMTS-4 (a disintegrin and metalloproteinase with thrombospondin-like motif-4) and -5 (ADAMTS-5) secreted by the chondrocytes degrade a surplus of matrix in OA (Heinegård & Saxne, 2011). In order to diminish the lysis of cartilage and thus to reduce OA progression, tissue inhibitors of metalloproteinases (TIMPs) can be over-expressed through gene therapy (Celiker et al., 2002; van der Laan et al., 2003).

Target cell	Transgene	Vector	Animal model	Reference
Chondrocytes	LacZ-neo	Retrovirus	Rabbit	Kang et al., 1997
	BMP-7	Adenovirus	Horse	Hidaka et al., 2003
	IGF-1	Plasmid	Rabbit	Madry et al., 2005
	bFGF	rAAV	Rabbit	Yokoo et al., 2005
	bFGF	Plasmid	Rabbit	Kaul et al., 2006
Synovial cells	LacZ-neo	Retrovirus	Rabbit	Bandara et al., 1992
	IL-1Ra IL-10	Retrovirus	Rabbit	Zhang et al., 2004
Perichondrium-derived stem cells	BMP-1 IGF-1	Adenovirus	Rat	Gelse et al., 2003
Bone-marrow-derived stem cells	CDMP1	Plasmid	Rabbit	Katayama et al., 2004
Fibroblasts	TGF-β	Retrovirus	Rabbit	Lee et al., 2001
Muscle-derived cells	LacZ	Retrovirus	Rabbit	Adachi et al., 2002

Table 2. *Ex vivo* gene delivery to various cell types in animal models for cartilage damage. Abbreviations: LacZ-neo=β-galaktosidase-neomycin phosphotransferase; BMP-7=bone morphogenic protein-7; IGF-1=insulin-like growth factor-1; bFGF=basic fibroblast growth factor; rAAV=recombinant adeno-associated virus; IL-1Ra=interleukin-1 receptor antagonist; IL-10=interleukin-10; CDMP1=cartilage-derived morphogenic protein 1; TGF-β=transforming growth factor β.

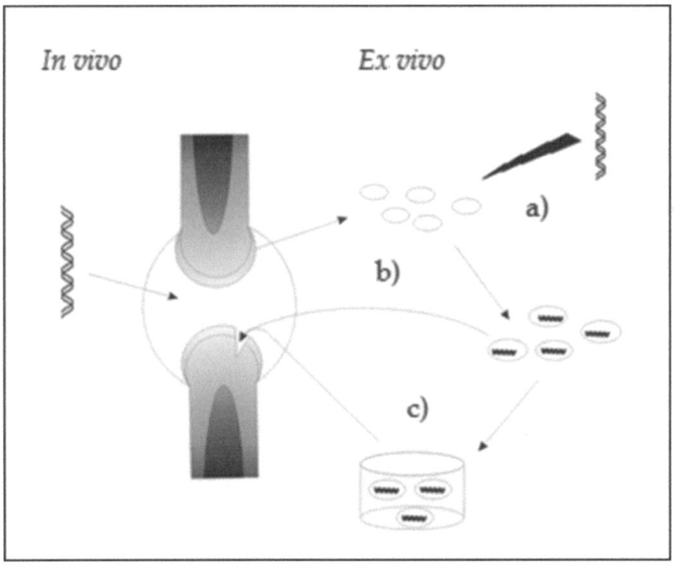

Fig. 1. *In vivo* and *ex vivo* gene transfers to the arthritic joint. *In vivo* gene delivery involves a direct injection of the transgenic vector, in the form of a naked DNA or coupled with a virus vehicle into the joint. In an *ex vivo* approach, gene transfer includes an intermediate step of transfection of the explanted, allogeneic cells (chondrocytes/synoviocytes) with the transgenic vector (a). The transfected cells can be injected directly into the joint (synoviocytes) or to the cartilage defect (chondrocytes) (b) or be embedded into a scaffold followed by the reimplantation into the cartilage lesion (c).

4.4 Selective anabolic gene products

While inhibition of catabolic pathways will diminish OA damage, it will not enhance repair of already degraded matrix. Therefore, gene products with anabolic functions are of special interest. These gene products comprise anabolic enzymes and growth factors that promote matrix synthesis and morphogenic mediators for chondrogenic differentiation. Matrix synthesis can be enhanced by expressing enzymes required for the synthesis of precursors of matrix constituents (J.N. Gouze et al., 2004). An overview of genes employed for OA gene therapy is provided in Table 3.

Candidate transgene	Effect	Reference
Anti-catabolic		
IL-1Ra	Blocks IL-1R on articular cells	Evans & Robbins, 1994
sIL-1R	Neutralizes secreted IL-1	Ghivizzani et al., 1998
sTNFR	Neutralizes secreted TNFα	Ghivizzani et al., 1998
IL-4	Down-regulates IL-1 and TNFα expression	Geurts et al., 2007; Rachakonda et al., 2008a; Woods et al., 2001
IL-10	Down-regulates IL-1 and TNFα expression	Amos et al., 2006; Müller et al., 2008; Zhang et al., 2004
IL-13	Anti-inflammatory action	Nabbe et al., 2005
TIMPs	Matrix proteinase inhibitor	Celiker et al., 2002; van der Laan et al., 2003
Anabolic		
IGF-1	Chondrocyte growth factor	Madry et al., 2002
TGF-β	Chondrocyte growth factors	Lafeber et al., 1997; Watson et al., 2010
BMPs	Chondrocyte growth factors	Hidaka et al., 2003
bFGF	Chondrocyte growth factor	Madry et al., 2004
SOX-9	Transcription factor	Cucchiarini et al., 2007
GFAT	Enhances matrix synthesis	J.N. Gouze et al., 2004
GlcAT-I	Enhances matrix synthesis	Venkatesan et al., 2004

Table 3. Examples of candidate transgenes for OA gene therapy. Abbreviations: IL-1Ra=Interleukin-1 receptor antagonist; sIL-1R=soluble IL-1 receptor; sTNFR=soluble tumour necrosis factor-α receptor; IL-4, -10, -13=interleukin-4,-10,-13; TIMPs=tissue inhibitors of metalloproteinases; IGF-1=insulin like growth factor 1; TGF-β=transforming growth factor β; BMPs=bone morphogenic proteins; bFGF = basic fibroblast growth factor; SOX-9=sex-determining region Y box 9; GFAT=glutamine fructose-6 phosphate aminotransferase; GlcAT-I= β1,3-glucuronosyltransferase-I.

4.5 Viral gene transfer

Viruses provide a natural system for horizontal gene transfer into a variety of cells. Several virus types (given below) infect mammalian cells and are adopted as vehicles for gene transfer. Retroviral transfection systems derived from Moloney murine leukaemia oncoretrovirus and others require dividing cells for infection and integration and have therefore been used mainly in *ex vivo* transfection (Evans et al., 2005) and occasionally *in vivo* (Ghivizzani et al., 1997). Retroviruses insert parts of their genome non-specifically into the host cell DNA, thus enabling stable transfection of the cells but carry the risk of insertional mutagenesis.

Lentiviruses, derived from the human immunodeficiency virus, are able to infect resting-state cells with high efficiency, show low immunogenicity and can integrate transgenes into the cell DNA. To avoid possible insertion mutagenesis, non-integrating lentiviruses have been developed which maintain the high transduction efficiency (Philpott & Thrasher, 2007) and can be used for *in vivo* and *ex vivo* transduction of articular cells (E. Gouze et al., 2007).

Adenoviruses readily transduce dividing and non-dividing cells. The integration frequency of adenoviral genome into host DNA is very low (Harui et al., 1999), and engineered replication deficient adenoviruses enhance biosafety. Many adenoviruses, however, elicit immune responses from the patient, which excludes them from *in vivo* approaches. To circumvent their immunogenicity, either adenovirus strains which normally infect different host species are used, or immunogenic viral proteins are deleted from the constructs (Evans et al., 2001). Adeno-associated viruses have low immunogenicity, are small in size and can carry only small gene constructs. They possibly penetrate the cartilage matrix and could therefore transduce chondrocytes *in vivo* (Madry et al., 2003).

In general, viral gene transfer is highly efficient. Synovial cells can be transduced *in vivo,* and chondrocytes *ex vivo* with high transduction rates. Drawbacks of viral systems are biosafety issues, the need of extra cell lines for virus generation and propagation, and special plasmids for viral delivery. Therefore, several non-viral methods are used parallel to viral approaches (Capito & Spector, 2007; Thomas et al., 2003).

4.6 Non-viral gene transfer

Non-viral gene transfer delivers plasmid DNA into the target cells with selected chemical and physical methods. In general, non-viral methods are less elaborate than the generation of transduction viruses. All non-viral methods achieve transient transfection (Welter et al., 2004).

The most common method uses non-ionic or cationic lipids to form DNA-lipid particles. These particles are taken up by the cell and transcribed after transfer into the nucleus. Several compounds are available, which transfect cells with variable efficiencies (Madry et al., 2000). Many protocols for *ex vivo* gene transfer with lipofection are established despite of the drawback of relatively low transfection efficiency. The cytotoxicity of most transfection agents causes limited damage to target cells and thus this method is not suitable for *in vivo* use. Intra-articular injection of naked DNA plasmids without addition of liposomal agents is also feasible for synoviocyte transfection (Sant et al., 1998). On the other hand, electroporation achieves high transfection rate and does not need cytotoxic chemicals (Welter et al., 2004). By applying intra-articular DNA injection and external electric pulses to knee joints, *in vivo* transfection of articular chondrocytes can be achieved (Grossin et al., 2003). Binding plasmid DNA to magnetic microparticles allows the complexes to be forced into cells by strong directional magnetic fields and does not require cytotoxic transfection reagents. This approach has been used on chondrocytes in monolayer (Plank et al., 2003), but its feasibility *in vivo* has not been tested yet. A selection of viral and non-viral gene transfer procedures are compiled in Table 4.

Gene transfer method	Efficiency	Reference
Viral		
Retrovirus	Low transduction efficiency *in vivo*, integrating	Evans et al., 2005
Lentivirus	High transduction efficiency of dividing and non-dividing cells, integrating	E. Gouze et al., 2002
Adenovirus	Immunogenic, high transduction efficiency	Ghivizzani et al., 1998
AAV	Moderate transduction efficiency *in vivo*, only small ORFs as transgenes	Jorgensen & Apparailly, 2010
Non-viral		
Lipofection	Cytotoxic, varying transfection efficiency, low cost	Madry et al., 2005
Electroporation	Efficient, high equipment costs	Welter et al., 2004
Matrix bound DNA	Long lasting, low transfection efficiency	Capito & Spector, 2007

Table 4. Comparison of gene transfer methods for articular gene therapy. Abbreviations: AAV=adeno-associated viruses; ORFs=open reading frames.

5. Tissue-engineered scaffolds for ACT

In the context of OA, repair of cartilage surface defects through biological regeneration and transplantation of various tissues or cells have been investigated (Goehring et al., 2010; Stoop, 2008). The technology of scaffold-free ACT pioneered by Brittberg and colleagues has been widely applied to repair small cartilage lesions. Herein, a biopsy is taken from non-weight-bearing regions of cartilage; the chondrocytes are enzymatically extracted, expanded in monolayer culture, and then injected beneath a periosteal flap sutured over the cartilage lesion (Brittberg et al., 1994). This strategy has been used to treat thousands of patients worldwide and offers a transient but practical solution for cartilage repair.

Porous 3-dimensional scaffolds are increasingly used to facilitate cellular attachment and at the same time provide superior mechanical properties. This technique is particularly useful given the lack of cell retention when cell suspensions are directly transplanted at the cartilage defect site. It also reduces potential donor site morbidity associated with procedures that utilize a periosteal flap to increase cellular retention (Brittberg et al., 1994). A wide range of materials have been produced to serve as scaffolds for cartilage repair. Generally they can be classified into three categories: natural, synthetic and biosynthetic materials (Goehring et al., 2010; Langer & Tirrell, 2004; Stoop, 2008). In the following paragraphs, we will highlight some of the important scaffolds from these categories.

5.1 Natural scaffold materials

Natural materials are composed of native biocompounds which mimick the natural surface for cell adhesion and maintain the required physiological environment. In addition, these materials (i) are non-toxic, (ii) follow a physiological biodegrading mechanism and (iii) are used to produce scaffolds for cartilage tissue-engineering (Hunziker, 2002; Stoop, 2008).

Collagen-based biomaterials are widely used in clinical practice and have been employed as carriers for chondrocytes (Wakitani et al., 1998) and mesenchymal stem cells (MSCs) (Im et al., 2001). Collagen type I hydrogels resemble hyaline cartilage. They are biodegradable, elicit no inflammation and can be metabolized by MSCs through the action of endogenous collagenases. Rat-tail extracted, collagen type I has been recently developed to construct scaffolds termed cartilage regeneration system (CaReS; Amedrix, Esslingen, Germany). It has been reported that patellofemoral transplantation of CaReS scaffolds for two years showed a significant improvement in cartilage repair in patients (Andereya et al., 2007) resulting in complete defect filling with superior quality repair tissue (Welsch et al., 2010).

Both fibrinogen and its polymer fibrin have been shown to play major roles in healing osteochondral defects (Shapiro et al., 1993), but owing to the exceedingly high concentrations and protein densities, the glue impeded rather than facilitated cell invasion, thus limiting its use (Brittberg et al., 1994). Hyaluronic acid is a non-sulphated glycosaminoglycan (GAG) that makes up a large part of cartilage extracellular matrix. In its unmodified form, it has a high biocompatibility and plays an important role in determining the biophysical microenvironment for chondrocyte growth and proliferation (Poole et al., 1990).

Cell-seeded agarose hydrogels enhance the matrix elaboration upon dynamic deformational loading (Häuselmann et al., 1994). Despite its suitability for implantation, the non-degradable nature of the gel limits its application in tissue-engineering. Alginate, a naturally derived polysaccharide gel, has been successfully shown to support cell retention and the chondrocytic phenotype by maintaining cell shape through encapsulation (Guo et al., 1989; Häuselmann et al., 1994; Rai et al., 2009). On the other hand, its inferior biomechanical properties as well as concerns over its immunogenicity have raised biocompatibility issues (Kulseng et al., 1999). Alginates are easy to use and suitable for the repair of small cartilage defects but fragile during surgery.

5.2 Synthetic scaffold materials

Many synthetic scaffolds commonly used in cartilage tissue-engineering are fabricated using poly(α-hydroxy acid) polymers such as poly-L-lactide, polyglycolic acid and their copolymers poly-DL-lactide-co-glycolide and poly-ϵ-caprolactone (Li et al., 2006; Nöth et al., 2002). They offer optimal fibre diameter, pore size, degradation time and reproducibility in production. The major advantages associated with the use of synthetic polymers are their design flexibility and elimination of disease transmission. Disadvantages of some synthetic polymers are the potential increase in local pH resulting from acidic degradation products, excessive inflammatory responses and poor clearance and chronic inflammation associated with these high molecular weight polymers (Stoop, 2008).

5.3 Biosynthetic scaffold materials

In recent years, a wide array of novel biosynthetic materials has been developed based on natural materials such as silk or cellulose and synthetic materials such as poly(1,8-octanediol citrate) or poly(ether ester) copolymer scaffolds. In addition, numerous attempts have been sought to optimize scaffold properties by combining several different materials. For example, scaffolds have been produced from gelatine, hyaluronic acid and chondroitin-6-sulphate and mixed with fibrin glue or polylactic-co-glycolic acid. To support bone as well as cartilage formation, hydroxyapatite was combined with chitosan to produce scaffolds that allow the treatment of osteochondral defects. Conversely, most of these developments show promise for future clinical application, so far they have mainly been investigated using *in vitro* systems or at the most, in animal models. Translation of these developments to the clinical and commercial setting will take longer (Stoop, 2008).

6. Obstacles and challenges in clinical application of gene therapy

Gene therapy for OA has been described extensively for the last twenty years and a large body of impressive preclinical safety and efficacy information has been documented (Bandara et al., 1992; Trippel et al., 2004). Despite this fact, only a few clinical trials of this therapeutic strategy have been conducted mainly due to scientific, technological, financial and sociological hurdles (Evans et al., 2011). A single phase II study has been reported recently and this slow pace indicates the unlikelihood of gene therapy to become clinically available in the near future (Mease et al., 2010). One of the most serious reason for the current slow progress in gene therapy research in OA (and RA) lies in the widespread public scepticism with anything relating to genes. The term gene is simply not understood by the average citizen and any genetic intervention in research has a priori a negative connotation. Fitting with this general attitude, regulatory bodies demand extremely hard safety precautions with any genetic intervention with patients which leads to an explosion of cost and duration for the development of these very promising therapies.

Nonetheless, this should not disappoint gene therapy researchers. Despite its slow progress, gene therapy promises to fulfil unmet needs in the treatment of OA and allied joint disorders and therefore has a bright future in the long run. It will eventually offer a focussed, local and perhaps personalized therapy avenue which may well cover the non-responders to the conventional treatment of joint disorders which in the case of RA amount to a substantial percentage (Gibbons & Hyrich, 2009). Furthermore, by applying local gene therapy it will certainly be possible to avoid the widely observed side-effects that occur with the present therapeutics.

Another leading challenge facing gene therapy today is the improvement of current vectors and this area continues to be another limiting factor in gene therapy applications. Even in the field of viral vectors, attempts have been made to combine their application with immunomodulating agents (Ikeda et al., 2000), still obvious problems exist with this approach (Zhou et al., 2004). Similarly, in the area of non-viral gene transfer, researchers are generating new transfection methods/strategies with a number of new products becoming commercially available every year (Donkuru et al., 2010; Haag et al., 2009; Madeira et al., 2011). Yet, an ideal agent that satisfies the requirements for application with the relevant target cells for OA gene therapy is not in sight.

Although the tissue-engineering scaffolds described above are becoming increasingly popular due to the high standards of cellular attachment and mechanical stability, their role in a pro-inflammatory environment in arthritic condition raises some doubts and has not been completely evaluated. An effective therapy of OA in the context of inflammation, however, may be achieved through genetic modification of suitable target cells present in the scaffolds to deliver therapeutic transgenes to the site of disease. Below we elaborate on the choice of cells that can be utilized in this approach and on the question which are the best vehicles for gene delivery mechanism as well as the type of scaffolds for engineering cartilage defects.

7. Controlled expression from "Smart Transplants"

As we all know that the conventional gene therapy has many potential limitations and therefore the need of customized gene therapy arises. The customized form of gene therapy could be defined as a therapy in which autologous cells are genetically modified by species-specific genes under the control of endogenous and disease-responsive elements and made clinically applicable by seeding in the scaffolds. As these scaffolds harbour cells that deliver therapeutic proteins in a fine-tuned manner to the defect site based on the severity of inflammation in the joint, we termed them smart transplants. Each component of smart transplants has been summarized below and is depicted in Figure 2.

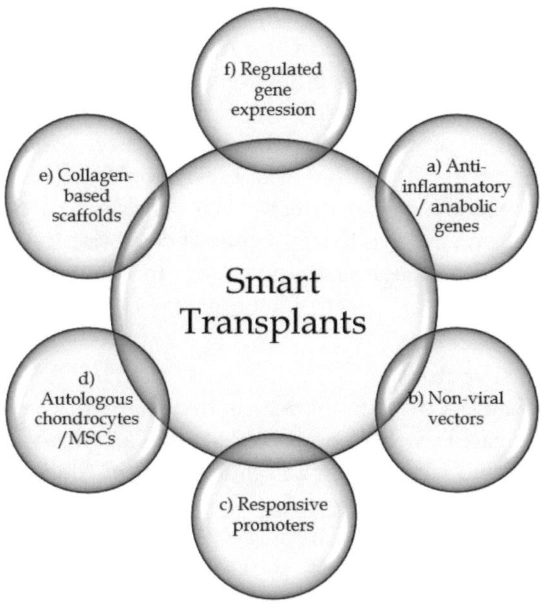

Fig. 2. A diagrammatic sketch showing the components of the smart transplant approach favoured by our research unit for future clinical application in veterinary as well as human medicine. Through recombinant DNA technology, (a) anti-inflammatory (IL-4) and/or anabolic (IGF-1) genes (a) are cloned with non-viral vectors (b) and endogenous responsive elements like COX-2 (c). Then the gene/vector cassette is introduced into autologous chondrocytes or MSCs (d) through an efficient transfection approach. The conditioned cells are finally seeded into collagen scaffolds (e) and finally implanted into the defected joint. Here it should secure a fine-tuned and regulated expression (f) of therapeutic proteins at the time when they are needed, i.e. when inflammatory mediators dominate the surrounding milieu.

7.1 Selection of genes for OA gene therapy

Though various biological factors have been independently identified as necessary for reducing inflammation or promoting regeneration in the diseased joint, the most promising therapeutic agents are those that modulate the activities of the pro-inflammatory cytokines IL-1β and TNFα (Fukui et al., 2003; M.B. Goldring, 1999; Martel-Pelletier et al., 1999). Several (anti-inflammatory) agents have been tested that suppress the production of pro-inflammatory mediators (Fernandes et al., 2002). Among these IL-4 (Woods et al., 2001), IL-10 (Amos et al., 2006), and IL-13 (Jovanovic et al., 1998) are of utmost significance in the context of OA. IL-4 compared to IL-10, has a higher potential to inhibit IL-1β (Rachakonda et al., 2008a, 2008b) and only IL-4 (not IL-10) can induce the production of IL-1Ra (Relic et al., 2001). Further, IL-4 can antagonize the effects of TNFα by inducing down-regulation and shedding of both forms of TNFα receptors while IL-13 failed to produce such effects (Manna & Aggarwal 1998) and unlike IL-4, it does not appear to directly regulate the growth of T_H2-type cells (Chomarat & Banchereau, 1998).

OA – particularly in its later stages – is characterized by inflammation and catabolism going side by side (M.B. Goldring & S.R. Goldring, 2007; Pelletier et al., 2001). Therefore, simultaneous expression of both anti-inflammatory and regenerative (anabolic) genes should be taken into consideration. One of the main anabolic mediators, which naturally aids in the protection of cartilage from regular wear and tear, is insulin-like growth factor-1 (IGF-1). IGF-1 is known to maintain homeostasis in articular cartilage by stimulating the synthesis of cartilage matrix proteins noted by an increased production of aggrecan and type II collagen (Manning et al., 2010). IL-4 and IGF-1 would offer a more complete therapy to combat the different aspects of the disease. We consider the dual expression of both proteins and surmise that an effective therapy should comprise the expression of both anti-inflammatory cytokines and cartilage anabolic factors to counteract the effects of catabolic mediators.

7.2 Selection of non-viral vectors

The most worrisome weakness of gene therapy is that many of the immunological defence systems which normally tackle wild-type infections are activated against the vectors and new transgene products might be recognized as foreign. In the past, great advances have been made to create new systems for the efficient production of gene-deleted less immunogenic vectors. These include the improvements such as expansion of the repertoire of vector tropisms and the evasion of pre-existing immune responses through the development of alternative viral serotypes (Hill et al., 1999; Thomas et al., 2003). Non-viral gene delivery is potentially safer than virus-mediated delivery with the exception of a few promising applications, such as vaccines. However, non-viral systems are, at the present, limited by their relatively low transfer efficiency (Thomas et al., 2003). Nevertheless, we prefer the use of non-viral vectors because of their higher safety level.

There is still a tremendous amount of work to be done in gene therapy research. We have encountered many obstacles so far, and will probably encounter more, but these obstacles are not insurmountable. By continuing to identify and address potential hurdles and by maintaining a strong focus on improving vectors and delivery protocols, gene therapy will eventually play a significant role in the treatment of severe inflammatory joint diseases.

7.3 Selection of suitable target cells

The most obvious source for cells that can regenerate cartilage is the tissue itself. Chondrocytes are the cells which reside within and retain and remodel this tissue (M.B. Goldring, 2006). They represent a homogenous population with limited (cell) number and tend to rapidly de-differentiate upon expansion *in vitro* with a complete loss of phenotype. Adequate tissue repair strategies may require specific cellular targeting to the site of injury as retention and engraftment of transplanted cells are inadequate. Besides clinically applied tissue-specific chondrocytes, undifferentiated bone-marrow origin MSCs are of special interest as promising candidates due to multiple advantages over the conventional chondrocytes (Pittenger et al., 1999). These advantages include, for instance, the trophic production of bioactive factors to initiate endogenous regenerative activities in OA (Nöth et al., 2008), their anti-inflammatory and immunosuppressive properties (Jorgensen& Apparailly, 2010) and their capacity to differentiate into chondrocytes.

7.4 Regulation of gene expression

Most gene therapy protocols involve constitutive delivery of therapeutic genes due to the transient nature of expression. In such instances, efficient gene transfer, expression, or stability have encountered limitations in preclinical and clinical applications mainly due to pleiotropic effects of the inducer, low-level basal expression and toxicity of the inducing agents. However, a non-toxic regulation of transgene expression may offer an effective means to control the expression levels of proteins with a narrow therapeutic index such as cytokines and hormones. Obviously, it would be most desirable to control the expression of therapeutic proteins in a disease-dependent manner. This would add considerably to the safety level of the gene therapy application. Incidentally, constitutive over-expression of transgenes typically would lead to detrimental effects under disease conditions. Therefore, regulation of gene expression is warranted. We have previously designed and reported a self-limiting promoter construct that expresses an anti-inflammatory gene only in the presence of inflammation (Patent: PCT/EP 2008/061408 published as US-2010-0255572-A1). The use of this construct for the expression of anti-inflammatory genes allows the production of a therapeutic gene product that is controlled by the severity of the disease. The effectiveness of this promoter construct for combating inflammation makes it a suitable candidate for the development of a new local gene therapy strategy for the treatment of OA (Rachakonda et al., 2008a). Furthermore, the ability to effectively control gene expression should also facilitate gene therapy studies because it will permit the expression of therapeutic genes and subsequently proteins to be regulated within the host. Thus, the application of inflammation-regulated therapeutic gene expression in arthritis conditions increases the efficiency of gene therapy by self-limiting the transgene.

Such elegant approaches have been adopted by applying disease-regulated promoters in a number of published reports (Cui et al., 2006; Godbey & Atala, 2003; Meynier de Salinelles et al., 2002; Miagkov et al., 2002; Rygg et al., 2001; Uhlar et al., 1997; Varley et al., 1995). Elements of the IL-1 and IL-6 promoter or of the COX-2 promoter, which are activated under inflammatory conditions, should up-regulate the transcription of transgenes such as IL-4 during acute OA and decrease expression rates after cessation of inflammation (Geurts et al., 2007; Rachakonda et al., 2008a). These self-regulating approaches may lead to safer stable transplants, which smartly react to the OA status of the joint.

7.5 Selection of suitable scaffolds

The selection of suitable scaffolds represents an important step to restore the damaged cartilage. Therefore, the selection of a suitable matrix composition may stabilize the transplant and support the regenerative process. Furthermore, the delivery of therapeutic genes will be more effective in a matrix that provides suitable protection, since the target cell population must often be exposed to factors throughout the entire course of repair, or at least for an extended period of time. An increased retention at treatment sites could also enable regenerative tissue-forming cells to migrate to the area of injury and to proliferate and differentiate. In addition, the materials should be biodegradable and remodel as the new cartilage forms and replaces the original construct. These matrix materials could be combined with other types of carriers, which release active factors into the environment as they disperse or are degraded without providing any matrix function.

In this regard, the matrix should be non-toxic, non-adhesive and non-stimulatory for inflammatory cells such as lymphocytes, macrophages and neutrophils. Furthermore, any matrix material needs to be non-immunogenic since immunological attack to this material (then serving as an antigen) would be detrimental to tissue regeneration. The topography and material properties of natural scaffolds should also support the differentiation of MSCs. Finally, the scaffolds should be easy to handle during surgery thereby allowing the fixation of the transplant into the implant site with ease. From our experience rat tail collagen-based scaffolds have a number of advantages along these lines.

8. Preliminary data on "Smart Transplants"

It has been shown previously that chondrocytes in scaffolds are susceptible to inflammatory mediators (Kuroki et al., 2005; Rai et al., 2008). This scenario indirectly raises a question on the validity of ACT into cartilage lesions surrounded by progressive inflammation (Hennerbichler et al., 2008). In order to address this problem, we validated the inducible expression of IL-4 in chondrocytes (Rachakonda et al., 2008a, 2008b) and in a chondrocyte-based, 3-dimensional inflammation model (Rai et al., 2011). The main objective was to examine whether IL-4 produced within scaffolds can down-regulate inflammation and recoup extracellular matrix synthesis in the face of inflammation. We believe that this was the first study of its type to assess the use of cytokine-therapy devoid of viral vectors in a 3-dimensional *in vitro* inflammation model.

Mature canine chondrocytes were conditioned through transient transfection using pcDNA3.1.IL-4 (constitutive) or pCOX-2.IL-4 (cytokine-responsive) plasmids. Conditioned cells were seeded in alginate microspheres and rat-tail collagen type I matrix (CaReS) to generate two types of tissue-engineered scaffolds, alginate beads and CaReS-matrices containing engineered chondrocytes. Inflammation was induced in the packed chondrocytes through addition of recombinant IL-1β plus TNFα into the culture medium. Harvested cells and culture media were analysed by various assays to monitor the anti-inflammatory and regulatory (anabolic) properties of IL-4 (Rai et al., 2011).

The data obtained proved that IL-4 was expressed at sufficient levels to effectively down-regulate inflammation in both types of scaffolds. This indicated that both scaffolds containing conditioned chondrocytes allowed unrestricted diffusion of cytokines in and out of the cells and through the matrix network into the surrounding culture medium. It was shown that IL-4 was able to successfully down-regulate several pro-inflammatory cytokines, matrix degrading enzymes and various catabolic end products such as nitric oxide and prostaglandin. Further, the biochemical assessment of the levels of collagen and sulphated GAG also indicated the anabolic net effect of IL-4 on chondrocytes.

One of the important characteristics of our approach is the ability of the pCOX-2.IL-4 construct to deliver the therapeutic gene (in this case IL-4) only upon stimulation with exogenous IL-1β and TNFα. Thereby the expression of IL-4 is controlled through the severity of inflammation as defined by the presence of pro-inflammatory cytokines (Figure 3).

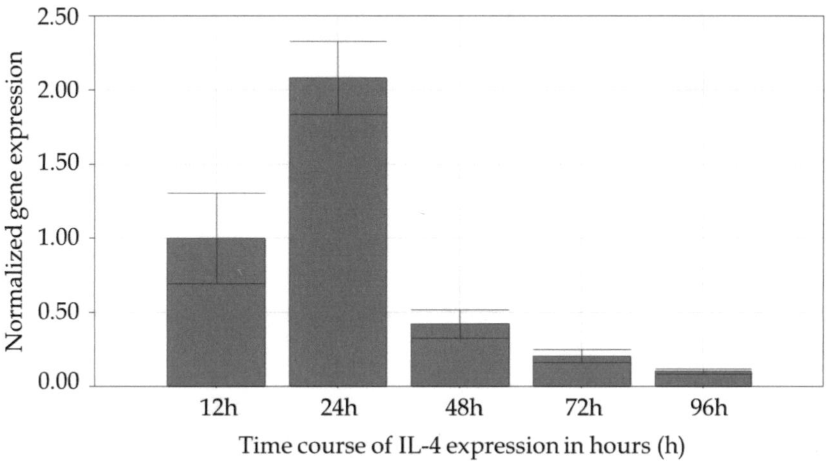

Fig. 3. Control of IL-4 expression through inflammatory mediators via the COX-2 promoter. **Experimental setup:** Conditioned chondrocytes (transfected with COX-2.IL-4) in scaffolds (CaReS) were stimulated by a 96 h exogenous treatment with IL-1β and TNFα. Thereafter the cells were re-isolated from the scaffolds and the expression levels of IL-4 assessed by qRT-PCR over time. The results show that after inflammatory induction IL-4 reaches peak levels at 24 hours followed by downregulation. **Interpretation:** Since endogenous pro-inflammatory mediators IL-1β and TNFα are both reduced under the influence of the regulatory action of IL-4 (data not shown, compare Manning et al., 2010 & Rai et al., 2011), the induction of the inflammation sensitive COX-2 promoter will also be attenuated. Since the IL-4 gene is transcribed under the control of this promoter, its own expression will eventually fade out. **Take home:** In smart transplants therapeutic genes under the control of the COX-2 promoter will only be expressed when inflammatory mediators are present close to the defective joint area. Thus, local therapy occurs only when it is needed - it is simply smart.

Since chondrocytes were conditioned by transfection prior to the generation of scaffolds, we coined a new term for this type of approach: ACCT (autologous conditioned cell therapy). Thus, therapeutic expression only occurs in a clearly defined condition, i.e. when the "conditioned" cells present in the scaffold "sense" inflammation in their surroundings.
We have also worked on the dual expression of IL-4 and IGF-1 in chondrocytes (Manning et al., 2010) because this approach potentially offers a more complete therapy to combat the different aspects of OA. The use of multiple genes could better alleviate the signs and symptoms characteristic for the disease process. Extension of this strategy to other suitable genes or combination of genes could in the future provide a better outlook to effectively heal OA. Ideally, if the cytokine-responsive matrices described above do work in the patient as they do *in vitro*, a promising strategy for the treatment of OA may emerge in the future.
Without any doubt, future therapy trials will have to occur to validate this novel approach.

9. Summary and future perspectives

OA affects a huge population of elderly. Recent progress in the understanding of OA pathophysiology has facilitated the development of therapeutic strategies aimed specifically at effectively retarding the disease process. Unfortunately most therapeutic efforts appear to have been directed either to temporal pain relief, or to the repair of OA-related cartilage lesions. As a final resort total joint replacement through surgery will be necessary. Gene therapy still has many pitfalls. The use of viral vectors and the unrestricted expression of transgenes are still subject to unanswered safety questions posed by the regulatory authorities. Nevertheless, it is tempting to speculate that an effective stimulation of cartilage regeneration paralleled by an inhibition of inflammation must be the key objectives of new therapeutic approaches. The negative impact of gene therapy can be overcome if it is suitably improved in each of its components. The first and foremost component of gene therapy is the vector. Viral vectors can be replaced by non-viral vectors regardless of which therapeutic genes they orchestrate and what expression levels may be achieved. Further, the promoter placed upstream of the therapeutic gene should be disease-dependent. In OA it should be inflammation dependent – like a COX-2 promoter that is always up-regulated when IL-1β and TNFα are up in the joint. Because IL-1β and TNFα drive OA progression and cartilage degradation, they become an important target in OA. Thus, genes like IL-4 and IGF-1 not only can coup with these pro-inflammatory cytokines, they also help to rebuild the normal cartilage tissue architecture.

For the delivery of suitable therapeutic genes in a non-viral approach, the selection of target cells is very important. Nature has provided the cartilage with only one cell type i.e. chondrocytes. In our opinion they are the best choice for transplantation in cartilage-related problems. But owing to their rapid differentiation into fibroblasts and lower cell number from a limited area of cartilage, stem cells may offer an important alternative in the future. Cell transplantation will require assembly for their implantation in the joint for which a wide-array of scaffolds is available. Whenever conditioned cells are involved that produce therapeutic proteins the best scaffolds are those that provide free diffusion of biological agents in and out.

To this end, we have established the applicability and usefulness of cell-seeded scaffolds *in vitro*. We cloned IL-4 downstream of a COX-2 promoter and transfected chondrocytes with the COX-2.IL-4 construct. The chondrocytes were then seeded into collagen type I scaffolds. To test the regulated expression of IL-4, a model of inflammatory arthritis was simulated by adding IL-1β and TNFα to the culture medium overlaying chondrocytes that were previously transfected (conditioned). Through the nuclear factor kappa B (NFκB) pathway IL-1β and TNFα up-regulated COX-2 which drove the expression of downstream IL-4. IL-4 in turn down-regulated multiple pro-inflammatory cytokines (e.g. IL-1β and TNFα), enzyme mediators and their catabolites and up-regulated the matrix molecules. Once the expression of IL-1β and TNFα dropped, COX-2 stopped the expression of IL-4 through a negative feedback loop mechanism (compare Figure 3). In this way the cells which were conditioned and incorporated within the scaffold, delivered the therapeutic effects of proteins in a coordinated and controlled manner. Our preliminary data form *in vitro* experiments are promising in many respects. It is realized that future therapy trials will have to reveal, whether ACCT with scaffolds containing conditioned cells will satisfy expectations as an effective approach.

The future of gene therapy as a viable medical application can be summarized in the words phrased by French Anderson in 1998: "Despite our present lack of knowledge, gene therapy will almost certainly revolutionize the practice of medicine over the next 25 years. In every field of medicine, the ability to give the patient therapeutic genes offers extraordinary opportunities to treat, cure and ultimately prevent a vast range of diseases that now plague mankind"(Anderson, 1998). Impressive progress has been made thus far, but nevertheless it seems we need the remaining 12 years to see where we stand.

10. References

Abramson, S.B. & Yazici, Y. (2006). Biologics in Development for Rheumatoid Arthritis: Relevance to Osteoarthritis. *Advanced Drug Delivery Reviews*, Vol.58, No.2, (May 2006), pp. 212-225, ISSN 0169-409X

Adachi, N., Sato, K., Usas, A., Fu, F.H., Ochi, M., Han, C.W., Niyibizi, C. & Huard, J. (2002). Muscle-derived, Cell-based *Ex Vivo* Gene Therapy for Treatment of Full-thickness Articular Cartilage Defects. *Journal of Rheumatology*, Vol.29, No.9, (September 2002), pp. 1920-1930, ISSN 0315-162X

Amos, N., Lauder, S., Evans, A., Feldmann, M. & Bondeson, J. (2006). Adenoviral Gene Transfer into Osteoarthritis Synovial Cells using the Endogenous Inhibitor IκBα Reveals that most, but not all, Inflammatory and Destructive Mediators are NFκB Dependent. *Rheumatology*, Vol.45, No.10, (October 2006), pp. 1201-1209, ISSN 1462-0324

Andereya, S., Maus, U., Gavenis, K., Müller-Rath, R., Miltner, O., Mumme, T. & Schneider, U. (2007). First Clinical Experiences with a Novel 3D Collagen Gel (CaReS) for the Treatment of Focal Cartilage Defects in the Knee. *Zeitschrift für Orthopädie und Ihrer Grenzgebiete*, Vol.144, No.3, (May-June 2007), pp. 272-280, ISSN 0044-3220

Anderson, W.F. (1998). Human Gene Therapy. *Nature*, Vol.392, No.S6679, (April 1998), pp. 25-30, ISSN 1476-4687

Bandara, G., Robbins, P.D., Georgescu, H.I., Mueller, G.M., Glorioso, J.C. & Evans, C.H. (1992). Gene Transfer to Synoviocytes: Prospects for Gene Treatment of Arthritis. *DNA & Cell Biology*, Vol.11, No.3, (April 1992), pp. 227-231, ISSN 1044-5498

Brittberg, M., Lindahl, A., Nilsson, A., Ohlsson, C., Isaksson, O. & Peterson, L. (1994). Treatment of Deep Cartilage Defects in the Knee with Autologous Chondrocyte Transplantation. *New England Journal of Medicine*, Vol.331, No.14, (October 1994), pp. 889-895, ISSN 0028-4793

Buckwalter, J.A., Martin, J.A. & Brown, T.D. (2006). Perspectives on Chondrocyte Mechanobiology and Osteoarthritis. *Biorheology*, Vol.43, No.3-4, (September 2006), pp. 603-609, ISSN 0006-355X

Capito, R.M. & Spector, M. (2007). Collagen Scaffolds for Non-viral IGF-1 Gene Delivery in Articular Cartilage Tissue-engineering. *Gene Therapy*, Vol.14, No.9, (May 2007), pp. 721-732, ISSN 0969-7128

Celiker, M.Y., Ramamurthy, N., Xu, J.W., Wang, M., Jiang, Y., Greenwald, R. & Shi, Y.E. (2002). Inhibition of Adjuvant-induced Arthritis by Systemic Tissue Inhibitor of Metalloproteinases-4 Gene Delivery. *Arthritis & Rheumatism*, Vol.46, No.12, (December 2002), pp. 3361-3368, ISSN 0004-3591

Chomarat, P. & Banchereau, J. (1998). Interleukin-4 and Interleukin-13: Their Similarities and Discrepancies. *International Reviews of Immunology,* Vol.17, No.1-4, (January 1998), pp. 1-52, ISSN 0883-0185

Clouet, J., Vinatier, C., Merceron, C., Pot-vaucel, M., Maugars, Y., Weiss, P., Grimandi, G. & Guicheux, J. (2009). From Osteoarthritis Treatments to Future Regenerative Therapies for Cartilage. *Drug Discovery Today,* Vol.14, No.19-20, (October 2009), pp. 913-925, ISSN 1359-6446

Cucchiarini, M. & Madry, H. (2005). Gene Therapy for Cartilage Defects. *Journal of Gene Medicine,* Vol.7, No.12, (December 2005), pp. 1495-1509, ISSN 1099-498X

Cucchiarini, M., Thurn, T., Weimer, A., Kohn, D., Terwilliger, E.F. & Madry, H. (2007). Restoration of the Extracellular Matrix in Human Osteoarthritic Articular Cartilage by Over-expression of the Transcription Factor SOX-9. *Arthritis & Rheumatism,* Vol.56, No.1, (January 2007), pp. 158-167, ISSN 0004-3591

Cui, X., Yang, S.C., Sharma, S., Heuze-Vourc'h, N. & Dubinett, S.M. (2006). IL-4 Regulates COX-2 and PGE2 Production in Human Non-small Cell Lung Cancer. *Biochemical & Biophysical Research Communications,* Vol.343, No.4, (May 2006), pp. 995-1001, ISSN 0006-291X

Di Cesare, P.E., Frenkel, S.R., Carlson, C.S., Fang, C. & Liu, C. (2006). Regional Gene Therapy for Full-thickness Articular Cartilage Lesions using Naked DNA with a Collagen Matrix. *Journal of Orthopaedic Research,* Vol.24, No.5, (May 2006), pp. 1118-1127, ISSN 0736-0266

Donkuru, M., Badea, I., Wettig, S., Verrall, R., Elsabahy, M. & Foldvari, M. (2010). Advancing Nonviral Gene Delivery: Lipid- and Surfactant-based Nanoparticle Design Strategies. *Nanomedicine,* Vol.5, No.7, (September 2010), pp. 1103-1127, ISSN 1743-5889

Dougados, M. (2006). Symptomatic Slow-acting Drugs for Osteoarthritis: What are the Facts? *Joint Bone Spine,* Vol.73, No.6, (December 2006), pp. 606-609, ISSN 1297-319X

Evans, C.H. & Robbins, P.D. (1994). The Interleukin-1 Receptor Antagonist and its Delivery by Gene Transfer. *Receptor,* Vol.4, No.1, (Spring 1994), pp. 9-15, ISSN 1052-8040

Evans, C.H., Ghivizzani, S.C., Oligino, T.A. & Robbins, P.D. (2001). Future of Adenoviruses in the Gene Therapy of Arthritis. *Arthritis Research,* Vol.3, No.3, (n.d. 2001), pp. 142-146, ISSN 1465-9905

Evans, C.H., Gouze, J.N., Gouze, E., Robbins, P.D. & Ghivizzani, S.C. (2004). Osteoarthritis Gene Therapy. *Gene Therapy,* Vol.11, No.4, (February 2004), pp. 379-389, ISSN 0969-7128

Evans, C.H., Robbins, P.D., Ghivizzani, S.C., Wasko, M.C., Tomaino, M.M., Kang, R., Muzzonigro, T.A., Vogt, M., Elder, E.M., Whiteside, T.L., Watkins, S.C. & Herndon, J.H. (2005). Gene Transfer to Human Joints: Progress toward a Gene Therapy of Arthritis. *Proceedings of the National Academy of Sciences of the United States of America,* Vol.102, No.24, (June 2005), pp. 8698-8703, ISSN 0027-8424

Evans, C.H., Ghivizzani, S.C. & Robbins, P.D. (2009). Gene Therapy of the Rheumatic Diseases: 1998 to 2008. *Arthritis Research & Therapy,* Vol.11, No.1, (January 2009), pp. 209, ISSN 1478-6354

Evans, C.H., Ghivizzani, S.C. & Robbins, P.D. (2011). Getting Arthritis Gene Therapy into the Clinic. *Nature Reviews Rheumatology*, Vol.7, No.4, (April 2011), pp. 244-249, ISSN 1759-4790

Fernandes, J.C., Tardif, G., Martel-Pelletier, J., Lascau-Coman, V., Dupuis, M., Moldovan, F., Sheppard, M., Krishnan, B.R. & Pelletier, J.P. (1999). *In Vivo* Transfer of Interleukin-1 Receptor Antagonist Gene in Osteoarthritic Rabbit Knee Joints. Prevention of Osteoarthritis Progression. *American Journal of Pathology*, Vol.154, No.4, (April 1999), pp. 1159-1169, ISSN 0002-9440

Fernandes, J.C., Martel-Pelletier, J. & Pelletier, J.P. (2002). The Role of Cytokines in Osteoarthritis Pathophysiology. *Biorheology*, Vol.39, No.1-2, (January 2002), pp. 237-246, ISSN 0006-355X

Frisbie, D.D., Ghivizzani, S.C., Robbins, P.D., Evans, C.H. & McIlwraith, C.W. (2002). Treatment of Experimental Equine Osteoarthritis by *In Vivo* Delivery of the Equine Interleukin-1 Receptor Antagonist Gene. *Gene Therapy*, Vol.9, No.1, (January 2002), pp. 12-20, ISSN 0969-7128

Fukui, N., Zhu, Y., Maloney, W.J., Clohisy, J. & Sandell, L.J. (2003). Stimulation of BMP-2 Expression by Pro-inflammatory Cytokines IL-1 and TNFα in Normal and Osteoarthritic Chondrocytes. *The Journal of Bone & Joint Surgery (America)*, Vol.85, No.3, (August 2003), pp. 59-66, ISSN 1535-1386

Gelse, K., von der Mark, K., Aigner, T., Park, J. & Schneider, H. (2003). Articular Cartilage Repair by Gene Therapy using Growth Factor–producing Mesenchymal Cells. *Arthritis & Rheumatism*, Vol.48, No.2, (February 2003), pp. 430-441, ISSN 0004-3591

Geurts, J., Arntz, O.J., Bennink, M.B., Joosten, L.A., van den Berg, W.B. & van de Loo, F.A. (2007). Application of a Disease-regulated Promoter is a Safer Mode of Local IL-4 Gene Therapy for Arthritis. *Gene Therapy*, Vol.14, No.23, (December 2007), pp.1632-1638, ISSN 0969-7128

Ghivizzani, S.C., Lechman, E.R., Tio, C., Mulé, K.M., Chada, S., McCormack, J.E., Evans, C.H. & Robbins, P.D. (1997). Direct Retrovirus-mediated Gene Transfer to the Synovium of the Rabbit Knee: Implications for Arthritis Gene Therapy. *Gene Therapy*, Vol.4, No.9, (September 1997), pp. 977-982, ISSN 0969-7128

Ghivizzani, S.C., Lechman, E.R., Kang, R., Tio, C., Kolls, J., Evans, C.H. & Robbins, P.D.(1998). Direct Adenovirus-mediated Gene Transfer of Interleukin-1 and Tumour Necrosis Factor-alpha Soluble Receptors to Rabbit Knees with Experimental Arthritis hasLocal and Distal Anti-arthritic Effects. *Proceedings of the National Academy of Sciences of the United States of America*, Vol.95, No.8, (April 1998), pp. 4613-4618, ISSN 0027-8424

Gibbons, L.J. & Hyrich, K.L. (2009). Biologic Therapy for Rheumatoid Arthritis: Clinical Efficacy and Predictors of Response. *BioDrugs*, Vol.23, No.2, (April 2009), pp. 111-124, ISSN 1173-8804

Godbey, W.T. & Atala, A. (2003). Directed Apoptosis in COX-2-overexpressing Cancer Cells through Expression-targeted Gene Delivery. *Gene Therapy*, Vol.10, No.17, (August 2003), pp. 1519-1527, ISSN 0969-7128

Godfrey, D.R. (2005). Osteoarthritis in Cats: ARetrospective Radiological Study. *The Journal of Small Animal Practice*,Vol.46, No.9, (September 2005), pp. 425-429, ISSN 0022-4510

Goehring, A.R., Lübke, C., Kaps, C., Häupl, T., Pruss, A., Perka, C., Sittinger, M. & Ringe, J. (2010). Tissue-engineered Cartilage of Porcine and Human Origin as In Vitro Test System in Arthritis Research. *Biotechnology Progress*, Vol.26, No.4, (July-August 2010), pp. 1116-1125, ISSN 1520-6033

Goldring, M.B. (1999). The Role of Cytokines as Inflammatory Mediators in Osteoarthritis: Lessons from Animal Models. *Connective Tissue Research,* Vol.40, No.1, (January 1999), pp. 1-11, ISSN 0300-8207

Goldring, M.B. (2001). Anticytokine Therapy for Osteoarthritis. *Expert Opinion on Biological Therapy*, Vol.1, No.5, (September 2001), pp. 817-829, ISSN 1471-2598

Goldring, M.B. (2006). Update on the Biology of the Chondrocyte and New Approaches to Treating Cartilage Diseases. *Best Practice & Research: Clinical Rheumatology*, Vol.20, No.5, (October 2006), pp. 1003-1025, ISSN 1521-6942

Goldring, M.B. & Goldring, S.R.(2007). Osteoarthritis. *Journal of Cellular Physiology*, Vol.21, No.3, (December 2007), pp. 626-634, ISSN 0021-9541

Gouze, E., Pawliuk, R., Pilapil, C., Gouze, J.N., Fleet, C., Palmer, G.D., Evans, C.H., Leboulch, P. & Ghivizzani, S.C. (2002). *In Vivo* Gene Delivery to Synovium by Lentiviral Vectors. *Molecular Therapy*, Vol.5, No.4, (April 2002), pp. 397-404, ISSN 1525-0016

Gouze, E., Gouze, J.N., Palmer, G.D., Pilapil, C., Evans, C.H. & Ghivizzani S.C. (2007). Transgene Persistence and Cell Turnover in the Diarthrodial Joint: Implications for Gene Therapy of Chronic Joint Diseases. *Molecular Therapy*, Vol.15, No.6, (June 2007), pp. 1114-1120, ISSN 1525-0016

Gouze, J.N., Gouze, E., Palmer, G.D., Kaneto, H., Ghivizzani, S.C., Grodzinsky, A.J. & Evans, C.H. (2004). Adenovirus-mediated Gene Transfer of Glutamine: Fructose-6-phosphate Amidotransferase Antagonizes the Effects of Interleukin-1β on Rat Chondrocytes. *Osteoarthritis & Cartilage*, Vol.12, No.3, (March 2004), pp. 217-224, ISSN 1063-4584

Grossin, L., Cournil-Henrionnet, C., Mir, L.M., Liagre, B., Dumas, D., Etienne, S., Guingamp, C., Netter, P. & Gillet, P. (2003). Direct Gene Transfer into Rat Articular Cartilage by *In Vivo* Electroporation. *The FASEB Journal*, Vol.17, No.8, (May 2003), pp. 829-835, ISSN 0892-6638

Grossin, L., Cournil-Henrionnet, C., Pinzano, A., Gaborit, N., Dumas, D., Etienne, S., Stoltz, J.F., Terlain, B., Netter, P., Mir, L.M. & Gillet, P. (2006). Gene Transfer with HSP 70 in Rat Chondrocytes Confers Cytoprotection *In Vitro* and during Experimental Osteoarthritis. *The FASEB Journal*, Vol.20, No.1, (January 2006), pp. 65-75, ISSN 0892 6638

Guo, J., Jourdian, G. & Maccallum, D.K. (1989). Culture and Growth Characteristic of Chondrocytes Encapsulated in Alginate Beads. *Connective Tissue Research,* Vol.19, No.2-4, (n.d. 1989), pp. 277-285, ISSN 1607-8438

Haag, J., Voigt, R., Soeder, S. & Aigner, T. (2009). Efficient Non-viral Transfection of Primary Human Adult Chondrocytes in a High-throughput Format. *Osteoarthritis & Cartilage,* Vol. 17, No.6, (June 2009), pp. 813-817, ISSN 1063-4584

Habib, G.S., Saliba, W. & Nashashibi, M. (2010). Local Effects of Intra-articular Corticosteroids. *Clinical Rheumatology*, Vol.29, No.4, (April 2010), pp. 347-356, ISSN 0770-3198

Harui, A., Suzuki, S., Kochanek, S. & Mitani, K. (1999). Frequency and Stability of Chromosomal Integration of Adenovirus Vectors. *Journal of Virology*, Vol.73, No.7, (July 1999), pp. 6141-6146, ISSN 0022-538X

Häuselmann, H.J., Fernandes, R.J., Mok, S.S., Schmid, T.M., Block, J.A., Aydelotte, M.B., Kuettner, K.E., Eugene, J.M. & Thonar, E.J. (1994). Phenotypic Stability of Bovine Articular Chondrocytes after Long-term Culture in Alginate Beads. *Journal of Cell Science*, Vol.107, No.1, (January 1994), pp. 17-27, ISSN 1477-9137

Heinegård, D. & Saxne, T. (2011). The Role of the Cartilage Matrix in Osteoarthritis. *Nature Reviews Rheumatology*, Vol.7, No.1, (January 2011), pp. 50-56, ISSN 1759-4790

Hennerbichler, A., Rosenberger, R., Arora, R., Hennerbichler, D. (2008). Biochemical, Biomechanical and Histological Properties of Osteoarthritic Porcine Knee Cartilage: Implications for Osteochondral Transplanation. *Archives of Orthopaedeic & Trauma Surgery*,Vol.128, No.1, (January 2008), pp. 61-70, ISSN 0936-8051

Hidaka, C., Goodrich, L.R., Chen, C.T., Warren, R.F., Crystal, R.G. & Nixon, A.J. (2003). Acceleration of Cartilage Repair by Genetically Modified Chondrocytes Over-expressing Bone Morphogenetic Protein-7. *Journal of Orthopaedic Research*, Vol.21, No.4, (July 2003), pp. 573-583, ISSN 0736-0266

Hill, C.L., Bieniasz, P.D. & McClure, M.O. (1999). Properties of Human Foamy Virus Relevant to its Development as a Vector for Gene Therapy. *The Journal of General Virology*, Vol.80, No.8, (August 1999), pp. 2003-2009, ISSN 0022-1317

Hotz-Behofsits, C.M., Walley, M.J, Simpson, R. & Bjarnason, I.T. (2003). COX-1, COX-2 and the Topical Effect in NSAID-induced Enteropathy. *Inflammopharmacology*, Vol.11, No.4 (n.d. 2003), pp. 363-370, ISSN 0925-4692

Hsieh, J.L., Shen, P.C., Shiau, A.L., Jou, I.M., Lee, C.H., Wang, C.R., Teo, M.L. & Wu, C.L. (2010). Intra-articular Gene Transfer of Thrombospondin-1 Suppresses the Disease Progression of Experimental Osteoarthritis. *Journal of Orthopaedic Research*, Vol.28, No.10, (October 2010), pp. 1300-1306, ISSN 0736-0266

Hunziker, E.B. (2002). Articular Cartilage Repair: Basic Science and Clinical Progress. A Review of the Current Status and Prospects. *Osteoarthritis & Cartilage*, Vol.10, No.6, (June 2002), pp. 432-463, ISSN 1063-4584.

Ikeda, K., Wakimoto, H., Ichikawa, T., Jhung, S., Hochberg, F.H., Louis, D.N. & Chiocca, E.A. (2000). Complement Depletion Facilitates the Infection of Multiple Brain Tumors by an Intravascular, Replication-Conditional Herpes Simplex Virus Mutant. *Journal of Virology*, Vol.74, No.10, (May 2000), pp. 4765-4775, ISSN 0022-538X

Im, G.I., Kim, D.Y., Shin, J.H., Hyun, C.W.& Cho, W.H. (2001). Repair of Cartilage Defect in the Rabbit with Cultured Mesenchymal Stem Cells from Bone-marrow. *The Journal of Bone & Joint Surgery (British)*, Vol.83, No.2, (March 2001), pp. 289-294, ISSN 0301-620X

Innes, J.F. & Clegg, P. (2010). Comparative Rheumatology: What can be Learnt from Naturally Occurring Musculoskeletal Disorders in Domestic Animals? *Rheumatology*,Vol.49, No.6, (June 2010), pp. 1030-1039, ISSN 1462-0324

Johnston, S.A. (1997). Osteoarthritis. Joint Anatomy, Physiology, and Pathobiology. *The Veterinary Clinics of North America: Small Animal Practice,* Vol.27, No.4, (July 1997), pp. 699-723, ISSN 0195-5616

Jorgensen, C. & Apparailly, F. (2010). Prospects for Gene Therapy in Inflammatory Arthritis. *Best Practice & Research: Clinical Rheumatology,* Vol.24, No.4, (August 2010), pp. 541-552, ISSN 1521-6942

Jovanovic, D., Pelletier, J.P., Alaaeddine, N., Mineau, F., Geng, C., Ranger, P. & Martel-Pelletier, J. (1998). Effect of IL-13 on Cytokines, Cytokine Receptors and Inhibitors on Human Osteoarthritis Synovium and Synovial Fibroblasts. *Osteoarthritis & Cartilage,* Vol.6, No.1, (January 1998), pp. 40-49, ISSN 1063-4584

Kang, R., Marui, T., Ghivizzani, S.C., Nita, I.M., Georgescu, H.I., Suh, J.K., Robbins, P.D. & Evans, C.H. (1997). *Ex Vivo* Gene Transfer to Chondrocytes in Full-thickness Articular Cartilage Defects: A Feasibility Study. *Osteoarthritis & Cartilage,* Vol.5, No.2, (March 1997), pp. 139-143, ISSN 1063-4584

Katayama, R., Wakitani, S., Tsumaki, N., Morita, Y., Matsushita, I., Gejo, R. & Kimura, T. (2004). Repair of Articular Cartilage Defects in Rabbits using CDMP1 Gene Transfected Autologous Mesenchymal Cells Derived from Bone Marrow. *Rheumatology,* Vol.43, No.8, (August 2004), pp. 980-985, ISSN 1462-0324

Katz, J.N., Brandon, E.E. & Gomoll, A.H.(2010). Surgical Management of Osteoarthritis. *Arthritis Care & Research,* Vol.62, No.9, (September 2010), pp. 1220-1228, ISSN 2151-464X

Kaul, G., Cucchiarini, M., Arntzen, D., Zurakowski, D., Menger, M.D., Kohn, D., Trippel, S.B. & Madry, H. (2006). Local Stimulation of Articular Cartilage Repair by Transplantationof Encapsulated Chondrocytes Over-expressing Human Fibroblast Growth Factor-2 (FGF-2) *In Vivo. Journal of Gene Medicine,* Vol.8, No.1, (January 2006), pp. 100-111, ISSN 1099-498X

Kulseng, B., Skjak-Braek, G., Ryan, L., Andersson, A., King, A., Faxvaag, A. & Espevik, T. (1999). Transplantation of Alginate Microcapsules: Generation of Antibodies against Alginates and Encapsulated Porcine Islet-like Cell Clusters. *Transplantation,* Vol.67, No.7, (April 1999), pp. 978-984, ISSN 1534-0608

Kuroki, K., Stoker, A.M. & Cook, J.L. (2005). Effects of Proinflammatory Cytokines on Canine Articular Chondrocytes in a Three-dimensional Culture. *American Journal of Veterinary Research,* Vol.66, No.7, (July 2005), pp. 187-196, ISSN 0002-9645

Lafeber, F.P., van Roy, H.L., van der Kraan, P.M., van den Berg, W.B. & Bijlsma, J.W. (1997). Transforming Growth Factor-beta Predominantly Stimulates Phenotypically Changed Chondrocytes in Osteoarthritic Human Cartilage. *The Journal of Rheumatology,* Vol.24, No.3, (March 1997), pp. 536-542, ISSN 0315-162X

Langer, R. & Tirrell, D.A. (2004). Designing Materials for Biology and Medicine. *Nature,* Vol.428, No.6982, (April 2004), pp. 487-492, ISSN 1476-4687

Lee, K.H., Song, S.U., Hwang, T.S., Yi, Y., Oh, I.S., Lee, J.Y., Choi, K.B. & Kim, S.J. (2001). Regeneration of Hyaline Cartilage by Cell-mediated Gene Therapy using

Transforming Growth Factor-β1-producing Fibroblasts. *Human Gene Therapy*, Vol.12, No.14, (September 2001), pp. 1805-1813, ISSN 1043-0342

Li, W.J., Jiang Y.J. & Tuan, R.S. (2006). Chondrocyte Phenotype in Engineered Fibrous Matrix is Regulated by Fiber Size. *Tissue Engineering*, Vol.12, No.7, (July 2006), pp. 1775-1785, ISSN 2152-4955

Liao, Y.H., Jones, S.A., Forbes, B., Martin, G.P. & Brown, M.B. (2005). Hyaluronan: Pharmaceutical Characterization and Drug Delivery. *Drug Delivery*, Vol.12, No.6, (November-December 2005), pp. 327-342, ISSN 1071-7544

Madeira, C., Ribeiro, S.C., Pinheiro, I.S., Martins, S.A., Andrade, P.Z., da Silva, C.L. & Cabral, J.M. (2011). Gene delivery to human bone marrow mesenchymal stem cells by microporation. *Journal of Biotechnology*, Vol.151, No.1, (January 2011), pp. 130-136, ISSN 0168-1656

Madry, H. & Trippel, S.B. (2000). Efficient Lipid-mediated Gene Transfer to Articular Chondrocytes. *Gene Therapy*, Vol.7, No.4, (February 2000), pp. 286-291, ISSN 0969-7128

Madry, H., Padera, R., Seidel, J., Langer, R., Freed, L.E., Trippel, S.B. & Vunjak-Novakovic, G. (2002). Gene Transfer of a Human Insulin-like Growth Factor 1 cDNA Enhances Tissue-engineering of Cartilage. *Human Gene Therapy*, Vol.13, No.13, (September 2002), pp. 1621-1630, ISSN 1043-0342

Madry, H., Cucchiarini, M., Terwilliger, E.F. & Trippel, S.B. (2003). Recombinant Adeno-associated Virus Vectors Efficiently and Persistently Transduce Chondrocytes in Normal and Osteoarthritic Human Articular Cartilage. *Human Gene Therapy*, Vol.14, No.4, (March 2003), pp. 393-402, ISSN 1043-0342

Madry, H., Emkey, G., Zurakowski, D. & Trippel, S.B. (2004). Over-expression of Human Fibroblast Growth Factor-2 Stimulates Cell Proliferation in an *Ex Vivo* Model of Articular Chondrocyte Transplantation. *The Journal of Gene Medicine*, Vol.6, No.2, (February 2004), pp. 238-245, ISSN 1099-498X

Madry, H., Kaul, G., Cucchiarini, M., Stein, U., Zurakowski, D., Remberger, K., Menger, M.D., Kohn, D. & Trippel, S.B. (2005). Enhanced Repair of Articular Cartilage Defects *In Vivo* by Transplanted Chondrocytes Over-expressing Insulin-like Growth Factor-1 (IGF-1). *Gene Therapy*, Vol.12, No.15, (August 2005), pp. 1171-1179, ISSN 0969-7128

Manna, S.K. & Aggarwal, B.B. (1998). Interleukin-4 Down-regulates both Forms of TumourNecrosis Factor Receptor and Receptor-mediated Apoptosis, NF-kappa B, AP-1, and c-Jun N-terminal Kinase. Comparison with Interleukin-13. *Journal of Biological Chemistry*, Vol.273, No.50, (December 1998), pp. 33333-33341, ISSN 1083-351X

Manning, K., Rachakonda, P.S., Rai, M.F. & Schmidt, M.F. (2010). Co-expression of Insulin-like Growth Factor-1 and Interleukin-4 in an *In Vitro* Inflammatory Model. *Cytokine*, Vol.50, No.3, (June 2010), pp. 297-305, ISSN 1043-4666

Martel-Pelletier, J., Alaaeddine, N. & Pelletier, J.P. (1999). Cytokines and their Role in the Pathophysiology of Osteoarthritis. *Frontiersin Bioscie*nce, Vol.4, No.D, (October 1999), pp. 694-703, ISSN 1093-9946

Martel-Pelletier, J. & Pelletier, J.P. (2007). Inflammatory Factors Involved in Osteoarthritis, In: *Osteoarthritis, Inflammation & Degradation: A Continuum*, J. Buckwalter, M. Lotz & J.F. Stolz, (Eds.), 3-13, IOS Press, ISBN 978-1-58603-773-4, Amsterdam, Netherlands

Mease, P.J., Wei, N., Fudman, E.J., Kivitz, A.J., Schechtman, J., Trapp, R.G., Hobbs, K.F., Greenwald, M., Hou, A., Bookbinder, S.A., Graham, G.E., Wiesenhutter, C.W., Willis, L., Ruderman, E.M., Forstot, J.Z., Maricic, M.J., Dao, K.H., Pritchard, C.H., Fiske, D.N., Burch, F.X., Prupas, H.M.,Anklesaria, P. & Heald, A.E. (2010). Safety, Tolerability, and Clinical Outcomes after Intra-articular Injection of a Recombinant Adeno-associated Vector Containing a Tumour Necrosis Factor Antagonist Gene: Results of a Phase 1/2 Study. *The Journal of Rheumatology*, Vol.37, No.4, (April 2010) pp. 692-703, ISSN 1499-2752

Meynier de Salinelles, V., Berenbaum, F., Jacques, C., Salvat, C., Olivier, J.L., Béréziat, G., Raymondjean, M. & Massaad, C. (2002). Design of a Chimeric Promoter induced by Pro-inflammatory Mediators in Articular Chondrocytes. *FEBS Letters*, Vol.518, No.1-3, (May 2002), pp. 67-71, ISSN 0014-5793

Miagkov, A.V., Varley, A.W., Munford, R.S. & Makarov, S.S. (2002). Endogenous Regulation of a Therapeutic Transgene Restores Homeostasis in Arthritic Joints. *Journal of Clinical Investigation*, Vol.109, No.9, (May 2002), pp. 1223-1229, ISSN 0021-9738

Minas, T., Gomoll, A.H., Solhpour, S., Rosenberger, R., Probst, C., Bryant, T. (2010). Autologous Chondrocyte Implantation for Joint Preservation in Patients with Early Osteoarthritis. *Clinical Orthopaedic & Related Research*,Vol.468, No.1, (January 2010), pp. 147-157, ISSN 0009-921X

Müller, R.D., John, T., Kohl, B., Oberholzer, A., Gust, T., Hostmann, A., Hellmuth, M., Laface, D., Hutchins, B., Laube, G., Veh, R.W., Tschoeke, S.K., Ertel, W. & Schulze-Tanzil, G. (2008). IL-10 Over-expression Differentially Affects Cartilage Matrix Gene Expression in Response to TNF-alpha in Human Articular Chondrocytes*In Vitro*. *Cytokine*, Vol.44, No.3, (December 2008), pp. 377-385, ISSN 1043-4666

Nabbe, K.C., van Lent, P.L., Holthuysen, A.E., Sloëtjes, A.W., Koch, A.E., Radstake, T.R. & van den Berg, W.B. (2005). Local IL-13 Gene Transfer Prior to Immune-complex Arthritis Inhibits Chondrocyte Death and Matrix-metalloproteinase-mediated Cartilage Matrix Degradation Despite Enhanced Joint Inflammation. *Arthritis Research & Therapy*, Vol.7, No.2, (January 2005), pp. R392-R401, ISSN 1478-6362

Nöth, U., Tuli, R., Osyczka, A.M., Danielson, K.G. & Tuan, R.S. (2002).*In Vitro*Engineered Cartilage Constructs Produced by Press-coating Biodegradable Polymer with Human Mesenchymal Stem Cells. *Tissue Engineering*, Vol.8, No.1, (n.d. 2002), pp.131-144, ISSN 2152-4955

Nöth, U., Steinert, A.F. & Tuan, R.S. (2008). Technology Insight: Adult Mesenchymal Stem Cells for Osteoarthritis Therapy. *Nature Clinical Practice: Rheumatology*, Vol.4, No.7, (July 2008), pp. 371-380, ISSN 1745-8382

Park, J.Y., Pillinger, M.H. & Abramson, S.B. (2006). Prostaglandin E2 Synthesis and Secretion: The Role of PGE2 Synthases. *Clinical Immunology*, Vol.119, No.3, (June 2006), pp. 229-240, ISSN 1521-6616

Parker, D.A., Beatty, K.T., Giuffre, B., Scholes, C.J.&Coolican, M.R. (2011). Articular Cartilage Changes in Patients with Osteoarthritis after Osteotomy. *The American Journal of Sports Medicine,* Vol.39, No.5, (May 2011), ISSN 0363-5465

Pelletier, J.P., Caron, J.P., Evans, C., Robbins, P.D., Georgescu, H.I., Jovanovic, D., Fernandes, J.C. & Martel-Pelletier, J. (1997). *In Vivo* Suppression of Early Experimental Osteoarthritis by Interleukin-1 Receptor Antagonist using Gene Therapy. *Arthritis & Rheumatism,* Vol.40S, No.6, (June 1997), pp. 1012-1019, ISSN 0004-3591

Pelletier, J.P., Martel-Pelletier, J. & Abramson, S.B. (2001). Osteoarthritis, an Inflammatory Disease: Potential Implication for the Selection of New Therapeutic Targets. *Arthritis & Rheumatism,* Vol.44, No.6, (June 2001), pp. 1237-1247, ISSN 00043591

Peterson, L., Brittberg, M., Kiviranta, I., Akerlund, E.L.& Lindahl, A. (2002). Autologous Chondrocyte Transplantation. Biomechanics and Long-term Durability. *The American Journal of Sports Medicine,* Vol.30, No.1,(January-February 2002), pp. 2-12, ISSN 0363-5465

Philpott, N.J. & Thrasher, A.J. (2007). Use of Non-integrating Lentiviral Vectors for Gene Therapy. *Human Gene Therapy,* Vol.18, No.6, (June 2007), pp. 483-489, ISSN 1043-0342

Pittenger, M.F., Mackay, A.M., Beck, S.C., Jaiswal, R.K., Douglas, R., Mosca, J.D., Moorman, M.A., Simonetti, D.W., Craig, S. & Marshak, D.R. (1999). Multilineage Potential of Adult Human Mesenchymal Stem Cells. *Science,* Vol.284, No.5411, (April 1999), pp. 143-147, ISSN 1095-9203

Plank, C., Schillinger, U., Scherer, F., Bergemann, C., Rémy, J.S., Krötz, F., Anton, M.,Lausier, J. & Rosenecker, J. (2003). The Magnetofection Method: Using Magnetic Force to Enhance Gene Delivery. *Biological Chemistry,*Vol.384, No.5, (May 2003), pp. 737-747, ISSN 0021-9258.

Poole, C.A., Honda, T., Skinner, S.J., Schofield, J.R., Hyde, K.F. & Shinkai, H. (1990). Chondrons from Articular Cartilage (II): Analysis of the Glycosaminoglycans in the Cellular Microenvironment of Isolated Canine Chondrons. *Connective Tissue Research,* Vol.24, No.3-4, (n.d. 1990), pp. 319-330, ISSN 1607-8438

Rachakonda, P.S., Rai, M.F. & Schmidt, M.F. (2008a). Application of Inflammation Responsive Promoter for an *In Vitro* Arthritis Model. *Arthritis & Rheumatism,*Vol. 58, No. 7, (July 2008), pp. 2088-2097, ISSN 0004-3591

Rachakonda, P.S., Rai, M.F., Manning, K. & Schmidt, M.F. (2008b). Expression of Canine Interleukin-4 in Canine Chondrocytes Inhibits Inflammatory Cascade through STAT6. *Cytokine,* Vol.44, No.1, (October 2008), pp. 179-184, ISSN 1043-4666

Rai, M.F., Rachakonda, P.S., Manning, K., Vorwerk, B., Brunnberg, L., Kohn, B. & Schmidt M.F. (2008). Quantification of Cytokines and Inflammatory Mediators in a Three-dimensional Model of Inflammatory Arthritis. *Cytokine,* Vol.42, No.1, (April 2008), pp. 8–17,ISSN 1043-4666

Rai, M.F., Rachakonda, P.S., Manning, K., Palissa, C., Sittinger, M., Ringe, J. & Schmidt, M.F. (2009). Molecular and Phenotypic Modulation of Primary and Immortalized Canine Chondrocytes in Different Culture Systems. *Research in Veterinary Science,* Vol.87, No.3, (December 2009), pp. 399-407,ISSN 0034-5288

Rai, M.F., Graeve, T., Twardziok, S. & Schmidt, M.F. (2011). Evidence for Regulated Interleukin-4 Expression in Chondrocyte-scaffolds Under *In Vitro* Inflammatory Conditions. (submitted)

Relic, B., Guicheux, J., Mezin, F., Lubberts, E., Togninalli, D., Garcia, I., van den Berg, W.B. & Guerne, P.A. (2001). IL-4 and IL-13, but not IL-10, Protect Human Synoviocytes from Apoptosis. *The Journal of Immunology,* Vol.166, No.4, (February 2001), pp. 2775-2782, ISSN 0022-1767

Rygg, M., Uhlar, C.M., Thorn, C., Jensen, L.E., Gaughan, D.J., Varley, A.W., Munford, R.S., Göke, R., Chen, Y. & Whitehead, A.S. (2001). *In Vitro* Evaluation of an Enhanced Human Serum Amyloid A (SAA2) Promoter-regulated Soluble TNF Receptor Fusion Protein for Anti-inflammatory Gene Therapy. *Scandinavian Journal of Immunology,* Vol.53, No.6, (June 2001), pp. 588-595, ISSN 1365-3083

Sandell, L.J. & Aigner, T. (2001). Articular Cartilage and Changes in Arthritis. An Introduction: Cell Biology of Osteoarthritis. *Arthritis Research,* Vol.3, No.2, (January 2001), pp.107-113, ISSN 1465-9905

Sant, S.M., Suarez, T.M., Moalli, M.R., Wu, B.Y., Blaivas, M., Laing, T.J. & Roessler, B.J. (1998). Molecular Lysis of Synovial Lining Cells by *In Vivo* Herpes Simplex Virus-thymidine Kinase Gene Transfer. *Human Gene Therapy,* Vol.9, No.18, (December 1998), pp. 2735-2743, ISSN 1043-0342

Scarpignato, C. & Hunt, R.H. (2010). Nonsteroidal Antiinflammatory Drug-related Injury to the Gastrointestinal Tract: Clinical Picture, Pathogenesis, and Prevention. *Gastroenterology Clinics of North America,* Vol.39, No.3, (September 2010), pp. 433-464, ISSN 0889-8553

Shapiro, F., Koide, S. & Glimcher, M.J. (1993). Cell Origin and Differentiation in the Repair of Full-thickness Defects of Articular Cartilage. *The Journal of Bone & Joint Surgery (America),* Vol.75, No.4, (April 1993), pp. 532-553, ISSN 1535-1386

Stoop, R. (2008). Smart Biomaterials for Tissue-engineering. *Injury,* Vol.39, No.S1, (April 2008), pp. S77-S87, ISSN 0020-1383

Thomas, C.E., Ehrhardt, A. & Kay, M.A. (2003).Progress and Problems with the Use of Viral Vectors for Gene Therapy. *Nature Review Genetics,* Vol.4, No.5, (May 2003), pp. 346-358, ISSN 1471-0064

Trippel, S.B., Ghivizzani, S.C. & Nixon, A.J. (2004).Gene-based Approaches for the Repair of Articular Cartilage. *Gene Therapy,*Vol.11, No.4, (February 2004), pp. 351-359, ISSN 1476-5462

Trumble, T.N., Trotter, G.W., Oxford, J.R., McIlwraith, C.W., Cammarata, S., Goodnight, JL., Billinghurst, R.C. & Frisbie, D.D. (2001). Synovial Fluid Gelatinase Concentrations and Matrix Metalloproteinase and Cytokine Expression in Naturally Occurring Joint Disease in Horses. *American Journal of Veterinary Research,*Vol.62, No.9, (September 2001), pp. 1467-1477, ISSN 0002-9645

Tuli, R., Li, W.J. & Tuan, R.S. (2003). Current State of Cartilage Tissue-engineering. *Arthritis Research & Therapy,* Vol.5, No.5, (August 2003), pp. 235-238, ISSN 1478-6354

Uhlar, C.M., Grehan, S., Steel, D.M., Steinkasserer, A. & Whitehead, A.S. (1997). Use of the Acute Phase Serum Amyloid A2 (SAA2) Gene Promoter in the Analysis of Pro- and Anti-inflammatory Mediators: Differential Kinetics of SAA2 Promoter Induction by

IL-1 beta and TNF-alpha Compared to IL-6. *Journal of Immunological Methods,* Vol.203, No.2, (April 1997), pp. 123-130, ISSN 0022-1759

van der Laan, W.H., Quax, P.H., Seemayer, C.A., Huisman, L.G., Pieterman, E.J., Grimbergen, J.M., Verheijen, J.H., Breedveld, F.C., Gay, R.E., Gay, S., Huizinga, T.W. & Pap, T. (2003). Cartilage Degradation and Invasion by Rheumatoid Synovial Fibroblasts is Inhibited by Gene Transfer of TIMP-1 and TIMP-3. *Gene Therapy,* Vol.10, No.3, (February 2003), pp. 234-242, ISSN 0969-7128

Varley, A.W., Coulthard, M.G., Meidell, R.S., Gerard, R.D. & Munford, R.S. (1995). Inflammation-induced Recombinant Protein Expression *In Vivo* Using Promoters from Acute-phase Protein Genes. *Proceedings of the National Academy of Sciences of the United States of America,* Vol.92, No.12, (June 1995), pp. 5346-5350, ISSN 0027-8424

Venkatesan, N., Barré, L., Benani, A., Netter, P., Magdalou, J., Fournel-Gigleux, S. & Ouzzine, M. (2004). Stimulation of Proteoglycan Synthesis by Glucuronosyltransferase-I Gene Delivery: A Strategy to Promote Cartilage Repair. *Proceedings of the National Academy of Sciences of the United States of America,* Vol.101, No.52, (December 2004), pp. 18087-18092, ISSN 0027-8424

Wakitani, S., Goto, T., Young, R.G., Mansour, J.M., Goldberg, V.M. & Caplan, A.I. (1998). Repair of Large Full-thickness Articular Cartilage Defects with Allograft Articular Chondrocytes Embedded in a Collagen Gel.*Tissue Engineering,* Vol.4, No.4, (Winter 1998), pp. 429-444, ISSN 2152-4955

Watson, R.S., Gouze, E., Levings, P.P., Bush, M.L., Kay, J.D., Jorgensen, M.S., Dacanay, E.A., Reith, J.W., Wright, T.W. & Ghivizzani, S.C. (2010). Gene Delivery of TGF-β1 Induces Arthrofibrosis and Chondrometaplasia of Synovium *In Vivo. Laboratory Investigation,* Vol.90, No.11, (November 2010), pp. 1615-1627, ISSN 0023-6837

Wei, L., de Bri, E., Lundberg, A. & Svensson, O. (1998). Mechanical Load and Primary Guinea Pig Osteoarthrosis. *Acta OrthopaedicaScandinavica,*Vol.69, No.4, (August 1998), pp. 351-357, ISSN 0001-6470

Welsch, G.H., Mamisch, T.C., Zak, L., Blanke, M., Olk, A., Marlovits, S. & Trattnig, S. (2010). Evaluation of Cartilage Repair Tissue after Matrix-associated Autologous Chondrocyte Transplantation Using a Hyaluronic-based or a Collagen-based Scaffold with Morphological MOCART Scoring and Biochemical T2Mapping: Preliminary Results. *The American Journal of Sports Medicine,* Vol.38, No.5, (May 2010), pp. 934-942, ISSN 0363-5465

Welter, J.F., Solchaga, L.A. & Stewart, M.C. (2004). High-efficiency Non-viral Transfection of Primary Chondrocytes. *Methods in Molecular Medicine,* Vol.100, No.X, (July 2004), pp. 129-146, ISSN 1543-1894

Wolf, A.D. & Pfleger, B. (2003). Burden of Major Musculoskeletal Conditions. *Bulletin of the World Health Organization,* Vol.81, No.9, (November 2003), pp. 646-656, ISSN 0042-9686

Wolfe, M.M., Lichtenstein, D.R. & Singh, G. (1999). Gastrointestinal Toxicity of Nonsteroidal Antiinflammatory Drugs. *The New England Journal of Medicine,* Vol.340, No.24, (June 1999), pp. 1888-1899, ISSN 0028-4793

Woods, J.M., Katschke, K.J., Volin, M.V., Ruth, J.H., Woodruff, D.C., Amin, M.A., Connors, M.A., Kurata, H., Arai, K., Haines, G.K., Kumar, P. & Koch, A.E. (2001). IL-4

Adenoviral Gene Therapy Reduces Inflammation, Pro-inflammatory Cytokines, Vascularization, and Bony Destruction in Rat Adjuvant-induced Arthritis. *The Journal of Immunology*, Vol.166, No.2, (January 2001), pp. 1214-1222, ISSN 0022-1767

Yokoo, N., Saito, T., Uesugi, M., Kobayashi, N., Xin, K.Q., Okuda, K., Mizukami, H., Ozawa, K. & Koshino, T. (2005). Repair of Articular Cartilage Defect by Autologous Transplantation of Basic Fibroblast Growth Factor Gene–transduced Chondrocytes with Adeno-associated Virus Vector. *Arthritis & Rheumatism*, Vol.52, No.1, (January 2005), pp. 164-170, ISSN 0004-3591

Zhang, X., Mao, Z. & Yu, C. (2004). Suppression of Early Experimental Osteoarthritis by Gene Transfer of Interleukin-1 Receptor Antagonist and Interleukin-10. *Journal of Orthopaedic Research*, Vol.22, No.4, (July 2004), pp. 742-750, ISSN 0736-0266

Zhou, H.S., Liu, D.P. & Liang, C.C. (2004) Challenges and Strategies: The Immune Responses in Gene Therapy. *Medicinal Research Reviews*, Vol.24, No.6, (November 2004), pp. 748-761, ISSN 1098-1128

10

Gene Therapy Challenges in Arthritis

Denys Anne, Thiolat Allan,
Boissier Marie-Christophe and Bessis Natacha
Université Paris 13; Bobigny
France

1. Introduction

1.1 From systemic to intra-articular gene therapy

The first experiments of gene therapy (GT) in arthritis were done in the mid- nineties.
Arthritis is a chronic, inflammatory disease responsible for joint inflammation and destruction resulting in an imbalance between pro-inflammatory and anti-inflammatory cytokines production. Moreover, we know that bone destruction is more active than bone regeneration. Therefore, there are different ways of targeting the disease. At the moment, there are three classes of drugs commonly used:

1. Non-steroidal Anti-inflammatory Agents (NSAIDs),
2. corticoids,
3. Disease Modifying Anti-rheumatic Drugs (DMARDS).

Biotherapies have been used for a decade. These treatments restore the balance of many functions such as the immune system and the bone metabolism. Agents used in biotherapy include recombinant proteins, monoclonal antibodies, growth factors, and vaccines. The efficiency of these treatments depends on the stage of the disease. Serious side effects and infrequent persistent remission are known as drawbacks. Furthermore, the systemic administration of immune regulator can affect several immune responses and trigger infections.
The objectives using gene therapy in arthritis are mainly 1) to obtain a therapeutic quantity of therapeutic molecule without side effects, 2) to get a long expression of the therapeutic molecule without multi injections, 3) to target the joint specifically resistant to the usual treatment (Fiocco & Punzi, 2011).
Arthritis models are still being used to improve gene therapy strategies: for instance we use induced arthritis models such as collagen induced arthritis (CIA) in mice developing sub-chronic poly arthritis or adjuvant induced arthritis or spontaneous models such as Tumour Necrosis Factor (TNF) transgenic mice.
Our team who had the first results in 1996 has seen many changes over the years in its approach due to scientific progress. Our first gene therapy experiments used the *ex vivo* strategy (using autolog transfected cells (immortalized fibroblast from DBA/1 mice) or heterolog transfected cells (xenogenic fibroblasts from Chinese hamster ovary (CHO) with plasmid encoding murine IL-4 or IL-13); then the viral vectors experiments were used until the risk of using this methods arose (Bessis et al., 1996). We also used a non viral vector as plasmid (Bloquel et al., 2004, 2007; Saidenberg-Kermanach et al., 2003). Several teams tried

to optimize the transfer of plasmid whereas others tried to improve the safety of viral vectors.
In order to decrease the risk of a systemic diffusion of the transgene and to target the joint which might not respond to the usual treatment we have developed a local intra-articular (i.a) gene delivery strategy.
It is important to note that i.a strategy has been the only choice for the two existing clinical trials using GT in patients with rheumatoid arthritis.
One of the two trials has been done using an adeno- associated virus (AAV) 2 encoding the human soluble Tumour necrosis factor receptor type I (hTNFR-Is) fused to the Fc fragment of human IgG1. The TNF-α binds the soluble TNFR-Is instead of binding the cell membrane receptor. The second clinical trial used cells transfected with a retroviral vector encoding IL-1Ra which binds the membrane receptor of IL-1 and prevents the binding of IL-1.
In this chapter, we will show the methods evaluated in arthritis models for the gene therapy challenges in rheumatoid arthritis.

1.2 Intra-articular gene therapy

Knees are formed of four bones (Femur, Tibia, fibula, patella) surrounded by a membrane called synovium. It produces the synovial fluid which lubricates and nourishes the bones and the cartilage. In rheumatoid arthritis, the synovium is overrun by white blood cells which produce inflammatory molecules as TNF-α, IL-1-β, IFN-γ. Intra-articular GT consists of a therapeutic gene injection in the articular space to allow a local production of the therapeutic molecule. In mice, the needle is placed in the middle of the patella (seen through the skin after having shaved the knee) as far as the femur, and gently withdraw the needle to allow the gene to mix with the synovial fluid. The uncertainty of this method is to find out which cells are being targeted. Synoviocytes, osteoclasts, osteoblasts, chondrocytes are interesting targets because synoviocytes are able to produce pro-inflammatory cytokines, osteoclasts are responsible for the bone degradation, the osteoblasts allow the bone regeneration and chondrocytes are responsible for formation, maintenance, and repair of articular cartilage.
Intra-articular treatments are currently used for patients with RA such as corticoids which are injected locally. The new approach by gene therapy is a challenge in rheumatology. Intra- articular GT allows to reduce the number of injections, the quantity of therapeutic molecules and to target the joint resisting the usual treatment (Bessis & Boissier, 2003).

2. From *ex vivo* to *in vivo* gene transfer

Two strategies have been assessed in order to introduce the gene into the joint: 1) the gene has been introduced into the cells before their injection into the joint (*ex vivo* gene therapy) or 2) the gene has been injected directly into the joint (*in vivo* gene therapy).

2.1 *Ex vivo* gene therapy

The choice of the *ex vivo* gene strategy requires to choose the cell type which must be transfected. It seems clear that using autolog cells are more effective than using heterolog cells. To regulate immune response in inflammatory diseases such as rheumatoid arthritis, cells presenting antigen (CPA) (dendritic cells, macrophages or B cells) are good candidates. However, it is difficult to transfect these cells *in vivo* therefore using *ex vivo* gene therapy is more feasible. CPA are interesting in the *ex vivo* strategy because they are able to reach the inflamed area such as an arthritic joint where they interact with T cells to regulate immune response (Burke, 2003; Kim et al., 2006; Stoop et al., 2010). They are also able to migrate in the spleen and the lymph node to regulate the immune response (Ahrens et al., 2005; Kim et al., 2001).

Dendritic cells (DC) can direct the differentiation of T cell from Th0 towards Th1, Th17 or Th2. The activity of Th1 cells is predominant in animal model of autoimmune diseases such as RA at the expense of Th2 cells. Genetically modified DC allow to direct cell differentiation towards Th2 cells which have a therapeutic effect in decreasing Th1 activity.

In collagen induced arthritis (CIA), intravenous (i.v) injection of DC transfected with anti inflammatory cytokines (IL-4) can decrease the inflammation. After the injection, cells have been found 6h later in the lymph node and the spleen but not in other tissues or organs such as muscle, heart, lung and kidney. Transfected DC migrate to the secondary lymphoid organ where they modulate the T cell activity. These T cells produced less IFNγ than T cells from splenocytes of untreated mice. This shows that the injection of DC –IL-4 has directed T cells from Th0 to Th2 rather than to Th1 type (Kim et al., 2001).

On the other hand, DC transfected with adenovirus encoding FasL are able to induce T cell apoptosis in a specific manner. According to the authors it seemed that it was more efficient to direct T cells towards apoptosis than to direct them towards Th2 differentiation (Okamoto et al., 1998).

More recently, the discovery of small interfering RNA (siRNA) has allowed a change of strategy (Fire et al., 1998). Instead of introducing a gene into DC to increase expression of the transgene, DC can be transfected with a siRNA which will block the production of a pathogenic molecule.

It is known that CD40, CD80 and CD86 are important in the regulation of T cell activity by DC. From these data, Zheng et al. have studied the efficiency of DC transfected with siRNA targeting CD40, CD80 and CD86 in CIA. The i.a injection of transfected DC in mice resulted in less bone destruction and a reduced number of immune cells (neutrophils and mononuclear cells) infiltrating the joint (Zheng et al., 2010).

As described, DC are good cell candidates for *ex vivo* GT. The knowledge of their differentiation and their capacity to modulate the immune response has allowed the improvement of the therapeutic effect of genetically modified DC.

The new challenge now is to use regulatory T cells (Treg). Their suppressive activity on T cells effectors and their implication in tolerance process could be used in GT. The first study using T reg has shown that it was difficult to transfect these cells. Recently, Hombach et al. have demonstrated that primary T reg cells stimulated via the complex TCR/CD3 and the co-stimulatory molecule CD28 improve the gene transfer in these cells. It is important to note that the stimulation and the transfection have no effect on the properties of these cells (Hombach et al., 2009). From these data, Wright et al. have assessed the therapeutic potential of Treg transfected with TCR specific of antigen in arthritis induced adjuvant (AIA) model. They showed that primary Treg cells transfected with specific TCR and T CD4+ transfected with specific TCR and Foxp3 are able to reduce the disease (cartilage destruction and inflammation) (Wright et al., 2009).

Apart from DC and Treg cells, others such as mesenchymal cells, autolog fibroblasts or human like fibroblasts extract from human joints have also been used in arthritis models. The choice of the cell type depends on the immune response targeted, the feasibility to transfect them and the way to administer them: subcutaneously (s.c), i.v or in the joint. Several teams now develop a local *ex vivo* gene therapy to increase the number of therapeutic cells in the inflamed target and to regulate locally the imbalance of the immune system or the bone metabolism.

The i.a strategy using *ex vivo* gene therapy has been studied in a big animal eg a rhesus monkey in CIA. Skin autolog fibroblasts from the animal and xenogenic CHO were transfected with a plasmid encoding LacZ then grafted in the synovium. This study showed that labelling in the joint grafted with autolog fibroblasts was stronger compared with the labelling in the joint grafted with heterolog cells CHO. The accessibility of these autolog fibroblasts is a serious advantage (Bessis et al., 2007).

Fibroblast-Like Synoviocytes (FLS) are the largest type of cells in the synovium and therefore they are more interesting to treat inflammation in the joint. In RA, they are partly responsible for the inflammation in producing pro-inflammatory cytokines. Their pro-inflammatory activity depends on their environment. *Ex vivo* GT was discussed because FLS are not easy to transfect and their access is difficult. However several teams showed the efficiency to use these cells to treat AIA (Adriaansen et al., 2006; Yamamoto et al., 2003).

Synovial Mesenchymal stem cells which are also in the synovium are more attractive than FLS because they are more accessible and they expand easily. They are used more specifically in the case of cartilage repair but the advantages mentioned above could be interesting to treat the inflammation and the destruction of cartilage (Horie et al., 2009).

To conclude on the type of cells used in *ex vivo* i.a GT, it is important to note that cells have to be transfected easily, extracted easily and have a good adhesion with the local joint environment.

Despite *ex vivo* GT being more complex than direct gene injection one of the clinical trials used *ex vivo* gene therapy. In this trial, autolog fibroblasts have been infected with a retroviral vector encoding IL-1Ra (Evans et al., 2005). Then, these cells have been injected in the joint. Wehling et al have published the first result of this strategy in 2009 (Wehling et al., 2009). Due to the serious secondary effects which happened in another unrelated protocol at the time of the trial, the team only injected two patients instead of six. Furthermore, they used the same retroviral vector backbone (MFG) which was the problem. The transfected cells have been injected in 3 metacarpophalangial joints in the hand. An intra-patient control system has been done with injection of autologous non transfected cells. For the first patient, the joint receiving 3.10^6 cells was less painful than the joint receiving 10^6 cells. Surprisingly, the pain in the joint receiving untransfected cells was reduced too. This first patient noticed an improvement as early as the day after the surgery whereas the second patient was less responding. She only noticed an improvement two to three weeks after surgery. Moreover she felt a slight pain improvement in the untreated joint. So, the feasibility was proven, however two surgical procedures are needed: one to take the autologous synoviocytes out and the second one to transplant these transfected cells. Evans et al. noticed that synoviocytes are able to produce IL-1Ra after three passages. This result shows the stability of the transfection. It is an important property which keeps the production of the therapeutic transgene for a long time (Wehling et al., 2009).

2.2 *In vitro* gene transfer progresses

Pioneers of the gene therapy were convinced that they could use viruses to bring a therapeutic gene into the cells (Hill & Hillova, 1972; Sambrook et al., 1968). For a long time, researchers have been using the property of the viruses to get into the cells naturally. However it was the risk of using these viruses which urged the researchers to find a non viral strategy. But early studies have shown the difficulty to transfect cells with non viral vectors. New vectors and new vectorisation methods had to be developed.

Calcium phosphate was one of the first methods used to transfect mammalian cells with DNA. Calcium phosphate and plasmid are able to co precipitate which allows DNA uptake into the cells. Cationic lipid and polymer have the same property. *In vitro* transfection reagents using different carrier molecules are now commercially available and have the advantage of being reproducible to always give the same results. Furthermore, using these reagents, fewer procedures are needed than in classical transfection methods. Calcium phosphate, polymer were used to transfect cells with non viral vectors but later on, they were used to increase the transfection with viral vectors such as adenovirus (Lee & Welsh, 1999).

A second method using electricity was set up in the nineties: electroporation and nucleofection are two examples (Gresch et al., 2004). With these technical strategies, electroporation and nucleofection, many more cell types can be used in GT. As a summary, the pulsed electric fields using electroporators modify the membrane potential resulting in breakdown of the lipid bilayer to form pores. These modifications are reversible and temporary. First of all, the vector encoding gene of interest and cells are mixed with a specific transfection buffer in a specific plate. Then, electric fields are applied. The choice of the waveform is an important step. Generators used to apply current can deliver two types of waveforms: an exponential decay waveform and a square waveform. However, it is important to note that: 1) the square waveform increases the temperature which leads to the death of the cells whereas the exponential decay waveform avoids overheating. 2) Furthermore, with the square form, the medium of the culture can change the transfection efficiency whereas the medium culture has less effect using exponential decay waveform (Lambert et al., 1990). The first electroporators were made to transfect DC or macrophage. But the number of cells transfected and their viability were limited. To transfect cells using the electroporator, the cells are put in a chamber where they received high electrical field to create transient pores in the cell membrane. A high number of cells and a high quantity of plasmid must be used to obtain a significant quantity of cells transfected.

Despite the progress of the electroporation the high percentage of death cell remained consequent. Another method called nucleofector has been applied. This apparatus increases the efficiency of the transfection and survival rate of the transfected cells compared with the classical protocol using lipofectamine or electroporation. Nucleofection has a better reproducibility than using electroporation. A review reports the efficiency of the gene transfer in different primary cell types and cell lines by nucleofection (Gresch et al., 2004). The lower primary cell type transfected was the human B cells and the lower cell line transfected was PC12 cells. It seems that the variation is not due to the transfection method but it depends on the preparation of the cells (human B cells and PC12 cells) and the donor of cells in the case of primary cells. Despite using electroporator or nucleofectors it is still difficult to transfect cells with a large plasmid (14.7 kb). Further studies are needed to improve the transfection of the cells with a larger plasmid. The improvement of electroporators which can deliver different voltages during the transfection and the improvement of the electrodes could improve the transfection (Cepurniene et al., 2010; Rebersek et al., 2007).

Furthermore, plasmid mobility is not well known. Authors are studying the role of electrophoresis in plasmid traffic in the cells to increase the DNA transfer (Cepurniene et al., 2010; Mir, 2009).

Electroporation involves several parameters: the form of the wave as seen above, the voltage (low or high) and the duration of each pulse applied. According to the parameters used, both following effects can be observed: a thermal effect and electrochemical effects. Whereas pulse duration using microseconds or milliseconds has been used for a long time in order to destabilize the membrane and to involve the penetration of chemical agents (bleomycin) or DNA, the efficacy of this method using nanosecond is now being studied. The overheating created when electric pulses are applied is a drawback of the electroporation. Therefore duration could be limited to avoid this increase of heat and using nanoseconds could avoid the rise of temperature. Silve et al. explained the advantages and the limits in using nanoseconds in the book called Advanced Electroporation Techniques in Biology and Medicine (Silve et al., 2010).

With technical improvements primary cells such as synoviocytes can be transfected easily.

Electroporation provides transfection efficiency, minimizes cell death in decreasing the quantity of the vector injected.

Despite the technical progress, the success of the *ex vivo* GT in arthritis models and the success of the first clinical trial in rheumatoid arthritis, the strategy remains difficult for patients who have to undergo two surgery procedures. This approach is still being used although other teams have focused their research on the *in vivo* GT.

2.3 *In vivo* gene therapy

In RA models, two methods can be used according to expected results: 1) to obtain a systemic effect on systemic immune disorders, 2) to obtain a local effect targeting the inflamed joint.

Systemic effects of a transgene are obtained after an intravenous (i.v), a subcutaneous (s.c) or an intra-peritoneal injection. However, drawbacks of the systemic injection have been reported:

1. there are side effects due to the lack of control of the diffusion of the transgene,
2. the immunogenicity or pro-inflammatory effects of vectors (Cottard et al., 2004; Ji et al., 1999; Zaiss & Muruve, 2005)
3. the need to inject a high dose of a vector in order to get an effective dose of therapeutic molecule.

In vivo gene therapy, via i.m injection of the vectors in arthritis models has been studied thoroughly (Bloquel et al., 2007; Chen S.Y. et al., 2009; Denys et al., 2010). The muscular cells have the advantage of being non-dividing cells, easy to access and they produce the protein encoded by the transgene for a long time (more than 6 months) (Bloquel et al., 2004). The efficiency of the transfection depends on the vector and the maturation of the muscle (Moisset & Tremblay, 2001). Indeed, viral vectors use viral membrane receptors to infect the cells. But as the cells get older they are less able to produce these receptors (Feero et al., 1997). In the case of non viral vectors we will see in section 2-5 that different methods have been studied to improve the transfection.

Initially, i.m injection was used to treat muscular disorders and to have a systemic secretion of a therapeutic molecule. In RA, the i.m injection is not totally adapted because the target is the joint. Besides, molecules injected in the muscle have less possibility to reach the joint than to diffuse in the body. Intra articular GT has also been suggested for the first time in 1992 (Bandara et al., 1993). The advantage of this injection was very quickly identified: 1) easy access to the joint 1) less quantity of vectors, 2) less risk of side effects because no or less vector and transgene diffusion, 3) high number of cells so high potential of cells to be transfected, 4) the FLS have a low mitotic rate ensuring a fairly long expression of the transgene. The efficiency of gene transfer using a systemic or a local injection has been compared. Kim et al. demonstrated that the adenoviral vector encoding IL-4 injected intravenously or in the joint decreased the inflammation and the destruction of the bone and the cartilage in established CIA. The quantity of the vector injected was respectively 10^9 and 5.10^8 (Kim et al., 2000). Adenoviruses and Adeno-Associated-viruses (AAV) have been frequently used to work locally. However, as mentioned before, it seems important to develop a non viral strategy safer than a viral strategy. We studied the efficiency of the i.a gene transfer in CIA using a plasmid encoding mTNFR-Is. The knees of mice treated with this plasmid showed a decrease of both inflammation and destruction and there was no systemic effect (Denys et al., 2010). Examples of joint inflammation and bone destruction are illustrated in Fig. 1.

Although a "comparative study on intra-articular versus systemic gene electrotransfer in experimental arthritis" showed that i.m injection of plasmid (pVAX2) encoding IL-10 decreased the development of the disease, the i.a injection had no effect. In this study, contrary to all expectations, 1) the quantity of the plasmid injected in the joint (100µg) was higher than the quantity injected in the muscle (25µg), 2) i.a injection had no effect (Khoury et al., 2006) . The difference between the two could come from the transgene: the TNF-α could play a role locally whereas IL10 does not show the importance of the choice of the target. In our study, the expression of the transgene after i.a gene transfer was shorter than after i.m injection which is an important drawback. The higher production is about 7-8 days after the i.a injection. It decreased rapidly and was undetectable 14 days later (Bloquel et al., 2007; Denys et al., 2010; Khoury et al., 2006). We have shown that a second injection of a plasmid encoding msTNFR can allow a new expression of the transgene. However, the level of msTNFR obtained after the second injection was lower than the level obtained after the first injection may be because of a limited capacity of the cells to integrate the plasmid (Bloquel et al., 2007).

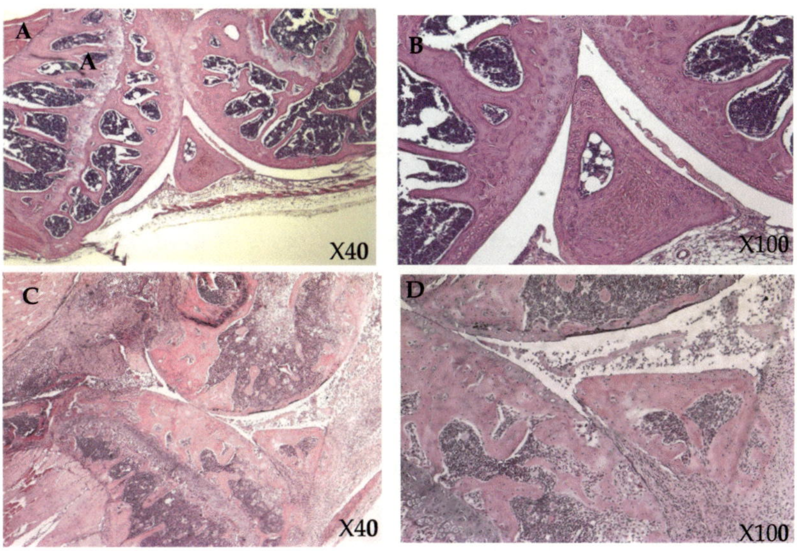

Fig. 1. Examples illustrating histological analysis of knee's inflammation and destruction. Haemalun/Eosin staining. (A-B) msTNFR-Is treated mice; aspect of normal synovial and normal cartilage. (C-D) Saline-treated mouse: inflammation and cartilage destruction of the knees.

A recent clinical trial using *in vivo* i.a strategy has been performed. An adeno-associated virus type 2 expressing TNF-α antagonist was injected in the knee of arthritic patients. These patients received a second injection either 12 or 30 weeks when necessary. Twelve adverse events and 2 deaths were reported after the second injection (Evans, 2010). The involvement of the vector in the pathogenecity has been rejected because this vector has been identified as a "good" vector and has been used in others studies (Boissier et al., 2007; Mueller & Flotte, 2008; Wu et al., 2006). In this study, viral genome was detectable in the blood as well as in the synovium where it remained longer. Therefore, this study has shown not only the feasibility but also the risk of i.a gene therapy.

This accident reminds us of the Jesse Gelsinger's case which shows the difficulty to select patients. This accident encourages researchers to improve the non viral gene transfer to be used safely in future treatments for humans and to improve the choice of patients' exclusion criteria.

2.4 Contralateral effect of *ex vivo* and *in vivo* gene therapy

It is important to underline that i.a injections could have a therapeutic effect in treated and untreated joints. The contralateral effect doesn't depend on :

1. the strategy using *ex vivo* or *in vivo* (Kim et al., 2002; Kim et al., 2005; Whalen et al., 1999)
2. the vector injected *in vivo* because it was observed using viral vector, adenovirus, adeno-associated virus and non viral vector (Chan et al., 2002; Ghivizzani et al., 1998; Van De Loo & Van Den Berg, 2002),
3. the model of arthritis because it is observed in CIA, AIA and Streptococcal Cell wall (SCW)-induced arthritis (Chan et al., 2002; Kim et al., 2005; Lechman et al., 2003),
4. species as observed in rabbits , in rats , in mice and also in human clinical trials (Chan et al., 2002; Ghivizzani et al., 1998; Van De Loo & Van Den Berg, 2002; Wehling et al., 2009).

The reason of the contralateral effect with *in vivo* gene transfer is not well known. However, authors have suggested that migration of APC in the case of *ex vivo* strategy might be responsible for that particular effect (Kim et al., 2002). Indeed, studies have showed before that these cells are able to travel to other sites of inflammation or secondary lymphoid tissues such as lymph nodes (Kim et al., 2000; Lechman et al., 1999; Morita et al., 2001).

In the case of *in vivo* gene strategy, local dendritic cells might be infected by the vector and they migrate to regulate the inflammation in the front paws or in the contralateral paw. We cannot control this distant effect at the moment therefore this property could be interesting to develop. It would be a serious advantage to be able to treat all the joints with the diffusion of the protein encoded by the transgene without the diffusion of the vector.

2.5 Technical strategies to improve *in vivo* gene therapy in rheumatoid arthritis

The first *in vivo* non viral gene delivery consisted in a single injection of the vector. However, the size of the DNA and anionic charges surrounding the DNA block the efficacy of the endocytosis. Mechanical, chemical or electrical approaches are being developed to improve gene delivery. We focused our description only on the methods used in arthritis models.

Liposomes

Liposomes are molecules which have been used for the last three decades and have become more and more performing. They were first used *in vitro* and the improvement in their safety allowed them to be used for *in vivo* gene therapy to carry nucleic acids (DNA or RNAi).

They are microbubbles of lipids which are anionic, cationic or zwitterion. The composition of the liposomes can vary and their interaction with cells depends on this composition (Ropert, 1999). Cationic Liposomal carrier has been considered as a good potential to facilitate molecule internalisation in cells because they have similarities with the cell plasma membrane. The advantages of liposomes in GT have first been described in the *ex vivo* gene transfer: liposomes involve the adhesion of packaged nucleic acids to the cell surface, then the internalisation of them by endocytosis. They also confer a protection against DNase. Studies have shown that Cationic liposomes increase the transfection by 3 fold in the skeletal muscle (Felgner, 1996). However, *in vivo*, some drawbacks were reported following liposomes nucleic acids complex injection in the serum. Liposomes DNA complex also called lipoplexes could be responsible for a toxicity action and/or an inflammatory action. Therefore, they could limit the biodistribution. Advantages and drawbacks of Cationic liposomes used *in vivo* gene transfer have been described in the human gene therapy journal (Felgner, 1996).

In arthritis models, lipoplexes are used to carry siRNA. Khoury et al. also used siRNA targeting pro-inflammatory cytokines as TNF-α, IL-1β, IL6 and IL-18 (Khoury et al., 2006; Khoury et al., 2008). They have noted that the i.v simultaneous injection of the three lipoplexes blocking IL-1β, IL-6 and IL-18 has curative and preventive effects (Khoury et al., 2008).

Other teams have targeted the immune cells rather than the pro-inflammatory cytokines in CIA. Indeed, the development of rheumatoid arthritis depends on the interaction between T cells and CPA. Adreakos et al. used lipoplexes able to block CD40/CD40L interaction. Authors have developed a liposome compatible with the *in vivo* GT called amphotenic liposome which facilitates the encapsulation, the blood circulation and the cell release from an endosome (Andreakos et al., 2009). This liposome has been injected intravenously at the onset of the disease. It releases CD40 anti sense which prevents the CD40 expression on T cells. The improvement of the clinical signs of the disease was noticed only 24h after the treatment. Furthermore, the efficacy on all paws was noted 10 days after the first injection of liposomes.

Electrotransfer

Electric fields were first used *in vitro* as seen in section 2-2. Since then, they have been used in cancerology. The strategy called electrochemotherapy helps the endocytosis of drugs in tumour cells. The first application was conducted in the 1990's on subcutaneous and cutaneous tumours (Gilbert et al., 1997; Mir et al., 1991; Titomirov et al., 1991).

Besides, electric fields have been used to transfer genes into cells. This strategy called electrotransfer (ET) has also been used to kill tumour cells or to force the liver and then later on the muscles to produce therapeutic molecules (Aihara & Miyazaki, 1998; Heller et al., 1996; Rols et al., 1998).

The action of electric fields *in vivo* is the same as the *ex vivo* electroporation:

1. pore formation in the cell plasma membrane,
2. penetration of the vector into the cells.

The development of the i.m gene therapy using ET has been a major advance in genes transfer (Miyazaki & Miyazaki, 2008). The stability of the transgene expression between individual subjects was a very major advance of this method.

In 1998, Mir et al. have published the parameters which give an efficient and a reproducible muscle cells transfection. Furthermore, they obtained a temporary permeabilization of the cells and of many survival cells (Mir et al., 1998).
The generator used for the ET delivers square waves. The current is transmitted to the target via electrodes which are two parallel stainless steel plates, their size depending on the target. Fig.2. shows the position of the electrodes for the knee's elecrotransfer (A) or for muscle's electrotransfer (B).

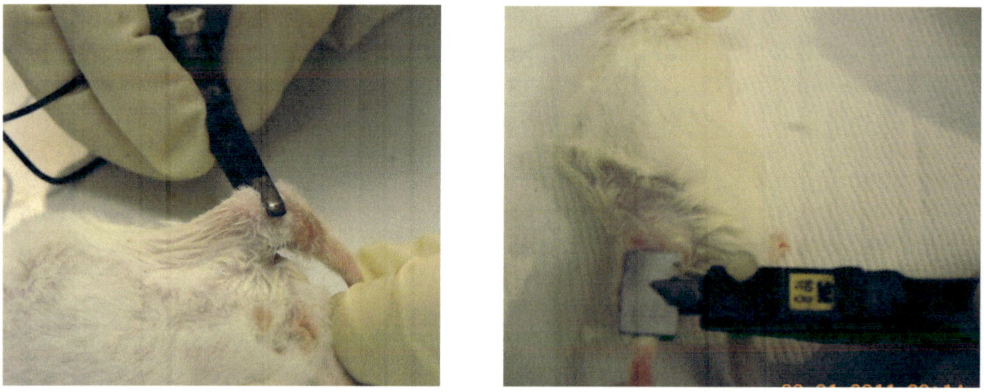

A B

Fig. 2. Electrotransfer to mouse knee or muscle. DNA electrotransfer was performed with a square wave electroporation system. The current is transmitted to the target via electrodes which are two parallel stainless steel plates, their size depending on the target. A. Electrotransfer to mouse knee: the pair of electrodes was placed on either side of the knees and then 12 electric pulses were applied during 20ms. B. Electrotransfer to mouse muscle : the pair of electrodes was placed on either side of the muscle and then 8 electric pulses were applied during 20ms.

In arthritis models, conventional parameters are used to deliver genes in the muscles: 8 pulses for 20ms at low voltage (100-200V) for 1cm between the electrodes with a frequency of 1Hz. The parameters are changed to deliver genes into the joint: 12 pulses for 20ms at 250V/cm with a frequency of 2Hz (Denys et al., 2010; Khoury et al., 2006). It is interesting to note that the parameters of the ET can be better controlled in using mathematical modelling or *in vivo* test (Miklavcic et al., 2000). The parameters programmed in the electroporator are set for a unique position of the electrodes. However, during the ET, it is known that the muscle contracts and electrodes move. As a result there is a decrease of the permeabilization responsible for a decrease of the efficiency of the ET. Cukjati et al have described a method controlled by a computer which adapts the parameters according to the changes of the movement of the electrodes to achieve the permeabilization at the end of the pulses (Cukjati et al., 2007).
Despite the results with the application of low voltage (100-200V) and long duration (20ms), it seems that high and then low voltage must be applied: 1) to permeabilize the cells and 2) to promote the DNA transfer. These two steps have been described in several studies (Andre & Mir, 2010; Hojman, 2010; Satkauskas et al., 2005) . The following elements play a role in the transfer of DNA in the cells: 1) the electric pulses, 2) the structure of the DNA, 3) the composition of the buffer in which the DNA is diluted, 4) the physiology of the muscle.

The damages and the physiological modifications on muscular fibres have been studied after electrotransfer. The parameters used can alter the muscular fibres temporarily (Gissel, 2010; Hojman, 2010; Tevz et al., 2008). When we used a high voltage for 20ms, we did not notice any fibrosis (Bloquel et al., 2004).
Mir et al have studied the ionic flux, apoptosis marker expression and muscular function after ET using different combinations of pulses. As explained by the authors, the effects depend on the combinations (Hojman et al., 2008).
On the other hand, Peng et al. noted that the vector could be integrated not only by mature muscle cells but also by satellite cells after electrotransfer. These satellite cells replace the damaged muscular cells. Their transfection seems important in order to have a long expression of the transgene (Peng et al., 2005).
Besides the role of the pulse on the efficiency, let's not forget the electrodes configuration and composition.
Two types of electrodes can be used: invasive or non invasive electrodes. In arthritis models we used non invasive electrodes as described before. Other electrodes have been constructed according to the target. Gothelf and Gelth have described different types of electrodes used for skin electrotransfer (Gothelf & Gehl, 2010). Invasive electrodes have been a great evolution for transfected skin and tumours as they release the pulses directly into the tissue. The voltage used with these electrodes is less than the voltage used with non invasive electrodes because the current must go through several barriers before reaching its target (Liu & Huang, 2002). However, a huge step in invasive electrode is the set up of the syringe electrodes. They are formed with two electrodes, one of them being used to inject the DNA.
Syringe electrodes have originally been developed to treat neuronal diseases such as Alzheimer disease but it also opens a potential application in i.a gene therapy (Li et al., 2010). Intra articular ET showed therapeutic effects in arthritis models (Bloquel et al., 2007; Denys et al., 2010). However the application of non invasive electrodes on both sides of the joint is not always controlled which could explain some individual differences in the results.
Therefore, *in vivo* ET depends on the chosen electrodes, on the electric parameters applied and on the tissue composition. It can be difficult to determine the optimal electric parameters for a type of electrodes in a specific tissue. Numerical modelling described by Zupanic et al. can determine the optimum parameters" for ET in muscular tissue". (Zupanic et al., 2010). This approach can be used for different tissues.

Nanoparticles vectors

Chitosan is a nanoparticle charged positively capable of binding anionic nucleic acids. Furthermore, it is biocompatible, and remains small after nucleic acids binding (Takka & Gurel, 2010). In CIA, Howard et al. demonstrated that i.p injection of chitosan containing anti TNF-α siRNA delayed the arthritis development by targeting peritoneal activated macrophages (Howard et al., 2009).
In the rat AIA, the IL1-Ra-chitosan-folate complex (nanoparticles complex) decreased the inflammation and the destruction of the joints (Fernandes et al., 2008). Shi et al. have performed this strategy using hydrodynamic injections of the nanoparticles-complex in the vein of the hind paws. They became aware of the smaller size of the circumference of the ankles in rats treated than in non treated rats (Shi et al., 2011). A study shows the efficiency of i.a injection of other nanoparticles (atecollagen) associated to a double-stranded miRNA-15 in the arthritis development. As a result, authors noted a successful transfection of the

synovium cells and the downregulation of Bcl2 which is the target of the miRNA-15. Despite an incomplete action on the disease, the i.a injection of miRNA carried by atecollagen opens new perspectives to simultaneously administer several miRNA (Nagata et al., 2009).

3. Progress and prospects on the structure of naked nucleic acids and viruses to treat rheumatoid arthritis

This section focuses on the most important technological modifications concerning naked nucleic acids and viruses in order to increase their efficiency in arthritis models.

3.1 Plasmids

Plasmid DNA expression has been hampered by a low level of transfection and the short time of the expression of the transgene. Several changes have been made to improve its safety, its internalisation in the cells, its translocation in the nucleus and its integration (Conese et al., 2004; Gill et al., 2009; Lam & Dean, 2010). Plasmids are also: 1) reduced (minicircle DNA) 2) deprived of the bacteria resistant gene 3) deprived of its CpG motifs.

Studies showed that minicircles produce the transgene for a longer time than when it is produced from the conventional plasmid (Mayrhofer et al., 2009). Different elements explain this advantage:

1. minicircles have a supercoiled form that will protect the DNA from degradation by enzymes
2. minicircles have less CpG sequence motifs which are usually responsible for an immune response destroying the plasmids (Bloquel et al., 2004; Mayrhofer et al., 2009)
3. minicircles are small facilitating their penetration in the cells.

Despite these advantages, a few studies have demonstrated their therapeutic efficiency in RA(Chen Z.Y. et al., 2003; Stenler et al., 2009) . Some teams are focusing mainly on the improvement of their purification; others are trying to improve the efficiency of the plasmid. Researchers replaced CpG by other sequence motifs or by removing the resistance gene to antibiotics (Kay et al., 2010; Mayrhofer et al., 2008).

For a long time, the genes making cells or bacteria resistant to specific antibiotics have been the only way to select and isolate the cells / bacteria containing them. However, once the genes spread into the germs, these germs become resistant to antibiotics and are impossible to eradicate. Therefore, the scientists tried to construct plasmids without these genes and with a conditional replication origin (Marie et al., 2010; Soubrier et al., 1999).

Besides, further improvements are expected in order to have more plasmids translocated in the nucleus. Lan et al have described these approaches as well as the inclusion of transcription factor-binding sites for a cell-specific delivery (Lam & Dean, 2010).

3.2 siRNA

RA is characterized by an uncontrolled increase of the production of inflammatory cytokines (TNF-α, IL-1β, IL-6), an uncontrolled production of enzymes destroying cartilages and bones (metalloproteases). First of all, treatments and studies have targeted these pathogenic molecules. Then, the emergence of siRNA and small hairpin RNA offer the possibility to prevent the production of the pathogenic molecules. However these naked nucleic acids are unstable and are rapidly damaged by enzymes. Different approaches have been used to enhance their stability, to protect them against nuclease degradation, to perform their ability to penetrate in the cells (Khoury et al., 2006; Shim & Kwon, 2010). The therapeutic effect in arthritis models has been demonstrated in blocking TNF-α by an i.a injection of siRNA and by an i.p injection (Howard et al., 2009; Schiffelers et al., 2005). The systemic injection of siRNA has been possible through the development of nanoparticles lipoplexes (Courties et al., 2011; Khoury et al., 2006). Another delivery approach has been developed using a cream containing siRNA (Takanashi et al., 2009). It targeted the osteopontin produced by macrophages and activated T cells. After application, osteopontin has been found reduced in the serum and siRNA ameliorate symptoms of the disease. Using a cream to deliver siRNA is an interesting new technology because this method acts locally without an invasive injection.

3.3 Viral gene therapy development in rheumatoid arthritis

The most common vectors used in RA are adenoviruses (AdV), retroviruses (oncoviruses and lentivirus) and recombinant adeno-associated viruses (rAAV). They have attractive characteristics for human GT (Bessis & Boissier, 2003; Cavazzana-Calvo et al., 2010; Herzog et al., 2010).

In 1985, for the first time, Roeschler et al. have injected an AdV encoding LacZ in the knees of rabbits. Authors showed that AdV are able to transfect both types A and B synoviocytes throughout the articular and periarticular knees (Roessler et al., 1993). Their use as a vector for gene delivery is limited due to the inflammatory effect and/or because they can be quickly lost when they transfect dividing cells. Researchers tried to construct AdV without viral sequences. The first result showed that the yield was weaker than for the first generation. Furthermore the process is difficult (Kochanek et al., 2001). Other modifications have been made to decrease the immunogenicity and to increase the stability and the specificity (Nayak & Herzog, 2010; Tang et al., 2010). Indeed, AdV under control of inducible promoter (human telomerase reverse transcriptase) can lyse synoviocytes which contain active telomerase in a rat CIA model. Furthermore authors noticed a replication of the AdV in the arthritic joints but not in the non- arthritic ones (Chen S.Y. et al., 2009). The ability of the AdV to target specifically pathogenic cells (without reaction against normal cells) is an important property to be developed for gene therapy in patients.

Retroviruses (RV) are divided into two classes. The first class called oncoretrovirus, used commonly, is derived from Monkey Murine Leukaemia oncoretrovirus. They are less adapted for i.a *in vivo* GT than AdV but the feasibility and safety of the *ex vivo* gene strategy has been demonstrated in patients RA (Wehling et al., 2009). The second class called lentivirus is able to easily transfect cells and then to produce the transgene for a long time. Several studies have shown that an i.a injection of lentivirus (encoding therapeutic molecules) decreases the development of arthritis in animal models (Gouze et al., 2003; Wang et al., 2010; Zondervan et al., 2008). Furthermore, lentivirus [encoding both a therapeutic molecule (galectin 1) and the shRNA of (galectin 3)] has been injected in the joint of arthritic mice (Wang et al., 2010). The joints injected with the lentivirus are less inflamed and show less bone degradation. Furthermore the angiogenesis seems lower in treated mice than in untreated mice. However, authors noted a lower vessel density.

RA is a disease developed from imbalance between pro and anti inflammatory mechanisms. This approach is also interesting because it shows the feasibility to target molecules playing an opposite role in the development of the pathology.

Recombinant adeno-associated viruses (rAAV) are non pathogenic and are able to produce the transgene for a long time. They exist under different serotypes, including eight characterized ones which differ by their ability to transfect specific tissues. The serotype rAAV2 has been used in several clinical trials including the local treatment of RA (Mueller & Flotte, 2008). In the last few years, serotype 5 has been defined as a "good" vector to target the synovial tissue (Apparailly et al., 2005; Boissier et al., 2007). However, autoantibodies production directed against AAV are responsible for neutralization of rAAV (Cottard et al., 2000) . Boutin et al. have published the titer of Immunoglobulin G subclasses produced against each serotype in humans (Boutin et al., 2010). These results and the knowledge of the efficiency of Serotypes 5 to transfect synovium demonstrate that rAAV5 may be an ideal candidate for i.a gene therapy in RA. Furthermore, the integration of an inducible promoter is encouraging in order to target a specific inflamed tissue (Apparailly et al., 2002; Yang et al., 2010).

Using rAAV is limited because the production strategy is long, difficult and only gives a poor performance. Different processes have been followed to increase the yield and answer the requirements for clinical trials (Negrete & Kotin, 2008; Wright, 2008). For a long time rAAV have been produced from mammalian adherent cells restricting the production of large doses which prevents in turn limits a higher number of clinical trials and a commercial production. Another system avoiding the usual limit for producing rAAV has been developed. This system uses insect cells and baculoviruses vector. This experiment carries on in order to increase the yield whilst reducing the complexity of the system (Mena et al., 2010; Negrete & Kotin, 2008). Aslandi et al. have also established a stable insect cell line containing helper genes necessary for the production of vectors. These genes will only be active when the cells are transfected with baculovirus. The system has improved the yield and the protocol to produce rAAV (Aslanidi et al., 2009).

4. Development of specific regulated promoters

There are two classes of promoters: constitutive (viral and eukariotic) and inducible. Among constitutive viral vectors, Cytomegalovirus (CMV) is the most used promoter in mammalian expression systems because it allows a high level of gene expression. However, its expression is regulated by a large variety of stimuli which can cause an uncontrolled production of the transgene.

Different inducible promoters under the control of molecules such as antibiotics have been developed to target tumours or specific tissues (Robson & Hirst, 2003). For the first time Bakker et al. showed the feasibility to use an inducible adenovirus vector made up of 2-component promoters. The promoters have sites for Nuclear factor kappa B binding and are activated by pro-inflammatory cytokines. Authors have injected this vector in the joint of mice immunized with collagen. They noticed an improvement in the treated and untreated paws. They have obtained the same result in using the adenovirus encoding IL-1Ra under the control of CMV (Bakker et al., 2002). In order to get a more specific inducible therapeutic action of vectors, it is possible to use bioinformatic. Geurts et al. have elaborated a system to design proximal-promoters aiming at to RA (Geurts et al., 2009) . Therefore, inflammation responsive promoters provide a huge progress in rheumatoid arthritis gene therapy because this disease is characterized by temporary acute flares.

5. Conclusion

The studies described in this chapter show the advances in gene transfer and its applications in RA. The clinical trials applied on RA patients demonstrate:

1. that gene therapy is not only appropriate for monogenic diseases but also for multigenic diseases
2. the feasibility of the strategy
3. that progress must carry on in the years to come to become more efficient.

Each strategy (*ex vivo* and *in vivo*), each vector and each target have their advantages and drawbacks. Experimental protocols have improved the efficiency, the safety, of Gene therapy involving the development of clinical trials in RA patients. Three startegies of GT have been been tried : 1) RA-FLS genetically modified (by RV encoding IL-1Ra *ex vivo*) before i.a injection , 2) i.a injection of plasmid encoding the Herpes simples virus thymidine kinase , 3) i.a injection of AAV2 encoding hTNFRs (table 1).

Trial Country	Vector	Transgene	Date approved	Status
Canada	Adeno-associated virus	TNFR-Fc Ig fusion gene	2004	Closed
Germany	retrovirus	IL-1Ra		open
USA	retrovirus	IL-1Ra	1995	closed
	plasmid	HSV-TK	1998	closed
	Adeno-associated virus	TNFR-Fc Ig fusion gene	2003	closed
	Adeno-associated virus	TNFR-Fc Ig fusion gene	2005	open

Table 1. Gene therapy clinical trial in rheumatoid arthritis in the world. Three countries only have attempted RA gene therapy clinical trials (Edelstein, 2011).

Furthermore, the knowledge acquired on the mechanisms of the disease increases the number of possible targets. The recent studies on signalisation pathway offer the opportunity for new therapeutic strategies.

Other promising therapeutic systems must be developed to combine researches in biology, chemistry and engineering.

6. References

Adriaansen, J., Vervoordeldonk, M. J., Vanderbyl, S., de Jong, G. & Tak, P. P. (2006). A novel approach for gene therapy: engraftment of fibroblasts containing the artificial chromosome expression system at the site of inflammation. *J Gene Med*, Vol. 8, No. 1, pp. 63-71.

Ahrens, E. T., Flores, R., Xu, H. & Morel, P. A. (2005). *In vivo* imaging platform for tracking immunotherapeutic cells. *Nat Biotechnol*, Vol. 23, No. 8, pp. 983-987.

Aihara, H. & Miyazaki, J. (1998). Gene transfer into muscle by electroporation *in vivo*. *Nat Biotechnol*, Vol. 16, No. 9, pp. 867-870.

Andre, F. M. & Mir, L. M. (2010). Nucleic acids electrotransfer *in vivo*: mechanisms and practical aspects. *Curr Gene Ther*, Vol. 10, No. 4, pp. 267-280.

Andreakos, E., Rauchhaus, U., Stavropoulos, A., Endert, G., Wendisch, V., Benahmed, A. S., Giaglis, S., Karras, J., Lee, S., Gaus, H., Bennett, C. F., Williams, R. O., Sideras, P. & Panzner, S. (2009). Amphoteric liposomes enable systemic antigen-presenting cell-directed delivery of CD40 antisense and are therapeutically effective in experimental arthritis. *Arthritis Rheum*, Vol. 60, No. 4, pp. 994-1005.

Apparailly, F., Millet, V., Noel, D., Jacquet, C., Sany, J. & Jorgensen, C. (2002). Tetracycline-inducible interleukin-10 gene transfer mediated by an adeno-associated virus: application to experimental arthritis. *Hum Gene Ther*, Vol. 13, No. 10, pp. 1179-1188.

Apparailly, F., Khoury, M., Vervoordeldonk, M. J., Adriaansen, J., Gicquel, E., Perez, N., Riviere, C., Louis-Plence, P., Noel, D., Danos, O., Douar, A. M., Tak, P. P. & Jorgensen, C. (2005). Adeno-associated virus pseudotype 5 vector improves gene transfer in arthritic joints. *Hum Gene Ther*, Vol. 16, No. 4, pp. 426-434.

Aslanidi, G., Lamb, K. & Zolotukhin, S. (2009). An inducible system for highly efficient production of recombinant adeno-associated virus (rAAV) vectors in insect Sf9 cells. *Proc Natl Acad Sci U S A*, Vol. 106, No. 13, pp. 5059-5064.

Bakker, A. C., van de Loo, F. A., Joosten, L. A., Arntz, O. J., Varley, A. W., Munford, R. S. & van den Berg, W. B. (2002). C3-Tat/HIV-regulated intraarticular human interleukin-1 receptor antagonist gene therapy results in efficient inhibition of collagen-induced arthritis superior to cytomegalovirus-regulated expression of the same transgene. *Arthritis Rheum*, Vol. 46, No. 6, pp. 1661-1670.

Bandara, G., Mueller, G. M., Galea-Lauri, J., Tindal, M. H., Georgescu, H. I., Suchanek, M. K., Hung, G. L., Glorioso, J. C., Robbins, P. D. & Evans, C. H. (1993). Intraarticular expression of biologically active interleukin 1-receptor-antagonist protein by *ex vivo* gene transfer. *Proc Natl Acad Sci U S A*, Vol. 90, No. 22, pp. 10764-10768.

Bessis, N., Boissier, M. C., Ferrara, P., Blankenstein, T., Fradelizi, D. & Fournier, C. (1996). Attenuation of collagen-induced arthritis in mice by treatment with vector cells engineered to secrete interleukin-13. *Eur J Immunol*, Vol. 26, No. 10, pp. 2399-2403.

Bessis, N. & Boissier, M. C. (2003). Vectors for gene therapy of joint disorders. *Joint Bone Spine*, Vol. 70, No. 6, pp. 471-473.

Bessis, N., Lemeiter, D., Laroche, L., Fournier, C., Huizinga, T., Brok, H., t Hart, B. & Boissier, M. C. (2007). Engraftment of cutaneous fibroblasts within synovial membrane in a nonhuman primate: short-term results. *Joint Bone Spine*, Vol. 74, No. 1, pp. 48-51.

Bloquel, C., Bessis, N., Boissier, M. C., Scherman, D. & Bigey, P. (2004). Gene therapy of collagen-induced arthritis by electrotransfer of human tumor necrosis factor-alpha soluble receptor I variants. *Hum Gene Ther*, Vol. 15, No. 2, pp. 189-201.

Bloquel, C., Fabre, E., Bureau, M. F. & Scherman, D. (2004). Plasmid DNA electrotransfer for intracellular and secreted proteins expression: new methodological developments and applications. *J Gene Med*, Vol. 6 Suppl 1, No. pp. S11-23.

Bloquel, C., Denys, A., Boissier, M. C., Apparailly, F., Bigey, P., Scherman, D. & Bessis, N. (2007). Intra-articular electrotransfer of plasmid encoding soluble TNF receptor variants in normal and arthritic mice. *J Gene Med*, Vol. 9, No. 11, pp. 986-993.

Boissier, M. C., Lemeiter, D., Clavel, C., Valvason, C., Laroche, L., Begue, T. & Bessis, N. (2007). Synoviocyte infection with adeno-associated virus (AAV) is neutralized by human synovial fluid from arthritis patients and depends on AAV serotype. *Hum Gene Ther*, Vol. 18, No. 6, pp. 525-535.

Boutin, S., Monteilhet, V., Veron, P., Leborgne, C., Benveniste, O., Montus, M. F. & Masurier, C. (2010). Prevalence of serum IgG and neutralizing factors against adeno-associated virus (AAV) types 1, 2, 5, 6, 8, and 9 in the healthy population:

implications for gene therapy using AAV vectors. *Hum Gene Ther*, Vol. 21, No. 6, pp. 704-712.

Burke, B. (2003). Macrophages as novel cellular vehicles for gene therapy. *Expert Opin Biol Ther*, Vol. 3, No. 6, pp. 919-924.

Cavazzana-Calvo, M., Hacein-Bey-Abina, S. & Fischer, A. (2010). [Ten years of gene therapy: thoughts and perspectives]. *Med Sci (Paris)*, Vol. 26, No. 2, pp. 115-118.

Cepurniene, K., Ruzgys, P., Treinys, R., Satkauskiene, I. & Satkauskas, S. (2010). Influence of plasmid concentration on DNA electrotransfer *in vitro* using high-voltage and low-voltage pulses. *J Membr Biol*, Vol. 236, No. 1, pp. 81-85.

Chan, J. M., Villarreal, G., Jin, W. W., Stepan, T., Burstein, H. & Wahl, S. M. (2002). Intraarticular gene transfer of TNFR:Fc suppresses experimental arthritis with reduced systemic distribution of the gene product. *Mol Ther*, Vol. 6, No. 6, pp. 727-736.

Chen, S. Y., Shiau, A. L., Shieh, G. S., Su, C. H., Lee, C. H., Lee, H. L., Wang, C. R. & Wu, C. L. (2009). Amelioration of experimental arthritis by a telomerase-dependent conditionally replicating adenovirus that targets synovial fibroblasts. *Arthritis Rheum*, Vol. 60, No. 11, pp. 3290-3302.

Chen, Z. Y., He, C. Y., Ehrhardt, A. & Kay, M. A. (2003). Minicircle DNA vectors devoid of bacterial DNA result in persistent and high-level transgene expression *in vivo. Mol Ther*, Vol. 8, No. 3, pp. 495-500.

Conese, M., Auriche, C. & Ascenzioni, F. (2004). Gene therapy progress and prospects: episomally maintained self-replicating systems. *Gene Ther*, Vol. 11, No. 24, pp. 1735-1741.

Cottard, V., Mulleman, D., Bouille, P., Mezzina, M., Boissier, M. C. & Bessis, N. (2000). Adeno-associated virus-mediated delivery of IL-4 prevents collagen-induced arthritis. *Gene Ther*, Vol. 7, No. 22, pp. 1930-1939.

Cottard, V., Valvason, C., Falgarone, G., Lutomski, D., Boissier, M. C. & Bessis, N. (2004). Immune response against gene therapy vectors: influence of synovial fluid on adeno-associated virus mediated gene transfer to chondrocytes. *J Clin Immunol*, Vol. 24, No. 2, pp. 162-169.

Courties, G., Baron, M., Presumey, J., Escriou, V., van Lent, P., Scherman, D., Cantagrel, A., van den Berg, W. B., Jorgensen, C., Apparailly, F. & Davignon, J. L. (2011). Cytosolic phospholipase A2alpha gene silencing in the myeloid lineage alters development of Th1 responses and reduces disease severity in collagen-induced arthritis. *Arthritis Rheum*, Vol. 63, No. 3, pp. 681-690.

Cukjati, D., Batiuskaite, D., Andre, F., Miklavcic, D. & Mir, L. M. (2007). Real time electroporation control for accurate and safe *in vivo* non-viral gene therapy. *Bioelectrochemistry*, Vol. 70, No. 2, pp. 501-507.

Denys, A., Thiolat, A., Descamps, D., Lemeiter, D., Benihoud, K., Bessis, N. & Boissier, M. C. (2010). Intra-articular electrotransfer of mouse soluble tumour necrosis factor receptor in a murine model of rheumatoid arthritis. *J Gene Med*, Vol. 12, No. 8, pp. 659-668.

Edelstein, M. (2007). Gene therapy Clinical worldwide trial provided by Journal of Gene Medicine, In : Wyley InterScience, 2011, Available from: http://www.wiley.com/legacy/wileychi/genmed/clinical/

Evans, C. (2010). Arthritis gene therapy trials reach phase II. *J Rheumatol*, Vol. 37, No. 4, pp. 683-685.

Evans, C. H., Robbins, P. D., Ghivizzani, S. C., Wasko, M. C., Tomaino, M. M., Kang, R., Muzzonigro, T. A., Vogt, M., Elder, E. M., Whiteside, T. L., Watkins, S. C. & Herndon, J. H. (2005). Gene transfer to human joints: progress toward a gene therapy of arthritis. *Proc Natl Acad Sci U S A*, Vol. 102, No. 24, pp. 8698-8703.

Feero, W. G., Rosenblatt, J. D., Huard, J., Watkins, S. C., Epperly, M., Clemens, P. R., Kochanek, S., Glorioso, J. C., Partridge, T. A. & Hoffman, E. P. (1997). Viral gene delivery to skeletal muscle: insights on maturation-dependent loss of fiber infectivity for adenovirus and herpes simplex type 1 viral vectors. *Hum Gene Ther*, Vol. 8, No. 4, pp. 371-380.

Felgner, P. L. (1996). Improvements in cationic liposomes for *in vivo* gene transfer. *Hum Gene Ther*, Vol. 7, No. 15, pp. 1791-1793.

Fernandes, J. C., Wang, H., Jreyssaty, C., Benderdour, M., Lavigne, P., Qiu, X., Winnik, F. M., Zhang, X., Dai, K. & Shi, Q. (2008). Bone-protective effects of nonviral gene therapy with folate-chitosan DNA nanoparticle containing interleukin-1 receptor antagonist gene in rats with adjuvant-induced arthritis. *Mol Ther*, Vol. 16, No. 7, pp. 1243-1251.

Fiocco, U. & Punzi, L. (2011). "Are there any evidences for using the intra-articular TNF-alpha blockade in resistant arthritis?" *Joint Bone Spine*, Vol. No. pp.

Fire, A., Xu, S., Montgomery, M. K., Kostas, S. A., Driver, S. E. & Mello, C. C. (1998). Potent and specific genetic interference by double-stranded RNA in Caenorhabditis elegans. *Nature*, Vol. 391, No. 6669, pp. 806-811.

Geurts, J., Joosten, L. A., Takahashi, N., Arntz, O. J., Gluck, A., Bennink, M. B., van den Berg, W. B. & van de Loo, F. A. (2009). Computational design and application of endogenous promoters for transcriptionally targeted gene therapy for rheumatoid arthritis. *Mol Ther*, Vol. 17, No. 11, pp. 1877-1887.

Ghivizzani, S. C., Lechman, E. R., Kang, R., Tio, C., Kolls, J., Evans, C. H. & Robbins, P. D. (1998). Direct adenovirus-mediated gene transfer of interleukin-1 and tumor necrosis factor alpha soluble receptors to rabbit knees with experimental arthritis has local and distal anti-arthritic effects. *Proc. Natl. Acad. Sci. USA.*, Vol. 95, No. pp. 4613-4618.

Gilbert, R. A., Jaroszeski, M. J. & Heller, R. (1997). Novel electrode designs for electrochemotherapy. *Biochim Biophys Acta*, Vol. 1334, No. 1, pp. 9-14.

Gill, D. R., Pringle, I. A. & Hyde, S. C. (2009). Progress and prospects: the design and production of plasmid vectors. *Gene Ther*, Vol. 16, No. 2, pp. 165-171.

Gissel, H. (2010). Effects of varying pulse parameters on ion homeostasis, cellular integrity, and force following electroporation of rat muscle *in vivo*. *Am J Physiol Regul Integr Comp Physiol*, Vol. 298, No. 4, pp. R918-929.

Gothelf, A. & Gehl, J. (2010). Gene electrotransfer to skin; review of existing literature and clinical perspectives. *Curr Gene Ther*, Vol. 10, No. 4, pp. 287-299.

Gouze, E., Pawliuk, R., Gouze, J. N., Pilapil, C., Fleet, C., Palmer, G. D., Evans, C. H., Leboulch, P. & Ghivizzani, S. C. (2003). Lentiviral-mediated gene delivery to synovium: potent intra-articular expression with amplification by inflammation. *Mol Ther*, Vol. 7, No. 4, pp. 460-466.

Gresch, O., Engel, F. B., Nesic, D., Tran, T. T., England, H. M., Hickman, E. S., Korner, I., Gan, L., Chen, S., Castro-Obregon, S., Hammermann, R., Wolf, J., Muller-

Hartmann, H., Nix, M., Siebenkotten, G., Kraus, G. & Lun, K. (2004). New non-viral method for gene transfer into primary cells. *Methods*, Vol. 33, No. 2, pp. 151-163.

Heller, R., Jaroszeski, M., Atkin, A., Moradpour, D., Gilbert, R., Wands, J. & Nicolau, C. (1996). *In vivo* gene electroinjection and expression in rat liver. *FEBS Lett*, Vol. 389, No. 3, pp. 225-228.

Herzog, R. W., Cao, O. & Srivastava, A. (2010). Two decades of clinical gene therapy--success is finally mounting. *Discov Med*, Vol. 9, No. 45, pp. 105-111.

Hill, M. & Hillova, J. (1972). Virus recovery in chicken cells tested with Rous sarcoma cell DNA. *Nat New Biol*, Vol. 237, No. 71, pp. 35-39.

Hojman, P., Gissel, H., Andre, F. M., Cournil-Henrionnet, C., Eriksen, J., Gehl, J. & Mir, L. M. (2008). Physiological effects of high- and low-voltage pulse combinations for gene electrotransfer in muscle. *Hum Gene Ther*, Vol. 19, No. 11, pp. 1249-1260.

Hojman, P. (2010). Basic principles and clinical advancements of muscle electrotransfer. *Curr Gene Ther*, Vol. 10, No. 2, pp. 128-138.

Hombach, A. A., Kofler, D., Rappl, G. & Abken, H. (2009). Redirecting human CD4+CD25+ regulatory T cells from the peripheral blood with pre-defined target specificity. *Gene Ther*, Vol. 16, No. 9, pp. 1088-1096.

Horie, M., Sekiya, I., Muneta, T., Ichinose, S., Matsumoto, K., Saito, H., Murakami, T. & Kobayashi, E. (2009). Intra-articular Injected synovial stem cells differentiate into meniscal cells directly and promote meniscal regeneration without mobilization to distant organs in rat massive meniscal defect. *Stem Cells*, Vol. 27, No. 4, pp. 878-887.

Howard, K. A., Paludan, S. R., Behlke, M. A., Besenbacher, F., Deleuran, B. & Kjems, J. (2009). Chitosan/siRNA nanoparticle-mediated TNF-alpha knockdown in peritoneal macrophages for anti-inflammatory treatment in a murine arthritis model. *Mol Ther*, Vol. 17, No. 1, pp. 162-168.

Ji, L., Bouvet, M., Price, R. E., Roth, J. A. & Fang, B. (1999). Reduced toxicity, attenuated immunogenicity and efficient mediation of human p53 gene expression *in vivo* by an adenovirus vector with deleted E1-E3 and inactivated E4 by GAL4-TATA promoter replacement. *Gene Ther*, Vol. 6, No. 3, pp. 393-402.

Kay, M. A., He, C. Y. & Chen, Z. Y. (2010). A robust system for production of minicircle DNA vectors. *Nat Biotechnol*, Vol. 28, No. 12, pp. 1287-1289.

Khoury, M., Bigey, P., Louis-Plence, P., Noel, D., Rhinn, H., Scherman, D., Jorgensen, C. & Apparailly, F. (2006). A comparative study on intra-articular versus systemic gene electrotransfer in experimental arthritis. *J Gene Med*, Vol. 8, No. 8, pp. 1027-1036.

Khoury, M., Louis-Plence, P., Escriou, V., Noel, D., Largeau, C., Cantos, C., Scherman, D., Jorgensen, C. & Apparailly, F. (2006). Efficient new cationic liposome formulation for systemic delivery of small interfering RNA silencing tumor necrosis factor alpha in experimental arthritis. *Arthritis Rheum*, Vol. 54, No. 6, pp. 1867-1877.

Khoury, M., Escriou, V., Courties, G., Galy, A., Yao, R., Largeau, C., Scherman, D., Jorgensen, C. & Apparailly, F. (2008). Efficient suppression of murine arthritis by combined anticytokine small interfering RNA lipoplexes. *Arthritis Rheum*, Vol. 58, No. 8, pp. 2356-2367.

Kim, S. H., Evans, C. H., Kim, S., Oligino, T., Ghivizzani, S. C. & Robbins, P. D. (2000). Gene therapy for established murine collagen-induced arthritis by local and systemic adenovirus-mediated delivery of interleukin-4. *Arthritis Res*, Vol. 2, No. 4, pp. 293-302.

Kim, S. H., Kim, S., Evans, C. H., Ghivizzani, S. C., Oligino, T. & Robbins, P. D. (2001). Effective treatment of established murine collagen-induced arthritis by systemic administration of dendritic cells genetically modified to express IL-4. *J Immunol*, Vol. 166, No. 5, pp. 3499-3505.

Kim, S. H., Lechman, E. R., Kim, S., Nash, J., Oligino, T. J. & Robbins, P. D. (2002). *Ex vivo* gene delivery of IL-1Ra and soluble TNF receptor confers a distal synergistic therapeutic effect in antigen-induced arthritis. *Mol Ther*, Vol. 6, No. 5, pp. 591-600.

Kim, S. H., Lechman, E. R., Bianco, N., Menon, R., Keravala, A., Nash, J., Mi, Z., Watkins, S. C., Gambotto, A. & Robbins, P. D. (2005). Exosomes derived from IL-10-treated dendritic cells can suppress inflammation and collagen-induced arthritis. *J Immunol*, Vol. 174, No. 10, pp. 6440-6448.

Kim, S. H., Bianco, N., Menon, R., Lechman, E. R., Shufesky, W. J., Morelli, A. E. & Robbins, P. D. (2006). Exosomes derived from genetically modified DC expressing FasL are anti-inflammatory and immunosuppressive. *Mol Ther*, Vol. 13, No. 2, pp. 289-300.

Kochanek, S., Schiedner, G. & Volpers, C. (2001). High-capacity 'gutless' adenoviral vectors. *Curr Opin Mol Ther*, Vol. 3, No. 5, pp. 454-463.

Lam, A. P. & Dean, D. A. (2010). Progress and prospects: nuclear import of nonviral vectors. *Gene Ther*, Vol. 17, No. 4, pp. 439-447.

Lambert, H., Pankov, R., Gauthier, J. & Hancock, R. (1990). Electroporation-mediated uptake of proteins into mammalian cells. *Biochem Cell Biol*, Vol. 68, No. 4, pp. 729-734.

Lechman, E. R., Jaffurs, D., Ghivizzani, S. C., Gambotto, A., Kovesdi, I., Mi, Z., Evans, C. H. & Robbins, P. D. (1999). Direct adenoviral gene transfer of viral IL-10 to rabbit knees with experimental arthritis ameliorates disease in both injected and contralateral control knees. *J Immunol*, Vol. 163, No. 4, pp. 2202-2208.

Lechman, E. R., Keravala, A., Nash, J., Kim, S. H., Mi, Z. & Robbins, P. D. (2003). The contralateral effect conferred by intra-articular adenovirus-mediated gene transfer of viral IL-10 is specific to the immunizing antigen. *Gene Ther*, Vol. 10, No. 24, pp. 2029-2035.

Lee, J. H. & Welsh, M. J. (1999). Enhancement of calcium phosphate-mediated transfection by inclusion of adenovirus in coprecipitates. *Gene Ther*, Vol. 6, No. 4, pp. 676-682.

Li, Y., Wang, J., Liu, J. & Liu, F. (2010). A novel system for *in vivo* neprilysin gene delivery using a syringe electrode. *J Neurosci Methods*, Vol. 193, No. 2, pp. 226-231.

Liu, F. & Huang, L. (2002). A syringe electrode device for simultaneous injection of DNA and electrotransfer. *Mol Ther*, Vol. 5, No. 3, pp. 323-328.

Marie, C., Vandermeulen, G., Quiviger, M., Richard, M., Preat, V. & Scherman, D. (2010). pFARs, plasmids free of antibiotic resistance markers, display high-level transgene expression in muscle, skin and tumour cells. *J Gene Med*, Vol. 12, No. 4, pp. 323-332.

Mayrhofer, P., Blaesen, M., Schleef, M. & Jechlinger, W. (2008). Minicircle-DNA production by site specific recombination and protein-DNA interaction chromatography. *J Gene Med*, Vol. 10, No. 11, pp. 1253-1269.

Mayrhofer, P., Schleef, M. & Jechlinger, W. (2009). Use of minicircle plasmids for gene therapy. *Methods Mol Biol*, Vol. 542, No. pp. 87-104.

Mena, J. A., Aucoin, M. G., Montes, J., Chahal, P. S. & Kamen, A. A. (2010). Improving adeno-associated vector yield in high density insect cell cultures. *J Gene Med*, Vol. 12, No. 2, pp. 157-167.

Miklavcic, D., Semrov, D., Mekid, H. & Mir, L. M. (2000). A validated model of *in vivo* electric field distribution in tissues for electrochemotherapy and for DNA electrotransfer for gene therapy. *Biochim Biophys Acta*, Vol. 1523, No. 1, pp. 73-83.

Mir, L. M., Belehradek, M., Domenge, C., Orlowski, S., Poddevin, B., Belehradek, J., Jr., Schwaab, G., Luboinski, B. & Paoletti, C. (1991). [Electrochemotherapy, a new antitumor treatment: first clinical trial]. *C R Acad Sci III*, Vol. 313, No. 13, pp. 613-618.

Mir, L. M., Bureau, M. F., Rangara, R., Schwartz, B. & Scherman, D. (1998). Long-term, high level *in vivo* gene expression after electric pulse-mediated gene transfer into skeletal muscle. *C R Acad Sci III*, Vol. 321, No. 11, pp. 893-899.

Mir, L. M. (2009). Nucleic acids electrotransfer-based gene therapy (electrogenetherapy): past, current, and future. *Mol Biotechnol*, Vol. 43, No. 2, pp. 167-176.

Miyazaki, S. & Miyazaki, J. (2008). *In vivo* DNA electrotransfer into muscle. *Dev Growth Differ*, Vol. 50, No. 6, pp. 479-483.

Moisset, P. A. & Tremblay, J. P. (2001). Gene therapy: a strategy for the treatment of inherited muscle diseases? *Curr Opin Pharmacol*, Vol. 1, No. 3, pp. 294-299.

Morita, Y., Yang, J., Gupta, R., Shimizu, K., Shelden, E. A., Endres, J., Mule, J. J., McDonagh, K. T. & Fox, D. A. (2001). Dendritic cells genetically engineered to express IL-4 inhibit murine collagen-induced arthritis. *J Clin Invest*, Vol. 107, No. 10, pp. 1275-1284.

Mueller, C. & Flotte, T. R. (2008). Clinical gene therapy using recombinant adeno-associated virus vectors. *Gene Ther*, Vol. 15, No. 11, pp. 858-863.

Nagata, Y., Nakasa, T., Mochizuki, Y., Ishikawa, M., Miyaki, S., Shibuya, H., Yamasaki, K., Adachi, N., Asahara, H. & Ochi, M. (2009). Induction of apoptosis in the synovium of mice with autoantibody-mediated arthritis by the intraarticular injection of double-stranded MicroRNA-15a. *Arthritis Rheum*, Vol. 60, No. 9, pp. 2677-2683.

Nayak, S. & Herzog, R. W. (2010). Progress and prospects: immune responses to viral vectors. *Gene Ther*, Vol. 17, No. 3, pp. 295-304.

Negrete, A. & Kotin, R. M. (2008). Strategies for manufacturing recombinant adeno-associated virus vectors for gene therapy applications exploiting baculovirus technology. *Brief Funct Genomic Proteomic*, Vol. 7, No. 4, pp. 303-311.

Okamoto, K., Asahara, H., Kobayashi, T., Matsuno, H., Hasunuma, T., Kobata, T., Sumida, T. & Nishioka, K. (1998). Induction of apoptosis in the rheumatoid synovium by Fas ligand gene transfer. *Gene Ther*, Vol. 5, No. 3, pp. 331-338.

Peng, B., Zhao, Y., Lu, H., Pang, W. & Xu, Y. (2005). *In vivo* plasmid DNA electroporation resulted in transfection of satellite cells and lasting transgene expression in regenerated muscle fibers. *Biochem Biophys Res Commun*, Vol. 338, No. 3, pp. 1490-1498.

Rebersek, M., Faurie, C., Kanduser, M., Corovic, S., Teissie, J., Rols, M. P. & Miklavcic, D. (2007). Electroporator with automatic change of electric field direction improves gene electrotransfer in-vitro. *Biomed Eng Online*, Vol. 6, No. pp. 25.

Robson, T. & Hirst, D. G. (2003). Transcriptional Targeting in Cancer Gene Therapy. *J Biomed Biotechnol*, Vol. 2003, No. 2, pp. 110-137.

Roessler, B. J., Allen, E. D., Wilson, J. M., Hartman, J. W. & Davidson, B. L. (1993). Adenoviral-mediated gene transfer to rabbit synovium *in vivo*. *J Clin Invest*, Vol. 92, No. 2, pp. 1085-1092.

Rols, M. P., Delteil, C., Golzio, M., Dumond, P., Cros, S. & Teissie, J. (1998). *In vivo* electrically mediated protein and gene transfer in murine melanoma. *Nat Biotechnol*, Vol. 16, No. 2, pp. 168-171.

Ropert, C. (1999). Liposomes as a gene delivery system. *Braz J Med Biol Res*, Vol. 32, No. 2, pp. 163-169.

Saidenberg-Kermanach, N., Bessis, N., Deleuze, V., Bureau, M., Scherman, D. & Boissier, M.-C. (2003). Efficacy of interleukin-10 gene electrotransfer into skeletal muscle in mice with collagen-induced arthritis. *J Gene Med*, Vol. 5, No. 2, pp. 164-171.

Sambrook, J., Westphal, H., Srinivasan, P. R. & Dulbecco, R. (1968). The integrated state of viral DNA in SV40-transformed cells. *Proc Natl Acad Sci U S A*, Vol. 60, No. 4, pp. 1288-1295.

Satkauskas, S., Andre, F., Bureau, M. F., Scherman, D., Miklavcic, D. & Mir, L. M. (2005). Electrophoretic component of electric pulses determines the efficacy of *in vivo* DNA electrotransfer. *Hum Gene Ther*, Vol. 16, No. 10, pp. 1194-1201.

Schiffelers, R. M., Xu, J., Storm, G., Woodle, M. C. & Scaria, P. V. (2005). Effects of treatment with small interfering RNA on joint inflammation in mice with collagen-induced arthritis. *Arthritis Rheum*, Vol. 52, No. 4, pp. 1314-1318.

Shi, Q., Wang, H., Tran, C., Qiu, X., Winnik, F. M., Zhang, X., Dai, K., Benderdour, M. & Fernandes, J. C. (2011). Hydrodynamic delivery of chitosan-folate-DNA nanoparticles in rats with adjuvant-induced arthritis. *J Biomed Biotechnol*, Vol. 2011, No. pp. 148763.

Shim, M. S. & Kwon, Y. J. (2010). Efficient and targeted delivery of siRNA *in vivo*. *Febs J*, Vol. 277, No. 23, pp. 4814-4827.

Silve, A., Villemejane, J., Joubert, V., Ivorra, A. & Mir, L. M. (2010). Advanced Electroporation Techniques in Biology and Medicine,In:*Nanosecond Pulsed Electric Field Delivery to Biological Samples: Difficulties and Potential Solutions*.James C. Lin, pp CRC press, 9781439819067

Soubrier, F., Cameron, B., Manse, B., Somarriba, S., Dubertret, C., Jaslin, G., Jung, G., Caer, C. L., Dang, D., Mouvault, J. M., Scherman, D., Mayaux, J. F. & Crouzet, J. (1999). pCOR: a new design of plasmid vectors for nonviral gene therapy. *Gene Ther*, Vol. 6, No. 8, pp. 1482-1488.

Stenler, S., Andersson, A., Simonson, O. E., Lundin, K. E., Chen, Z. Y., Kay, M. A., Smith, C. I., Sylven, C. & Blomberg, P. (2009). Gene transfer to mouse heart and skeletal muscles using a minicircle expressing human vascular endothelial growth factor. *J Cardiovasc Pharmacol*, Vol. 53, No. 1, pp. 18-23.

Stoop, J. N., Harry, R. A., von Delwig, A., Isaacs, J. D., Robinson, J. H. & Hilkens, C. M. (2010). Therapeutic effect of tolerogenic dendritic cells in established collagen-induced arthritis is associated with a reduction in Th17 responses. *Arthritis Rheum*, Vol. 62, No. 12, pp. 3656-3665.

Takanashi, M., Oikawa, K., Sudo, K., Tanaka, M., Fujita, K., Ishikawa, A., Nakae, S., Kaspar, R. L., Matsuzaki, M., Kudo, M. & Kuroda, M. (2009). Therapeutic silencing of an endogenous gene by siRNA cream in an arthritis model mouse. *Gene Ther*, Vol. 16, No. 8, pp. 982-989.

Takka, S. & Gurel, A. (2010). Evaluation of chitosan/alginate beads using experimental design: formulation and *in vitro* characterization. *AAPS PharmSciTech*, Vol. 11, No. 1, pp. 460-466.

Tang, B., Cullins, D. L., Zhou, J., Zawaski, J. A., Park, H., Brand, D. D., Hasty, K. A., Gaber, M. W., Stuart, J. M., Kang, A. H. & Myers, L. K. (2010). Modulation of collagen-induced arthritis by adenovirus-mediated intra-articular expression of modified collagen type II. *Arthritis Res Ther*, Vol. 12, No. 4, pp. R136.

Tevz, G., Pavlin, D., Kamensek, U., Kranjc, S., Mesojednik, S., Coer, A., Sersa, G. & Cemazar, M. (2008). Gene electrotransfer into murine skeletal muscle: a systematic analysis of parameters for long-term gene expression. *Technol Cancer Res Treat*, Vol. 7, No. 2, pp. 91-101.

Titomirov, A. V., Sukharev, S. & Kistanova, E. (1991). *In vivo* electroporation and stable transformation of skin cells of newborn mice by plasmid DNA. *Biochim Biophys Acta*, Vol. 1088, No. 1, pp. 131-134.

van de Loo, F. A. & van den Berg, W. B. (2002). Gene therapy for rheumatoid arthritis. Lessons from animal models, including studies on interleukin-4, interleukin-10, and interleukin-1 receptor antagonist as potential disease modulators. *Rheum Dis Clin North Am*, Vol. 28, No. 1, pp. 127-149.

Wang, C. R., Shiau, A. L., Chen, S. Y., Cheng, Z. S., Li, Y. T., Lee, C. H., Yo, Y. T., Lo, C. W., Lin, Y. S., Juan, H. Y., Chen, Y. L. & Wu, C. L. (2010). Intra-articular lentivirus-mediated delivery of galectin-3 shRNA and galectin-1 gene ameliorates collagen-induced arthritis. *Gene Ther*, Vol. 17, No. 10, pp. 1225-1233.

Wehling, P., Reinecke, J., Baltzer, A. W., Granrath, M., Schulitz, K. P., Schultz, C., Krauspe, R., Whiteside, T. W., Elder, E., Ghivizzani, S. C., Robbins, P. D. & Evans, C. H. (2009). Clinical responses to gene therapy in joints of two subjects with rheumatoid arthritis. *Hum Gene Ther*, Vol. 20, No. 2, pp. 97-101.

Whalen, J. D., Lechman, E. L., Carlos, C. A., Weiss, K., Kovesdi, I., Glorioso, J. C., Robbins, P. D. & Evans, C. H. (1999). Adenoviral transfer of the viral IL-10 gene periarticularly to mouse paws suppresses development of collagen-induced arthritis in both injected and uninjected paws. *J Immunol*, Vol. 162, No. 6, pp. 3625-3632.

Wright, G. P., Notley, C. A., Xue, S. A., Bendle, G. M., Holler, A., Schumacher, T. N., Ehrenstein, M. R. & Stauss, H. J. (2009). Adoptive therapy with redirected primary regulatory T cells results in antigen-specific suppression of arthritis. *Proc Natl Acad Sci U S A*, Vol. 106, No. 45, pp. 19078-19083.

Wright, J. F. (2008). Manufacturing and characterizing AAV-based vectors for use in clinical studies. *Gene Ther*, Vol. 15, No. 11, pp. 840-848.

Wu, Z., Asokan, A. & Samulski, R. J. (2006). Adeno-associated virus serotypes: vector toolkit for human gene therapy. *Mol Ther*, Vol. 14, No. 3, pp. 316-327.

Yamamoto, A., Fukuda, A., Seto, H., Miyazaki, T., Kadono, Y., Sawada, Y., Nakamura, I., Katagiri, H., Asano, T., Tanaka, Y., Oda, H., Nakamura, K. & Tanaka, S. (2003). Suppression of arthritic bone destruction by adenovirus-mediated dominant-negative Ras gene transfer to synoviocytes and osteoclasts. *Arthritis Rheum*, Vol. 48, No. 9, pp. 2682-2692.

Yang, T., Duan, R., Cao, H., Lee, B. H., Xia, C., Chang, Z., Keith Tanswell, A. & Hu, J. (2010). Development of an inflammation-inducible gene expression system using helper-dependent adenoviral vectors. *J Gene Med*, Vol. 12, No. 10, pp. 832-839.

Zaiss, A. K. & Muruve, D. A. (2005). Immune responses to adeno-associated virus vectors. *Curr Gene Ther*, Vol. 5, No. 3, pp. 323-331.

Zheng, X., Suzuki, M., Ichim, T. E., Zhang, X., Sun, H., Zhu, F., Shunnar, A., Garcia, B., Inman, R. D. & Min, W. (2010). Treatment of autoimmune arthritis using RNA interference-modulated dendritic cells. *J Immunol*, Vol. 184, No. 11, pp. 6457-6464.

Zondervan, R., Xia, T., van der Meer, H., Storm, C., Kulzer, F., van Saarloos, W. & Orrit, M. (2008). Soft glassy rheology of supercooled molecular liquids. *Proc Natl Acad Sci U S A*, Vol. 105, No. 13, pp. 4993-4998.

Zupanic, A., Corovic, S., Miklavcic, D. & Pavlin, M. (2010). Numerical optimization of gene electrotransfer into muscle tissue. *Biomed Eng Online*, Vol. 9, No. pp. 66.

11

Gene Therapy Outcomes in Experimental Models of Inflammatory Arthritis

Charles J. Malemud
Department of Medicine, Division of Rheumatic Diseases, Case Western Reserve University School of Medicine & University Hospitals Case Medical Center, Cleveland, Ohio
USA

1. Introduction

During the past decade the development of medical therapies for the treatment of the inflammatory arthopathies such as rheumatoid arthritis (RA) was revolutionized by the development of disease modifying anti-rheumatic biological drugs (DMARBDs) (Ŝenolt et al., 2009). DMARBDs were first discovered to be effective by altering intracellular signaling pathways and those gene expressional events that have proven to be relevant to RA pathogenesis and progression through the use of experimental studies in pre-clinical *in vitro* testing systems (Malemud, 2010; Malemud & Miller, 2008, Malemud & Pearlman, 2009; Marone et al., 2008; Walker et al., 2006). Those DMARBDs that appeared to have significant modifying effects on immune deregulation were then shown to ameliorate arthritis by virtue of their capacity to delay the onset or reducing the severity of inflammatory arthritis in several well-validated small animal models of RA (Feely et al., 2009). Finally, those DMARBDs which proved to have disease-modifying effects in rodent models of RA were then assessed for their efficacy, tolerability and safety in human RA clinical trials (Gibbons & Hyrich, 2009). Those successful DMARBDs are now fully incorporated into RA treatment regimens in the clinical practice setting.

2. Animal models of RA

Animal models of human RA have proven to be critical for determining the potential efficacy of DMARBDs for subsequent use in the treatment of human RA. The DMARBDs that are now employed for RA therapy were always first tested in RA animal models where the molecular events governing the onset and progression of RA disease activity could be rigorously and longitudinally assessed (Wooley, 2008; Leung et al., 2010). The DMARBDs that targeted pro-inflammatory cytokines relevant to RA progression such as tumor necrosis factor-α (TNF-α), interleukin-1 (IL-1), IL-6, IL-12/IL-23 and IL-17 as well as other molecules whose activity correlated with progressive RA disease activity, such as CTLA-4 and CD20/CD-22 were shown to significantly modify the progression of inflammatory arthritis in mice (Finckh & Gabay, 2008).

3. The use of DMARBDs in RA

Despite improvement in the frequency of positive clinical responses in RA patients that have been obtained using DMARBDs when combined with immunosuppressive drugs such as methotrexate, the chronic use of DMARBDs in RA therapy has also revealed that serious adverse events typified by the onset of new infections, the development of refractoriness to DMARBDs as well as the long term specter of potential malignancies have also been documented (Salliot et al., 2009). These long-term treatment considerations have resulted in the need for a continuous stream of development of additional and hopefully novel RA therapies that specifically target molecules intimately involved in RA progression. One strategy that has been utilized for this purpose is the development of gene therapy for RA (Gaddy & Robbins, 2008; Jorgensen & Apparailly, 2010; Traister & Hirsh, 2008; Woods et al., 2008)

4. Gene therapy for RA

Over the past 7 years or so a considerable amount of research activity has been devoted to the development of gene therapeutic strategies that have resulted in 1) neutralization of the effects of IL-1 with an IL-1 receptor antagonist (IL-1-Ra) expression plasmid (Kim et al.; 2003); 2) elevating the levels of Th2 cytokines exemplified by IL-10 (Traister & Hirsh, 2008), IL-4 (Kageyama et al., 2004) and IL-13 (Nabbe et al., 2005); 3) suppression of Th1 cytokines such as IL-18 (Smeets et al., 2003) and IL-17, the latter by modification of the indoleamine 2,3-dioxygenase pathway (Chen et al., 2011); 4) blunting of TNF-α-stimulated signaling (Denys et al., 2010) and interferon-β activity (Adriaansen et al.; 2006); 5) up-regulation of the protein inhibitor of activated STAT1 (PIAS) activity by stimulating the capacity of small ubiquitin-like modifier E3 ligase (SUMO E3) to alter inhibitor of κB kinaseα (IKKα) phosphorylation (Liu & Shuai, 2008); 6) gene transfer of genetically modified chondrocytes into cartilage defects to promote cartilage regeneration (Steinert et al., 2008); and 7) promotion of adiponectin gene expression (Ebina et al., 2009). In addition, because new blood vessel formation is also intimately involved with perpetuating the chronic state of inflammation associated with RA, experimental gene therapy strategies designed to suppress the activity of pro-angiogenesis factors such as vascular endothelial growth factor (VEGF) (Afuwape et al., 2003) and Tie-2 (Chen et al., 2005) have also been earnestly pursued.

There also exists an elevated frequency of apoptotic cells in RA articular cartilage joints which is likely to contribute to diminished chondrocyte vitality (Malemud & Gillespie, 2005). By contrast, resistance to induction of apoptosis in RA synovial-like fibroblasts (Hutcheson & Perlman, 2008) and up-regulation of chemokines and adhesion molecules (Malemud & Reddy, 2008) are generally considered to be hallmarks of synovial tissue hyperplasia. Thus, apoptosis, chemokines and adhesion molecules may also be suitable targets for gene therapy strategies.

4.1 Novel gene therapy strategies and improvements in the delivery of gene constructs

Several gene therapy strategies have taken advantage of recent advances in silencing RNA (siRNA) technology (Aigner, 2008; Blagbrough & Zara, 2009; Li & Huang, 2008; Lu & Woodle, 2008). Thus, siRNA has already been employed to generate tolerogenic dendritic antigen-presenting cells (Khan et al., 2009; Zheng et al., 2010) or to "shut-down" pro-inflammatory cytokine production (Khoury et al., 2008). siRNAs have also been incorporated into a gene "cream" for delivery to inflamed synovial joints. This concept has already been used to regulate the biological activity of molecules such as osteopontin in a rodent model of RA (Takanashi et al., 2009).

Most importantly, vast improvements have occurred in developing new strategies for administering gene constructs. This has been achieved through the use of non-viral vectors (Adriaansen et al., 2006) adeno-associated viral (AAV) vectors (Tang et al., 2010) or lentiviral vectors (Gouze et al. 2002). In that regard, the development of useful vectors for preparing gene constructs has taken on greater significance in the field. Thus, these various approaches to delivering gene constructs of interest to synovial joints are likely to be critical because the improved administration of gene constructs and/or plasmids will be instrumental for future studies designed to regulate the activities of such RA-related molecules such as IL-17, IL-18, CD40/nuclear factor-κB, COT/Tpl-2 and extracellular matrix degrading proteinases to name just a few relevant targets for ameliorating inflammatory arthritis *in vivo* (Wisler et al., 2011).

The major emphasis in this chapter has been placed on systematically analyzing the recent advances since 2007-2008 when this field was last reviewed (Malemud, 2007; Woods et al., 2008; Dai et al., 2008). Thus, this review will focus its attention on several novel modalities for developing gene constructs as well as emerging strategies for delivering genes to inflamed synovial joints in the murine or rat Type II collagen-induced arthritis (CIA) model of RA (Wooley, 2008). This animal model of inflammatory arthritis is considered useful for the pre-clinical assessment of safety, tolerability and efficacy of gene constructs for their potential application to human RA.

5. Gene therapy in the CIA model

5.1 Pro-inflammatory and anti-inflammatory cytokines

The imbalance between pro-inflammatory cytokines such as IL-1, TNF-α and IL-6 and anti-inflammatory cytokines such as IL-4 and IL-10 have been shown to be a significant driving force in the progression of inflammation in animal models of arthritis and as such the gene targeting of these cytokines would be expected to alter the progress of arthritis severity (van de Loo & van den Berg, 2002). Thus, polarization of T-helper type 1 cells (T_h1) to T-helper type 2 cells (T_h2) in favor of T_h1 appears to be at the root cause of immune-mediated dysfunction in RA (Asquith & McInnes, 2007). In RA, T_h1/ T_h2 polarization appears to account, at least in part, for the skewed repertoire of pro-inflammatory cytokines to anti-inflammatory cytokines. This change appears to be coupled to the deficient production and/or activity of T_h2 cytokines, exemplified by IL-4 and IL-10, which may also account for accelerating the progression of RA. Additionally, the genesis of a specific T-cell subset, termed T_h17, also activates a key intracellular signaling pathway in RA, namely, JAK/STAT (Malemud, 2010). It has been postulated that activation of JAK/STAT signaling causes acute synovitis to progress into a chronic destructive arthritis (Khoury et al., 2008; Lubberts, 2008). It was not unexpected that gene therapy strategies employed in CIA have been directed at neutralizing the activity of IL-1, and/or TNF-α or towards augmenting the production of the anti-inflammatory cytokines, IL-4 and/or IL-10. Several of these studies have yielded some promising results.

There have been significant advances in suppressing the activity of TNF-α in several animal models of arthritis through targeted gene therapy. Thus, Adriaansen et al. (2007) showed that a recombinant AAV5 vector (rAAV5) encoding the NF-κB-TNFR1-Ig construct reduced paw swelling in the rat arthritis model which was accompanied not only by decreased levels of TNF-α, but also by reduced levels of IL-1β and IL-6 whereas the level of IL-10 was increased. These results suggested that a coupling mechanism between TNF-α and IL-1/IL-6 must be pertinent to arthritis progression in CIA if suppression of TNF-α gene expression resulted in lower levels of IL-1β/IL-6 and elevated levels of IL-10 as well. Importantly, the rAAV5 vector remained localized to the injected joint and no trace of rAAV5 was found in the periphery. The suppressive effect of a rAAV5 vector encoding TR1 fused to the F_c portion of mouse IgG1 (i.e. TNFRp55 extracellular domain-Ig) on inflammation was also seen in murine CIA (Khoury et al., 2007). In that study, there was a robust correlation between decreased levels of local TR1 and markers of inflammation that contributed to an overall reduction in the inflammation score.

Gould et al. (2007) employed a novel gene delivery system using plasmid vectors pGTLMIK and pGTTMIK from which luciferase and a dimeric TNF receptor were co-expressed in a doxycycline-regulated fashion, to show that administered GTTMIK delayed the onset of arthritis in murine CIA and the progression of inflammation as measured by reduced paw thickness. Additionally, the clinical score diminished but only when doxycycline was co-administered. The results of this study indicated that suppression of murine CIA could be achieved by inhibiting TNF-α-mediated events via gene expression-specific regulation. Inoue et al. (2009) used siRNAs which are double-stranded oligonucleotides that are designed to perfectly pair with the targeted mRNA in order to cause mRNA degradation to show that intra-articular delivery of TNF-α or IL1β-specific siRNAs reduced inflammation in rat CIA. The results of this study also showed that siRNA duplexes when administered *in vivo* to specifically degrade TNF-α, IL1β, IL-6 or receptor activator of nuclear factor κB ligand (RANKL) mRNA also reduced the level of these cytokines *in vitro*. RANKL is a key growth factor in osteoclast differentiation and bone destruction in inflammatory arthritis (Choi et al., 2009).

Finally, Lai Kwan Lam et al. (2008) employed siRNA technology using a lentivirus-regulated B-cell activating factor (Lv-shBAFF) to limit BAFF levels. BAFF is a critical molecule in RA because it promotes the survival of activated B-cells (Townsend et al., 2010). In this study, Lv-shBAFF suppressed BAFF production. However, and unexpectedly so, silencing of BAFF gene expression also reduced the activity of T_h17 cells as well as B-cell activity in murine CIA. The suppression of T_h17 cell-mediated activity was accompanied by reduced synovial tissue inflammation. Moreover, Lv-shBAFF reduced the percentage of mice developing CIA by around 50% and reduced the onset time for arthritic pathology. Of note, computer tomography scanning failed to detect any narrowing of the joint space or changes in bone erosions when mice with CIA who had had Lv-shBAFF administered were compared to mice with CIA who were injected with an LV vector expressing shRNA for β-actin. In accompanying *in vitro* studies, Lv-shBAFF inhibited dendritic cell maturation which could have been responsible for the suppression of T_h17 cell differentiation produced by Lv-shBAFF in CIA.

5.2 Signal transduction pathways

Gene targeting of the JAK/STAT and PI3K/Akt/PTEN/mTOR signal transduction pathways have been considered as an alternative to orally-administered enzyme inhibitors to suppress immune-mediated inflammation in animal models of arthritis (Camps et al.,

2005; Milici et al., 2008) as well as for inflammatory disorders in general (Ghigo et al., 2010). In that regard, Hildner et al. (2007) showed that targeting STAT4 by antisense phosphorothioate oligonucleotides reduced inflammation in murine CIA. In a correlative analysis (Hildner et al., 2007), STAT-4 deficient mice also developed significantly less severe arthritis than their wild-type counterparts. Further, T-cells recovered from the STAT-4 deficient mice produced less IL-6, TNF-α and IL-17. In another interesting study, adenoviral vectors encoding PTEN (AdPTEN) or β-galactosidase (AdLacZ) were injected directly into the joints of rats with CIA (Wang et al., 2008). AdPTEN was shown to reduce ankle circumference, articular cartilage degradation, radiographic and histology scores compared to rats with CIA injected with AdLacZ. AdPTEN also reduced microvessel density as well as VEGF and IL-1β levels while suppressing Akt activation. The suppressed activity of Akt correlated with a concomitant increase in the frequency of apoptotic cells in the arthritic ankle joints of rats with CIA. Taken together these results indicated that down-regulation of the PI3K/Akt/PTEN/mTor pathway by AdPTEN gene transfer could be an effective future strategy for not only suppressing the neoangiogenic response in synovial tissue that is a hallmark of joints with inflammatory arthritis (Szekanecz & Koch, 2008) but also as an alternative to using small molecule enzyme inhibitors in order to increase apoptosis in arthritic apoptosis-resistant synovial tissue (Hutcheson & Perlman, 2008).

5.3 T-cells, growth factors, metalloproteinase(s) and assorted other gene targets

T-cell receptor (TCR) gene transfer was originally proposed as a novel approach for use in antigen-specific immunotherapy (Fujio et al., 2006). Thus, in lupus-prone NZB/W F1 mice, nucleosome-specific TCRs and CTLA4-Ig-transduced cells suppressed autoantibody production and the development of nephritis whereas in CIA, TCRs recovered from T-cells that accumulated in the affected arthritic joints combined with TNFR-Ig -transduced cells or TCRs in combination with Forkhead box p3 (Foxp3) transcription factor-transduced cells, the latter a marker of the regulatory T-cell phenotype (Haque et al., 2010) suppressed the progression of arthritis and reduced bone erosions (Fujio et al., 2007a, 2007b). These results indicated that the production of antigen-specific T-cells engineered to express specific functional genes could be a productive immunotherapeutic strategy for future considerations in the treatment of human autoimmunity and arthritis.

Several growth factors pertinent to the abnormal increase in microvascular density that is a characteristic of RA synovial tissue have been targeted by gene constructs, including, VEGF (Afuwape et al., 2003), Ang-1 and Tie-2 (Fielder & Augustin, 2006). Because increased levels of synovial tissue Tie-2 and Ang-1 were shown to correlate with aberrant neoangiogenesis in CIA (DeBusk et al. 2003), Chen et al. (2005) studied the extent to which arthritis in CIA could be regulated by a Tie-2 gene construct. Thus, the severity of arthritis was markedly reduced when an adenovirus vector containing a soluble Tie-2 receptor (Ad.ExTek) was locally administered after the onset of arthritis. In addition, Ad.ExTek protected mice with CIA against bony erosions, suppressed neoangiogenesis, reduced the level of RANKL, but did not suppress anti-Type II collagen antibody production. However, a search of the PubMed literature since 2007 did not reveal any current studies directed at targeting angiogenesis via either Ang-1 or Tie-2 gene therapy suggesting that a greater focus has been placed on defining a common thread such as PI3K/Akt/PTEN/mTor pathway activation as a way of regulating neoangiogenesis in CIA (Wang et al., 2008).

The failure of chondrocytes to respond to insulin-like growth factor-1 (IGF-1) has been proposed as one of the mechanisms that underlie the inefficient repair of articular cartilage in arthritis (van de Loo et al., 2008). Although the results of a study (Nixon et al., 2005) showed that synovial membrane co-transduced *in vitro* with an E1-deleted adenovirus vectors, one containing IGF-1 and the other IL-1 receptor antagonist (IL-1Ra) regulated by a cytomegalovirus promoter increased IGF-1 and IL-1Ra mRNA, an analysis as to the extent to which a gene strategy such as this one was capable of altering cartilage homeostasis in CIA was not performed. Thus, the more recent study results reported by Izal et al. (2008) becomes more significant because AAV-derived vectors containing IGF-1 increased secreted IGF-1 protein in cells infected with AAV-IGF-1 and increased cartilage protein synthesis 2 months after being locally administered into rats. However, this result could be not be reproduced in rats with CIA or in rats in which the arthritis was induced by mechanical injury indicating that AAV vectors capable of up-regulating the expression of IGF-1 *in vitro* was not an effective chondroprotective strategy.

Three additional targets for which gene therapy has been employed in experimental models of arthritis are worthy of comment. The down-regulation of MMP gene expression and inhibition of MMP activation are critical mechanisms for regulating cartilage and bone extracellular matrix degradation in RA (Zafarullah et al., 2008). Chia et al. (2008) employed the mouse model of CIA to show that the MMP-9 (92kDa gelatinase) gene was up-regulated in both the acute and chronic (late) stage of mouse CIA whereas elevated IL-1β gene expression was limited only to the acute stage of CIA. This result suggested that targeting MMP-9 by gene therapy could significantly limit the destruction of cartilage and bone extracellular matrix in CIA. Furthermore, because the activity of MMP-9 is regulated by neutrophil gelatinase-associated lipocalin (NGAL) which prevents the autocatalytic degradation of pro-MMP-9 (Gupta et al., 2007), NGAL synthesis could also be targeted by gene therapy to determine the extent to which down-regulating NGAL gene expression reduces the onset and/or severity of arthritis in CIA. Resistance to induction of apoptosis in RA synoviocytes results in perpetuating the inflammatory response in RA synovium for which several intracellular pathways that regulate the induction of apoptosis are known to converge contributing to RA pathogenesis and progression, including the development of pannus (Baier et al., 2003; Ospelt et al., 2004; Sweeney & Firestein, 2004; Malemud & Gillespie, 2005). Since it would be unlikely that inhibiting only one of these intracellular signaling pathways would induce apoptosis in RA synovium (Malemud, 2011), it was notable that Chen et al. (2009) showed that an E1B-55-kDa-deleted AV (Ad.GS1) driven by the human telomerase reverse transcriptase promoter induced cytolysis of human RA synovial fibroblasts and synoviocytes from rats with CIA *ex vivo*. Further, Ad.GS1 replicated only in arthritic rats where Ad.GS1 significantly reduced ankle size, the arthritis severity score, radiographic progression, and histological evidence of joint inflammation while also suppressing the expression of IL-1β, MMP-9 and prolyl-4-hydroxylase, the latter a marker of collagen biosynthesis (Kivirikko et al., 1989). Thus, Ad.GS1 was the first AV-vector driven by a telomerase promoter that was shown to ameliorate the severity of arthritis in CIA while also suppressing IL-1β and MMP-9, but with reduced collagen synthesis. The overall significance of Ad.GS1 in reducing prolyl-4-hydroxylase activity in RA cartilage and bone repair has not been completely elucidated. Finally, α-1-antitrypsin (AAT) belongs to a class of acute phase reactant proteins which is also well known as an anti-inflammatory protein with marked tissue protective characteristics. Whereas serum levels of AAT are generally altered in RA, AAT levels failed to correlate with the titer of rheumatoid factor but AAT did correlate with erythrocyte sedimentation rate (Cylwik et al., 2010). Further, AAT levels were closely related to RA clinical activity as measured by the Disease Activity Score-28 criteria.

Recently, Grimstein et al. (2010; 2011) showed that mice with CIA treated either with AAT or rAAV-AAT alone or in combination with doxycycline delayed the onset and reduced the severity of arthritis. The severity of arthritis in CIA was correlated with reduced levels of BAFF and with lower anti-collagen autoantibodies suggesting that a major target of AAT therapy in CIA was to suppress the activity of hyperactive B-cells.

6. Conclusions

Significant progress has been made in the potential for future medical therapies of RA to employ gene therapy. In that regard, a few gene therapy strategies have already been tested in cell cultures and pre-clinical animal models of arthritis most notability in the CIA model in mice and rats. Of note, several targets for gene therapy such as IL-1Ra, TNF-α, and IL-17 have already yielded DMARBDs or other forms of neutralizing compounds which are either currently being assessed in pre-clinical studies, tested in RA clinical trials or routinely used in the treatment of RA in clinical practice (Genovese et al., 2010; Finckh & Gabay, 2008; Gibbons & Hyrich, 2009; Ishiguro et al., 2011; Sênolt et al., 2009; Toh et al., 2010). However, the positive results obtained with various gene therapy strategies in cell cultures and/or in animal models of arthritis must always be cautiously interpreted as the previous supportive results with inhibitors of p38 kinase in arthritis animal models (Böhm et al., 2009; Hammaker & Firestein, 2010) which provided the impetus for the clinical testing of p38 kinase inhibitors proved to be disappointing in terms of clinical outcomes in human RA trials (Genovese, 2009). Thus, it remains to be seen if the biopharmaceutical industry will use pertinent targets for RA intervention such as IL-10, BAFF, MMP-9, etc. in gene therapy studies so that the effects of these gene constructs can be pre-clinically assessed. In addition, an increased attention to the potential negative biological effects of the viral vectors so commonly used to regulate the activity of these gene constructs must also take place. If no toxic or adverse effects occur in pre-clinical testing, then and only then should these gene constructs be further developed for their eventual assessment in RA.

7. Acknowledgments

Research in the Malemud laboratory is funded by Takeda Pharmaceuticals of North America and by Roche/Genentech. No further conflicts of interest relevant to this article were reported.

8. References

Adriaansen, J., Vervoordeldonk, M.J., Vanderbyl, S. et al. (2006) A novel approach for gene therapy: engraftment of fibroblasts containing the artificial chromosome expression system at the site of inflammation. *Journal of Gene Medicine* 8(1): pp. 63-71.

Adriaansen, J., Khoury, M., de Cortie C. J. et al. (2007) Reduction of arthritis following intra-articular administration of an adeno-associated virus serotype 5 expressing a disease-inducible TNF-blocking agent. *Annals of the Rheumatic Diseases* 66(9): pp. 1143-1150.

Afuwape, A. O., Feldmann, M. & Paleolog, E.M. (2003) Adenoviral delivery of soluble VEGF receptor (sFlt-1) abrogates disease activity in murine collagen-induced arthritis. *Gene Therapy* 10(23): pp.1950-1960.

Aigner, A. (2008) Cellular delivery in vivo of siRNA-based therapeutics. *Current Pharmaceutical Design* 14(34): pp. 3603-3619.

Asquith D. L. & McInnes, I. B. (2007) Emerging cytokine targets in rheumatoid arthritis. *Current Opinion in Rheumatology* 19(3): pp. 246-251.

Baier, A., Meineckel, I., Gay, S., Pap T. (2003) Apoptosis in rheumatoid arthritis. *Current Opinion in Rheumatology* 15(3): pp. 274-279.

Blagbrough, I. S. & Zara C. (2009) Animal models for target diseases in gene therapy—using DNA and siRNA delivery strategies. *Pharmaceutical Research* 26(1): pp. 1-18.

Böhm, C. Hayer, S., Kilian, A. et al. (2009) The α isoform of p38 kinase MAPK specifically regulates arthritic bone loss. *Journal of Immunology* 183(9): pp. 5938-5947.

Camps, M., Rückle, T, Ji H et al. (2005) Blockade of PI3Kγ suppresses joint inflammation and damage in mouse models of rheumatoid arthritis. *Nature Medicine* 11(9): pp. 936-943.

Chia, W.T., Chen, Y. W., Cheng, L. Y. et al. (2008) MMP-9 mRNA as a therapeutic marker in acute and chronic stages of arthritis induced by type II collagen antibody. *Journal of the Formosan Medical Association* 107(3): pp. 245-252.

Chen, S. Y., Shiau, A. L., Shieh, G. S. et al. (2009) Amelioration of experimental arthritis by a telomerase-dependent conditionally replicating adenovirus that targets synovial fibroblasts. *Arthritis & Rheumatism* 60(11): pp. 3290-3302.

Chen, S.Y., Wu, C.L., Lai, M.D. et al. (2011) Amelioration of rat collagen-induced arthritis through CD4+ T cells apoptosis and synovial interleukin-17 reduction by indoleamine 2, 3-dioxygenase gene therapy. *Human Gene Therapy* 22(2): pp. 145-154.

Chen, Y., Donnelly, E., Kobayashi, H. et al. (2005) Gene therapy targeting the Tie2 function ameliorates collagen-induced arthritis and protects against bone destruction. *Arthritis & Rheumatism* 52(5): pp.1585-1594.

Choi, Y., Arron, J. R., & Townsend, M. J. (2009) Promising bone-related therapeutic targets for rheumatoid arthritis. *Nature Reviews in Rheumatology* 5(10): pp. 543-548.

Cylwik, B., Chrostek, L., Gindzienska-Sieskiewicz, E. et al. (2010) Relationship between serum acute-phase proteins and high disease activity in patients with rheumatoid arthritis. *Advances in Medical Sciences* 55(1): pp. 80-85.

Dai K.R, Zhang, X. L., Shi, Q., & Fernandes, J. C. (2008) Gene therapy of arthritis and orthopaedic disorders: current experimental approaches in China and in Canada. *Expert Opinion on Biological Therapy* 8(9): pp. 1337-1346.

DeBusk, L. M., Chen, Y., Nishishita, J. et al. (2003) Tie2 receptor kinase, a major mediator of tumor necrosis factor-α-induced angiogenesis in rheumatoid arthritis. *Arthritis & Rheumatism* 48(9): pp. 2461-2471.

Denys, A., Thiolat A., Descamps D. et al. (2010) Intra-articular electrotransfer of mouse soluble tumour necrosis factor receptor in a murine model of rheumatoid arthritis. *Journal of Gene Medicine* 12(8): pp. 659-668.

Ebina, K., Oshima, K., Matsuda M. et al. (2009) Adenovirus-mediated gene transfer of adiponectin reduces the severity of collagen-induced arthritis in mice. *Biochemical & Biophysical Research Communications* 378(2): pp.186-191.

Feely, M.G., Erickson, A. & O'Dell, J.R. (2009) Therapeutic options for rheumatoid arthritis. *Expert Opinion on Pharmacotherapy* 10(13): pp.2095-2106.

Fielder, U. & Augustin, H. G. (2006) Angiopoietins: a link between angiogenesis and inflammation. *Trends in Immunology* 27(12): pp. 552-558.

Finckh, A. & Gabay, C. (2008) At the horizon of innovative therapy in rheumatology: new biological agents. *Current Opinion in Rheumatology* 20(3): pp. 269-275.

Fujio, K., Okamoto, A., Araki, Y. et al. (2006) Gene therapy of arthritis with TCR isolated from the inflamed paw. *Journal of Immunology* 177(11): pp. 8140-8147.

Fujio, K., Okamura, T., Okamoto, A., Yamamoto, K. (2007a) T cell receptor gene therapy for autoimmune diseases. *Annals of the New York Academy of Sciences* 1110: pp. 222-232.

Fujio, K., Okamura, T., Okamoto, A., Yamamoto, K. (2007b) T-cell receptor- and anti-inflammatory gene-modulated T cells as therapy for autoimmune disease. *Expert Reviews in Clinical Immunology* 3(6): pp. 883-890.

Gaddy, D. F. & Robbins, P.D. (2008) Current status of gene therapy for rheumatoid arthritis. *Current Rheumatology Reports* 10(5): pp. 398-404.

Genovese, M. C. (2009) Inhibition of p38: has the fat lady sung? *Arthritis & Rheumatism* 60(2): pp. 317-320.

Genovese, M. C., van den Bosch, F., Robertson, S. A. et al. (2010) LY2439821, a humanized anti-interleukin-17 monoclonal antibody, in the treatment of patients with rheumatoid arthritis; a phase I randomized, double-blind, placebo-controlled, proof-of-concept study. *Arthritis & Rheumatism* 62(4): pp. 929-939.

Ghigo, A., Damilano, F, Braccini, L. & Hirsch, E. (2010) PI3K inhibition in inflammation: toward tailored therapies for specific diseases. *Bioessays* 32(3): pp. 185-196.

Gibbons, L. J. & Hyrich, K. L. (2009) Biologic therapy for rheumatoid arthritis: clinical efficacy and predictors of response. *BioDrugs* 23(2): pp.111-124.

Gould, D., Yousaf, N., Fatah, R., Subang, M. C. & Chernajovsky, Y. (2007) Gene therapy with an improved doxycycline-regulated plasmid encoding a tumour necrosis factor-alpha inhibitor in experimental arthritis. *Arthritis Research & Therapy* 9(1): Pg. R7.

Gouze, E., Pawliuk, R., Pilapil, C. et al. (2002) In vivo gene delivery to synovium by lentiviral vectors. *Molecular Therapy* 5(4): pp. 397-404.

Grimstein, C., Choi, Y. K., Satoh, M. et al. (2010) Combination of alpha-1 antitrypsin and doxycycline suppresses collagen-induced arthritis. *The Journal of Gene Medicine* 12(1): pp. 35-44.

Grimstein, C., Choi, Y. K., Wasserfall, C.H. (2011) Alpha-1 antitrypsin protein and gene therapies decrease autoimmunity and delay arthritis development in mouse model. *Journal of Translational Medicine* 9: pp. 21.

Gupta K., Shukla M., Cowland J. B. et al. (2007) Neutrophil gelatinase-associated lipocalin (NGAL) is expressed in osteoarthritis and forms a complex with matrix metalloproteinase-9. *Arthritis & Rheumatism* 56(10): pp. 3326-3335.

Hammaker, D. & Firestein, G. S. (2010) "Go upstream, young man": lessons learned from the p38 saga. *Annals of the Rheumatic Diseases* 69 Suppl 1: pp. i77-i82.

Haque, R., Lei, F., Xiong, X., Wu, Y. & Song, J. (2010) FoxP3 and Bcl-xL cooperatively promote regulatory T cell persistence and prevention of arthritis development. *Arthritis Research & Therapy* 12(2): Pg. R66.

Hildner, K. M., Schirmacher, P., Atreya, I et al. (2007) Targeting of the transcription factor STAT4 by antisense phosphorothioate oligonucleotides suppresses collagen-induced arthritis. *Journal of Immunology* 178(6): pp. 3427-3436.

Hutcheson, J. C. & Perlman, H. (2008) Apoptotic regulators in RA. *Current Rheumatology Reviews* 4(4): pp. 254-258.

Inoue A., Takahashi. K. A., Mazda, O. et al. (2009) Comparison of anti-rheumatic effects of local RNAi-based therapy in collagen-induced arthritis rats using various cytokine genes as molecular targets. *Moderm Rheumatology* 19(2): pp. 125-133.

Ishiguro, A., Akiyama, T., Adachi, H., Inoue, J., Nakamura, Y. (2011) Therapeutic potential of anti-interleukin-17 aptamer. Suppression of interleukin-17A signaling and attenuation of autoimmunity in two mouse models. *Arthritis & Rheumatism* 63(2): pp. 455-466.

Izal, I., Acosta, C. A., Ripalda, P. et al. (2008) IGF-1 gene therapy to protect articular cartilage in a rat model of joint damage. *Archives of Orthopaedics & Trauma Surgery* 128(2): pp. 239-247.

Jorgensen, C. & Apparailly, F. (2010) Prospects for gene therapy in inflammatory arthritis. *Best Practice & Research in Clinical Rheumatology* 24(4): pp. 541-552.

Kageyama, Y., Koide, Y., Uchijima, M. et al. (2004) Plasmid encoding interleukin-4 in the amelioration of murine collagen-induced arthritis. *Arthritis & Rheumatism* 50(3): pp. 968-975.

Khan, S. Greenberg, J. D. & Bhardwaj, N. (2009) Dendritic cells as targets for therapy in rheumatoid arthritis. *Nature Reviews Rheumatology* 5(10): pp. 566-571.

Kim, J. M., Jeong, J. G., Ho, S. H. et al. (2003) Protection against collagen-indued arthritis by intramuscular gene therapy with an expression plasmid for the interleukin-1 receptor antagonist. *Gene Therapy* 10(8): pp. 1543-1550.

Kivirikko, K. I., Myllyla, R. & Pihlajaniemi, T. (1989) Protein hydroxylation: prolyl 4-hydroxylase, an enzyme with 4 cosubstrates and a multifunctional subunit. *The FASEB Journal* 3(5): pp. 1609-1617.

Khoury, M. Adriaansen, J., Vervoordeldonk, M. J. et al. (2007) Inflammation-inducible anti-TNF gene expression mediated by intra-articular injection of serotype 5 adeno-associated virus reduces arthritis. *Journal of Gene Medicine* 9(7): pp. 596-604.

Khoury, M., Courties, G., Fabre, S. et al. (2010) Adeno-associated virus type 5-mediated intraarticular administration of tumor necrosis factor small interfering RNA improves collagen-induced arthritis. *Arthritis & Rheumatism* 62(3): pp.765-770.

Khoury, M., Escriou, V., Courties G. et al. (2008) Efficient suppression of murine arthritis by combined anticytokine small interfering RNA lipoplexes. *Arthritis & Rheumatism* 58(8): pp. 2356-2367.

Lai Kwan Lam, Q., King Hung Koo, O., Zheng, B. J. & Lu, L. (2008) Local BAFF gene silencing suppresses Th17-cell generation and ameliorates autoimmune arthritis. *Proceedings of the National Academy of Sciences United States of America* 105(39): pp. 14993-14998.

Leung, P.S., Shu, S. A., Kenny, T.P., Wu, P. Y. & Tao, M. H. (2010) Development and validation of gene therapies in autoimmune diseases: Epidemiology to animal models. *Autoimmunity Reviews* 9(5): pp. A400-A405.

Li, S. D. & Huang, L. (2008) Targeted delivery of siRNA by nonviral vectors: lessons learned from recent advances. *Current Opinion on Investigational Drugs* 9(12): pp. 1317-1323.

Liu, B. & Shuai, K. (2008) Targeting the PIAS1 SUMO ligase pathway to control inflammation. *Trends in Pharmacological Sciences* 29(10): pp. 505-509.

Lu, P. & Woodle, M.C. (2008) Delivering small interfering RNA for novel therapeutics. *Methods in Molecular Biology* 437: pp. 93-107.

Lubberts, E. (2008) IL-17/Th17 targeting: on the road to prevent chronic destructive arthritis? *Cytokine* 41(2): pp. 84-91.

Malemud, C. J. (2007) Gene therapy for arthritis. *Gene Therapy and Molecular Biology* 11: pp. 27-36.

Malemud, C. J. (2010) Differential activation of JAK enzymes in rheumatoid arthritis and autoimmune disorders by pro-inflammatory cytokines: potential drug targets. *International Journal of Interferon, Cytokine and Mediator Research* 2: pp. 97-111.

Malemud C.J. (2011) Dysfunctional immune-mediated inflammation in rheumatoid arthritis dictates that development of anti-rheumatic disease drugs target multiple intracellular signaling pathways. *Anti-Inflammatory & Anti-Allergy Agents in Medicinal Chemistry* (In Press)

Malemud, C. J. & Gillespie, H. J. (2005) The role of apoptosis in arthritis. *Current Rheumatology Reviews* 1(1): pp. 131-142.

Malemud, C. J. & Miller, A. H. (2008) Pro-inflammatory cytokine-induced SAPK/MAPK and JAK/STAT in rheumatoid arthritis and the new anti-depression drugs. *Expert Opinion in Therapeutic Targets* 12(2): pp. 171-183.

Malemud, C. J. & Pearlman, E. (2009) Targeting JAK/STAT signaling pathway in inflammatory diseases. *Current Signal Transduction Therapy* 4: pp. 201-221.

Malemud, C. J. & Reddy, S. K. (2008) Targeting cytokines, chemokines and adhesion molecules in rheumatoid arthritis. *Current Rheumatology Reviews* 4(4): pp. 219-234.

Marone, R, Cmiljanovic V, Giese B. & Wymann MP. (2008) Targeting phosphoinositide-3-kinase: moving towards therapy. *Biochim Biophys Acta* 1784(1): pp. 159-185.

Milici, A. J., Kudlacz, E. M., Audoly, L., Zwillich, S., Changelian, P. (2008) Cartilage preservation by inhibition of Janus kinase 3 in two rodent models of rheumatoid arthritis. *Arthritis Research & Therapy* 10(1): Pg. R14.

Nabbe, K. C., van Lent, P.L., Holthuysen, A.E. et al. (2005) Local IL-13 gene transfer prior to immune-cartilage complex arthritis inhibits chondrocyte death and matrix-metalloproteinase-mediated cartilage matrix degradation despite enhanced joint inflammation. *Arthritis Research & Therapy* 7(2): pp. R392-R401.

Nixon, A. J., Haupt, J. L. Frisbie, D. D. et al. (2005) Gene-mediated restoration of cartilage matrix by combination insulin-like growth factor/interleukin-1 receptor antagonist therapy. *Gene Therapy* 12(2): pp. 177-186.

Ospelt, C., Neidhart, M., Gay, R. E., Gay, S. (2004) Synovial activation in rheumatoid arthritis. *Frontiers in Bioscience* 9: pp. 2323-2334.

Salliot, C., Dougados, M., & Gossec, L. (2009) Risk of serious infections during rituximab, abatacept and anakinra treatment for rheumatoid arthritis: meta-analysis of randomised placebo-controlled trials. *Annals of the Rheumatic Diseases* 68(1): pp. 25-32.

Ŝenolt, L., Vencovský, J., Pavelka, K., Ospelt, C., Gay, S. (2009) Prospective new biological therapies for rheumatoid arthritis. *Autoimmunity Reviews* 9(2): pp.102-107.

Szekanecz, Z. & Koch, A. E. (2008) Targeting angiogenesis in RA. *Current Rheumatology Reviews* 4(4): pp. 298-303.

Smeets, R.L., van de Loo, F.A., Arntz, O.J. et al. (2003) Adenoviral delivery of IL-18-binding protein C ameliorates collagen-induced arthritis in mice. *Gene Therapy* 10(12): pp.1004-1011.

Steinert, A.F., Nöth, U. & Tuan, R. S. (2008) Concepts of gene therapy for cartilage repair. *Injury* 39 Suppl 1: pp. S97-S113.

Sweeney, S. E. & Firestein, G. S. (2004) Rheumatoid arthritis: regulation of synovial inflammation. *The International Journal of Biochemistry & Cell Biology* 36(3): pp. 372-378.

Takanashi, M., Oikawa, K., Sudo, K. et al. (2009) Therapeutic silencing of an endogenous gene by siRNA cream in an arthritis model mouse. *Gene Therapy* 16(8): pp. 982-989.

Tang, B., Cullins, D. L., Zhou, J. et al. (2010) Modulation of collagen-induced arthritis by adenovirus-mediated intra-articular expression of modified collagen type II. *Arthritis Research & Therapy* 12(4): pg. R136.

Toh, M. L., Kawashima, M., Hot, A., Miossec, P., Miossec, P. (2010) Role of IL-17 in the Th1 systemic defects in rheumatoid arthritis through selective IL-12Rβ2 inhibition. *Annals of the Rheumatic Diseases* 69(8): pp. 1562-1567.

Townsend, M. J., Monroe, J. G. & Chan, A. C. (2010) B-cell targeted therapies in human autoimmune diseases: an updated perspective. *Immunological Reviews* 237(1): pp. 264-283.

Traister, R.S. & Hirsch, R. (2008) Gene therapy for arthritis. *Modern Rheumatology* 18(1): pp. 2-14.

van de Loo, F. A., Veenbergen, S., & van den Berg, W. B. (2008) Targeting growth factors in arthritis: a rational for restoring the IGF-1 response in chondrocytes. *Current Rheumatology Reviews* 4(4): pp. 266-277.

van de Loo, F. A. & van den Berg, W.B. (2002) Gene therapy for rheumatoid arthritis. Lessons from animal models, including studies on interleukin-4, interleukin-10, and interleukin-1 receptor antagonist as potential disease modulators. *Rheumatic Disease Clinics of North America* 28(1): pp. 127-149.

Walker, JG, Ahern, M. J. Coleman, M. et al. (2006) Expression of Jak3, STAT1, STAT4, and STAT6 in inflammatory arthritis: unique Jak3 and STAT4 expression in dendritic cells in seropositive rheumatoid arthritis. *Annals of the Rheumatic Diseases* 65(2): pp. 149-156.

Wang, C. R., Shiau, A. L., Chen, S. Y. et al. (2008) Amelioration of collagen-induced arthritis in rats by adenovirus-mediated PTEN gene transfer. *Arthritis & Rheumatism* 58(6): pp. 1650-1656.

Wisler, B. A., Dennis, J. E. & Malemud, C. J. (2011) New organ-specific pharmacological strategies interfering with signaling pathways in inflammatory disorders/autoimmune disorders. *Current Signal Transduction Therapy* – Supplement: Towards tailoring treatment – New organ-specific drug strategies interfering in signal pathway (in press)

Woods, J. M., Sitabkhan, Y. & Koch, A.E. (2008) Gene therapy for rheumatoid arthritis: recent advances. *Current Gene Therapy* 8(1): pp.24-41.

Wooley, P.H. (2008) Which animal models are best for testing novel RA therapies? *Current Rheumatology Reviews* 4(4): pp.277-287.

Zafarullah, M., Ahmad, R., El Mabrouk, M. et al. (2008) Inhibition of matrix metalloproteinases a a feasible therapeutic target in RA. *Current Rheumatology Reviews* 4(4): pp. 288-297.

Zheng, X., Suzuki, M., Ichim, T.E. et al. (2010) Treatment of autoimmune arthritis using RNA interference-modulated dendritic cells. *Journal of Immunology* 184(11): pp.6457-6464.

12

Gene Therapy Applications for Fracture Repair

Cassandra A. Strohbach[1], Donna D. Strong[2] and Charles H. Rundle[3]
[1]*Military Performance Division, U.S. Army Research Institute of Environmental Medicine, Natick, MA,*
[2]*VA Loma Linda HealthCare system, Research 151, Loma Linda, CA Department of Medicine, Biochemistry & Microbiology, Loma Linda University, Loma Linda, CA*
[3]*Musculoskeletal Disease Center, VA Loma Linda HealthCare system, Research 151, Loma Linda, CA, Department of Medicine, Loma Linda University, Loma Linda, CA, USA*

1. Introduction

Each year more than 15 million fractures are treated in the United States and billions of dollars are spent on the treatment musculoskeletal injuries (Brinker, 2004). Ten to fifteen percent of fractures fail to heal correctly resulting in non-union or delayed union healing (Einhorn 1995; Klamut et al., 2004; Pelled, et al., 2010). The underlying medical conditions, including osteoporosis, contributing to inadequate bone healing during fracture repair are numerous and have been previously reviewed (Komatsu and Warden, 2010; Evans, 2010). With regard to normal or impaired fracture repair, stimulation and/or acceleration of bone healing would yield considerable health and economic benefits. In orthopedics, there is great interest in reducing fracture healing time, increasing the rates of unions or complete regeneration and in being able to treat non-unions more successfully.

One non-traditional approach of accomplishing this is by applying gene therapy to alter the cellular and/or molecular milieu in areas in need of regeneration. Gene therapy could be used to increase the local concentration of osteoinductive molecules at the fracture site thereby stimulating healing at sites of non-union or accelerating union in the case of normal fracture healing. Regenerative genes that replace recombinant osteogenic proteins are attractive alternatives to the costly therapeutics now available in the clinic. Direct gene therapy should be regarded as the most straight forward approach to fracture repair and this approach will be the main focus of this review.

Gene therapy is a new frontier that incorporates the current scientific understanding of human physiology, cellular and molecular biology, and in some cases virology to develop new and more effective treatments for diseases and disorders. In some cases this involves direct correcting of defective genes and other times it is merely a means to enhance production of selected proteins for a specified period of time such as during the healing of a fractured bone. Although gene therapy was initially conceived to treat often lethal genetic disorders, its applications have expanded to non-lethal conditions such as non-union fractures and will one day be used to expedite normal human healing processes such as fracture repair.

2. Clinical treatment of bone fractures

Traditional approaches to treating fractures have varied according to the subject and their condition. Standard treatment for a simple or "green-stick" fracture is immobilization usually by the application of a cast for approximately 6 weeks. The decision of whether to surgically intervene in bone repair is dictated by developing circumstances. Obviously, one would not intervene in a younger patient without a severe injury or impaired healing. Additionally, in elderly patients, the risk of surgical stress to the subject might outweigh the potential benefits of surgical intervention. Bone repair clinically often involves the "wait and see" approach to healing, during which time physicians hope that the bone heals. Surgical intervention, despite the risks, is often necessary to deal with severe musculoskeletal injuries that accompany major trauma. These injuries often require surgical reduction of the fracture, involve significant soft tissue damage or infection, any of which can alter the surgical approach beyond that normally used for simple fractures.

There are also chronic situations of impaired healing in patients with health conditions in which surgery is risky, or in which it has failed, and that might benefit from novel molecular therapeutic approaches to improve healing. A variety of conditions present potential risks and benefits to fracture therapy, necessitating careful consideration of the need and the type of intervention. The application of gene therapy certainly could avoid some of the stress of the traditional and more invasive approaches such as surgical intervention. Additionally, with proper development, gene therapy could also be used to accelerate fracture repair and return to function in cases generally not deemed in need of surgical intervention.

3. Fracture repair

Fracture healing coordinates several molecular pathways and is initiated by the inflammatory response of the injury. There are generally four recognized stages of fracture repair that involve different processes of cell recruitment, proliferation, differentiation and remodeling (Fig. 1): 1) the infiltration of inflammatory cells to the wound, 2) intramembranous bone formation, 3) cartilage/endochondral bone formation by the cells of the soft callus, and 4) endochondral bone formation and remodeling of the fracture callus (Bolander, 1992; Franceschi, 2005). When a fracture is sustained, an inflammatory response occurs, recruiting granulocytes, polymorphonuclear neutrophils and macrophages that remove debris and microorganisms and release osteoinductive molecules. A hematoma is formed in response to platelet derived growth factor (PDGF), insulin-like growth factors (IGFs), tumor necrosis factor (TNF) and fibroblast growth factor-2 (FGF-2). Various growth factors stimulate periosteal cell proliferation and the differentiation of chondrocytes that compose fracture cartilage that eventually bridges the fracture gap with cartilage. Bone formation and resorption, mediated by osteoblasts and osteoclasts, respectively function to convert the cartilage to a woven, low-density (trabecular-type) bone that is subsequently remodeled to lamellar cortical bone of pre-fracture structural and functional integrity. The underlying physiological and biomechanical conditions that regulate the transition of the cells through the stages of healing affect the rate of fracture repair (Fig. 1).

Fracture repair involves the interplay of the well regulated interdependent processes of chondrogenesis and osteogenesis. These processes have been characterized by gene profiling of the regulated expression of numerous growth factors, growth factor receptors, cytokines and transcription factors (Hadjiargyrou et al., 2002; Li et al., 2005; Rundle et al., 2006; Bais et al., 2009). The effect of growth factors and other regulatory proteins on fracture repair have also been characterized by observational studies of fracture repair in normal animal subjects compared to those with genetically defined deficiencies, i.e., knockout mice. These approaches have identified candidate genes through protein and gene expression studies *in situ* or global studies in different models of fracture repair (Zhang, et al., 2002; Rundle, et al., 2006; Ota, et al., 2009; Komatsu, et al., 2010). Subsequent development of knockout mice deficient in the expression of the gene(s) has then established the functional significance of their expression during fracture healing, and key molecular pathways have been elucidated. In this way the study of various knockout mouse strains with different gene deficiencies has provided valuable information on molecular regulation of fracture repair. These studies have also revealed two other problems. There is considerable redundancy in the regulation of fracture repair, such that the predicted phenotype is often masked by the expression of genes with redundant functions. Also, these studies have been forced to adapt to the problem that several growth factors that cannot be compensated for are embryonic or perinatal lethal, and very difficult to use in bone repair studies on live animals. The fracture model has therefore been further adapted to use conditional knockout mice that express the gene of interest from a regulatable system, such as tamoxifen or tet-related regulation. In these cases the investment in the development of the mouse strain has to be considered, but these studies have nevertheless proven extremely valuable.

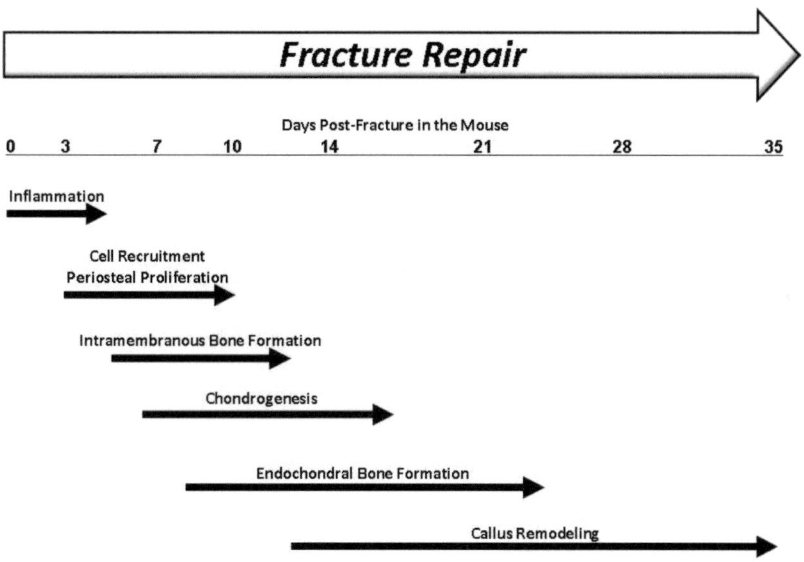

Fig. 1. Fracture repair. The time of appearance and duration of the different processes that regulate the stages of fracture callus development are shown. Bony union of the fracture callus in the mouse and the rat fracture models occurs during the fourth week of healing, and remodeling follows.

4. Bone development

The similarities between bone repair and bone formation extend to intramembranous bone and endochondral bone repair, two different types of bone that heal through the molecular mechanisms that were functional during their development. This concept is stated as "repair recapitulates development" and has been associated with bone, as it has with other tissues (Gerstenfeld et al., 2003; Bais et al., 2009). It is highly informative to view fracture repair in the context of the cells that mediate the development of the different types of bone during embryogenesis: osteoblast maturation for intramembranous bone repair and chondrocyte maturation and osteoblast maturation for endochondral bone repair. Both intramembranous and endochondral bone formation are observed during embryonic skeletal development and both of these processes of bone formation are recapitulated during fracture repair. As encountered with other tissues during healing, an examination of the molecular pathways of fracture repair has established that bone repair shares several similarities with embryonic bone formation.

4.1 Intramembranous bone formation

The flat bones of the skeleton are formed by membranous bone formation, and include the vertebrae and the bones of the skull vault, mandible, and scapula. In contrast to endochondral bone formation, in areas of intramembranous bone formation mesenchymal cells differentiate directly into osteoblasts without a cartilage intermediate. As the osteoblasts proliferate and differentiate they synthesize the osteoid that eventually mineralizes. During intramembranous bone formation, angiogenesis is essential and bone formation occurs in regions rich in blood vessels. Osteoblast development is promoted through the expression and reaction to the expression of different transcription factors and families of growth factors (Fig. 2).

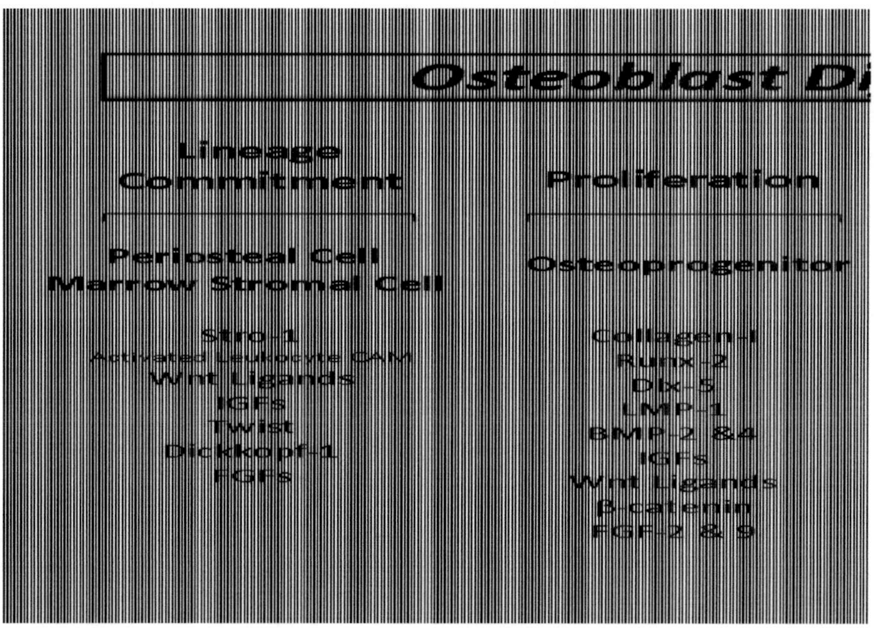

Fig. 2. Osteoblast development. Major transcription factors and growth factors that promote the different stages of osteoblast development are illustrated (adapted from Karsenty, 2009).

Bones of intramembranous origin heal entirely through intramembranous bone formation. Additionally, an endochondral bone fracture that is sufficiently stable can also heal entirely through a fracture callus formed by intramembranous bone formation, without a cartilage intermediate. Intramembranous bone formation also occurs in "gap" repair during direct bone healing, when woven bone bridges the injury between the ends of the cortical bone without any callus formation; that bone is subsequently remodeled to lamellar bone. This type of bone repair is the principle upon which distraction osteogenesis by the Ilizarov technique is based.

4.2 Endochondral bone formation

The long bones of the limbs, the ribs and vertebrae are all formed through endochondral bone formation. During embryonic development, in areas where the aforementioned bones are created, mesenchymal stem cells (MSCs) concentrate and create regions of high cell density that represent outlines of future bones. As MSCs within long bone structures differentiate, they proceed down the endochondral bone formation path. The cells either differentiate into bone-forming osteoblasts (Fig. 2) or differentiate into cartilage-forming chondrocytes (Fig. 3). This type of bone formation occurs in areas from which blood vessels are reduced or excluded. As endochondral bone formation proceeds, the proliferating chondrocytes in the avascular regions cease to proliferate and hypertrophy. At this point, blood vessels invade the hypertrophic cartilage and osteoblasts form bone around the hypertrophic chondrocytes, resulting in the formation of a primary ossification center. The hypertrophic cartilage is progressively replaced with (trabecular-type) woven bone of the bony fracture callus that is itself eventually remodeled to cortical bone to complete healing.

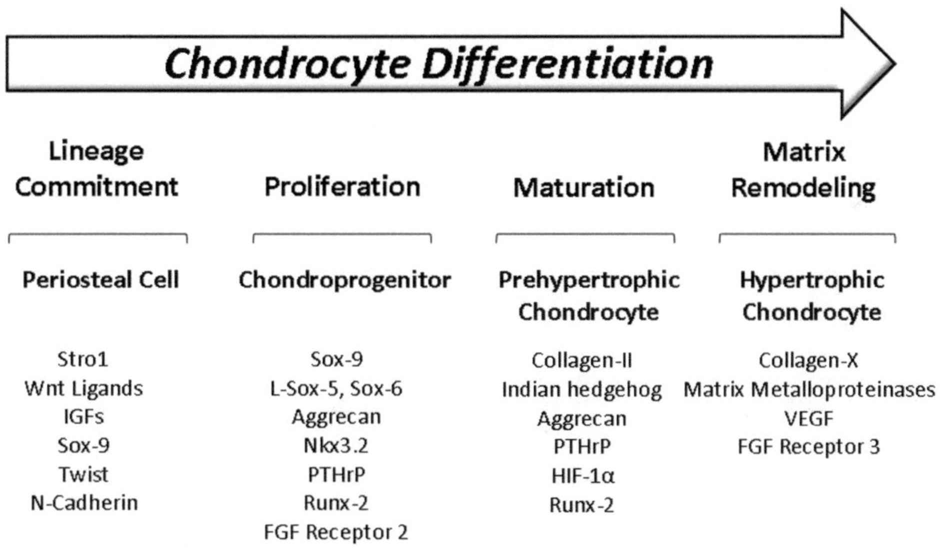

Fig. 3. Chondrocyte development. Major transcription factors and growth factors that promote the different stages of chondrocyte development are illustrated (adapted from de Crombrugghe and Akiyama, 2009; Kronenberg et al., 2009).

Two important tissue repair processes do differ from embryonic development: 1) inflammation and 2) angiogenesis. Inflammation characteristic of fracture repair is completely absent during bone development. Repair studies conducted *in utero* have introduced inflammation in an embryo and impaired embryonic tissue repair developed to the point where embryonic tissues uncharacteristically formed scars. These characteristics are important considerations for bone therapy, a tissue that does undergo an acute inflammatory phase mediated from the innate immune system that is necessary for fracture repair. However, evidence from T cell and B cell deficient mice has also suggested that even in the absence of an immune response, the adaptive immune system mediates an inflammation that can impede fracture repair, suggesting immune regulation of the pro- and anti-inflammatory cytokines (Toben et al., 2011). Additionally, bone therapy must also consider the sources of chronic or infectious inflammation that can impede healing and produce delayed healing or scarring. Therefore, inflammation offers the chance to regulate and promote an important early stage of healing that is distinct to tissue repair, but one in which poor regulation could ultimately severely impair healing. Studies on knockout mice have demonstrated the requirement for innate inflammatory cells and signaling molecules for efficient bone repair.

Angiogenesis, the development of new blood vessels from existing blood vessels, is characteristic of fracture repair, while vasculogenesis, the *de novo* development of blood vessels, is the mechanism by which the embryonic vasculature develops. Perfusion of the fracture callus vasculature in a rat femur osteotomy model revealed that the invasion of the vasculature in the healing fracture, while similar in structure and progression to the growth plate during development, did seem to display a variable spatial organization different from the linear orientation of the developmental growth plate (Mark et al., 2004). This might be due to the chondrocyte organization affected by the enlarged circumference of the fracture callus relative to the growth plate. Street et al. (2002) demonstrated that locally applied vascular endothelial growth factor (VEGF) promoted angiogenesis and bone healing in two different models of bone repair: mouse femur fractures that heal by endochondral bone formation, and in rabbit tibial unicortical defects that heal by intramembranous bone formation. These results establish that angiogenic factors are important in regulating the different types of bone repair and suggest that repair and development utilize the same growth factor families; it seems likely that they would also act through the same mechanisms. However, the regulation of angiogenesis involves several different families of growth factors, signaling molecules and extracellular matrix enzymes, and intervention to improve angiogenesis probably involves complex regulation that requires a detailed understanding, for dysregulated angiogenesis has been associated with cancer.

5. Development of gene therapy for fracture repair

5.1 Bone healing

For the description of the effects of therapeutic efficacy, of gene therapy, it is first important to agree on the definition of bone healing. The ultimate objective of bone repair is the bridging of the cortical defect with bone and the return to pre-fracture mechanical strength and function. An orthopedic definition of healing concludes that healing is successful when there is bridging of the cortical injury in three of four aspects when viewed by X-ray (the two cortices viewed in the anterior-posterior aspect, and those cortices viewed in the lateral-medial aspect). However, a definition often used to evaluate the healing of *in vivo* models of fracture repair for research purposes simply defines healing as the appearance of a bony callus over the cortical injury, a condition that will remodel to pre-fracture bone absent complicating factors, such as infection. Both definitions describe the same process, although at different stages. It is critical to develop atherapy that actually promotes bony union, rather than a therapy that simply produces a larger fracture callus. It is therefore necessary to evaluate the characteristics of the healing fracture to identify the target tissues or the particular defect, engineer the vehicle and select the transgene that provides the best opportunity for timely expression in the appropriate fracture tissues.

5.2 Source of cells

There has been considerable effort dedicated to identifying the source of the cells that contribute to the fracture callus tissues, and some debate as to whether the cells required for fracture callus development are derived from the circulation, as would be expected for stem cells, or whether they are derived from cells resident in the periosteum and bone marrow. The studies of Meyers et al. (2010) support mesenchymal stem cell (MSC) homing to the fracture site mediated by CXCR4 expression and that these cells contribute to healing. On the other hand, the experiments of Colnot et al. (2006, 2009) seem to indicate that the bone formation capacity of the fracture callus originates locally and support the periosteum as the primary source of cells for bone and cartilage formation in the fracture callus. Through bone marrow transplant studies, this work determined that the bone formation cells were derived from the recipient and not from the donor through the circulation; the inflammatory and osteoclast populations were derived from the donor through the circulation, which is in agreement with the hematopoietic origin of these lineages. Other studies demonstrated that the periosteum responded to chondrogenic stimulation by BMP-2 (Yu et al., 2010). Finally, these studies have established that while the endosteum has osteogenic potential, the periosteum possesses chondrogenic and osteogenic potential, evidence that bone formation potential is local in origin. Other populations of cells that are not derived from the periosteum are also required for fracture repair, most notably the inflammatory cells and osteoclasts that are derived from the hematopoietic cell repertoire and arrive at the fracture site through the bone marrow or the reforming periosteal circulation. This conclusion argues against developing a gene therapy with circulating multipotent stem cells as the primary source of cells for the repair of bone tissue. Whatever the defect, it is critical to identify and target the cell populations and the particular function that might be deficient.

If the periosteum is the tissue targeted for gene therapy in the clinic, the delivery approach and the vector/transgene combination must account for the morphology and the cellular composition of the periosteum during fracture healing. Immediately post-fracture, the most obvious time to use gene therapy to intervene to improve fracture repair, the periosteum is only a few layers of fibroblast and pre-osteoblast cells in thickness, making accurate therapeutic gene delivery possible but vector retention very difficult. Additionally, the periosteum is usually disrupted by fracture, and a significant interruption in the periosteum can impede the therapeutic application, as well as more significantly impair normal fracture repair. While the fracture periosteum thickens very rapidly in the initial stages of fracture repair, the therapy must be applied to dividing cells to disperse the therapy in the callus that forms. This problem is addressed by using a targeting system that can best transfect the resident cells present in the tissue at that time, such as a Murine Leukemia Virus (MLV)-based vector or an electroporated non-viral vector that would transduce or transfect the cells that proliferate in the first few days post-fracture (Iwaki et al., 1997). The therapy can then be propagated throughout the fracture tissues as the host cells proliferate (Rundle et al., 2003). The choice of vector for a particular stage of healing is therefore very important.

Cells derived from the circulation are commonly thought to be MSC in origin or function, are attracted to the fracture site and subsequently proliferate to become soft tissue. Another concern with stem cells is that the probability of transformation to a cancerous state appears to be more characteristic than with other types of cells. Stem cells have great potential for fracture therapy, but their contributions to the fracture tissues and their responses to manipulations as therapeutic vehicles must be carefully considered.

5.3 Growth factor genes

A considerable effort has been expended in determining the genes that are critical at different stages of repair for the healing process. Gene therapy attempts to intervene with factors that improve the normal healing process. The skeletal gene therapy strategies to date have targeted the osteoblasts, osteogenic progenitors, chrondrogenic progenitors and other cells within the fracture repair region.

To begin to identify appropriate target genes that might be used to accelerate healing, several laboratories subjected mRNA isolated from different aspects of fracture repair to gene profiling procedures to gain insight to the molecular pathways regulating each situation, including the stages of fracture repair (Hadjiargyrou et al., 2002; Li et al., 2005; Rundle et al., 2006) and the expression of genes of current therapeutic interest, such as stem cell genes (Bais et al., 2009). A variety of genes, involved in activation and repression, were discovered to participate in each stage of the repair process and suggest therapeutic candidates for fracture repair, but the first target genes selected for fracture therapy were those that influenced the rate of osteoblast differentiation and thus bone formation (Fig. 2).

5.4 Fracture model

Fracture models have taken different paths for research purposes: 1) genetic models to describe the functional importance of a gene or gene pathway for healing, and 2) procedural manipulations that examine mechanisms of healing or model clinical situations for the evaluation of therapeutic intervention.

Intramembranous bone repair models have modeled bone repair on those bones that undergo intramembranous bone formation, often using a rodent calvarial defect model. In this case, a defect of a critical size that will not heal without intervention is produced in the calvaria and viral or cell-mediated therapy applied on a scaffold (Gysin et al., 2002; Pelled et al., 2010). These models have been successful in promoting the healing of the critical size defect and show great potential for developing therapy to repair skull and facial injuries, or conditions resulting from birth defects or cancer.

Endochondral bone repair models have become the most common model for bone repair, traditionally using rodents. The rat has been the preferred model for pharmacological studies, and the femur fracture model was originally developed in the rat (Bonnarens and Einhorn, 1984). The phases of endochondral bone healing in rodents have been characterized in detail in numerous reviews, but the initial description of endochondral bone healing in the rat (Bolander, 1992) is still the standard of fracture callus development to which impaired healing is compared and by which therapy is evaluated (Fig. 2).

The development of genetically defined (knockout) mouse strains has necessitated adaptation of the rat model to the mouse. There is an obvious problem with the size of the animal model; because the mouse tibia was larger than other limb bones and more accessible for surgery, tibial fracture models were developed first (Hiltunen et al., 1993).

This model is used quite often, but the variable architecture of the tibia makes fracture production and healing more variable, and fracture calluses usually present with some asymmetry. The mouse femur has a much more consistent architecture, and although smaller and very close to the body and therefore more difficult to surgically manipulate, the mouse femur facture model has been used. Fracture repair studies also tend to be driven by the availability of the desired mouse strain and whether it is viable to serve as a subject of bone repair. This problem has necessitated the development of conditional knockout mouse strains as described above. To add to the difficulties of fracture analysis, the genetic background of the mouse strain under study can impact healing, and result in variations in callus size and tissue content that should be considered when analyzing bone development and fracture repair in knockout mice (Jepsen et al., 2008). Even with consistent fractures and bone architecture, differences in fracture repair can be subtle, especially among strains of knockout mice. Traditional approaches using X-ray examination to visualize the fracture callus have been confined to fracture production, or at best preliminary screening of healing. It is necessary to refine analysis techniques to improve the sensitivity. In this respect, micro-CT analysis of fracture repair has become invaluable (Morgan et al., 2009; Bouxsein et al., 2010). The disadvantage here is that the soft tissue callus is excluded from the analysis, so that conclusions on fracture repair are limited to bone formation. However, recent adaptations of the micro-CT have resolved differences in the vasculature of osteopontin knockout mice, a powerful application for evaluating angiogenesis in bone repair (Duvall et al., 2007). Histomorphometry is also used quite frequently to evaluate soft and hard fracture callus tissues with high resolution (Gerstenfeld et al., 2005).

The development of the even more challenging models of fracture repair that one would expect to encounter in a clinical situation has emphasized the study of surgical segmental defects. Recently, investigations have characterized endochondral bone formation during fracture healing in response to delayed stabilization, or when stabilization of the fracture is reduced or delayed (Miclau et al., 2007). Although the periosteum is disrupted during the standard closed fracture model, it is severely interrupted in these models. The periosteum is a critical source of cells for fracture repair; segmental cortical bone graft transplantations from ROSA 26A mice demonstrated that approximately 70% of the recipient graft was derived from the donor, as observed by β-galactosidase staining. Moreover, the donor cell transplants mediated BMP-2 therapy that improved segmental defect vascularization and healing (Zhang et al., 2005). A recent study demonstrated that a periosteal covering was necessary for healing a segmental defect in a "trabecular" metal cylinder implant to the femur diaphysis of the goat. In the absence of a periosteum, the implant lacked the bone ingrowth associated with healing (Bullens et al., 2010). Whether on not the periosteum is the main source of cells for fracture repair, impaired fracture repair with periosteal resection indicates that it is a major mediator of fracture callus development. Other approaches have induced ischemia through femoral artery resection which demonstrated the importance of the circulation to fracture repair (Lu et al., 2007). These models produce significantly delayed or non-union fracture healing. Evaluation of PTH therapy in an open rat femur fracture model revealed that it was not as successful as in the closed fracture model (Tagil et al., 2010), indicating that fracture therapy cannot be extrapolated to all clinical conditions.

5.5 Delivery of therapy to the fracture model

The delivery of gene therapy can be critical for the success of bone repair. Without injury, the periosteum consists of only a few cell layers of osteoblasts and fibroblasts. Its development into a fracture callus is dramatic. However, at the time of fracture and for a few days thereafter, the periosteum presents a small target for accurate application of the vector and transformation of the resident cells. The two options that exist for the delivery of therapy to a rodent fracture are percutaneous applications to the bone surface, and intramedullary injections. Most of our fracture therapy has utilized percutaneous injections. Injections of a radio-opaque contrast dye soon after fracture (Fig. 4A) established that even small volumes applied percutaneously leak from the periosteal surface into the surrounding tissues (Fig. 4B). The percutaneous application to the lateral aspect of the mouse femur fracture limited transgene expression to that aspect of the fracture callus. Intramedullary injections can distribute the injection around the fracture circumference, but leakage into the supra-periosteal tissues still occurs. The vector can facilitate transformation of the target tissues; in the case of rapidly proliferating periosteal cells in early fracture healing (Iwaki et al, 1997), transgene expression was propagated quite well from the MLV-based vector following percutaneous injection (Roe et al., 1993). The efficiency of delivery might also be compensated for by the transgene; a BMP transgene produced heterotopic bone in the surrounding tissue (Rundle et al., 2003), while a Cyclooxygenase (COX)-2 transgene did not (Rundle et al., 2008). Hence, the choice of vector and transgene can compensate for some of the difficulties in accurate delivery of the therapy and growth factor genes are discussed below with the gene therapy vectors they utilized for gene transduction and expression.

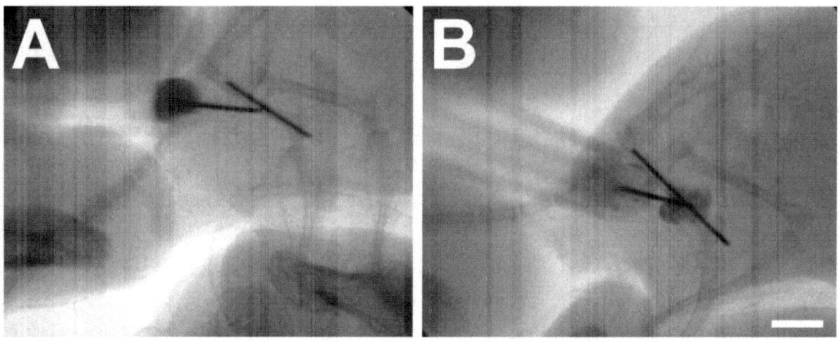

Fig. 4. Fracture therapy delivery by lateral percutaneous injection to the mouse femur fracture site. To illustrate the delivery technique, a radio-opaque contrast dye is injected and tracked by fluoroscopy. The injection needle is placed on the fracture at midshaft, and 25 ul of the dye injected. The intramedullary stabilizing pin of this model is visible perpendicular to the needle. (A) Immediately before injection. (B) Immediately after injection. Scale bar = 5 mm.

6. Vectors for fracture therapy

6.1 Viral vectors

Because there are several significant advantages to viral vectors, they are by far the most extensively studied vector for gene therapy. Viral vectors possess the ability to transduce their DNA into a variety of cells. They are relatively easy and cheap to produce and some will integrate into the host genomic DNA. The two main types of viral vectors used for *in vivo* fracture repair gene therapy are adenoviruses and retroviruses (Klamut et al., 2004; Evans, 2010; Pelled et al., 2010).

Adenoviruses are double-stranded DNA viruses that do not generally insert into the genome of the host cell but remain extrachromosomal. Adenoviruses are highly efficient in that they have a wide host cell range, transduction is followed by rapid transgene expression and they can transduce dividing and non-dividing cells; but these vectors provide only transient gene expression because they do not integrate into genomic DNA. Direct injection of a transgene into the fracture site in small and large animal models, performed percutaneously, was accomplished using adenoviral vectors encoding bone morphogenetic proteins (BMPs), vascular endothelial growth factor (VEGF) and other growth factors (Evans, 2010). Adenovirus directed BMP-2, BMP-4, and BMP-6 have all been reported to stimulate bone formation when directly injected at the fracture site (Baltzer et al., 2000a; Baltzer et al., 2000b; Chen et al., 2002; Bertone et al., 2004). However, in some models adenovirus directed BMP delayed healing (Egermann et al., 2006) and even when enhanced healing is reported, it is often accompanied by ectopic bone formation in the musculature, which is counterproductive. Clinical trials with adenoviral vectors have indicated that these vectors stimulate an immune response and this feature impedes the repair process and opportunities for multiple applications. Thus, adenoviral vectors have not yet been used successfully and are unlikely to be used in the clinic to accelerate fracture repair.

Adeno-associated vectors (AAV) are single stranded-DNA viruses that do not integrate readily into the host-cell genome but are capable of transducing a number of cell types whether they are dividing or not. Problems with producing the virus in large quantities, the small transgene carrying capacity and other technological considerations have limited the use of this vector for gene therapy applications. However, AAVs have been incorporated into Gene Activated Matrices (GAMs) to reduce their immune response and to effectively deliver a gene therapeutic to a bone defect. AAV in a GAM (collagen implant) transduced host cells surrounding the implant and led to remodeling of the allograft and replacement with bone (Koefoed et al., 2005; Evans, 2010).

Retroviruses are RNA viruses and therefore in order to replicate they must integrate into the host DNA. Retroviruses are highly regarded as orthopedic vectors because they possess the ability to transduce osteoblasts, bone marrow stromal cells, chondrocytes, and muscle-derived stem cells. Retroviruses transduce a variety of cells with high efficiency; they are highly stable; they have a large transgene capacity (i.e., more than 8kb of genomic information can be incorporated into the cassette), are easy to construct, do not elicit an immune response and expression of the transgene is robust and persistent because of DNA integration. However, there is a risk of insertional mutagenesis which is discussed below. Although retroviruses can only infect dividing cells (Roe et al., 1993), this disadvantage can make them efficient vectors for expressing transgenes during wound repair (Fig. 5).

Certain growth factors or signaling molecules that act early in the normal fracture repair process (BMP-4, COX-2, LMP-1) stimulate bone formation in small animal fracture models using retroviral gene therapy (Rundle et al., 2003; Rundle et al., 2008; Strohbach et al., 2008). Studies with single growth factor gene therapy with retroviral vectors in closed fractures in the rat femur fracture model demonstrated that retroviral-based gene therapy produced specific effects on fracture healing, and was even capable of improving it. A MLV-based vector expressing a hybrid BMP-2/4 gene that increased BMP-4 secretion, and therefore osteogenesis, was the first retroviral-based gene therapy studied by our group. Post-fracture administration of the MLV-BMP-4 vector to the rat femur fracture periosteum produced a dramatic enhancement of hard callus bone formation when compared to controls, with results somewhat similar to the BMP-2 protein administrations in a similar study (Einhorn et al., 2003). No evidence of viral vector expression in extraskeletal tissues was detected, suggesting that transfection was limited to the injury. MLV-based retroviral FGF-2 vectors were also tested for enhancement of fracture repair. FGF-2 has been proposed to function through cell proliferation, and recombinant FGF therapy had demonstrated increased callus size (Nakajima et al., 2001). FGF-2 gene therapy stimulated proliferation of periosteal and adjacent cells of the soft callus but did not lead to the development of hard callus or accelerate bony bridging (unpublished data). Therefore, FGF alone is not an ideal therapeutic candidate, but FGF could potentially be used in a combination therapy to enhance the early formation of cartilage callus if combined with a transgene that would enhance the subsequent ossification of the cartilage callus. Studies introducing single growth factor genes into a fracture site have generally shown an augmentation of hard and soft callus formation without improved bony union of bone tissues at the fracture gap, as determined by X-ray examination.

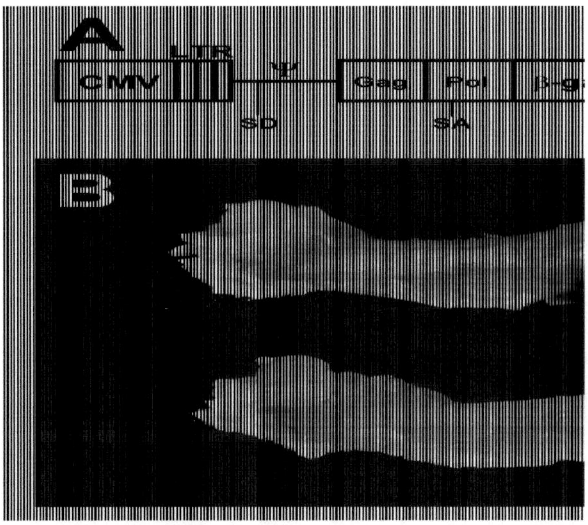

Fig. 5. Retroviral vector transgene expression in fracture tissues. The MLV-based vector construct expressed a β-galactosidase transgene. Femur fractures were harvested at 7 days post-fracture and stained for β-galactosidase expression. Injections were performed at one day post-fracture as described in Fig. 4. Staining revealed β-galactosidase transgene expression on the lateral aspect of the fracture callus (dark spot, upper bone). The lower fracture received a negative control gene expressed from the same vector and injected in the same manner. Scale bar = 5 mm.

Retroviral-based COX-2 gene therapy for fracture repair did differ from other transgene therapies. COX-2 is the rate limiting enzyme in the synthesis of prostaglandins during tissue repair. The COX-2 product Prostaglandin-E_2 induces the expression of multiple osteogenic growth factors, stimulates osteogenesis and supports cortical and trabecular bone formation, angiogenesis, and reduces apoptosis. COX-2 expression increases the osteoblastic potential of MSCs and supports osteoblast differentiation. COX-2 deficient mice also demonstrated that COX-2 was essential for the fracture repair process (Simon et al., 2002; Zhang et al., 2002). To prepare a retroviral gene therapeutic, the COX-2 gene was manipulated to remove sequences that destabilize mRNA, AU-rich elements (AREs) in the 3'translated region, to increase mRNA half-life. In addition, the Kozak sequence was modified to improve translation. The COX-2 expressing retrovirus was injected 24 hours after fracture to target proliferating cells at the fracture site to maximize the number of cells that were transduced within the fracture tissue. COX-2 expression did not produce inflammation at the fracture site, nor were systemic effects of prostaglandin production observed. The COX-2 gene was expressed in osteoblasts and other cells at the fracture site. Unlike BMP-2 and FGF-2 that were expressed from retroviral vectors, application of the COX-2 retroviral vector accelerated bony union of the callus tissues and hence improved healing of the fractured bone, possibly through angiogenic mechanisms (Rundle et al., 2008). Similar results were observed in PTH treatments in the rat femur fracture, although unlike COX-2 gene therapy, this approach required repeated applications of PTH (Alkhiary et al., 2005).

Lim Mineralizing Protein (LMP)-1 was also examined for its therapeutic efficacy. LMP-1 is an osteogenic factor that is a part of the BMP pathway and is a critical regulator of osteoblast differentiation. It is especially novel because it is an intracellular factor, unlike most transgenes utilized in gene therapy which are secreted soluble factors. Therefore, the effects of LMP-1 gene therapy are limited to the cells that are transduced by the retrovirus, an important consideration if the target cells of the host tissue are limited. LMP-1 affects osteoblast differentiation by binding to Smurf1, an E3 ligase, preventing it from ubiquitinating BMP-activated Smads and Runx2 and targeting them for proteosomal degradation (Boden et al., 1998; Sangadala et al., 2006). The LMP-1 retroviral gene therapeutic contained the human LMP-1 coding region and an optimized Kozak sequence which was ligated into the 6.8-kb CSLA retroviral backbone. LMP-1 expressing retrovirus (Fig. 6A) was injected 24 hours post-fracture. Immunohistochemistry of the fracture callus at 21 days revealed LMP-1 expression in chondroblasts and osteoblasts. Radiographs demonstrated bridging of the fracture callus at 21 days in LMP-1 treated animals and not in control animals (Fig. 6B). Additionally, the bone mineral content at the fracture site was increased in LMP-1 treated animals and these findings demonstrated that injection of the LMP-1 retroviral vector enhanced fracture healing (Strohbach et al., 2008).

Direct injection of MLV-based vectors have been used extensively in gene therapy studies including those described above, and are generally successful (Evans, 2010). However, there is a risk of insertional mutagenesis associated with each type of retrovirus (Mitchell, et al., 2004; Lewinski et al., 2006). Such mutagenesis has been conclusively demonstrated in MLV-based gene therapy for the Interleukin-2 receptor gamma chain deficiency in Severe Combined Immunodeficiency (SCID)-X1 (Howe et al., 2008) where transduction of cells led to the development of a clonal T cell acute lymphocytic leukemia. The leukemia was caused by retroviral integration near to proto-oncogenes, although other genetic abnormalities unrelated to the vector also contributed. The majority of gene therapy applications with lentiviral vectors have been *ex vivo*, because of this vector's association with the human immunodeficiency virus. Repair of bone defects treated with syngeneic rat bone marrow cells transduced with lentiviral vectors expressing BMPs have been compared to repair with cells transduced with adenoviral vectors (Hsu, et al., 2007; Miyazaki, et al., 2008; Virk, et al., 2008). Prolonged therapeutic BMP expression provided with the lentiviral vector in a critical sized femoral defect model provided superior repair associated with regional gene therapy than that observed with adenoviral vectors (Hsu et al., 2007; Virk, et al., 2008). In a spinal fusion model, MSCs expressing BMP after lentiviral transfer induced more abundant bone within the spinal fusion mass then cells transduced with adenovirus. Cells transduced with lentivirus or adenovirus expressing BMP both outperformed recombinant BMP protein therapy (Miyazaki, et al., 2008). Both the MLV-based and the lentiviral-based retroviral vectors have displayed characteristic preferences for integration sites, with the MLV-based vector integration associated with transcription start regions and lentiviral vector integration associated with sites of active gene transcription (Mitchell et al., 2004). Studies with chimeric viruses demonstrated that these characteristics were determined, at least for MLV, by the integrase and gag proteins (Lewinsky et al., 2006). This tendency toward activation of adjacent genes could also be minimized by the removal of segments of the U3 enhancer sequence of the viral long terminal repeat, although this step necessitated further modification of the vector to maximize its production (Jang et al., 2011).

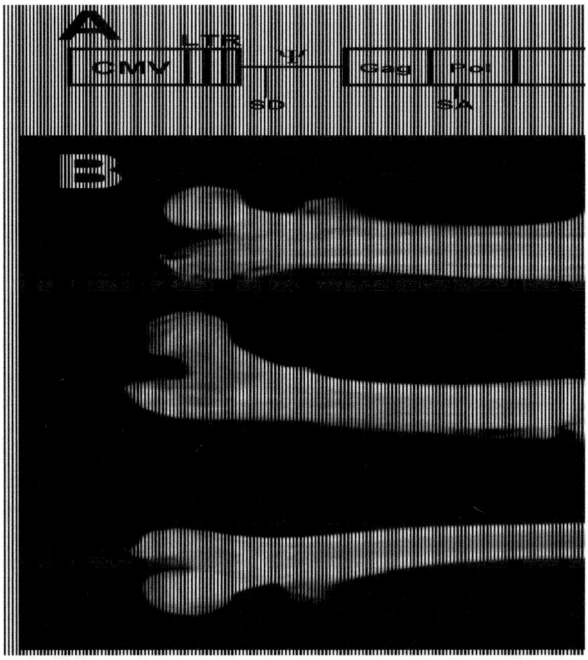

Fig. 6. LMP-1 gene therapy in the rat femur fracture. The MLV-based vector construct expressed a LMP-1 transgene. (B) Percutaneous injections were performed at one day post-fracture to the lateral and medial aspects of the fracture site. X-rays examination at 21 days post-fracture revealed that the LMP-1 transgene promoted bone formation that bridged the fracture gap (top). The control transgene injected in the same manner did not promote bone formation and healing appeared normal (middle). The unfractured contralateral bone (bottom) is presented for comparison. Scale bar = 10 mm.

Obviously, in spite of having the pathologic elements of the genome engineered so that they are absent from the vector, again lentiviral vectors suffer from the association with human immunodeficiency virus (HIV) in public opinion. Given this association, patients might explore other therapeutic options, even for severe or chronic clinical conditions. Because of their efficiency for gene transduction and expression, their ease of use and the number of studies in which they have been utilized, the viral vectors will probably continue to be used mainly for experimental purposes. Problems with viral vector safety could be obviated by the development of efficient non-viral gene therapy vectors for gene therapy in bone (Pountos et al., 2010). Progress towards this goal is discussed below.

6.2 Cell vectors

Using cells as a method of gene therapy can be looked at in two broad categories: use of stem cells or somatic cells. When stem cells were first discovered, there was great hope from the scientific community for the untold potential that these cells possessed. However, with the scientific hope came public concern. These concerns have been somewhat alleviated with the discovery of adult stem cells. Orthopedic gene therapy with adult stem cells has focused on the use of mesenchymal stem cells (MSCs). MSCs can be found in the bone marrow and obtained by a relatively simple bone marrow biopsy. After biopsy the cells can be expanded in culture and then used to treat the same individual that they were taken from. The advantage of this approach is that there is little risk of an immune response as the cells are unaltered and genetically identical to the individual they are being implanted into. However, there are a few fairly obvious disadvantages of this approach. First, a bone marrow biopsy is painful and there is a risk of infection. Second, and more importantly, if the individual from which the cells were taken has a defect in the healing process at the molecular level, use of their bone marrow MSCs (BMSCs) to treat a non-union fracture would not likely provide a benefit. A major limitation for BMSCs in allogeneic applications is, of course, the immune response, which could eliminate the possibility of further applications, including those from donors who share a significant portion of the original donor haplotype, much as has been observed in clinical transfusions.

Delivering osteogenic transgenes or cells with transgenes in a minimally invasive way remains the goal for development of clinical therapeutics. MSCs expressing BMP-2, TGF-β1, LMP-1, IGF-I, growth and differentiation factor (GDF)-5 have been shown to enhance bone, cartilage and tendon repair. Delivering osteogenic transgenes or cells with transgenes in a minimally invasive way remains the goal for development of clinical therapeutics. The use of allogeneic cells or *ex vivo* gene delivery may be attractive with regard to safety but would dramatically increase the cost of the gene therapy. MSC and skin fibroblasts may be able to differentiate into osteoblasts and chondrocytes, but difficulties with the isolation of large quantities of genetically modified cells and with the choice of cell scaffold material to seed genetically modified cells is likely to impede the development of these approaches.

Use of BMSCs for *ex vivo* based gene therapy for fracture and bone repair has been explored and provided some encouraging results in animal models. Transduction of BMSCs with BMPs prior to implantation at a fracture site stimulates bone formation. These cells become incorporated into the endochondral fracture callus (Gamradt et al., 2006). Furthermore, combination therapy of more than one BMP such as BMP-2 and BMP-7 or BMP-4 was shown to produce cooperative interactions that enhance bone regeneration. Transduction of MSCs with BMP-2/7 or BMP-4/7 demonstrated enhanced osteogenesis (Zhao et al, 2005). Likewise, combination therapy of BMP-2 and BMP-7 transduction of cells implanted into a cranial defect enhanced healing (Koh et al., 2008). Combination therapy of VEGF and BMP-6 transduction of osteoprogenitor cells has also shown preliminary promising results for future fracture repair studies (Cui et al., 2010). In addition to BMPs, one study found that cells transduced with IGF-I injected post-fracture resulted in accelerated progression toward complete fracture healing as measured by percent of mineralized callus and mineralized matrix compared to controls (Shen et al., 2002). However, no functional structural testing was done to determine if IGF-I transduced cell application actually restored mechanical integrity more quickly.

A newly explored source of MSCs is from human adipose tissue. Adipose-derived stromal cells (ADSCs) are very similar to BMSCs but ADSCs have the advantage of being more readily accessible and harvesting does not involve a highly painful procedure like a bone marrow biopsy (Kawai et al., 2009). Preliminary studies of the use of ADSCs to stimulate bone formation and fracture repair are promising. Non-transduced ADSCs transplanted into the fracture site in a rat model enhanced fracture repair when compared to transplanted fibroblasts or placebo (Shoji et al., 2010). ADSCs transduced with adenoviral BMP-2 implanted on a collagen-ceramic carrier inserted into a critical sized femoral defect demonstrated induced bone formation, which was not observed with untransduced ADSCs (Peterson et al., 2005). ADSCs expressing BMP-2 implanted in a critical size defect stimulated bone formation and healing far beyond control treatment (Li et al., 2007).

Additionally, muscle-derived stem cells (MDSCs) have been used in *ex vivo* gene therapy for repair of bone defects. Therapies for bone repair using MDSCs all involve manipulation of the BMP pathway, generally overexpression of BMP-2 or BMP-4 because they are such potent osteogenic factors. Implantation of MDSCs transduced with BMP-2 using either an adenoviral or retroviral vector stimulate bone formation in critical-size defect mouse models (Lee et al., 2001; Lee et al., 2002). Likewise, transduction of MDSCs with BMP-4 as an *ex vivo* cellular therapy to stimulate bone formation was effective in rodent models (Wright et al., 2002; Shen et al., 2004). Furthermore, combination therapy of VEGF and BMP-2 or BMP-4 overexpressing MDSCs accelerates bone healing in a skull defect mouse model (Peng et al., 2005).

Skin fibroblasts, a somatic cell, have also been explored as a potential cellular vector for *ex vivo* mediated gene therapy to enhance bone formation. When transduced with a retroviral vector for Runx-2, skin fibroblasts seeded on collagen scaffolds and implanted into mice demonstrated the capability to mineralize *in vivo* (Phillips and Garcia, 2008). Although easier to obtain than bone marrow cells, the problem of immunological reaction remains if these cells are isolated from allogeneic donors.

Hematopoietic cells offer an additional vehicle for bone therapy. Hematopoietic stem cells have been enriched for Sca-1+ expression and modified using a MLV-based viral vector to express FGF-2. These cells efficiently engrafted into the bone marrow and expressed FGF-2 that produced a dramatic increase in endosteal bone formation (Hall et al., 2007). This study supports a role for hematopoietic cells in gene therapy, at least for the bone marrow. In addition, this approach might be invaluable for prevention of fractures in osteoporotic patients, because their effect of increasing bone mineral density in conditions such as osteoporosis could dramatically reduce the incidence of fractures.

6.3 Non-viral plasmid vectors

Adenoviral, AAV, retroviral, and lentiviral based gene therapies have proven effective in fracture repair, but safety issues inherent with use of these therapeutics in clinical trials have not been resolved. A current focus of gene therapy is the development of non-viral plasmid vectors. There are several reasons for this. First, plasmid vectors do not insert into the genome of the cell into which they are introduced, and there is no risk of insertional mutagenesis. Second, non-viral plasmid vectors are not immunogenic, and there is minimal risk of a host immune response. Third, plasmids are being developed that possess specific expression time-frames and have cellular specificity (i.e., they will only be expressed in restricted target cell populations even if transfected into tissues). Non-viral vectors, such as plasmid vectors and linear DNA, have the potential to provide a much safer form of gene therapy, but they have not been optimized for the clinic to provide therapeutic levels of gene expression for a sufficient time period, at least in tissues other than muscle.

Historically, Gene Activated Matrices (GAMs) were developed with non-viral (plasmid) vectors to heal bone (Bonadio, 1999). The first GAM was a collagen sponge with plasmid

DNA containing the parathyroid hormone (PTH) 1-34 transgene. The strategy was to transfect *in situ* host cells that invaded the collagen sponge that was saturated with plasmid DNA that had been placed in the bone defect. Although shown to be effective in a rodent implant model (Bonadio, 1999; Geiger, et al., 2005), this therapeutic approach has not been further developed for extensive use in the clinic.

Currently, the major disadvantage of non-viral plasmid vectors for gene therapy is low transfection efficiency. The most widely utilized method of non-viral plasmid transfection is lipid-based or other soluble mediators that cause alterations in the cellular membrane allowing for introduction of the plasmid into a cell. More recently, electroporation has been explored in combination with plasmid vectors possessing DNA nuclear entry sequences. Efficient delivery of non-viral plasmids in muscle, cornea, lung, smooth muscle and vasculature (Dean et al., 2003, 2005; Zhou and Dean, 2007) has been achieved. However, expression of transgene from the plasmid vector continues for only 3-7 days, a time frame achieved with adenoviral vectors. With respect to bone repair, electroporation of a BMP-9 expression plasmid into a collagen sponge implant healed a murine radial segmental defect (Kimelman-Bleich et al., 2010). This result is quite promising for the future of non-viral gene therapy in the clinic, although few such studies have been performed to date.

Clinical trials have not been conducted with non-viral agents that stimulate fracture repair, however, phase I and II clinical trials with injections of FGF-1 in the pCOR DNA plasmid-based gene delivery system (called NV1FGF, Soubrier et al., 1999) into muscle provides an effective therapy for peripheral vascular disease and induces therapeutic angiogenesis (Baumgartner, et al., 2008). NV1FGF restored capillary and arteriolar density in animal models of hind limb ischemia. In phase II clinical trials, NV1FGF effectively increased FGF-1 mRNA and circulating protein levels, and reduced the number of amputations and deaths of subjects with critical limb ischemia (Maulik, 2009). These studies provide proof of concept that minimally toxic plasmid vectors are capable of providing therapeutic levels of a type of growth factor (FGF-1) that might also stimulate fracture repair. Because this vector is already undergoing clinical trials and has demonstrated minimal toxicity, it is well positioned to enter clinical trials for bone healing. These studies have served as an impetus to develop non-viral plasmid-based vectors for fracture repair.

There are several barriers to plasmid-based gene therapies in most tissues other than muscle. These include low levels of gene transfer and expression *in vivo* when targeting genes into non-replicating or slowly replicating cells. However, movement of DNA into the nucleus remains the crucial step for gene transfer and expression in non-dividing and slowly dividing cells. Early during fracture repair, periosteal cells and MSCs derived from the marrow proliferate to provide chondrogenic and osteoblastic lineage cells to repair the fracture, and a window of opportunity for application of a viral gene therapeutic was identified. We found that this same rapidly dividing cell population is also an excellent target for non-viral gene therapy if used in conjunction with *in vivo* electroporation. With regard to enhancing vector delivery and therapeutic gene expression, our group and others have focused on modifying plasmid DNA by incorporating a copy of a DNA Targeting Sequence (DTS) from the SV40 enhancer into a plasmid vector to increase nuclear entry of the DNA delivered into the cytoplasm following electroporation (Fig. 7A,B). This method has been shown to increase gene delivery and expression in muscle, blood vessels, lung and cornea tissue *in vivo* (Li, et al., 2001; Dean et al, 2003; Young, et al. 2003; Dean et al., 2005; Zhou and Dean 2007).

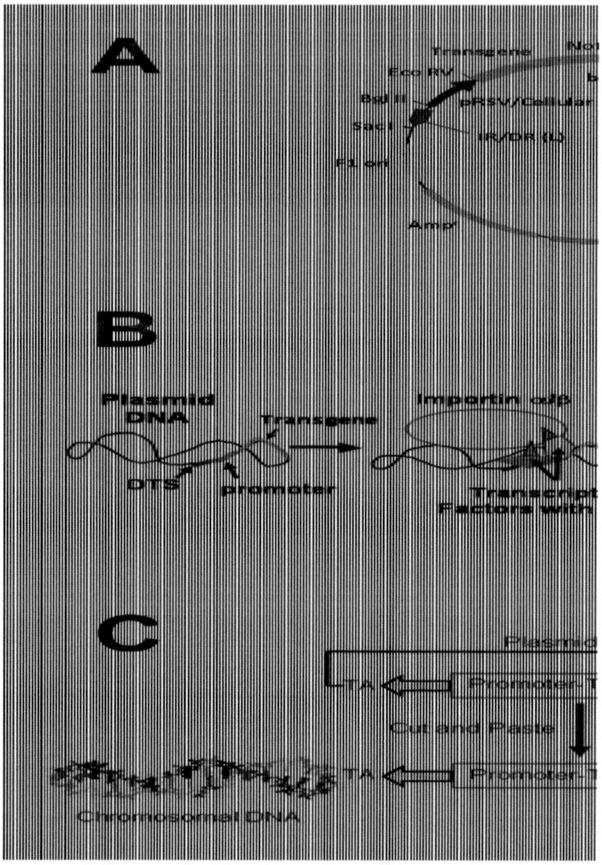

Fig. 7. Development of non-viral plasmid vectors for fracture repair. (A) A non-viral plasmid proposed for fracture repair contains two robust nonspecific viral promoters (RSV and CMV) that drive expression of the transgene and the *Sleeping Beauty* transposase, respectively. The *Sleeping Beauty* transposon (Harris, et al., 2002) stimulates transgene integration and increases the duration of transgene expression. The RSV promoter can be replaced with a cell specific promoter for cell-specific expression (Type I collagen promoter or osteocalcin promoter to target osteoblasts or a Type II collagen promoter to target chondrocytes). A SV40 DTS is inserted in the Sal I site to direct nuclear entry to enhance delivery to the nucleus and expression of the transgene. (B) For nuclear entry, natural transcription factors bind to gene promoter and enhancer regions that are present on the plasmid DNA. The transcription factors have nuclear localization signals (NLSs) that protect the plasmid DNA and facilitate its movement into the nucleus. Translocation to the nucleus requires the NLSs bind to the nuclear import machinery (importin α/β) and move the DNA/protein complex through the nuclear pore complex (NPC) into the nucleus, where it is stably integrated and transcribed. (C) Once plasmid DNA is delivered to the nucleus, transgenes are expressed and the SB transposase is produced. SB transposition of a therapeutic gene and promoter from the plasmid to the chromosome occurs with integration only into genomic regions with TA-base pairs. Insertion of the transgene and promoter extends expression until attenuated by cellular silencing mechanisms that ultimately limit transgene expression.

Lack of tissue specificity also remains a significant safety problem with currently developed non-viral therapies. The SV40 DNA nuclear targeting sequences (DTS) have supported nuclear import of plasmid DNA in a number of cells, but several laboratories have discovered that some promoter sequences undergo cell specific DNA nuclear import (Dean, 2005). The smooth muscle gamma actin (SMGA) promoter (Miller and Dean, 2008; Young, et al., 2003), the endothelial cell flk-1 (receptor) promoter, human surfactant protein C (SP-C) promoter (Degiulio, et al., 2010) and the collagen-Iα2 promoter (Strong, et al., 2006) all undergo nuclear import in restricted cell popultions. Thus, these cell-specific plasmid nuclear import sequences have the potential to provide targeted and enhanced gene expression in specific cells when incorporated into clinically tested nonviral vectors.

To increase the duration of *in vivo* transgene expression from both adenoviral and plasmid vectors that do not integrate into the host genome, the Tcl/mariner family of transposable elements (Izsvak et al., 2010) has been utilized. The Sleeping Beauty element undergoes cut-and paste transposition through a DNA intermediate (Fig. 7C). This process requires Sleeping Beauty transposase (SB) expression and short direct-repeat sequences in the transposon terminal inverted repeats that bracket the transgene and TA rich target regions in chromatin. SB transposase expression allows plasmid-based and adenovirus based transposons to integrate stably into chromatin and provide long-term transgene expression *in vivo* (Yant, et al., 2002). This system has been used to transduce human CD34+ stem/progenitor cells and achieve long-term transgene expression (Sumiyoshi, et al., 2009). Thus, this system can be used to integrate genes into stem/progenitor cells and to maintain pluripotency and could find use in fracture repair. However, insertional mutagenesis of the transgene might also become enough of a safety issue to delay clinical application.

7. Acknowledgements

Our research summarized in this review was funded by a US Congressional Appropriation and an Assistance Award from the United States Army (Award No. DAMD-17-03-2-0021) to the Musculoskeletal Disease Center at the VA Loma Linda Health Care System and by the National Medical Testbed which was funded by cooperative agreement number DAMD-17-97-2-7016. The opinions or assertions contained herein are the views of the authors and should not be assumed to reflect official policy or endorsement by the US Army, US Department of Defense or US Department of Veterans Affairs. All of our work was performed in facilities provided by the Department of Veterans Affairs.

8. Conclusion

Gene therapy for fracture repair has continually evolved over the last decade. Potential gene therapeutics now range from plasmid vectors placed in collagen supports, adenoviral vectors used in supports or in direct injections, direct retrovirus injections, *ex vivo* MSC therapies and electroporation mediated delivery of enhanced plasmid vectors. During this evolution, effective therapeutic genes have been identified based on an increased understanding of regulatory pathways involved during different stages of the fracture repair process. Based on perceived safety issues, non-viral and cell based therapeutics have recently received more attention and will likely be the vector of choice in the future. Recent studies engineering plasmid vectors to overcome problems with efficient delivery to non-dividing cells in tissues, inefficient DNA transport to the nucleus, and to increase cell specificity suggest that gene therapy for fracture repair has a bright future.

9. Reference

Alkhiary, Y.M., Gerstenfeld, L.C., Krall, E., Westmore, M., Sato, M., Mitlak, B.H. & Einhorn, T.A. (2005). Fracture-healing by systemic administration of recombinant human parathyroid hormone (PTH $_{1-34}$). *J. Bone Joint Surg.* Vol.A-87, pp. 731-741.

Bais, M., McLean, J., Sebastiani, P., Young, M., Wigner, N., Smith, T., Kotton, D.N., Einhorn, T.A., & Gerstenfeld, L.C. (2009). Transcriptional analysis of fracture healing and the induction of embryonic stem cell-related genes. *PLoS ONE* Vol.4, pp. e5393.

Baltzer, A.W., Lattermann, C., Whalen, J.D., Ghivizzani, S., Wooley, P., Krauspe, R., Robbins, P.D. & Evans, C.H. (2000a). Potential role of direct adenoviral gene transfer in enhancing fracture repair. *Clin. Orthop. Relat. Res.* Vol.379, pp. S120-S125.

Baltzer, A.W.A., Lattermann, C, Whalen, J.D., Wooley, P. Weiss, K., Grimm, M, Ghivizzani, S.C., Robbins, P.D. & Evans, C.H. (2000b). Genetic enhancement of fracture repair: healing of an experimental segmental defect by adenoviral transfer of the BMP-2 gene. *Gene Ther.* Vol.7, pp. 734- 739.

Baumgartner, I., Chronos, N., Comerota, A., Henry T., Pasquet, J-P., Finiels, F., Caron, A., Dedieu, J-F., Pilsudski, R. & Delaère, P. (2009). Local gene transfer and expression following intramuscular administration of FGF-1 plasmid DNA in patients with critical limb ischemia. *Mol. Ther.* Vol.17, pp. 914–921.

Bertone, A.L., Pittman, D.D., Bouxsein, M.L., Li, J., Clancy, B., & Seeherman H.J. (2004). Adenoviral-mediated transfer of human BMP-6 gene accelerates healing in a rabbit ulnar osteotomy model. *J. Orthop. Res.* Vol.22, pp. 1261-1270.

Boden, S.D., Liu, Y., Hair, G.A., Helms, J.A., Hu, D., Racine, M., Nanes, M.S. & Titus, L. (1998). LMP-1, a LIM-domain protein, mediates BMP-6 effects on bone formation. *Endocrinology* Vol.139, pp. 5125-5134.

Bolander, M.E. (1992). Regulation of fracture repair by growth factors. *Proc. Soc. Exp. Biol. Med.* Vol.200, pp. 165-170.

Bouxsein, M.L., Boyd, S.K., Christiansen, B.A., Guldberg, R.E., Jepsen, K.J. & Muller, R. (2010). Guidelines for assessment of bone microstructure in rodents using micro-computed tomography. *J. Bone Miner. Res.* Vol.25, pp. 1468-1486.

Bonadio, J. (1999). Localized, direct plasmid gene delivery *in vivo*: prolonged therapy results in reproducible tissue regeneration. Nature Med. Vol.5, pp. 753-759.

Bonnarens, F. & Einhorn, T.A. (1984). Production of a standard closed fracture in laboratory animal bone. *J. Orthop. Res.* Vol.2, pp. 97-101.

Brinker, M.R. & O'Connor, D.P. (2004). The incidence of fractures and dislocations referred for orthopaedic services in a capitated population. *J. B one Joint. Surg.* Vol.A-86, pp. 290-297.

Bullens, P.H.J., Schreuder, H.W.B., de Waal Malefijt, M.C., Verdonschot, N. & Buma, P. (2010). The presence of periosteum is essential for the healing of large diaphyseal segmental bone defects reconstructed with trabecular metal: A study in the femur of goats. *J. Biomed. Mater. Res. Part B: Appl. Biomater.* Vol.92B, pp. 24-31.

Chen, Y., Cheung, K.M., Kung, H.F., Leong, J.C., Lu, W.W. & Luk, K.D. (2002). In vivo new bone formation by direct transfer of adenoviral-mediated bone morphogenetic protein-4 gene. *Biochem. Biophys. Res. Commun.* Vol.298, pp. 121-127.

Colnot, C., Huang, S. & Helms, J.A. (2006). Analyzing the cellular contribution of bone marrow to fracture healing using bone marrow transplantation in mice. *Biochem. Biophys. Res. Commun.* Vol.350, pp. 557-561.

Colnot, C. (2009). Skeletal cell fate decisions within periosteum and bone marrow during bone regeneration. *J. Bone Miner. Res.* Vol.24, pp. 274-282.

Cui, F., Wang, X., Liu, X., Dighe, A.S., Balian, G. & Cui, Q. (2010). VEGF and BMP-6 enhance bone formation mediated by cloned mouse osteoprogenitor cells. *Growth Factors* Vol.28, pp. 306-317.

Dean, D.A., Machado-Aranda, D., Blair-Parks, K., Yeldani, A.V. & Young, J.L. (2003). Electroporation as a method for high-level non-viral gene transfer to the lung. *Gene Ther.* Vol.10, pp. 1608-1615.

Dean, D.A., Strong, D.D. & Zimmer, W.E. (2005). Nuclear entry of non-viral vectors. *Gene Ther.* Vol.12, pp. 881-890.

De Crombrugghe, B. & Akiyama, H. (2009). Transcriptional control of chondrocyte differentiation, In: *The Skeletal System*, O. Pourquie, ed., pp. 147-170. Cold Spring Harbor Laboratory Press, ISBN 978-0-87969-825-6, Cold Spring Harbor, NY.

Degiulio, J.V., Kaufman, C.D., & Dean, D.A. (2010). The SP-C promoter facilitates alveolar type II epithelial cell-specific plasmid nuclear import and gene expression. *Gene Ther.* Vol.17, pp. 541-549.

Duvall, C.L., Taylor, W.R., Weiss, D., Wojtowicz, A.M. & Guldberg, R.E. (2007). Impaired angiogenesis, early callus formation, and late stage remodeling in fracture healing of osteopontin-deficient mice. *J. Bone Miner. Res.* Vol.22, pp. 286-297.

Egermann, M., Lill, C.A., Griesbeck, K., Evans, C.H., Robbins, P.D., Schneider E. & Baltzer, A.W. (2006). Effect of BMP-2 gene transfer on bone healing in sheep. *Gene Ther.* Vol.13, pp. 1290-1299.

Einhorn, T.A., Majeska, R.J., Mohaideen, A., Kagel, E.M., Bouxsein, M.L., Turek, T.J. & Wozney, J.M. (2003). A single percutaneous injection of recombinant human bone morphogenetic protein-2 accelerates fracture repair. *J. Bone Joint Surg.* Vol.A-85, pp. 1425-1435.

Einhorn, T.A. (1995). Enhancement of fracture healing. J. Bone Joint Surg. A-77, pp. 940-956.

Evans, C.H. (2010). Gene therapy for bone healing. Expert Reviews in Molecular Medicine. Vol.12, pp.1-17.

Franceschi, R.T. (2005). Biological approaches to bone regeneration by gene therapy. *J. Dent. Res.* Vol.84, pp. 1093-1103.

Gamradt, S.C., Abe, N., Bahamonde, M.E., Lee, Y.P., Nelson, S.D., Lyons, K.M. & Lieberman, J.R. (2006). Tracking expression of virally mediated BMP-2 in gene therapy for bone repair. *Clin. Orthop. Relat. Res.* Vol.450, pp. 238-245.

Geiger, F., Bertram, H., Berger, I., Lorenz, H., Wall, O., Eckhardt, C., Simank, H.G. & Richter, W. (2005). Vascular endothelial growth factor gene-activated matrix (VEGF165-GAM) enhances osteogenesis and angiogenesis in large segmental bone defects. *J. Bone Miner. Res.* Vol.20, pp. 2028-2035.

Gerstenfeld, L.C., Cullinane, D.M., Barnes, G.L., Graves, D.T. & Einhorn, T.A. (2003). Fracture healing as a post-natal developmental process: molecular, spatial, and temporal aspects of its regulation. *J. Cell Biochem.* Vol.88, pp. 873-884.

Gerstenfeld, L.C., Wronski, T.J., Hollinger, J.O. & Einhorn T.A. (2005). Application of histomorphometric methods to the study of bone repair. *J. Bone Miner. Res.* Vol.20, pp. 1715-22.

Gysin, R., Wergedal, J.E., Sheng, M.H-C., Kasukawa, Y., Miyakoshi, N., Chen, S-T., Peng, H., Lau, K-H.W., Mohan, S. & Baylink, D.J. (2002). Ex vivo gene therapy with stromal cells transduced with a retroviral vector containing the BMP4 gene completely heals critical size calvarial defect in rats. *Gene Ther.* Vol.9, pp. 991-999.

Hadjiargyrou, M., Lombardo, F., Zhao, S., Ahrens, W., Joo, J., Ahn, H., White, D.W., & Rubin, C.T. (2002) Transcriptional Profiling of Bone Regeneration. J. Biol. Chem. Vol.277, pp. 30177-30182.

Hall, S.L., Lau, K-H.W., Chen, S-T, Wergedal, J.E., Srivastava, A., Klamut, H., Sheng, M.H-C., Gridley D.S., Mohan, S. & Baylink, D.J. (2007). Sca-1+ hematopoietic cell-based gene therapy with a modified FGF-2 increased endosteal/trabecular bone formation in mice. *Mol. Ther.* Vol.15, pp. 1181-1889.

Harris, J.W., Strong, D.D., Amoui, M., Baylink, D.J. & Lau, K.H. (2002). Construction of a Tc1-like transposon sleeping beauty-based gene transfer plasmid vector for generation of stable transgenic mammalian cell clones. *Anal. Biochem.* Vol.310, pp. 15-26.

Hiltunen, A., Vuorio, E. & Aro, H.T. (1993). Standardized experimental fracture in the mouse tibia. *J. Orthop. Res.* Vol.11, pp. 305-312.

Howe, S.J. Mansour, M.R., Schwarzwaelder, K., Bartholomae, C., Hubank, M., Kempski, H., Brugman, M.H., Pike-Overzet, K., Chatters, S.J., de Ridder, D., Gilmour, K.C. Adams, S., Thornhill, S.I., Parsley, K.L., Staal, F.J.T., Gale, R.E., Linch, D.C., Bayford, J., Brown, L., Quaye, M., Kinnon, C., Ancliff, P., Webb, D.K., Schmidt, M., von Kalle, C., Gaspar, H.B. & Thrasher, A.J. (2008). Insertional mutagenesis combined with acquired somatic mutations causes leukemogenesis following gene therapy of SCID-X1 patients. *J. Clin. Invest.* Vol.9, pp. 3143-3150.

Hsu, W.K., Sugiyama, O., Park, S.H., Conduah, A., Feeley, B.T., Liu, N.q., Krenek, L., Virk, M.S., An, D.S., Chen, I.S., & Liberman, J.R. (2007). Lentiviral-mediated BMP-2 gene transfer enhances healing of segmental femoral defects in rats. Bone. Vol. 40, pp. 931-938.

Iwaki, A., Jinguishi, S., Oda, Y., Izumi, T., Shida, J.I., Tsuneyoshi, M. & Sugioka, Y. (1997). Localization and quantification of proliferating cells during rat fracture repair: Detection of proliferating cellular nuclear antigen by immunohistochemistry. *J. Bone Miner. Res.* Vol.12, pp. 96-102.

Izsvak, Z, Hackett, P.B., Cooper L.J.N.& Ivics, Z. (2010). Translating Sleeping Beauty transposition into cellular therapies: Victories and challenges. Bioessays. Vol. 32, pp. 756-767.

Kawai, M., Devlin, M.J. & Rosen, C.J. (2009). Fat targets for skeletal health. *Nat. Rev. Rheumatol.* Vol.5, pp. 365-372.

Klamut, H.J., Chen, S.-T., Lau, K.-H. W., & Baylink, D.J. (2004). Progress toward skeletal gene therapy. Critical Rev in Eukaryotic Gene Expression, Vol.14, pp. 89-136.

Jang, J., Lee, J-T., Lee, K., Kim, S., Kim, J.Y., Yoon, K. & Kim, S. (2011). Development of murine leukemia virus-based retroviral vectors with a minimum possibility of *cis*-activation. *Gene Ther.* Vol.18, pp. 240-249.

Jepsen, K.J., Price, C., Silkman, L.J., Nicholls, F.H., Nasser, P., Hu, B., Hadi, N., Alapatt, M., Stapleton, S.N., Kakar, S., Einhorn, T.A. & Gerstenfeld, L.C. (2008). Genetic variation in the patterns of skeletal progenitor cell differentiation and progression during endochondral bone formation affects the rate of fracture healing. *J. Bone Miner. Res.* Vol.23, pp. 1204-1216.

Karsenty, G. (2009). Transcriptional control of osteoblast differentiation, In: *The Skeletal System*, O. Pourquie, ed., pp. 205-218. Cold Spring Harbor Laboratory Press, ISBN 978-0-87969-825-6, Cold Spring Harbor, NY.

Kimelman-Bleich, N., Pelled, G., Ziberman, Y., Kallai, I., Mizrahi, O., Tawackali W., Gazit Z. & Gazit, D. (2010). Targeted gene-and-host progenitor cell therapy for nonunion bone fracture repair. *Mol. Ther.* Vol.19, pp. 53-59

Koefoed, M., Ito, H., Gromov, K., Reynolds, D.G., Awad, H.A., Rubery, P.T., Ulrich-Vinther, M., Soballe, K., Guldberg, R.E., Lin, A.S., O'Keefe, R.J., Zhang, X. & Schwarz, E.M. (2005). Biological effects of rAAV-caALK2 coating on structural allograft healing. *Mol. Ther.* Vol.12, pp. 212-218.

Koh, J.T., Zhao, Z., Wang, Z., Lewis, I.S., Krebsbach, P.H. & Franceschi, R.T. (2008). Combinatorial gene therapy BMP2/7 enhances cranial bone regeneration. *J. Dent. Res.* Vol.87, pp. 845-849.

Komatsu, D.E. & Warden, S.J. (2010). The control of fracture healing and its therapeutic targeting: Improving upon nature. *J Cell. Biochem.* Vol.109, pp. 302-311.

Kronenberg, H.M., McMahon, A.P., & Tabin, C.J. (2009). Growth factors and chondrogenesis, In: *The Skeletal System*, O. Pourquie, ed., pp. 171-204. Cold Spring Harbor Laboratory Press, ISBN 978-0-87969-825-6, Cold Spring Harbor, NY.

Lee, J.Y., Musgrave, D., Pelinkovic, D., Fukushima, K., Cummins, J., Usas, A., Robbins, P., Fu, F.H. & Huard, J. (2001). Effect of bone morphogenetic protein-2-expressing muscle-derived cells on healing of critical-sized bone defects in mice. *J. Bone Joint Surg.* Vol.A-83, pp. 1032-1039.

Lee, J.Y., Peng, H., Usas, A., Musgrave, D., Cummins, J., Pelinkovic, D., Jankowski, R., Ziran, B., Robbins, P. & Huard, J. (2002). Enhancement of bone healing based on *ex vivo* gene therapy using human muscle-derived cells expressing bone morphogenetic protein 2. *Hum. Gene. Ther.* Vol.13, pp. 1201-1211.

Lewinski, M.K., Yamashita, M., Emerman, M., Ciuffi, A., Marshall, H., Crawford, G., Collins, F., Shinn, P., Leipzig, J., Hannenhalli, S., Berry, C.C., Ecker, J.R. & Bushman, F.D. (2006). Retroviral DNA integration: Viral and cellular determinants of target-site selection. *PLoS Pathog.* Vol.2, pp. e60.

Li, S., MacLaughlin, F.C., Fewell, V.G., Gondo, M., Wang, J., Nicol, F., Dean, D.A. & Smith, L.C. (2001). Muscle-specific enhancement of gene expression by incorporation of SV40 enhancer in the expression plasmid. *Gene Ther.* Vol.8, pp. 494-497.

Li, X., Quigg, R.J., Zhou, J., Ryaby, J.T. & Wang, H. (2005). Early signals for fracture healing. *J. Cell. Biochem.* Vol.95, pp. 189-205.

Li, H., Dai, K., Tang, T., Zhang, X., Yan, M. & Lou, J. (2007). Bone regeneration by implantation of adipose-derived stromal cells expressing BMP-2. *Biochem. Biophys. Res. Commun.* Vol.356, pp. 836-842.

Lu, C., Miclau, T., Hu D. & Marcucio, R.S. (2007). Ischemia leads to delayed-union during fracture healing: A mouse model. *J. Orthop. Res.* Vol.25, pp. 51-61.

Mark, H., Penington, A., Nannmark, U., Morrison, W. & Messina, A. (2004). Microvascular invasion during endochondral ossification in experimental fractures in rats. *Bone* Vol.35, pp. 535-542.

Maulik, N. (2009). NV1FGF, a pCOR plasmid-based angiogenic gene therapy for the treatment of intermittent claudication and critical limb ischemia. *Curr. Opin. Investig. Drugs* Vol.10, pp. 259-268.

Miclau, T., Lu, C., Thompson, Z., Choi, P., Puttlitz, C., Marcucio, R. & Helms, J.A. (2007). The effects of delayed stabilization on fracture healing. *J. Orthop. Res.* Vol.25, pp. 1552-1558.

Miller, A.M. & Dean, D.A. (2008). Cell-specific nuclear import of plasmid DNA in smooth muscle requires tissue-specific transcription factors and DNA sequences. *Gene Ther.* Vol.15, pp. 1107-1115.

Mitchell, R.S., Beitzel, B.F., Schroder, A.R.W., Shinn, P., Chen, H., Berry, C.C., Ecker, J.R. & Bushman, F.D. (2004). Retroviral DNA integration: ASLV, HIV, MLV show distinct target site preferences. *PLoS Biol.* Vol.2, pp. e234.

Miyazaki, M., Sugiyama, O., Zou, J., Yoon, S.H., Wei, F., Morishita, Y., Sintuu, C., Virk, M.S., Liverman, J.R. & Wang, J.C. (2008). Comparison of lentiviral and adenoviral gene therapy for spinal fusion in rats. Spine. Vol. 33, pp. 1410-1407.

Morgan, E.F., Mason, Z.D., Chien, K.B., Pfeiffer, A.J., Barnes, G.L., Einhorn, T.A. & Gerstenfeld, L.C. (2009). Micro-computed tomography assessment of fracture healing: Relationships among callus structure, composition and mechanical function. *Bone* Vol.44, pp. 335-344.

Myers, T.J., Granero-Molto, F., Longobardi, L., Li, T., Yan, Y. & Spagnoli, A. (2010) Mesenchymal stem cells at the intersection of cell and gene therapy. Expert Opin Biol Ther. Vol.12, pp. 1663-1679.

Nakajima, F., Ogasawara, A., Goto, K., Moriya, H., Ninomiya, Y., Einhorn, T.A. & Yamazaki, M. (2001). Spatial and temporal gene expression in chondrogenesis during fracture healing and the effects of basic fibroblast growth factor. *J. Orthop. Res.* Vol.19, pp. 935-944.

Ota, N., Takaishi, H., Kosaki, N., Takito, J., Yoda, M., Tohmonda, T., Kimura, T., Okada, Y., Yasuda, H., Kawaguchi, H., matsumoto, M., Chiba, K., Ikegami, H. & Toyama, Y. (2009). Accelerated cartilage resorption by chrondroclasts during bone fracture healing in osteoprotegerin-deficient mice. Endocrinology Vol. 150, pp. 4823-4834.

Pelled, G., Ben-Arav, A., Hock, C., Reynolds, D.D., Yazici, C., Zibeman, Y., Gazit, Z., Awad, H., Gazit, D. & Schwarz, E.M. (2010). Direct gene therapy for bone regeneration: gene delivery, animal models and outcome measures. *Tissue Eng. Part B Rev.* Vol.1, pp. 13-20.

Peng, H., Usas, A., Olshanski, A., Ho, A.M., Gearhart, B., Cooper, G.M. & Huard, J. (2005). VEGF improves, whereas sFlt1 inhibits, BMP2-induced bone formation and bone healing through modulation of angiogenesis. *J. Bone Miner. Res.* Vol.20, pp. 2017-2027.

Peterson, B., Zhang, J., Iglesias, R., Kabo, M., Hendrick, M., Benhaim, P. & Lieberman, J.R. (2005). Healing of critically sized femoral defects using genetically modified mesenchymal stem cells from human adipose tissue. *Tissue Eng.* Vol.11, pp. 120-129.

Phillips, J.E. & Garcia, A.J. (2008). Retroviral-mediated gene therapy for the differentiation of primary cells into a mineralizing osteoblastic phenotype. *Methods Mol. Bio.* Vol.433, pp. 333-354.

Pountos, I., Georgouli, T., Kontakis, G. & Giannoudis, P.V. (2010). Efficacy of minimally invasive techniques for enhancement of fracture healing: evidence today. *Int. Orthop.* Vol.34, pp. 3-12.

Roe, T.Y., Reynolds, T.C., Yu, G. & Brown, P.O. (1993). Integration of murine leukemia virus DNA depends on mitosis. *EMBO J.* Vol.12, pp. 2099-2108.

Rundle, C.H., Miyakoshi, N., Kasukawa, Y., Chen, S-T, Sheng, M.H.-C., Wergedal, J.E., Lau, K.-H. W. & Baylink, D.J. (2003). In vivo bone formation in fracture repair induced by direct retroviral-based gene therapy with bone morphogenetic protein-4. *Bone* Vol.32, pp. 591-601.

Rundle, C.H., Wang, H., Yu, H., Chadwick, R.B., Davis, E.I., Wergedal, J.E., Lau, K-H.W., Mohan, S., Ryaby, J.T. & Baylink, D.J. (2006). Microarray analysis of gene expression during the inflammation and endochondral bone formation stages of rat femur fracture repair. *Bone* Vol.38, pp. 521-529.

Rundle, C.H., Strong, D.D., Chen S-T., Linkhart, T.A., Sheng, M.H.-C., Wergedal, J.E., Lau, K-H.W. & Baylink, D.J. (2008). Retroviral-based gene therapy with cyclooxygenase-2 promotes the union of bony callus tissues and accelerates fracture healing in the rat. *J. Gene Med.* Vol.10, pp. 229-241.

Sangadala, S., Boden, S.D., Viggeswarapu, M., Liu, Y. & Titus, L. (2006). LIM mineralization protein-1 potentiates bone morphogenetic protein responsiveness via a novel interaction with Smurf1 resulting in decreased ubiquitination of Smads. *J. Biol. Chem.* Vol.281, pp. 17212-17219.

Shen, H.C., Peng, H., Usas, A., Gerhart, B., Cummins, J., Fu, F.H. & Huard, J. (2004). Ex vivo gene therapy-induced endochondral bone formation: comparison of muscle-derived stem cells and different subpopulations of primary muscle-derived cells. *Bone* Vol.34, pp. 982-992.

Shen, F.H., Visger, J.M., Balian, G., Hurwitz, S.R. & Diduch, D.R. (2002). Systemically administered mesenchymal stromal cells transduced with insulin-like growth factor-I localize to a fracture site and potentiate healing. *J. Orthop. Trauma* Vol.16, pp. 651-659.

Shoji, T., Ii, M., Mifune, Y., Matsumoto, T., Kawamoto, A., Kwon, S.M., Kuroda, T., Kuroda, R., Kurosaka, M. & Asahara, T. (2010). Local transplantation of human multipotent adipose-derived stem cells accelerates fracture healing via enhanced osteogenesis and angiogenesis. *Lab Invest.* Vol.90, pp. 637-649.

Simon, A.M., Manigrasso, M.B. & O'Connor, J.P. (2002). Cyclo-oxygenase 2 function is essential for bone fracture healing. *J. Bone Miner. Res.* Vol.17, pp. 963-976.

Soubrier, F. Cammeron, B., Manse, B., Somarriba, S., Dubertret, C.,Jaslin, G., Jung, G., La Caer, C., Dang, D., Mouvvault, J.M., Scherman, D., Mayaux, J.F. &Crouzet, J. (1999). pCOR: A new design of plasmid vectors for nonviral gene therapy. *Gene Ther.* Vol.6, pp.1482-1488.

Strohbach, C.A.., Rundle, C.H., Wergedal, J.E., Chen, S-T., Linkhart, T.A., Lau, K.-H.W. & Strong, D.D. (2008). LMP-1 Retroviral gene therapy influences osteoblast differentiation and facture repair: A preliminary study. *Calcif. Tissue Int.* Vol.83, pp. 202-211.

Street, J., Bao, M., deGuzman, L., Bunting, S., Peale, F.V., Jr., Ferrara, N., Steinmetz, H., Hoeffel, J., Cleland, J.L., Daugherty, A., van Bruggen, N., Redmond, H.P., Carano, R.A.D. & Filvaroff, E.H. (2002). Vascular endothelial growth factor stimulates bone repair by promoting angiogenesis and bone turnover. *Proc. Natl. Acad. Sci. USA* Vol.99, pp. 9656-9661.

Strong, D.D., Linkhart, T.A. & Dean, D.A. (2006). Cell specific molecule and method for importing DNA into osteoblast nuclei. *U.S. Patent Application* 11/410,579.

Sumiyoshi, T., Holt, N.G., Hollis, R.P., Ge, S., Cannon, P.M. Crooks, G.M. & Kohn, D.B. (2009). Stable transgene expression in primitive human CD34+ hematopoietic stem/progenitor cells, using the Sleepinig Beauty transposon system. *Hum. Gene Ther.* Vol.20, pp. 1607-1626.

Tagil, M., McDonald, M.M., Morse, A., Peacock, L., Mikulec, K., Amanat, N., Godfrey, C. & Little, D.G. (2010). Intermittent PTH(1-34) does not increase union rates in open rat femoral fractures and exhibits attenuated anabolic effects compared to closed fracture. *Bone* Vol.46, pp. 852-859.

Toben, D., Schroeder, I., El Khassawna, T., Hehta, M., Hoffman, J-E., Frisch, J-T., Schell, H., Lienau, J., Serra, A., Radbruch, A. & Duda, G.N. (2011). Fracture healing is accelerated in the absence of the adaptive immune system. *J. Bone Miner. Res.* Vol.26, pp. 113-124.

Virk, M.S., Conduah, A., Park, S.H., Liu, N., Sugiyama, O., Cuomo, A., Kang, C. & Liberman, J.R. (2008). Influence of short-term adenoviral vector and prolonged lentiviral vector mediated bone morphogenetic protein-2 expression on the quality of bone repair in a rat femoral defect model. Bone. Vol. 42, pp. 921-931.

Wright, V., Peng, H., Usas, A., Young, B., Gearhart, B., Cummins, J. & Huard, J. (2002). BMP4-expressing muscle-derived stem cells differentiate into osteogenic lineage and improve bone healing in immunocompetent mice. *Mol. Ther.* Vol.6, pp. 169-178.

Yant, S.R., Ehrhardt, A., Mikkelsen, J.G., Meuse, L., Pham, T. & Kay, M.A. (2002). Transposition from a gutless adeno-transposon vector stabilized transgene expression *in vitro*. *Nature Biotech.* Vol.20, pp. 999-1005.

Young, J.L. Benoit, J.N. & Dean, D.A. (2003). Effect of a DNA nuclear targeting sequence on gene transfer and expression of plasmids in the intact vasculature. *Gene Ther.* Vol.10, pp. 1465-1470.

Yu, Y.Y., Lieu, S., Lu, C. & Colnot, C. (2010). Bone morphogenetic protein 2 stimulates endochondral ossification by regulating periosteal cell fate during bone repair. *Bone* Vol.47, pp. 65-73.

Zhang, X. Schwarz, E.M., Young, D.A., Puzas, J.E., Rosier, R.N. & O'Keefe, R.J. (2002). Cyclooxygenase-2 regulates mesenchymal cell differentiation into the osteoblast lineage and is critically involved in bone repair. *J. Clin. Invest.* Vol.109, pp. 1405-1415.

Zhang, X., Wie, C., Lin, A.S.P., Ito, H., Awad, H., Lieberman, J.R., Rubery, P.T., Schwarz, E.M., O'Keefe, R.J. & Guldberg, R.E. (2005). Periosteal progenitor cell fate in segmental cortical bone graft transplantations: Implications for functional tissue engineering. J. Bone Miner. Res. Vol.20, pp. 2124-2137.

Zhao, M., Zhao, Z., Koh, J.T., Jin, T. & Franceschi, R.T. (2005). Combinatorial gene therapy for bone regeneration: cooperative interactions between adenovirus vectors expressing bone morphogenetic proteins 2, 4, and 7. *J. Cell Biochem.* Vol.95, pp. 1-16.

Zhou, R. & Dean, D.A. (2007). Gene transfer of interleukin 10 to the murine cornea using electroporation. Exp. Biol. Med. Vol. 232, pp. 362-369.

13

Ex Vivo Gene Therapy for Spinal Fusion

Takashi Kaito, Stephanie S. Ngo and Jeffrey C. Wang
University of California, Los Angeles
USA

1. Introduction

When instability of the lumbar spine causes persistent pain or neurological impairment, it is usually treated by spinal fusion. Unfortunately, despite the development of spinal instrumentation such as pedicle screws, rods and intervertebral cages, nonunion rates are still close to 15%. Autogenous bone grafting has been the gold standard as the bone graft material of choice, however, its use has several disadvantages, such as a limited supply and a reasonable percentage of donor site problems. For these reasons, alternative sources of bone grafting materials or replacements have been explored and developed. One possibility is the use of bone morphogenetic proteins (BMPs), which belong to the transforming growth factor (TGF) superfamily and are known to be capable to eliciting new bone formation can provide an alternative to bone grafting (Reddi et al., 1998, Khan et al., 2002, Vaccaro et al., 2002, Veillette et al., 2007). Three types of BMP- based bone tissue engineering have been tried to date: cell therapy involving the transplantation of autogenous mesenchymal cells differentiated by BMP, gene therapy involving the transduction of genes encoding BMPs into cells at the repair site (Kaito et al, 2005), and cytokine therapy involving recombinant BMP and carriers that retain and release BMP as needed. Of the three types of BMP-based bone tissue engineering techniques, cytokine therapy has received significant attention. Several kinds of combination with cytokine and carriers were reported (Khan et al., 2004). However, uncontrolled release of high dose BMP has been known to cause inflammation, soft tissue edema, and unintended bone formation (Carlisle et al., 2005, Mroz et al., 2010). An alternative to recombinant proteins, is the use of novel methods and gene transfer techniques to achieve bone formation in the spine. Gene therapy is ideal for orthopaedic use because, in most cases, local and transient expression of osteogenic factors is necessary for bone formation (Helm et al., 2000). Regional gene therapy for spinal fusion is an attractive option to treat multi-operated unstable spines where osteogenic cells, blood supply and bone stock are limited (Wang et al., 2003).

The recent progress in molecular biology, genetics, and stem cell biology demonstrate that gene therapy for spinal fusion could result in effective bone formation by sustained and controlled release of osteogenic factors (Yoon et al., 2004). *Ex vivo* gene therapy, which is the combination of gene therapy and cell therapy, is currently the most fascinating areas of orthopedic research and surgery. In this chapter, the authors summarize the latest research in *ex vivo* gene therapy for spinal fusion and discuss the clinical implications of these treatments.

2. *Ex vivo* gene therapy

Regional gene therapy is ideal for spinal fusion because local and transient expression of osteogenic factors is necessary for bone formation, compared to systemic genetic disorders in which consistent and systemic expression of specific genes are required (Baltzer et al., 2004). Therefore, there is more flexibility with respect to the use of vectors for treatment of these problems and it may stave off the side effects associated with the current use of high dose and uncontrolled release of recombinant BMPs (Mroz et al., 2010). Regional gene therapy can be employed via either an *in vivo* or an *ex vivo* approach. In an *in vivo* technique, the vector is delivered directly to the target site. The advantage of the *in vivo* approach is that it involves only one step. The disadvantages of this technique are that it is more difficult to transduce cells *in vivo*, and one cannot select the target cells that will be transduced. Reports of successful fusion using the *in vivo* approach have been mostly reported in athymic rats (Alden TD et al., 1999). On the other hand, in an *ex vivo* approach, the vector is delivered into harvested cells. The transduced cells are then implanted into a specific regeneration site. The advantage of the *ex vivo* technique is that there is an increased transduction efficiency and safety as compared to when performed *in vitro*. In addition, the transduced mesenchymal stem cells (MSCs) could act not only as a production plant for osteogenic factors, but also as a source of osteogenic cells. The *ex vivo* technique also allows for attachment of a desirable carrier material which can act as an osteoconductive scaffold (Oakes DA et al., 2000). The disadvantage of this strategy is that this approach is more labor intensive, and therefore may not be cost-effective (Phillips et al., 2005).

3. Vectors for gene delivery

3.1 Non-viral vectors

Vectors may be classified broadly as either viral (Kootstra et al., 2003) or non-viral (Li S et al., 2001). Non-viral vectors are easy to handle, chemically more stable than viruses and have no limit as to the size of the genetic materials that can be introduced into the cell. However their use is limited because the transfection efficiency is low and the duration of expression of the protein product tends to be short due partly to the episomal nature of the transgene. Non-viral gene delivery includes direct injection of naked DNA, direct injection or liposomal transfection of plasmids and particle-mediated gene transfer (i.e.; gene gun). Plasmids are circular DNA initially found in bacteria and work to acquire resistance to antibiotics. They are usually used in combination with cationic liposomes or scaffolds to form what has been termed the "gene activated matrix" (GAM) (Fang et al., 1996). A particle-mediated transfer (gene gun) is a projection of a metallic particle coated with DNA by electrical charge or gas pressure into the target cells. The disadvantage of this technique is transient and limited gene expression and toxicity caused by metal particles (Benn et al., 1996). Despite many advantages such as the ability to transfer a large amount of DNA, a decreased risk of insertion into the host DNA and no incitement of immune response (repeat administration is possible), the low gene transduction rate and short-time gene expression are limiting the use of these non-viral vectors. Current investigations are attempting to overcome these limitations.

3.2 Viral vectors

Currently, the most efficient vectors are utilize viruses. Viral vectors are usually designed so that genes required for viral replication are replaced by a specific therapeutic gene of interest. The resulting recombinant vector is replication incompetent. However, they are still able to deliver genetic material directly to a cell's nucleus efficiently, and then the cellular machinery can produce the therapeutic protein coded by the introduced genetic material. Vectors vary in the efficiency of gene transfer, the genetic carrying capacity, ease of production, and reactions with host immunity (Khan et al., 2000, Alden et al., 2002, Evans et al., 2004, Nishida et al., 2008).

3.2.1 Retrovirus

Retroviral vectors have single-stranded RNA and have been derived from oncoretroviruses such as the murine leukemia virus (MLV). The advantage of using a retroviral vector is that it transduces the genes into the host chromosomes very efficiently and reliably during cell division (Miller DG et al., 1990). Therefore the integrated genes are passed on to subsequent daughter cells, giving the gene the potential for lifelong expression. However, this integration may occur only during cell division, thus, only highly proliferative cells can be transduced with retroviral vectors. Therefore, it may not be suitable for *in vivo* direct injection. Some of the major disadvantages of retroviral vectors are the low infectivity, instability of their virions, a limited capacity of genetic materials (~8kb) and risk of oncogenesis by the insertion of genetic materials (Li et al., 2002). There have also been concerns about the potential ability of the recombinant retroviruses to convert into replication competent viruses.

3.2.2 Adenovirus

The most commonly tested viral delivery vehicle for gene therapy for bone healing has been the adenovirus. Adenoviruses are double-stranded DNA viruses with a genome size of approximately 35kilobases. The genetic material is inserted into the nucleus in an episomal state, and not integrated within the host chromosome. The viral genome is divided into immediate early genes, early genes, and late genes according to the time during which the genes are expressed. First-generation adenoviral vectors often have deleted the E1and E3 region which necessary for virus replication and can accommodate up to 8kb of foreign DNA (Lai et al., 2002). Recombinant adenoviral vectors can be produced at high levels, transfer genes to both dividing cells and non-dividing cells efficiently, and maintain more genetic material than other viruses (Gugala et al., 2003). The transgene remains episomal so that the therapeutic gene expression is stopped when the genetically modified cell divides. This episomal nature reduces the risk of insertional mutagenesis. The main disadvantage of the adenovirus is the high immunogenic potential. The humoral and cellular immune responses can actually remove the transduced cells, resulting in decreased gene expression (McCoy et al., 1995). Also, the immunologic memory established against the viral vector by the initial exposure limits the ability to give a second administration of gene therapy. Newer formulations of adenovirus vectors have undergone removal of many viral antigens to minimize this challenge and the so-called gutless vectors have virtually no adenovirus genes to minimize these responses (Hammerschmidt et al., 1999). As another approach for this immunological response, transient immunosuppression using cyclophosphamide has been shown to improve BMP expression after BMP adenoviral vector gene therapy (Okubo et al., 2000, Kim et al., 2003). Lieberman et al used *ex vivo* adenoviral gene transfer to create BMP-2 producing bone marrow cells for the delivery of BMP-2 to heal a critical-sized femoral segmental defect in a rat model (Lieberman et al., 1998). The genetically modified cells were implanted with inactivated demineralized bone matrix as a substrate. At two months, 92% of the defects healed radigraphically, and there was no significant difference in biomechanical testing between the group that had been treated with genetically modified cells and those that had been treated with rhBMP-2 alone. Their results showed that BMP-2 producing bone marrow cells created by means of adenoviral gene transfer produced sufficient proteins to heal a segmental femoral defect in a rat model.

3.2.3 Adeno associated virus

Adeno-associated viruses (AAVs) are a defective single stranded parvovirus (requires a helper virus such as adenovirus or herpes simplex virus for replication) that integrates its genetic material into a specific site located on chromosome 19 which can minimize the risk of insertional mutagenesis (Monahan et al., 2000). The virus infects a wide variety of dividing and non-dividing cells with high efficiency and little inflammatory response. Also, long-term gene expression has been reported in several tissues types. The disadvantages of AAVs are the difficulty in the virus production and limited titers of virus which can be generated (Kotin et al., 1994).

3.2.4 Herpes virus

Herpes viruses are double-stranded DNA viruses that can cause significant human pathology, including cold sores and encephalitis. Gene therapy studies using herpes viral vectors typically use genetically modified herpes simplex Type 1 (HSV-1). Herpes viral vectors have the advantage of being able to accommodate up to 40 kb of foreign DNA, and can be used to a variety of cell populations with limited toxicity (Evans et al., 1997). However, the disadvantage is that HSVs are highly immunogenic.

3.2.5 Lentivirus

Whereas retroviruses can only infect dividing cells, lentiviruses such as the human immunodeficiency virus type 1 (HIV-1) can also infect non-proliferating cells. What could be termed the third-generation lentivirus conserves only three (gag, pol, and rev) of the nine genes present in the genome of the original HIV-1. This eliminates the possibility that a wild -type virus will be reconstituted through recombination and create room for a relatively large gene delivery. Lentiviral-based gene transfer provides improved delivery, integration, and expression of target genes *in vitro* as well as *in vivo*. Furthermore, lentiviruses are capable of inserting into the host genome ensuring prolonged gene expression with a limited host immune response (Feeley et al., 2006). However, safety issues of HIV-based vectors are a major concern when adapting these vectors for clinical use (Bai et al., 2003, Dull et al., 1998, Zufferey et al., 1997, Zufferey et al., 1998).

4. Osteoinductive factors for *ex vivo* gene therapy

4.1 BMPs

BMPs comprise a large and diverse family, and many may have a distinct role not only in the cascade of bone morphogenesis but also in orchestrating tissue architecture throughout the body. More than 20 BMPs have been identified in humans and rodents (Bragdon B et al., 2011). Signal transduction of BMPs consists of interaction with both type-1(BMPR-1) and type-2(BMPR-2) BMP receptors, phospholylation of the GS domain of BMPR-1 by BMPR-2, phosphorylation of Smad1/5/8, and the translocation of the Smad1/5/8 partnering with the Smsd4 to the nucleus to activate the transcription for BMP-response genes (Reddi et al., 2001, Bragdon B et al., 2011). To date, most attempts at gene therapy to achieve spinal fusion have involved transfection with various BMPs (Li et al., 2003). Among BMPs, BMP-2 and BMP-7 have been the most extensively studied, both in animal studies and in clinical trials of spinal fusion. Recently, some combinations of BMPs have been demonstrated to have a synergic effect on bone formation (Israel et al., 1996, Zhu et al., 2004, Zhao et al., 2005).

4.2 LIM

LIM mineralization protein-1 (LMP-1) is an intracellular LIM-domain protein that is directly involved in osteoblast differentiation. LMP-1 also appears to elicit the increased synthesis of BMPs. Unlike a BMP, which is a secreted protein that binds to cell-surface receptors to initiate a response, LMP-1 is an intracellular signaling molecule and must be synthesized inside cells to exert its osteoinductive effects. Thus, the use of LMP-1 to form bone must involve the techniques of gene therapy to deliver the cDNA inside the cells and result in the synthesis of LMP-1 protein in situ (Cha et al., 2003, Pola et al., 2004).

4.3 NELL-1

NELL-1 (NEL-like molecule-1; NEL[a protein strongly expressed in neural tissue encoding epidermal growth factor like domain]) is a novel growth factor believed to specifically target cells committed to the osteochondral lineage. NELL-1 was isolated and characterized in craniosynostosisi patients as specifically upregulated within prematurely fusing sutures (Zhang et al., 2002). The phenotype of the *Nell-1* transgenic overexpression mouse revealed cranial suture overgrowth similar to human craniosynostosis, suggesting a distinct role for Nrll-1 in bone formation. Conversely, a mouse model with mutated RNU-induced alleles, including Nell-1, resulted in cranial and other vertebral skeletal defects (Desai et al., 2006). In committed osteoblasts, Nell-1 upregulation accelerates osteogenic differentiation and bone formation. Interestingly, human NELL-1 was reported to be directly regulated by Cbfa1/Runx2, confirming its osteochondral specificity (Truong S et al., 2007). Additionally, co-administration to C2C12 myoblasts with AdBMP-2 and AdNell-1 showed a synergistic effect on osteogenic differentiation as detected by alkaline phosphatase activity and osteopontin production. Importantly, Nell-1 alone did not induce osteogenic differentiation of myoblasts.

5. Cells combined with *ex vivo* gene therapy

MSCs from adult tissues present fewer ethical and tumorigenicity problems in their use than embryonic stem (ES) cells. These MSCs have demonstrated not only self-renewal ability but also "plasticity" meaning they have the ability to differentiate into phenotypes not restricted to the tissue from which they are derived (Augello et al., 2010). Another key feature of these MSCs is their rapid expansion *in vitro* without loss of progenitor characteristics. Various sources of MSCs that could be used for *ex vivo* gene therapy include bone marrow, muscle and adipose tissue (Lee et al., 2008, Gottfried et al., 2008). In clinical practice, the most widely used source of MSCs is bone marrow. The advantages of using bone marrow are the technique to collect them from the iliac crest is simple and is associated with the least morbidity. However, the problem of low MSC concentration upon harvest (1 in 10,000 cells) have led to an interest in adipose derived stem cells as they have been shown to have a higher prevalence (1 in 4,000 cells). The multipotentiality of adipose-derived stem cells (ADSCs) has been demonstrated *in vivo* and they have been shown to differentiate to bone cells in reaction to BMP signaling (Zuk et al., 2001, Zuk et al., 2010, Zuk et al., 2011). Hsu et al. reported that stem cells from human adipose cell transfected with AdBMP-2 can work as cellular delivery vehicles in an athymic rat posterolateral spine fusion model (Hsu et al., 2008). Miyazaki et al. have compared the osteogenic and osteoinductive ability between human bone marrow stem cells and human adipose derived stem cells for adenovirus mediated *ex vivo* gene therapy in an athymic rat spinal fusion model and demonstrated that both cells have similar ability for inducing new bone and spinal fusion (Miyazaki et al., 2008)

6. Spinal fusion by *ex vivo* gene therapy

6.1 BMP-2 *ex vivo* gene therapy

Riew et al attempted to prolong the bone-inducing effect of BMP-2 using an adenoviral vector carrying the human BMP-2 gene to transduce marrow-derived mesenchymal stem cells in New Zealand White rabbits. In their model, they isolated and expanded bone marrow mesenchymal cells from the resected ribs. Immunocytochemistry was used to show that approximately 80% of mesenchymal cells could be modified genetically to overexpress BMP-2 protein by treatment with an adenoviral vector encoding human BMP-2 (AdBMP-2). A similar efficiency of gen e transfer was shown with the control vector encoding a marker gene β-galactosidase (Adβ-gal). Four weeks after rib harvest, the rabbits underwent spinal fusion at L5-6. Genetically modified mesenchymal stem cells loaded onto collagen sponges were placed between the transverse processes of L5 and L6 with AdBMP-2 transduced mesenchymal stem cells placed on the left side and the Adβ-gal cells on the right. After the second postoperative week, all rabbits were examined weekly using a radiograph. Of the five study rabbits, one showed radiographic evidence of new bone formation on the side implanted with AdBMP-2 at 5 weeks after surgery. No new bone was noted on the control Adβ-gal side. No new bone formation was observed on either side in the other four study rabbits. Rabbits were sacrificed 7 weeks after the operation, and histologic examination of the rabbit with new bone revealed mature bone with a trabecular structure. The authors concluded that it was possible to transduce mesenchymal stem cells with human BMP-2 gene so that the transformed cells could produce BMP-2 *in vivo* that would exert an osteoinductive effect (Riew et al., 1998). Riew et al also reported using *ex vivo* AdBMP-2 transduction to perform anterior spinal fusion on pigs. Bone marrow cells were harvested from a resected rib and were expanded. Cells were then incubated overnight with AdBMP-2. Anterior arthrodesis was performed by a thoracoscopic technique and the researchers reported a 100% fusion rate by histologic and radiologic evaluation for six of six disc spaces treated with AdBMP-2, whereas none of the controls fused (Riew et al., 2003).

Wang et al. compared single-level posterolateral spine fusion rates between rhBMP-2 with various carriers, bone marrow cells transduced for 48 hours with AdBMP-2 and iliac crest bone graft (ICBG) in rats. They reported higher fusion rates with *ex vivo* BMP-2 transduction as compared with autogenous ICBG. All of the animals treated with AdBMP-2 and rhBMP-2 achieved solid fusion masses at four weeks, whereas none of the control groups fused. Qualitatively, the *ex vivo* AdBMP-2-treated rats produced abundant trabecular fusion masses, whereas the rhBMP-2-treated rats exhibited thinner, lacelike trabecular fusion masses. The researchers concluded that *ex vivo* AdBMP-2 transduction produced solid posterolateral spinal fusion in rats and was superior to ICBG alone (Wang et al., 2003). The same group also reported that human bone marrow cells can be infected by AdBMP-2 and produce sufficient bone *in vivo* to fuse the lumbar spine in athymic rats (Peterson et al. 2005). Miyazaki et al. have compared lentiviral and adenoviral gene therapy. They had implanted a collagen sponge containing rat bone marrow cells transfected with either Lenti-BMP-2 or Adeno-BMP-2 and achieved solid fusion masses at eight weeks, whereas the new bone volume and levels fused are greater in the Lenti-BMP-2 treated group. They concluded that lentiviral gene therapy with BMP-2 shows great potential for application in various pathologies of the spine despite the fact that the safety of using lentiviral vectors and the side effects of prolonged BMP-2 production are required to be elucidated before the application of this technology in humans (Miyazaki et al., 2008).

6.2 BMP-7 *ex vivo* gene therapy

Hidaka et al. recently reported successful posterolateral spinal fusion in immune-competent rats in *ex vivo* study using rat bone marrow cells that were expanded for four weeks, then treated with AdBMP-7 or Adβ-gal for two hours. Three million cells were implanted with allograft bone at the L4-5 level using a paraspinal muscle-splitting approach. A β-galastosidase assay was performed in homogenetes of fusion masses harvested three, seven, and 14 days after surgery to evaluate the extent and duration of adenovirus mediated gene transfer in this model. The gene expression was maximal on day three, waning to background levels by 14 days. Additionally, with AdBMP-7 treatment, radiographic fusion rates were 70% and mechanical fusion rates were 80% versus 0% by either parameter in control groups at eight weeks after the index procedure. Fusion masses of AdBMP-7 treated spines had the microscopic appearance of normal trabecular bone and showed a 23-fold higher uptake of fluorochrome indicating increased bone formation. (Hidaka et al., 2003).

6.3 BMP-9 *ex vivo* gene therapy

Dumont et al. reported that human bone marrow mesenchymal stem cells were transduced with AdBMP-9 or Adβ-gal for 12hours and then, the cells (1 million cells/ml) were injected into the lumbar region with the use of fluoroscopic guidance in an athymic rat model. At eight weeks, the sites treated with the cells transduced AdBMP-9 showed copious bone formation, whereas the control injections showed no osteogenic activity. They did not mention about the fusion rate or bone volume of the newly induced bone (Dumont et al., 2002).

6.4 Combination of different BMPs

Although a variety of BMPs still are being investigated for their therapeutic potential, a combination of different BMPs and other growth factors may prove to be the most effective initiators of bone formation. The use of BMP2/7 and BMP4/7 heterodimers has demonstrated increased bone induction and compared with that of their homodimer counterparts (Israel et al., 1996). Zhu et al. reported that supernatants from the culture media of a producer cell (A549) co-transfected by AdBMP-2 and AdBMP-7 induced much higher osteocalcin expression and alkaline phosphatase activity in both C2C12 and MC3T3-E-1 cells than the supernatants from the cells transfected either AdBMP-2 or AdBMP-7 alone even though the concentration of the produced BMPs are much lower in the co-transfected group. They further demonstrated that co administration of AdBMP-2 and AdBMP-7 resulted in a significantly greater number of mechanically stable fusions ans also 2-fold higher mineralization rate and bone volume in the fusion mass versus single BMP gene transfer (co-administrated group; 73% fusion, AdBMP-2 group; 8% fusion and AdBMP-7 group 16% fusion (Zhu et al., 2004).

6.5 LIM

Although the exact mechanism of LMP-1 remains unclear, solid spinal fusions have been achieved in rat and rabbit models using *ex vivo* LMP-1-transduced bone marrow cells and buffy-coat blood cells.

Boden et al investigated the feasibility of achieving lumbar spine fusion by liposomal-mediated transfer of a different osteoinductive protein gene, the LIM mineralization protein-1 (LMP-1) gene. LMP-1 is an intracellular protein that plays a key role in the BMP-6 stimulation of osteoblasts. Because LMP-1 is an intracellular signaling molecule, the technique of gene therapy is best suited to deliver the LMP-1 cDNA within the cell. Marrow fibroblasts were isolated from the hind limbs of rats and transfected with a plasmid containing LMP-1 in the forward orientation (study group) or the reverse orientation (control group) using lipofection. Once the cells were transfected, they were soaked in a devitalized bone matrix carrier. 14 athymic rats were used. Implants were composed of a devitalized bone matrix carrier loaded with bone marrow cells transfected with either the LMP-1 gene (active) or the reverse LMP-1 (control). In the pilot phase, two rats received subcutaneous implants on the right (active) and left (control) sides of the chest. The same rats received implants to the lumbar (active) and received implants to the posterior thoracic (control) spine. In the experimental phase, 12 rats received active and control implants in the thoracic (T11-12) and lumbar (L5-6) spine. Rats that received bone marrow cells transfected with the active gene in the thoracic region and vice versa. Four weeks postoperation, all rats were sacrificed. The samples of the rats that received subcutaneous implants underwent high-definition radiographs and undecalcified histology. All thoracic and lumbar spines in the experimental group underwent assessment of fusion by manual palpation, radiography, and undecalcified histology. Examination of subcutaneous implants from the two pilot rats revealed complete bone formation with marrow and osteoblast-lined trabeculae on the active side (carrier plus marrow cells with active LMP-1 cDNA) with no bone formation on the control side (carrier plus marrow cells with reverse LMP-1 cDNA). The two lumbar spines of the pilot rats that were implanted with the active LMP-1 cDNA were completely fused, whereas the two thoracic control fusion sites that had been implanted with reverse LMP-1 cDNA failed to show new bone formation. In the experimental group, three of the 12 rats died of perioperative anesthetic complications. In the remaining nine rats, complete arthrodesis was shown manually, radiographically, and histologically in nine of nine (100%) sites receiving bone marrow cells transfected with inactive LMP-1 cDNA were fused. The authors concluded that the local delivery of LMP-1 cDNA to bone marrow cells was feasible and efficacious for enhancing spine arthrodesis.

Boden et al. reported solid posterior fusion in an athymic rat model using bone marrow cells transduced for two hours with AdLMP-1 in a demineralized bone matrix carrier (Boden et al., 1998). Viggeswarapu et al. showed bone marrow or buffy-coat cells transduced with AdLMP-1 for 10 minutes combined with demineralized bone matrix or collagen-ceramic-composite sponges induced posterolateral lumbar fusion in rabbits (Viggeswarapu et al., 2001).

6.6 Nell-1

Lu et al reported the osteoinductive properties of Nell-1 in rat spinal fusion model. Demineralized bone matrix (DBM) carriers containing either adenovirus coding for Nell-1 (AdNell-1) or Lac Z (AdLacZ) were implanted at the intertransverse process of L4-5 in athymic rats. After six weeks, direct application of adenoviral Nell-1 in a DBM carrier achieved significantly higher rates of spinal fusion over Lac Z controls: 60% Nell-1 versus 20% Lac Z by manual palpation and 70% Nell-1 versus 20% Lac Z by micoroCT and histology. Histological assessment of bone quality and maturity revealed more mature, higher quality bone in all the Nell-1 treated specimens relative to Lac Z at six weeks. They concluded that Nell-1, which is regulated by the master bone regulatory gene Runx2, may exert its effects more specifically in osteoblastic cells than BMPs which affects multiple cell types.

7. Conclusion and future direction

Spinal fusion will continue to be an important part of the surgical treatment of spinal pathology for the foreseeable future. Promising research in progress involves the understanding of the biology of bone formation (White et al., 2004) and the use of gene

Authors	Vector	Gene	cell	animal	Fusion rate	F/U weeks	carrier
Riew et al	adenovirus	BMP-2	Rat BMC	rabbits	20%	7	collagen
Boden et al	plasmid	LIM-1	Ratfibloblast	Athymic rats	100%	4	DBM
Peterson et al	adenovirus	BMP-2	Human BMC	Athymic rats	100%	12	CS
Wang et al	adenovirus	BMP-2	Rat BMC	rats	100%	8	DBM
Hsu et al	adenovirus	BMP-2	Human ADSC	Athymic rats	100%	12	CS
Miyazaki et al	lentivirus	BMP-2	Rat BMC	rats	100%	8	CS
Viggeswarapu et al	adenovirus	LIM-1	BCC PBC	rabbits	100%	5 4	DBM CCC
Hidaka et al	adenovirus	BMP-7	Rat BMC	rats	70%	8	allograft
Dumont et al	adenovirus	BMP-9	Human BMC	Athymic rats	N/A	8	none
Riew et al	adenovirus	BMP-2	Pig BMC	pigs	100%	6	none
Miyazaki et al	adenovirus lentivirus	BMP-2	Rat BMC	rats	100%	8	CS
Miyazaki et al	adenovirus	BMP-2	Human ADSC Human BMC	Athymic rats	100%	8	CS
Lu et al	adenovirus	Nell-1	none	Athymic rats	70%	6	DBM

BMC: bone marrow cell, ADSC: adipose derived stem cell, CCC: collagen-ceramic-composite, CS: collagen sponge, Buffy-coat cell: BCC, Peripheral blood cell: PBC

Table 1. Animal studies on *ex vivo* gene therapy for spinal fusion.

therapy or tissue engineering in facilitating the natural processes of a spinal fusion. A viral vector can be used to transfer a gene into human cells to produce various recombinant growth factors that may modify the fusion cascade both qualitatively and quantitatively. Viral vectors, particularly the adenovirus, may serve as transports for the material encoding osteogenic factors. However, significant advances need to be made in vector design for low immunogenetic potential, controlled gene expression techniques like tetracycline-regulated system, the way of preventing insertional mutagenesis, and tissue targeting before human clinical trials can be safely and successfully conducted.

8. References

Alden TD, Pittman DD, Beres EJ, et al. (1999) Percutaneous spinal fusion using bone morphonenetic protein-2 gene therapy. *Journal of Neurosurgery* 90 (1 Suppl), pp.109-114

Alden TD, Varady P, Kallmes DF, et al. (2002) Bone morphogenetic protein gene therapy. *Spine* 27 (165), pp.S87-S93

Augello A, Kurth TB, De Bari C. (2010) Mesenchymal stem cells: a perspective from *in vitro* cultures to *in vivo* migration and niches. *European Cells and Materials* 1 (20), pp.121-133

Bai Y, Soda Y, Izawa K, et al. (2003) Effective transduction and stable transgene expression in human blood cells by a third-generation lentiviral vector. *Gene Therapy* 10, pp.1446-1457

Baltzer AWA, Lieberman. (2004) Regional gene therapy to enhance bone repair. *Gene Therapy* 11 (4), pp.344-350

Benn SI, Whitsitt JS, Broadley KN, et al. (1996) Particle-mediated gene transfer with transforming growth factor bata 1 cDNA enhances wound repair in rats. *Journal of Clinical Investigation* 98, pp.2894-2902

Boden SD, Titus L, Hair G, et al. (1998) Lumbar spine fusion by local gene therapy with a cDNA encoding a novel osteoinductive protein (LMP-1). *Spine* 23 (23), pp.2486-2492

Bragdon B, Moseychuk O, Saldanha S, et al. (2011) Bone morphogenetic proteins: a critical review. *Cell Signal* 23(4), pp.609-620

Carlisle E, Fischgrund JS. (2005) Bone morphogenetic proteins for spinal fusion. *The Spine Journal* 5, pp.240S-249S

Cha CW, Boden SD. (2003) Gene Theray Applications for Spine Fusion. *Spine* 28 (15S), pp.S74-S84

Cowan CM, Jiang X, Hsu T, et al. (2007) Synergistic effects of Nell-1 and BMP-2 on the osteogenic differentiation of myoblasts. *Journal of Bone and Mineral Research* 22 (6), pp. 918-930

Desai J, Shannon ME, Johnson MD, et al. (2007) Nell-1 deficient mice have reduced expressiion of extrcellular matrix proteins causing cranial and vertebral defects. *Human Molecular Genetics* 15, pp.1329-1341

Dull T, Zufferey R, Kelly M, et al. (1998) A Third-Generation Lentivirus Vector with a Conditional Packaging System. *Journal of virology*, 72(11), pp. 8463-8471

Dumont RJ, Dayoub H, Li JZ, et al. (2002) *Ex vivo* bone morphogenetic protein-9 gene therapy using human mesenchymal stem cells induces spinal fusion in rodents. *Neurosurgery* 51 (5), pp.1239-1244

Evans CH, Ghivizzani SC, Robbins PD. (2004) Orthopaedic Gene Therapy, *Clinical Prthopaedics and related research* 429, pp.316-329

Evans C, Goins WF, Schmidt MC, et al. (1997) Progress in development of herpes simplex virus gene vectors for treatment of rheumatoid arthritis. *Advanced Drug Delivery Reviews* 27, pp.41-57

Fang J, Zhu YY, Smiley E., et al. (1996) Stimulation of new bone formation by direct transfer of osteogenic plasmid genes. *Proceedings of the National Academy of Sciences* 93, pp.5753-5758

Feeley BT, Conduah AH, Sugiyama O, et al. (2006) *In vivo* molecular imaging of adenoviral versus lentiviral gene therapy in two bone formation models. *Journal of Orthopaedic Research*, pp.1709-1721

Gottfried ON, Dailey AT. (2008) Mesenchymal stem cell and gene therapies for spinal fusion. *Neurosurgery* 63 (3), pp.380-392

Gugala Z, Olmsted-Davis EA, Gannon FH, et al. (2003) Osteoinduction by *ex vivo* adenovirus-mediated BMP-2 delivery is independent of cell type. *Gene Therapy* 10. Pp.1289-1296

Hammerschmidt DE. (1999) Development of a gutless vector. *Journal of Laboratory and Clinical medicine* 134 (3), C3

Helm GA, Alden TD, Sheehan JP, et al. (2000) Bone morphogenetic proteins and bone morphogenetic gene therapy in neurological surgery : a review. *Neurosurgery* 46 (5), pp.1213-1222

Hidaka C, Goshi K, Rawlins B, et al. (2003) Enhancement of Spine Fusion Using Combined Gene Theray and Tissue Engineering BMP-7 Expressing Bone Marrow Cells and Allograft Bone. *Spine* 28 (18), pp.2049-2057

Hsu WK, Wang JC, Liu NQ, et al. (2008) Stem cells from human fat as cellular delivery vehicles in an athymic rat posterolateral spine fusion model. *Journal of Bone and Joint Surgery* 90, pp.1043-1052

Israel DI, Nove , Kerns KM, et al. (1996) Heterodimeric bone morphogenetic proteins show enhanced activity *in vitro* and *in vivo*. *Growth Factors* 13, pp.291-300

Kaito T, Myoui A, Takaoka K, et al. (2005) Potentiation of the activity of bone morphogenetic protein-2 in bone regeneration by a PLA-PLG/hydroxyapatite composite. *Biomaterials* 26(1), pp.73-79

Khan SN, Hidaka C, Sandhu HS, et al. (2000) Gene therapy for spine fusion. *Tissue Engineering in Orthopedic Surgery* 31 (3), pp.473-484

Khan SN, Sandhu HS, Lane JM, et al. (2002) Bone morphogenetic proteins : relevance in spine surgery. *The Orthopedic Clinics of North America* 33, pp.447-463

Khan SN, Lane JM. (2004) Spinal fusion surgery : animal models for tissue-engineered bone constructs. *Biomaterials* 25, pp.1475-1485

Kim HS, Viggeswarapu M, Boden SDD, et al. (2003) Overcoming the immune response to permit *ex vivo* gene therapy for spine fusion with human type 5 adenoviral delivery of the LIM mineralization protein-1 cDNA. *Spine* 28 (3), pp.219-226

Kootstra NA, Verma IM. (2003) Gene therapy with viral vectors. *Annual Review of Pharmacology and Toxicology* 43, pp.413-439

Kotin RM. (1994) Prospects for the use of adeno-associated virus as a vector for human gene therapy. *Human Gene Therapy* 5, pp.793-801

Lai CM, Lai YK, Rakoczy PE, et al. (2002) Adenovirus and adeno-associated virus vectors. *DNA and Cell Biology* 21, pp. 895-913

Lee K, Chan CK, Patil N, et al. (2008) Cell therapy for bone regeneration-Bench to bedside. *Journal of Biomedical Material and Research* Part B, pp. 252-263

Li JZ, Li H, Sasaki T, et al. (2003) Osteogenic potential of five different recombinant human bone morphogenetic protein adenoviral vectors in the rat. *Gene Therapy* 10, pp.1735-1743

Li S, Ma Z. (2001) Nonviral gene therapy. *Current Gene Therapy* 1, pp.201-226

Li Z, Dullmann J, Schiedlmeier B, et al. (2002) Murine Leukemia induced by retroviral gene marking. *Science* 296, pp.497

Lieberman JR, Le LQ, Finermn GA, et al. Regional gene therapy with a BMP-2-producing murine stromal cell line induces heterotopic and orthotopic bone formation in rodents. *Journal of Orthopaedic Research* 16 (3), pp.330-339

Lu SS, Zhang, X, Soo C, et al. (2007) The osteoinductive properties of Nell-1 in a rat spinal fusion model. *The Spine Journal* 7, pp,50-60

McCoy RD, Davidson BL, Roessler BJ, et al. (1995) Expression of human interleukin-1 receptor antagonist in mouse lungs using a recombinant adenovirus: effects on vector-induced inflammation. *Gene Therapy* 2 (79, pp.437-442

Miller DG, Adam MA, Miller AD. (1990) Gene transfer by retrovirus vectors occurs only in cells that are actively replicating at the time of infection. *Journal of Molecular Cell Biology* 10, pp.4239-4242

Miyazaki M, Sugiyama O, Tow B, et al. (2008) The effects of lentiviral gene therapy with bone morphogenetic protein-2-producing bone marrow cells on spinal fusion in rats. *Journal of Spinal Disorder and Techniques* 21 (5), pp.372-379

Miyazaki M, Sugiyama O, Zou J, et al. (2008) Comparison of Lentiviral and Adenoviral gene Therapy for Spinal Fusion in Rats. *Spine* 33 (13), pp.1410-1417

Miyazaki M, Zuk PA, Zou J, et al. (2008). Comparison of Human Mesenchymal Stem Cells Derived From Adipose Tissue and Bone Marrow for *Ex Vivo* Gene Therapy in Rat Spinal Fusion Model, *Spine* 33 (8), pp.863-869

Monahan PE, Samulski RJ. (1999) AAV vectors: Is clinical success on the horizon? *Gene Therapy* 6, pp.904-912

Mroz TE, Wang JC, Hashimoto R, et al. (2010) Complications related to osteobiologics use in spine surgery: a systematic review. *Spine* 35 (9 Suppl), pp.S86-104

Nishida K, Suzuki T, Kakutani K, et al. (2008) Gene therapy approach for disc degeneration and associated spinal disorders. *European Spine Journal* 17 (Suppl 4), pp.S459-S466

Peterson B, Iglesias R, Zhang J, et al. (2005) Genetically modified human derived bone marrow cells for posterolateral lumbar spine fusion in athymic rats. *Spine* 30 (3), pp.283-290

Pola E, Gao W, Zhou Y, et al. (2004) Efficient bone formation by gene transfer of human LIM mineralization protein-3. *Gene Therapy* 11, pp.683-693

Oakes DA, Lieberman JR. (2000) Osteoinductive applications of regional gene therapy: *ex vivo* gene transfer. *Clinical Orthopaedics and Related Research* 379 Suppl, pp.S101-112

Okubo Y, Bessho K, Fujimura K, et al. (2000) Osteoinduction by bone morphogenetic protein-2 via adenoviral vector under transient immunosuppression. *Biochemical and Biophysical Research Communications* 267, pp.382-387

Phillips FM, Bolt PM, He TC, et al. (2005) Gene therapy for spinal fusion. *The Spine Journal* 5, pp250S-258S

Reddi AH. (1998) Role of morphogenetic proteins in skeletal tissue engineering and regeneration. *Nature Biotechnology* 16, pp.247-252

Reddi AH. (2001) Bone morphogenetic protein :from basic science to clinical applications. *Journal of Bone and Joint Surgery* 83-A, pp.S1-1-S1-6

Riew KD, Wright NM, Cheng SL, et al. (1998) Induction of bone formation using a recombinant adenoviral vector carrying the human BMP-2 gene in a rabbit spinal fusion model. *Calcified Tissue International* 63. Pp357-360

Riew KD, Lou J, Wright NM, et al. (2003) Thoracoscopic intradiscal spine fusion using a minimally invasive gene-therapy technique. *Journal of Bone and Joint Surgery* 85-A, pp.866-871

Truong S, Zhang X, Pathmanathan D, et al. (2007) Craniosynostosis-associated gene Nell-1 is regulated by Runx2. *Journal of Bone and Mineral Research* 122, pp.7-18

Vaccaro AR, Chiba K, Heller JG, et al. (2002) Bone grafting alternatives in spinal surgery. *The Spine Journal* 2, pp.206-215

Veillette CJH, Mckee MD. (2007) Growth factors - BMPs, DBMs, and buffy coat products :are there any proven differences amongst them ? Injury, *International Journal of the Care of the Injured* 38S1, pp.S38-S48

Viggeswarapu M, Boden SD, Liu Y, et al. (2001) Adenoviral delivery of LIM mineralization protein-1 induces new-bone formation *in vitro* and vivo. *Journal of Bone and Joint Surgery* 83-A, pp.364-376

Wang JC, Lanim LE, Campbell RA, et al. (2003) Effect of regional gene therapy with bone morphogenetic protein-2-producing bone marrow cells on spinal fusion in rats. *Journal of Bone and Joint Surgery* 85-A (5), pp.905-911

White AP, Weinstein MA, Patel TC, et al. (2004) Lumbar arthrodesis gene expression. *Clinical Orthopaedics and related research* 429, pp.330-337

Yoon ST, Boden SD. (2004). Spine fusion by gene therapy, *Gene therapy* 11, pp.360-367

Zhang X, Kuroda S, Carpenter D, et al. (2002) Craniosynostosis in transgenic mice overexpressing Nell-1. *Journal of Clinical Investigation* 110, pp.861-870

Zhao M, Zhao Z, Koh JT, et al. (2005) Combinatorial Gene Therapy for Bone Regeneration : Cooperative interactions between adenovirus vectors expressing bone morphogenetic priteins 2,4, and 7. *Journal of Cellular Biochemistry* 95, pp.1-16

Zhu W, Rawlins BA, Oachie-Adjei O, et al. (2004) Combined bone morphogenetic protein-2 and -7 gene transfer enhances osteoblastic differentiation and spine fusion in a rodent model. *Journal of Bone and Mineral Research* 19, pp.2021-2032

Zufferey R, Nagy D, Mandel RJ, et al. (1997) Multiply attenuated lentiviral vector achieves efficient gene delivery *in vivo*. *Nature Biotechnology* 15, pp.871-875

Zufferey R, Dull T, Mandel RJ, et al. (1998) Self-Inactivating Lentivirus Vector for Safe and Efficient *In Vivo* Gene Delivery. *Journal of Virology*, pp.9873-9880

Zuk PA. (2001) Multilineage cells from human adipose tissue : implications for cell-based therapies. *Tissue Engineering* 7 (2), pp.211-228

Zuk PA. (2010) The adipose-derived stem cell : looking back and looking ahead. *Molecular Biology of the Cell* 21, pp.1783-1787

Zuk PA. (2011) Viral transduction of adipose-derived stem cells. *Methods in Molecuar Biology* 702,pp.345-357

Part 3

Gene Therapy in Genitourinary System

14

Gene Therapy in Urology

Ratha Mahendran, Sin Mun Tham and Kesavan Esuvaranathan
Department of Surgery, Yong Loo Lin School of Medicine,
National University of Singapore
Singapore

1. Introduction

The application of gene therapy in the field of Urology is not limited to cancer therapy but is also being evaluated for non-cancer related bladder dysfunctions as well as erectile dysfunction (ED). This article will review the use of gene therapy for these conditions; the vectors used and limitations associated with different gene delivery systems and the attempts to overcome these shortcomings.

2. Bladder cancer

Bladder cancer is the 7th most common cancer worldwide. It has a natural history of superficial recurrences and local progression. It is estimated that within 18 months of first diagnosis approximately 50% of patients will have a recurrence (Anderson & Naish 2008). Thus there is a need for frequent monitoring of these patients. In the US the estimated life-time cost of therapy for bladder cancer patients with non-muscle invasive disease was US $21.03 million based on a Medicare database (Cooksley et al. 2008). The majority of this is spent on surveillance and the treatment of recurrences. Tumors occur on the luminal surface of the bladder and the architecture of the bladder permits topical intravesical therapies. The bladder is isolated from other organs and tissues and intravesical therapy permits contact with the entire internal surface of the bladder with minimal systemic side-effects.
The present gold standard therapy for superficial bladder cancers is immunotherapy with Mycobacterium bovis, Bacillus Calmette Guerin (BCG) following local transurethral resection of the bladder tumor (TURBT). BCG induces a mononuclear and neutrophilic infiltrate in the bladder wall which results in an inflammatory response as measured by cytokine production that causes sloughing of both tumor and normal cells (Herr and Morales 2008). The presence of IL-2, IL-8 and IL-18 in the urine of patients has been reported to correlate with response to therapy (Thalmann et al. 1997; Thalmann et al. 2000; Saint et al. 2003). Unfortunately, BCG has several shortcomings: it is a live vaccine and commonly causes side effects and occasionally septicemia. In addition some patients (20-42%) do not respond to therapy (Kamat and Lamm 2000). In place of BCG, recombinant cytokines such as IFN-γ, TNF-α, and IL-2 have been used in a number of clinical trials with encouraging results (Glazier et al. 1995; Den Otter et al. 1998; Stavropoulos et al. 2002). However, recombinant cytokines are costly, unstable in urine and have poor permeability

across the glycosaminoglycan (GAG) layer of the urothelium. Gene therapy is a natural alternative approach to ensure cytokine production in the bladder environment.

2.1 Viral transfection systems for bladder cancer

Initially replication defective viruses were generated with the sole purpose of gene delivery (Thomas et al. 2003). The viruses evaluated included: Adenovirus (type 2 and 5), Adeno-associated virus (*Parvoviridae* family), Herpes simplex virus, Retrovirus (Dumey et al. 2005), Canary pox virus and Vaccinia virus (Lee et al. 1994). Table 1 lists their characteristics.
However, because of the limited transduction capability of some viruses, replicating and conditionally replicating viruses were developed. These viruses amplify the transfection efficiency, as virus transduced cells produce more viruses that can infect the surrounding cells. Replication of wild type viruses also induces cytolysis of infected cells.

2.1.1 Limitations and Improvements

2.1.1.1 Non-specificity of transfection

Siemens *et al.* compared adeno-, canary pox and vaccinia viruses in terms of their ability to transfect tumor cells after intravesical delivery in a murine model of bladder cancer (Siemens et al. 2003). The vaccinia and avian pox viruses were better at transfecting tumor cells than adenoviruses but all three resulted in transfection of extravesical tissue (e.g. kidney, liver, spleen). In contrast Wood et al reported only sporadic extravesical transfection after intravesical adenovirus instillations (Wood et al. 1999).
To reduce non specific viral transduced gene expression, oncolytic adenoviruses have been engineered to express the E1A and E1B genes under the control of the uroplankin II gene promoter (Zhang et al. 2002; He et al. 2009) which limits expression to urothelial cells. Another strategy to target viral replication to tumor cells is to place the adenovirus E1A gene under the control of the telomerase promoter (Lanson et al. 2003), the midkine gene promoter (Terao et al. 2007) or the Cox-2 promoter (Shirakawa et al. 2004). All these genes are highly expressed in tumor cells.
Bladder cancer cells often over-express the epidermal growth factor receptor (EGFR) and targeting EGFR with bi-specific antibodies improved the delivery of adenovirus to cancer cells (van der Poel et al. 2002). A gammaretrovirus carrying a chimeric envelope protein containing a single chain variable fragment (scFv) antibody to the human epidermal growth factor receptor 2 (HER2) was shown to specifically target cells expressing Her2 (Tsai et al. 2010).

2.1.1.2 Transfection efficiency

The internal surface of the bladder is covered by uroplakin proteins and the GAG layer which together provide a barrier to transfection of urothelial cells. Agents that disrupt this protective layer such as ethanol, HCl, dodecyl-B-d-maltoside and sodium dodecyl sulphate have been shown to improve viral transduction of the bladder (Engler et al. 1999; Lin et al. 2002; Ramesh et al. 2004).
Though adenoviruses are the most popular viruses for gene therapy they require adhesion with the cellular coxsackie-adenoviral receptor (CAR) for transduction of mammalian cells. Neoplastic tissue unlike normal bladder cells have reduced CAR expression (Buscarini et al. 2007) as a result of epigenetic control mechanisms (Pong et al. 2003).

Virus	Transfection efficiency	Immunogenicity	DNA inserts	Gene expression
Adenovirus	High with CAR receptor	high	8kb	Transient expression, DNA remains episomal
Adeno-associated virus	Good, no receptor	low	4.5kb	Stable, DNA episomes found
Herpes simplex virus	High in neurons	high	>30kb	Stable in neurons and transient in others, episomal
Moloney murine leukemia virus	High in dividing cells	low	8kb	Stable expression, DNA integration into host genome Hematopoietic cells
Lentivirus	Non dividing cells	low	8kb	Stable expression, Integration in host chromosome,
Canary pox virus	Most cells	low	25kb	Transient expression, Viral DNA limited to cytoplasm
Vaccinia virus	Most cells	high	Up to 25kb	Transient expression, Viral DNA limited to cytoplasm

Table 1. Characteristics of viral vectors for gene therapy

To circumvent the need for receptor mediated uptake, polymers have been used to enhance adenovirus transfection of bladder cells (Kasman et al. 2009) or even small molecule excipients such as Syn3 (Connor et al. 2001; Yamashita et al. 2002; Nagabhushan et al. 2007). A recent study has shown that CAR receptor expression and thus adenoviral expression can be increased by treatment with histone deacetylase inhibitors (HDACI) such as trichostatin A and sodium phenylbutyrate (Sachs et al. 2004).

2.1.1.3 Previous Immunity

Vaccinia viruses have long been used in man as vaccines against smallpox. This raised the issue of whether previous immunization would block the effectiveness of these viruses as gene delivery vehicles. Intravesical instillation of vaccinia viruses was successfully demonstrated in pre-immunized mice (Lee et al. 1994). The immunogenicity of adenoviruses is a major limitation in most therapeutic strategies. However it may be advantageous in bladder cancer therapy where non-specific inflammation as a consequence of BCG instillation has been associated with tumor removal.

2.1.1.4 Promoter inactivation

Adenovirus genes expressed from a CMV promoter induced better gene expression than those expressed using a RSV promoter (Freund et al. 2000). But quite often the CMV promoter is inactivated *in vivo*. It has been found that adenoviral transfection together with HDAC inhibitor trichostatin or retinoic acid improved CMV promoter activity. Treatment with these drugs could improve and prolong adenoviral transgene expression (Gaetano et al 2000). The development of tissue specific promoters as described above may resolve this problem.

2.2 Non-viral transfection systems for bladder cancer

The strength and weakness of non-viral vectors is the transient expression of the delivered genes. For non-viral gene delivery the genes are encoded on plasmid DNA of bacterial origin. Non-viral delivery agents include liposomes (N-[1-(2,3-Dioleoyloxy)propyl]-N,N,N-trimethylammonium chloride, DOTAP), polyethylenimine (PEI), viral envelopes (with fusogenic properties) conjugated to liposomes (Hemagglutinating Virus of Japan (HVJ) liposomes), chitosans as well as physical means such as the use of an electrogun or ultrasound (Harimoto et al. 1998; Lawrencia et al. 2001; Ogawa et al. 2004; Bonnet et al. 2008; Tsai et al. 2009; Zaharoff et al. 2009). Plasmid DNA delivery systems result in cellular entry via the endosomes (Al-Dosari & Gao 2009). Endosomal escape is often difficult and when successful the plasmid DNA is mainly restricted to the cytoplasm. A small amount may make it to the nucleus and exist as episomal DNA molecules that can be lost during replication (Al-Dosari & Gao 2009). Besides the delivery agents, the plasmid DNA sequence can also modulate the efficiency of transfection as discussed below.

2.2.1 Limitations and Improvements

2.2.1.1 Promoter inactivation

It has been reported that the CMV promoter often used for plasmid gene expression does not always result in good gene expression (Loser et al. 1998) as a consequence of promoter inactivation. This can be overcome by using a HDAC inhibitor, as demonstrated with OSU-HDAC42 (Lai et al. 2010). An alternative strategy is to utilize tissue/cancer cell specific promoters such as the COX-2, H19 and human IGF2-P4 gene promoters (Ohana et al. 2002; Zhang et al. 2008; Amit & Hochberg 2010).

2.2.1.2 Transfection efficiency

The primary focus of improving plasmid DNA transfection is improving escape from the endosomes and this is achieved by developing new additives and lipoplexes or even polyplexes that use either acidification or osmotic pressure changes or membrane fusogenic molecules to allow DNA escape (Al-Dosari and Gao 2009). We developed a formulation comprised of DOTAP and Methyl-β-cyclodextrin solubilized cholesterol (MBC) that transfects urothelial cells *in vivo* within 2 hours of exposure. Transfection was confined to the bladder (Lawrencia et al. 2001) and occurred in the superficial and deeper layers of the urothelial tumours (Wu et al. 2003).

2.2.1.3 Specificity of plasmid expression and activity/duration

Antibodies have been used to target delivery of plasmids to tumor cells. ScFv antibody to Her-2 (Tsai et al. 2009) or transferrin have been demonstrated to successfully target plasmids to tumor cells (Pirollo et al. 2008). The latter strategy targets both primary and metastatic disease when delivered systemically. Targeting of plasmid DNA to the nucleus can also be induced by introducing mammalian transcription factor binding sites in the plasmid and this increased the duration of expression (Gill et al. 2009).

Plasmid DNA expression is transient because of the episomal nature of transfected DNA. In bladder cancer therapy this can be overcome by repeated intravesical instillations. Another strategy to improve gene expression is to add a scaffold matrix attachment region (S/MAR) to the plasmid DNA. S/MAR serve both to ensure prolonged gene expression, by reducing the silencing of plasmid DNA as well as to ensure plasmid DNA replication as episomes (Gill et al. 2009).

Integration of plasmid DNA into chromosomal DNA is achievable now. The techniques used include retroviral integrase (Tanaka et al. 1998), sleeping beauty (SB) transposons

(Hackett et al. 2010) or phage recombinase mediated integration (Olivares et al. 2002). Thus in the future a single intravesical instillation may be sufficient for prolonged therapeutic effects.

2.2.1.4 Liposome free delivery

For small molecules such as CpG oligodeoxynucleotides (ODN), intravesical delivery to urothelial cells can be achieved without a transfection agent (Ninalga et al. 2005). But plasmid DNA requires a delivery agent. Nanoparticles (10-100nm in size) with bound plasmid DNA are recognized by cell surface nucleolin on HeLa cells and this results in DNA transport to the nucleus (Chen et al. 2008) and avoidance of endosomal entrapment.

2.2.1.5 Inflammation

The CpG sequences on plasmid DNA induce inflammation that could reduce gene expression by either destruction of transfected cells or promoter inactivation (Yew et al. 2000). Minicircle DNA (mcDNA), are supercoiled DNA with only the therapeutic gene cassette. They are generated *in vivo* by site specific recombination in E coli and exhibit improved gene expression in terms of the level and duration of gene expression (Darquet et al. 1997).

2.3 Preclinical evaluation of genes and evolving gene therapy strategies

The different categories of genes used successfully in animal studies are listed in Table 2. Both Sub-cutaneous (sc) and orthotopic models of bladder cancer have been used to evaluate gene therapy. While the data from sc studies have shown the efficacy of the expressed genes, it is the orthotopic models that best reflect clinical disease and therapeutic gene delivery. In general regardless of the delivery system or gene delivered tumor growth reduction or even eradication has been reported in murine models of bladder cancer. Most therapeutic schedules used in the animal studies require repeated instillations of the gene delivery vehicle whether it is a viral or non-viral vector. However, a recent study of viral gene delivery of IFNα indicated that a high dose could reduce the need for increased intravesical instillations (Tao et al. 2006). Transfection using transposons may also reduce the need for repeated transfection of plasmid DNA.

New therapies aim to combine several strategies at once. These include the use of oncolytic viruses and immune modulation using GMCSF (Cozzi et al. 2001; Ramesh et al. 2006); wild type p53 and ribozyme erb-2 (Irie et al. 2006) and Rb94 or oncolytic viruses and chemotherapeutic drugs (Zhang et al. 2002; Pirollo et al. 2008). *In vitro* studies have shown that combining AdHSVTK, ganciclovir and chemotherapy may have therapeutic benefit (Freund et al. 2003). Further the beneficial effect of 5-FU and adenovirus cytosine deaminase gene therapy could be enhanced by irradiation (Zhang et al. 2003). Such multi-factor therapies may be better at eradicating tumor cells. Another strategy is to modify immune cells *in vitro* for cancer therapy. Dendritic cell manipulation by transfection with adenovirus carrying the survivin gene has been shown to induce cytotoxic T lymphocytes (CTLs) (Kikkawa et al. 2009).

2.4 Gene therapy clinical trials

Table 3 lists several Phase I trials that have been carried out for bladder cancer. However, results from only a few of these trials are published.

Therapy strategy	Genes	Dosage and cure rate	Reference
Cell cycle modulation	RB94	Adenovirus delivery and nanocomplex delivery, sc	(Xu et al. 1996; Pirollo et al. 2008)
	P53	VVp53, increased survival and some mice were cured	(Fodor et al. 2005)
	p53, P21,	Adp53 and p21 blocked tumor induction in transformed cells, sc	(McGarvey et al. 2001)
Immune modulation	IL2,	Liposome, 1 dose 40%;	(Horiguchi et al. 2000)
	GMCSF	Liposome, 6 doses, twice a week 50%	(Wu et al. 2004)
	TNF-α	Liposome, 6 doses, twice a week 50%	(Zang et al. 2004)
	IFN-γ	Co-administered with MBT-2 cells, reduced tumor growth	(Shiau et al. 2001)
	IFN-α	AdIFNα + Syn3, 2 doses, marked tumor reduction	(Benedict et al. 2004)
	IL12,	Ad.mIL-12 (10^9 PFU) 1 intratumoral injection, cured, sc	(Chen et al. 1997)
	IL12	Chitosan IL12, 4 doses 88-100% cured	(Zaharoff et al. 2009)
	IL12	Liposome IL12, 6 doses 0,3,5 and 10μg DNA, 25-37.5% cured	(Horinaga et al. 2005)
	CD40 Ligand,	Ad CD40L (10^9PFU) +clorpactin, 3 doses 60% cured	(Loskog et al. 2005)
	CpG	CpG ODN, 4 doses, increased survival	(Ninalga et al. 2005)
Prodrug activators,	Thymidine Kinase	Plasmid HSV-TK by electrogun + GCV, induced apoptosis in carcinogen induced rat tumor model	(Shibata et al. 2003)
		Ad HSVTK 3 x 10^8 PFU + GCV, >4 fold reduction in tumor growth, sc	(Sutton et al. 1997)
		Chemically induced bladder tumor, AdHSVTK + GCV, growth inhibited	(Akasaka et al. 2001)
Antisense therapy	bFGF,	Ad-bFGF-AS, Tumor growth significantly inhibited, sc	(Inoue et al. 2000)
	survivin + PLK-1	0.5-1mg/kg 4 doses, suppressed growth of tumors	(Seth et al. 2011)
	PCNA + Adp53	Reduced tumor growth, sc	(Zhu et al. 2003)
Oncolytic virus	HSV G207 + Nv1020	1x10^7 PFU, 3 doses, 61.5% and 83.3% cured respectively	(Cozzi et al. 2001)
	Ad E1B defective	AdE1AdB , tumor growth inhibition	(Wang et al. 2006)
Toxin delivery	Diphtheria toxin	Calcium phosphate percipitate of plasmid DNA, doses, 40% reduction in tumor eight, sc	(Ohana et al. 2002)
Enhancing Chemotherapy	Cytosine deaminase + etoposide + 5-FU	Ad-hTERT-CD 1x10^9PFU, 5-FC (200 mg/kg), etoposide (2 mg/kg), tumor growth reduced	(Shieh et al. 2006)
	PTEN + doxorubicin	AdMMAC, Reduced tumor growth, sc	(Tanaka and Grossman 2003)
	P53 + cisplantin	Combination better than either alone	(Miyake et al. 2000)
Anti-Angiogenesis	AAV Endostatin	1x10^{11} PFU, 6 doses, reduction in tumor growth, sc	(Pan et al. 2011)
Actin regulation	gelsolin	AdGSN 1x10 PFU, 3 doses, tumor suppression	(Sazawa et al. 2002)
Apoptosis	Caspace 3 + 9	PEI/DNA COX-2 driven gene expression with exogenous activation, 5 doses, tumor reduction better than BCG or celecoxcib	(Zhang and Godbey 2010)

sc –stands for sub-cutaneous models.

Table 2. Genes demonstrated to cause tumor reduction in murine models of bladder cancer.

Trial ID	Year	Country	Phase	Status	Vehicle	Gene (ref)
CA-0019	2005	Canada	I	Open	Adenovirus	CG0070 GMCSF
BE-0005	1998	Belgium	I	Closed	Poxvirus	Antigen MAGE-1.A1 and MAGE-3.A1
DE-0013	1997	Germany	I	Closed	Adenovirus	P53 and transduction enhancing agent (Kuball et al. 2002)
UK0057	2000	UK	I	Open	Adenovirus	E1B deleted
SE-0004/ NCT00891748	2006	Sweden	I/II	Closed	Adenovirus	Antigen, CTLA-4 (Malmstrom et al. 2010)
US-0145/ 9601-145	1996	USA	I	Closed	Adenovirus	Rb
US-0219/9710-219/ NCT00003167	1998	USA	I	completed	Adenovirus	P53 (Pagliaro et al. 2003)
US-0500/0110-500	2001	USA	I	Open	Adenovirus	HSV thymidine kinase and ganciclovir
US-0643/ 0404-643	2004	USA	I/II	Open	Adenovirus	CG0070, GMCSF
US-0581/0304-581	2003	USA	I	Active	Vaccinia, Fowl pox virus	GMCSF and CD80, ICAM1, LFA-3
US-0688/ 0501-688	2005	USA	I	Open	Adenovirus	SCH 721015 (IFNalpha 2b)
NCT00109655	2005	USA	I	Active not, recruiting	Adenovirus	Oncolytic (serotype 5) - CG0070
NCT00393809	2006	Israel	I/IIa	Completed	Plasmid	Diphtheria toxin (Sidi et al. 2008)
NCT00536588	2006	USA	I	completed	Adenovirus	SCH 721015
NCT00595088	2008	USA	2b	recruiting	PEI/plasmid	Intravesical DTA-H19
NCT00959868	2009	Canada	I	recruiting	oligo	OGX-427 (antisense hsp27)
NCT01162785	2010	USA	Ib	Not started	Adenovirus	SCH 721015 (rAd-IFN) and Syn-3,

Table 3. Clinical trials for bladder cancer gene therapy. NCT designation indicates data obtained from http://www.who.int/ictrp/en/;
Other alphabet and number designations are for data obtained from http://www.wiley.com/legacy/wileychi/genmed/clinical where the alphabets indicate country of registration and the numbers only designation are for data obtained from http://www.gemcris.od.nih.gov/Contents/GC_HOME.asp . Note some trials were registered on more than one web-site.

Information about completed, on-going and planned trials were obtained from the following sources: gene therapy clinical trials world wide web-site http://www.wiley.com/legacy/wileychi/genmed/clinical/; the clinical trials.gov, US National Institutes of Health and the Genetic Modification Clinical research Information System database http://www.gemcris.od.nih.gov/Contents/GC_HOME.asp and the World Health Organization International Clinical Trials registry platform portal http://www.who.int/ictrp/en/.

A Phase I trial on vaccinia virus instillation showed increased lymphocyte recruitment and the induction of an inflammatory response in the bladder (Gomella et al. 2001). There were no clinical manifestations of vaccinia toxicity indicating the safety and therapeutic potential of this virus as a gene therapy vector. Adenovirus delivery of p53 was also shown to successfully deliver p53 gene to bladder cells but there was no change in immunohistochemical detection of p53 in bladder tissue (Pagliaro et al. 2003). However, adenovirus therapy was safe and well tolerated (Pagliaro et al. 2003). Delivery of adenovirus carrying p53 with a transduction enhancing agent improved p53 gene delivery and protein expression was found in patient tissue samples (Kuball et al. 2002). Though higher doses of the virus were administered, no dose toxicity was observed (Kuball et al. 2002). Similarly no serious adverse effects were reported by Malmstrom et al. from a recently concluded Phase I/IIa trial using AdCD40L (Malmstrom et al. 2010). They observed gene transfer in biopsies and the infiltration of T lymphocytes (Malmstrom et al. 2010).

A plasmid was used to deliver the diphtheria toxin gene under the control of the H19 gene regulatory sequence in a Phase I/IIa trial for non-muscle invasive bladder cancer (Sidi et al. 2008). They reported mild toxicity and observed complete and partial response in some patients. Thus based on these Phase I trials, both non viral and viral vectors appear to be well tolerated in man.

Several new trials are either in progress or about to commence. These use non-viral and viral delivery vectors as listed in Table 3. A proposal for a Phase I trial for intravesical therapy in bladder cancer patients using plasmid DNA carrying the IFN-α gene and our liposome based delivery system is being evaluated by the Health Sciences Authority, Singapore.

2.5 Other urological malignancies

Though not covered here several clinical trials are on-going, evaluating gene therapy for prostate and renal cancers. In general the vectors and genes used are similar though tissue specific promoters may differ. Information on these trials can be obtained from the web-sites listed above. Unlike bladder cancer however, gene delivery to these tissues is not as simple. Thus tissue specific targeted gene expression has been developed. Another strategy is the use of macrophages transfected *ex vivo* with a plasmid carrying the E1A/B construct under the control of the hypoxia response element (HRE) as well as a replication competent adenovirus with the E1A under the control of the prostate specific antigen promoter. At the hypoxic tumor site the E1A protein is produced and the adenoviruses released infect tumor cells and cause their lysis (Muthana et al. 2011). Such a strategy prevents virus neutralization *in vivo*.

3. Non-cancer related urological problems

The bladder is made up of a reservoir and an outlet (bladder neck, urethra and urethral sphincter) whose activities are controlled by smooth and striated muscles. There are more patients with bladder dysfunctions related to its primary function of urine storage and voiding than cancer. These include: lower urinary tract symptoms (LUTS), interstitial cystitis (IC), overactive bladder (OAB), spinal cord injuries affecting micturition and urinary incontinence (UI). It is estimated that by 2018, some 2.3 billion people worldwide will be affected by at least one LUTS, OAB, UI and LUTS suggestive of bladder obstruction (Irwin et al. 2011). LUTS is an umbrella term that encompasses urine storage (increased frequency, at least one episode of nocturia per night, urgency and UI), voiding and post-micturition symptoms (Abrams et al. 2003). Another urological problem is erectile dysfunction (ED). Both LUTS and ED are increased with aging and in patients with diabetes (Brown et al. 2005). With the worldwide increase in the incidence of diabetes the incidence of these urological problems will increase.

Most current therapies for the above mentioned conditions are palliative rather than therapeutic. Gene therapy however, may provide a way to cure the disease and the recent review by Christ lists some of these strategies (Christ 2011). Most of the bladder related problems seem to be linked to muscle and neuronal defects and because of the latter the most common vectors used for animals studies of bladder dysfunctions are HSV vectors.

3.1 Urinary incontinence

Urinary incontinence is a general term used to cover three types of incontinence namely stress, urge and overflow (Chancellor et al. 2001). Stress incontinence occurs when the urinary sphincter muscle is unable to prevent urine leakage following jumping or coughing. This is more common in women than men. Treatment approaches include exercise, surgery and collagen injections into the sphincter muscle. Often multiple injections are required which adds to the cost of treatment and some patients are allergic to bovine collagen. Tissue engineering and *ex vivo* gene therapy are alternative therapeutic strategies that are being evaluated (Shokeir et al. 2010). Phase I trials of the delivery of autologous myoblasts and fibroblasts from muscle biopsies to female patients with stress incontinence have shown some benefit (Mitterberger et al. 2007). In mice, combining myoblast and gene therapy such as the ex vivo transformation of myoblasts with the VEGF gene resulted in improved volume and function of muscle cells (Delo et al. 2008).

Urge incontinence is characterized by increased urinary urgency and frequency caused by involuntary bladder contractions leading to uncontrollable urine leakage. One study has evaluated intravesical non-viral delivery of a cDNA for the K+ channel and showed that this resulted in increased K+ channels in the smooth muscle of the bladder and amelioration of bladder overactivity (Christ et al. 2001).

Overflow incontinence results from nerve damage such that patients cannot urinate. One common cause is diabetes related neuropathy. Diabetes related cystopathy is often irreversible and restoring bladder functions to diabetic patients is difficult (Sasaki et al. 2002). Animal studies have identified nerve growth factor (NGF) as a good candidate for gene therapy for diabetes induced incontinence (Apfel et al. 1994). HSV delivery of NGF increased NGF in the bladder wall and dorsal root ganglion and improved voiding function in streptozotocin (STZ) induced diabetic rats (Goins et al. 2001; Sasaki et al. 2004).

3.2 Interstitial cystitis/painful bladder syndrome

Interstitial cystitis or painful bladder syndrome occurs predominantly in females (Persu et al. 2010). It is believed to result from underlying inflammation in the bladder. It cannot be adequately treated by drugs and prolonged drug therapy can lead to dependency and tolerance to drugs that may require dose escalation to remain effective. Thus it is a candidate for gene therapy. Delivery of the preproenkephalin gene by HSV (Yokoyama et al. 2009) has been shown to be beneficial in reducing pain. A HSV vector carrying the ionotropic glycine receptor (GlyR) whose expression was induced by glycine had an analgesic effect (Goss et al. 2011). This vector when inoculated into the bladder wall of an inflammation model of IC/PBS in rats was activated by systemic glycine delivery.

3.3 Overactive bladder

Overactive bladder (OAB) is defined as "urinary urgency, usually accompanied by frequency and nocturia, with or without urgency urinary incontinence" (Haylen et al. 2010) Detrusor over activity is considered a single marker for OAB. It can occur as a result of spinal injury and could result in a lack of control of micturition. This has been demonstrated in animal models of spinal injury. HSV vector delivery of glutamic acid decarboxylase has shown benefit in a rat model of spinal injury (Miyazato et al. 2009; Miyazato et al. 2010).

3.4 Erectile dysfunction

Approximately 150 million men are projected to suffer from ED and the incidence of ED increases with age. Normal erectile function occurs as a result of 3 synergistic events namely: neurological mediated penial arterial inflow increase; cavernosal smooth muscle relaxation and restriction of venous outflow from the penis (Andersson & Wagner 1995). In ED one or more of these events may be impaired. The penis is an excellent candidate for gene therapy because it is easily accessible, has limited blood flow and a slow cellular turnover (Bivalacqua & Hellstrom 2001). Though therapy is available for erectile dysfunction there are a significant number of patients who do not respond to available therapy (Yoshimura et al. 2010). The recent review by Harraz et al. provides an excellent overview of gene therapy strategies used in animal models of ED that have been shown to resolve this problem (Harraz et al. 2010). Rather than reproducing that information only recent publications not included in that review are mentioned here. Over expression of the transient receptor potential (TRP) channels 6 (dominant negative) by transfection with a plasmid caused a decrease in calcium levels in the corporal smooth muscle and improved erectile function in diabetic rats (Jung et al. 2010). Using a STZ induced diabetes model to evaluate erectile dysfunction, it was found that implantation of mesenchymal stem cells transfected with VEGF improved erectile function compared to implantation of mesenchymal stem cells alone (Qiu et al. 2011).

3.5 Clinical trials

Only two clinical trials are listed on the http://www.gemcris.od.nih.gov/Contents/GC_HOME.asp for urological conditions unrelated to cancer. One is the Phase I trial for ED and the other is a trial for overactive bladder syndrome. Both trials used plasmid DNA carrying the calcium activated potassium channel (Melman et al. 2007). The results of the Phase I trial for ED indicate the safety of this delivery system.

4. Major issues and future prospects for gene therapy

One major issue is the safety of gene therapy in terms of its impact on the environment as well as long term safety in patients. Schenk-Braat et al found that only half of all registered clinical trials included viral shedding data (Schenk-Braat et al. 2007) and what data was available was primarily for the time after virus delivery and not at the time of delivery. These questions should also be raised for plasmid based gene therapy. Long term follow-up data on patients who have received gene therapy may further ameliorate the safety concerns of this therapy. This will result in gene therapy being more readily applied to other non-malignant conditions. The development of better plasmids and ways to integrate plasmids into the chromosome may lead to the greater use of plasmid rather than viral vectors for urological gene therapy.

MicroRNAs (MiRNA) are new targets for cancer therapy. These are small non-coding RNA molecules that bind to complementary sequences in the protein coding regions of mRNA and block their translation. Their expression levels vary in cancer and normal tissues (Catto et al. 2011). MiRNA-203 and MiRNA-221 have been shown to modulate the growth and apoptosis of human bladder cancer cell lines (Lu et al. 2010; Bo et al. 2011) and these could be new targets for therapy. Given the function of miRNA it is possible that these molecules could also be targets for non-cancer related bladder dysfunctions. This has not yet been explored and identifying such molecules may improve our knowledge of the development of these conditions.

5. Conclusion

The application of gene therapy for urological conditions is being evaluated in many preclinical disease models. In general the results obtained are encouraging and soon these therapies may move to Phase I trials.

6. References

Abrams, P., Cardozo, L., Fall, M., Griffiths, D., Rosier, P., Ulmsten, U., Van Kerrebroeck, P., Victor, A. and Wein, A. (2003) The standardisation of terminology in lower urinary tract function: report from the standardisation sub-committee of the International Continence Society. *Urology* 61, 37-49.

Akasaka, S., Suzuki, S., Shimizu, H., Igarashi, T., Akimoto, M. and Shimada, T. (2001) Suicide gene therapy for chemically induced rat bladder tumor entailing instillation of adenoviral vectors. *Jpn J Cancer Res* 92, 568-575.

Al-Dosari, M.S. and Gao, X. (2009) Nonviral gene delivery: principle, limitations, and recent progress. *AAPS J* 11, 671-681.

Amit, D. and Hochberg, A. (2010) Development of targeted therapy for bladder cancer mediated by a double promoter plasmid expressing diphtheria toxin under the control of H19 and IGF2-P4 regulatory sequences. *J Transl Med* 8, 134.

Anderson, B. and Naish, W. (2008) Bladder cancer and smoking. Part 4: efficacy of health promotion. *Br J Nurs* 17, 1340-1344.

Andersson, K.E. and Wagner, G. (1995) Physiology of penile erection. *Physiol Rev* 75, 191-236.

Apfel, S.C., Arezzo, J.C., Brownlee, M., Federoff, H. and Kessler, J.A. (1994) Nerve growth factor administration protects against experimental diabetic sensory neuropathy. *Brain Res* 634, 7-12.

Benedict, W.F., Tao, Z., Kim, C.S., Zhang, X., Zhou, J.H., Adam, L., McConkey, D.J., Papageorgiou, A., Munsell, M., Philopena, J., Engler, H., Demers, W., Maneval,

D.C., Dinney, C.P. and Connor, R.J. (2004) Intravesical Ad-IFNalpha causes marked regression of human bladder cancer growing orthotopically in nude mice and overcomes resistance to IFN-alpha protein. *Mol Ther* 10, 525-532.

Bivalacqua, T.J. and Hellstrom, W.J. (2001) Potential application of gene therapy for the treatment of erectile dysfunction. *J Androl* 22, 183-190.

Bo, J., Yang, G., Huo, K., Jiang, H., Zhang, L., Liu, D. and Huang, Y. (2011) microRNA-203 suppresses bladder cancer development by repressing bcl-w expression. *FEBS J* 278, 786-792.

Bonnet, M.E., Erbacher, P. and Bolcato-Bellemin, A.L. (2008) Systemic delivery of DNA or siRNA mediated by linear polyethylenimine (L-PEI) does not induce an inflammatory response. *Pharm Res* 25, 2972-2982.

Brown, J.S., Wessells, H., Chancellor, M.B., Howards, S.S., Stamm, W.E., Stapleton, A.E., Steers, W.D., Van Den Eeden, S.K. and McVary, K.T. (2005) Urologic complications of diabetes. *Diabetes Care* 28, 177-185.

Buscarini, M., Quek, M.L., Gilliam-Hegarich, S., Kasahara, N. and Bochner, B. (2007) Adenoviral receptor expression of normal bladder and transitional cell carcinoma of the bladder. *Urol Int* 78, 160-166.

Catto, J.W., Alcaraz, A., Bjartell, A.S., De Vere White, R., Evans, C.P., Fussel, S., Hamdy, F.C., Kallioniemi, O., Mengual, L., Schlomm, T. and Visakorpi, T. (2011) MicroRNA in Prostate, Bladder, and Kidney Cancer: A Systematic Review. *Eur Urol.*

Chancellor, M.B., Yoshimura, N., Pruchnic, R. and Huard, J. (2001) Gene therapy strategies for urological dysfunction. *Trends Mol Med* 7, 301-306.

Chen, L., Chen, D., Block, E., O'Donnell, M., Kufe, D.W. and Clinton, S.K. (1997) Eradication of murine bladder carcinoma by intratumor injection of a bicistronic adenoviral vector carrying cDNAs for the IL-12 heterodimer and its inhibition by the IL-12 p40 subunit homodimer. *J Immunol* 159, 351-359.

Chen, X., Kube, D.M., Cooper, M.J. and Davis, P.B. (2008) Cell surface nucleolin serves as receptor for DNA nanoparticles composed of pegylated polylysine and DNA. *Mol Ther* 16, 333-342.

Christ, G.J. (2011) Potential applications of gene therapy/transfer to the treatment of lower urinary tract diseases/disorders. *Handb Exp Pharmacol*, 255-265.

Christ, G.J., Day, N.S., Day, M., Santizo, C., Zhao, W., Sclafani, T., Zinman, J., Hsieh, K., Venkateswarlu, K., Valcic, M. and Melman, A. (2001) Bladder injection of "naked" hSlo/pcDNA3 ameliorates detrusor hyperactivity in obstructed rats in vivo. *Am J Physiol Regul Integr Comp Physiol* 281, R1699-1709.

Connor, R.J., Engler, H., Machemer, T., Philopena, J.M., Horn, M.T., Sutjipto, S., Maneval, D.C., Youngster, S., Chan, T.M., Bausch, J., McAuliffe, J.P., Hindsgaul, O. and Nagabhushan, T.L. (2001) Identification of polyamides that enhance adenovirus-mediated gene expression in the urothelium. *Gene Ther* 8, 41-48.

Cooksley, C.D., Avritscher, E.B., Grossman, H.B., Sabichi, A.L., Dinney, C.P., Pettaway, C. and Elting, L.S. (2008) Clinical model of cost of bladder cancer in the elderly. *Urology* 71, 519-525.

Cozzi, P.J., Malhotra, S., McAuliffe, P., Kooby, D.A., Federoff, H.J., Huryk, B., Johnson, P., Scardino, P.T., Heston, W.D. and Fong, Y. (2001) Intravesical oncolytic viral therapy using attenuated, replication-competent herpes simplex viruses G207 and Nv1020 is effective in the treatment of bladder cancer in an orthotopic syngeneic model. *FASEB J* 15, 1306-1308.

Darquet, A.M., Cameron, B., Wils, P., Scherman, D. and Crouzet, J. (1997) A new DNA vehicle for nonviral gene delivery: supercoiled minicircle. *Gene Ther* 4, 1341-1349.

Delo, D.M., Eberli, D., Williams, J.K., Andersson, K.E., Atala, A. and Soker, S. (2008) Angiogenic gene modification of skeletal muscle cells to compensate for ageing-induced decline in bioengineered functional muscle tissue. *BJU Int* 102, 878-884.

Den Otter, W., Dobrowolski, Z., Bugajski, A., Papla, B., Van Der Meijden, A.P., Koten, J.W., Boon, T.A., Siedlar, M. and Zembala, M. (1998) Intravesical interleukin-2 in T1 papillary bladder carcinoma: regression of marker lesion in 8 of 10 patients. *J Urol* 159, 1183-1186.

Dumey, N., Mongiat-Artus, P., Devauchelle, P., Lesourd, A., Cotard, J.P., Le Duc, A., Marty, M., Cussenot, O. and Cohen-Haguenauer, O. (2005) In vivo retroviral mediated gene transfer into bladder urothelium results in preferential transduction of tumoral cells. *Eur Urol* 47, 257-263.

Engler, H., Anderson, S.C., Machemer, T.R., Philopena, J.M., Connor, R.J., Wen, S.F. and Maneval, D.C. (1999) Ethanol improves adenovirus-mediated gene transfer and expression to the bladder epithelium of rodents. *Urology* 53, 1049-1053.

Fodor, I., Timiryasova, T., Denes, B., Yoshida, J., Ruckle, H. and Lilly, M. (2005) Vaccinia virus mediated p53 gene therapy for bladder cancer in an orthotopic murine model. *J Urol* 173, 604-609.

Freund, C.T., Tong, X.W., Block, A., Contant, C.F., Kieback, D.G., Rowley, D.R. and Lerner, S.P. (2000) Adenovirus-mediated suicide gene therapy for bladder cancer: comparison of the cytomegalovirus- and Rous sarcoma virus-promoter. *Anticancer Res* 20, 2811-2816.

Freund, C.T., Tong, X.W., Rowley, D., Engehausen, D., Frolov, A., Kieback, D.G. and Lerner, S.P. (2003) Combination of adenovirus-mediated thymidine kinase gene therapy with cytotoxic chemotherapy in bladder cancer in vitro. *Urol Oncol* 21, 197-205.

Gaetano, C., Catalano, A., Palumbo, R., Illi, B., Orlando, G., Ventoruzzo, G., Serino, F. and Capogrossi, M.C. (2000) Transcriptionally active drugs improve adenovirus vector performance in vitro and in vivo. *Gene Ther* 7, 1624-1630.

Gill, D.R., Pringle, I.A. and Hyde, S.C. (2009) Progress and prospects: the design and production of plasmid vectors. *Gene Ther* 16, 165-171.

Glazier, D.B., Bahnson, R.R., McLeod, D.G., von Roemeling, R.W., Messing, E.M. and Ernstoff, M.S. (1995) Intravesical recombinant tumor necrosis factor in the treatment of superficial bladder cancer: an Eastern Cooperative Oncology Group study. *J Urol* 154, 66-68.

Goins, W.F., Yoshimura, N., Phelan, M.W., Yokoyama, T., Fraser, M.O., Ozawa, H., Bennett, N.J., de Groat, W.C., Glorioso, J.C. and Chancellor, M.B. (2001) Herpes simplex virus mediated nerve growth factor expression in bladder and afferent neurons: potential treatment for diabetic bladder dysfunction. *J Urol* 165, 1748-1754.

Gomella, L.G., Mastrangelo, M.J., McCue, P.A., Maguire, H.J., Mulholland, S.G. and Lattime, E.C. (2001) Phase i study of intravesical vaccinia virus as a vector for gene therapy of bladder cancer. *J Urol* 166, 1291-1295.

Goss, J.R., Cascio, M., Goins, W.F., Huang, S., Krisky, D.M., Clarke, R.J., Johnson, J.W., Yokoyama, H., Yoshimura, N., Gold, M.S. and Glorioso, J.C. (2011) HSV Delivery of a Ligand-regulated Endogenous Ion Channel Gene to Sensory Neurons Results in Pain Control Following Channel Activation. *Mol Ther* 19, 500-506.

Hackett, P.B., Largaespada, D.A. and Cooper, L.J. (2010) A transposon and transposase system for human application. *Mol Ther* 18, 674-683.

Harimoto, K., Sugimura, K., Lee, C.R., Kuratsukuri, K. and Kishimoto, T. (1998) In vivo gene transfer methods in the bladder without viral vectors. *Br J Urol* 81, 870-874.

Harraz, A., Shindel, A.W. and Lue, T.F. (2010) Emerging gene and stem cell therapies for the treatment of erectile dysfunction. *Nat Rev Urol* 7, 143-152.

Haylen, B.T., de Ridder, D., Freeman, R.M., Swift, S.E., Berghmans, B., Lee, J., Monga, A., Petri, E., Rizk, D.E., Sand, P.K. and Schaer, G.N. (2010) An International Urogynecological Association (IUGA)/International Continence Society (ICS) joint report on the terminology for female pelvic floor dysfunction. *Neurourol Urodyn* 29, 4-20.

He, X.D., Wang, Z.P., Wei, H.Y., Zhou, Q., Wang, D.G., Tian, J.Q., Fu, S.J. and Rodriguez, R. (2009) Construction of urothelium-specific recombinant adenovirus and its inhibition in bladder cancer cell. *Urol Int* 82, 209-213.

Herr, H.W. and Morales, A. (2008) History of bacillus Calmette-Guerin and bladder cancer: an immunotherapy success story. *J Urol* 179, 53-56.

Horiguchi, Y., Larchian, W.A., Kaplinsky, R., Fair, W.R. and Heston, W.D. (2000) Intravesical liposome-mediated interleukin-2 gene therapy in orthotopic murine bladder cancer model. *Gene Ther* 7, 844-851.

Horinaga, M., Harsch, K.M., Fukuyama, R., Heston, W. and Larchian, W. (2005) Intravesical interleukin-12 gene therapy in an orthotopic bladder cancer model. *Urology* 66, 461-466.

Inoue, K., Perrotte, P., Wood, C.G., Slaton, J.W., Sweeney, P. and Dinney, C.P. (2000) Gene therapy of human bladder cancer with adenovirus-mediated antisense basic fibroblast growth factor. *Clin Cancer Res* 6, 4422-4431.

Irie, A., Matsumoto, K., Anderegg, B., Kuruma, H., Kashani-Sabet, M., Scanlon, K.J., Uchida, T. and Baba, S. (2006) Growth inhibition efficacy of an adenovirus expressing dual therapeutic genes, wild-type p53, and anti-erbB2 ribozyme, against human bladder cancer cells. *Cancer Gene Ther* 13, 298-305.

Irwin, D.E., Kopp, Z.S., Agatep, B., Milsom, I. and Abrams, P. (2011) Worldwide prevalence estimates of lower urinary tract symptoms, overactive bladder, urinary incontinence and bladder outlet obstruction. *BJU Int.*

Jung, J.H., Kim, B.J., Chae, M.R., Kam, S.C., Jeon, J.H., So, I., Chung, K.H. and Lee, S.W. (2010) Gene transfer of TRPC6 (dominant negative) restores erectile function in diabetic rats. *J Sex Med* 7, 1126-1138.

Kamat, A.M. and Lamm, D.L. (2000) Intravesical therapy for bladder cancer. *Urology* 55, 161-168.

Kasman, L.M., Barua, S., Lu, P., Rege, K. and Voelkel-Johnson, C. (2009) Polymer-enhanced adenoviral transduction of CAR-negative bladder cancer cells. *Mol Pharm* 6, 1612-1619.

Kikkawa, K., Fujii, R., Kuramoto, T., Mori, T., Inagaki, T., Kohjimoto, Y., Iwahashi, M., Yamaue, H. and Hara, I. (2009) Dendritic cells with transduced survivin gene induce specific cytotoxic T lymphocytes in human urologic cancer cell lines. *Urology* 74, 222-228.

Kuball, J., Wen, S.F., Leissner, J., Atkins, D., Meinhardt, P., Quijano, E., Engler, H., Hutchins, B., Maneval, D.C., Grace, M.J., Fritz, M.A., Storkel, S., Thuroff, J.W., Huber, C. and Schuler, M. (2002) Successful adenovirus-mediated wild-type p53 gene transfer in patients with bladder cancer by intravesical vector instillation. *J Clin Oncol* 20, 957-965.

Lai, M.D., Chen, C.S., Yang, C.R., Yuan, S.Y., Tsai, J.J., Tu, C.F., Wang, C.C., Yen, M.C. and Lin, C.C. (2010) An HDAC inhibitor enhances the antitumor activity of a CMV promoter-driven DNA vaccine. *Cancer Gene Ther* 17, 203-211.

Lanson, N.A., Jr., Friedlander, P.L., Schwarzenberger, P., Kolls, J.K. and Wang, G. (2003) Replication of an adenoviral vector controlled by the human telomerase reverse transcriptase promoter causes tumor-selective tumor lysis. *Cancer Res* 63, 7936-7941.

Lawrencia, C., Mahendran, R. and Esuvaranathan, K. (2001) Transfection of urothelial cells using methyl-beta-cyclodextrin solubilized cholesterol and Dotap. *Gene Ther* 8, 760-768.

Lee, S.S., Eisenlohr, L.C., McCue, P.A., Mastrangelo, M.J. and Lattime, E.C. (1994) Intravesical gene therapy: in vivo gene transfer using recombinant vaccinia virus vectors. *Cancer Res* 54, 3325-3328.

Lin, L.F., Zhu, G., Yoo, J.J., Soker, S., Sukhatme, V.P. and Atala, A. (2002) A system for the enhancement of adenovirus mediated gene transfer to uro-epithelium. *J Urol* 168, 813-818.

Loser, P., Jennings, G.S., Strauss, M. and Sandig, V. (1998) Reactivation of the previously silenced cytomegalovirus major immediate-early promoter in the mouse liver: involvement of NFkappaB. *J Virol* 72, 180-190.

Loskog, A.S., Fransson, M.E. and Totterman, T.T. (2005) AdCD40L gene therapy counteracts T regulatory cells and cures aggressive tumors in an orthotopic bladder cancer model. *Clin Cancer Res* 11, 8816-8821.

Lu, Q., Lu, C., Zhou, G.P., Zhang, W., Xiao, H. and Wang, X.R. (2010) MicroRNA-221 silencing predisposed human bladder cancer cells to undergo apoptosis induced by TRAIL. *Urol Oncol* 28, 635-641.

Malmstrom, P.U., Loskog, A.S., Lindqvist, C.A., Mangsbo, S.M., Fransson, M., Wanders, A., Gardmark, T. and Totterman, T.H. (2010) AdCD40L immunogene therapy for bladder carcinoma--the first phase I/IIa trial. *Clin Cancer Res* 16, 3279-3287.

McGarvey, T.W., Meng, R.D., Johnson, O., El-Deiry, W. and Malkowicz, S.B. (2001) Growth inhibitory effect of p21 and p53 containing adenoviruses on transitional cell carcinoma cell lines in vitro and in vivo. *Urol Oncol* 6, 155-162.

Melman, A., Bar-Chama, N., McCullough, A., Davies, K. and Christ, G. (2007) Plasmid-based gene transfer for treatment of erectile dysfunction and overactive bladder: results of a phase I trial. *Isr Med Assoc J* 9, 143-146.

Mitterberger, M., Marksteiner, R., Margreiter, E., Pinggera, G.M., Colleselli, D., Frauscher, F., Ulmer, H., Fussenegger, M., Bartsch, G. and Strasser, H. (2007) Autologous myoblasts and fibroblasts for female stress incontinence: a 1-year follow-up in 123 patients. *BJU Int* 100, 1081-1085.

Miyake, H., Hara, I., Hara, S., Arakawa, S. and Kamidono, S. (2000) Synergistic chemosensitization and inhibition of tumor growth and metastasis by adenovirus-mediated P53 gene transfer in human bladder cancer model. *Urology* 56, 332-336.

Miyazato, M., Sugaya, K., Goins, W.F., Wolfe, D., Goss, J.R., Chancellor, M.B., de Groat, W.C., Glorioso, J.C. and Yoshimura, N. (2009) Herpes simplex virus vector-mediated gene delivery of glutamic acid decarboxylase reduces detrusor overactivity in spinal cord-injured rats. *Gene Ther* 16, 660-668.

Miyazato, M., Sugaya, K., Saito, S., Chancellor, M.B., Goins, W.F., Goss, J.R., de Groat, W.C., Glorioso, J.C. and Yoshimura, N. (2010) Suppression of detrusor-sphincter dyssynergia by herpes simplex virus vector mediated gene delivery of glutamic acid decarboxylase in spinal cord injured rats. *J Urol* 184, 1204-1210.

Muthana, M., Giannoudis, A., Scott, S.D., Fang, H.Y., Coffelt, S.B., Morrow, F.J., Murdoch, C., Burton, J., Cross, N., Burke, B., Mistry, R., Hamdy, F., Brown, N.J., Georgopoulos, L., Hoskin, P., Essand, M., Lewis, C.E. and Maitland, N.J. (2011) Use of Macrophages to Target Therapeutic Adenovirus to Human Prostate Tumors. *Cancer Res* 71, 1805-1815.

Nagabhushan, T.L., Maneval, D.C., Benedict, W.F., Wen, S.F., Ihnat, P.M., Engler, H. and Connor, R.J. (2007) Enhancement of intravesical delivery with Syn3 potentiates interferon-alpha2b gene therapy for superficial bladder cancer. *Cytokine Growth Factor Rev* 18, 389-394.

Ninalga, C., Loskog, A., Klevenfeldt, M., Essand, M. and Totterman, T.H. (2005) CpG oligonucleotide therapy cures subcutaneous and orthotopic tumors and evokes protective immunity in murine bladder cancer. *J Immunother* 28, 20-27.

Ogawa, R., Kagiya, G., Feril, L.B., Jr., Nakaya, N., Nozaki, T., Fuse, H. and Kondo, T. (2004) Ultrasound mediated intravesical transfection enhanced by treatment with lidocaine or heat. *J Urol* 172, 1469-1473.

Ohana, P., Bibi, O., Matouk, I., Levy, C., Birman, T., Ariel, I., Schneider, T., Ayesh, S., Giladi, H., Laster, M., de Groot, N. and Hochberg, A. (2002) Use of H19 regulatory sequences for targeted gene therapy in cancer. *Int J Cancer* 98, 645-650.

Olivares, E.C., Hollis, R.P., Chalberg, T.W., Meuse, L., Kay, M.A. and Calos, M.P. (2002) Site-specific genomic integration produces therapeutic Factor IX levels in mice. *Nat Biotechnol* 20, 1124-1128.

Pagliaro, L.C., Keyhani, A., Williams, D., Woods, D., Liu, B., Perrotte, P., Slaton, J.W., Merritt, J.A., Grossman, H.B. and Dinney, C.P. (2003) Repeated intravesical instillations of an adenoviral vector in patients with locally advanced bladder cancer: a phase I study of p53 gene therapy. *J Clin Oncol* 21, 2247-2253.

Pan, J.G., Zhou, X., Zeng, G.W. and Han, R.F. (2011) Suppression of bladder cancer growth in mice by adeno-associated virus vector-mediated endostatin expression. *Tumour Biol* 32, 301-310.

Persu, C., Cauni, V., Gutue, S., Blaj, I., Jinga, V. and Geavlete, P. (2010) From interstitial cystitis to chronic pelvic pain. *J Med Life* 3, 167-174.

Pirollo, K.F., Rait, A., Zhou, Q., Zhang, X.Q., Zhou, J., Kim, C.S., Benedict, W.F. and Chang, E.H. (2008) Tumor-targeting nanocomplex delivery of novel tumor suppressor RB94 chemosensitizes bladder carcinoma cells in vitro and in vivo. *Clin Cancer Res* 14, 2190-2198.

Pong, R.C., Lai, Y.J., Chen, H., Okegawa, T., Frenkel, E., Sagalowsky, A. and Hsieh, J.T. (2003) Epigenetic regulation of coxsackie and adenovirus receptor (CAR) gene promoter in urogenital cancer cells. *Cancer Res* 63, 8680-8686.

Qiu, X., Sun, C., Yu, W., Lin, H., Sun, Z., Chen, Y., Wang, R. and Dai, Y. (2011) Combined Strategy of Mesenchymal Stem Cells Injection with VEGF Gene Therapy for the Treatment of Diabetes Associated Erectile Dysfunction. *J Androl.*

Ramesh, N., Ge, Y., Ennist, D.L., Zhu, M., Mina, M., Ganesh, S., Reddy, P.S. and Yu, D.C. (2006) CG0070, a conditionally replicating granulocyte macrophage colony-stimulating factor--armed oncolytic adenovirus for the treatment of bladder cancer. *Clin Cancer Res* 12, 305-313.

Ramesh, N., Memarzadeh, B., Ge, Y., Frey, D., VanRoey, M., Rojas, V. and Yu, D.C. (2004) Identification of pretreatment agents to enhance adenovirus infection of bladder epithelium. *Mol Ther* 10, 697-705.

Sachs, M.D., Ramamurthy, M., Poel, H., Wickham, T.J., Lamfers, M., Gerritsen, W., Chowdhury, W., Li, Y., Schoenberg, M.P. and Rodriguez, R. (2004) Histone deacetylase inhibitors upregulate expression of the coxsackie adenovirus receptor (CAR) preferentially in bladder cancer cells. *Cancer Gene Ther* 11, 477-486.

Saint, F., Kurth, N., Maille, P., Vordos, D., Hoznek, A., Soyeux, P., Patard, J.J., Abbou, C.C. and Chopin, D.K. (2003) Urinary IL-2 assay for monitoring intravesical bacillus Calmette-Guerin response of superficial bladder cancer during induction course and maintenance therapy. *Int J Cancer* 107, 434-440.

Sasaki, K., Chancellor, M.B., Goins, W.F., Phelan, M.W., Glorioso, J.C., de Groat, W.C. and Yoshimura, N. (2004) Gene therapy using replication-defective herpes simplex virus vectors expressing nerve growth factor in a rat model of diabetic cystopathy. *Diabetes* 53, 2723-2730.

Sasaki, K., Chancellor, M.B., Phelan, M.W., Yokoyama, T., Fraser, M.O., Seki, S., Kubo, K., Kumon, H., Groat, W.C. and Yoshimura, N. (2002) Diabetic cystopathy correlates with a long-term decrease in nerve growth factor levels in the bladder and lumbosacral dorsal root Ganglia. *J Urol* 168, 1259-1264.

Sazawa, A., Watanabe, T., Tanaka, M., Haga, K., Fujita, H., Harabayashi, T., Shinohara, N., Koyanagi, T. and Kuzumaki, N. (2002) Adenovirus mediated gelsolin gene therapy for orthotopic human bladder cancer in nude mice. *J Urol* 168, 1182-1187.

Schenk-Braat, E.A., van Mierlo, M.M., Wagemaker, G., Bangma, C.H. and Kaptein, L.C. (2007) An inventory of shedding data from clinical gene therapy trials. *J Gene Med* 9, 910-921.

Seth, S., Matsui, Y., Fosnaugh, K., Liu, Y., Vaish, N., Adami, R., Harvie, P., Johns, R., Severson, G., Brown, T., Takagi, A., Bell, S., Chen, Y., Chen, F., Zhu, T., Fam, R., Maciagiewicz, I., Kwang, E., McCutcheon, M., Farber, K., Charmley, P., Houston Jr, M.E., So, A., Templin, M.V. and Polisky, B. (2011) RNAi-based Therapeutics Targeting Survivin and PLK1 for Treatment of Bladder Cancer. *Mol Ther.*

Shiau, A.L., Lin, C.Y., Tzai, T.S. and Wu, C.L. (2001) Postoperative immuno-gene therapy of murine bladder tumor by in vivo administration of retroviruses expressing mouse interferon-gamma. *Cancer Gene Ther* 8, 73-81.

Shibata, M.A., Horiguchi, T., Morimoto, J. and Otsuki, Y. (2003) Massive apoptotic cell death in chemically induced rat urinary bladder carcinomas following in situ HSVtk electrogene transfer. *J Gene Med* 5, 219-231.

Shieh, G.S., Shiau, A.L., Yo, Y.T., Lin, P.R., Chang, C.C., Tzai, T.S. and Wu, C.L. (2006) Low-dose etoposide enhances telomerase-dependent adenovirus-mediated cytosine deaminase gene therapy through augmentation of adenoviral infection and transgene expression in a syngeneic bladder tumor model. *Cancer Res* 66, 9957-9966.

Shirakawa, T., Hamada, K., Zhang, Z., Okada, H., Tagawa, M., Kamidono, S., Kawabata, M. and Gotoh, A. (2004) A cox-2 promoter-based replication-selective adenoviral vector to target the cox-2-expressing human bladder cancer cells. *Clin Cancer Res* 10, 4342-4348.

Shokeir, A.A., Harraz, A.M. and El-Din, A.B. (2010) Tissue engineering and stem cells: basic principles and applications in urology. *Int J Urol* 17, 964-973.

Sidi, A.A., Ohana, P., Benjamin, S., Shalev, M., Ransom, J.H., Lamm, D., Hochberg, A. and Leibovitch, I. (2008) Phase I/II marker lesion study of intravesical BC-819 DNA plasmid in H19 over expressing superficial bladder cancer refractory to bacillus Calmette-Guerin. *J Urol* 180, 2379-2383.

Siemens, D.R., Crist, S., Austin, J.C., Tartaglia, J. and Ratliff, T.L. (2003) Comparison of viral vectors: gene transfer efficiency and tissue specificity in a bladder cancer model. *J Urol* 170, 979-984.

Stavropoulos, N.E., Hastazeris, K., Filiadis, I., Mihailidis, I., Ioachim, E., Liamis, Z. and Kalomiris, P. (2002) Intravesical instillations of interferon gamma in the prophylaxis of high risk superficial bladder cancer--results of a controlled prospective study. *Scand J Urol Nephrol* 36, 218-222.

Sutton, M.A., Berkman, S.A., Chen, S.H., Block, A., Dang, T.D., Kattan, M.W., Wheeler, T.M., Rowley, D.R., Woo, S.L. and Lerner, S.P. (1997) Adenovirus-mediated suicide gene therapy for experimental bladder cancer. *Urology* 49, 173-180.

Tanaka, A.S., Tanaka, M. and Komuro, K. (1998) A highly efficient method for the site-specific integration of transfected plasmids into the genome of mammalian cells using purified retroviral integrase. *Gene* 216, 67-76.

Tanaka, M. and Grossman, H.B. (2003) In vivo gene therapy of human bladder cancer with PTEN suppresses tumor growth, downregulates phosphorylated Akt, and increases sensitivity to doxorubicin. *Gene Ther* 10, 1636-1642.

Tao, Z., Connor, R.J., Ashoori, F., Dinney, C.P., Munsell, M., Philopena, J.A. and Benedict, W.F. (2006) Efficacy of a single intravesical treatment with Ad-IFN/Syn 3 is dependent on dose and urine IFN concentration obtained: implications for clinical investigation. *Cancer Gene Ther* 13, 125-130.

Terao, S., Shirakawa, T., Kubo, S., Bishunu, A., Lee, S.J., Goda, K., Tsukuda, M., Hamada, K., Tagawa, M., Takenaka, A., Fujisawa, M. and Gotoh, A. (2007) Midkine promoter-based conditionally replicative adenovirus for targeting midkine-expressing human bladder cancer model. *Urology* 70, 1009-1013.

Thalmann, G.N., Dewald, B., Baggiolini, M. and Studer, U.E. (1997) Interleukin-8 expression in the urine after bacillus Calmette-Guerin therapy: a potential prognostic factor of tumor recurrence and progression. *J Urol* 158, 1340-1344.

Thalmann, G.N., Sermier, A., Rentsch, C., Mohrle, K., Cecchini, M.G. and Studer, U.E. (2000) Urinary Interleukin-8 and 18 predict the response of superficial bladder cancer to intravesical therapy with bacillus Calmette-Guerin. *J Urol* 164, 2129-2133.

Thomas, C.E., Ehrhardt, A. and Kay, M.A. (2003) Progress and problems with the use of viral vectors for gene therapy. *Nat Rev Genet* 4, 346-358.

Tsai, Y.S., Shiau, A.L., Chen, Y.F., Tsai, H.T., Lee, H.L., Tzai, T.S. and Wu, C.L. (2009) Enhancement of antitumor immune response by targeted interleukin-12 electrogene transfer through antiHER2 single-chain antibody in a murine bladder tumor model. *Vaccine* 27, 5383-5392.

Tsai, Y.S., Shiau, A.L., Chen, Y.F., Tsai, H.T., Tzai, T.S. and Wu, C.L. (2010) Enhancement of antitumor activity of gammaretrovirus carrying IL-12 gene through genetic modification of envelope targeting HER2 receptor: a promising strategy for bladder cancer therapy. *Cancer Gene Ther* 17, 37-48.

van der Poel, H.G., Molenaar, B., van Beusechem, V.W., Haisma, H.J., Rodriguez, R., Curiel, D.T. and Gerritsen, W.R. (2002) Epidermal growth factor receptor targeting of replication competent adenovirus enhances cytotoxicity in bladder cancer. *J Urol* 168, 266-272.

Wang, H., Satoh, M., Abe, H., Sunamura, M., Moriya, T., Ishidoya, S., Saito, S., Hamada, H. and Arai, Y. (2006) Oncolytic viral therapy by bladder instillation using an E1A, E1B double-restricted adenovirus in an orthotopic bladder cancer model. *Urology* 68, 674-681.

Wood, M., Perrotte, P., Onishi, E., Harper, M.E., Dinney, C., Pagliaro, L. and Wilson, D.R. (1999) Biodistribution of an adenoviral vector carrying the luciferase reporter gene following intravesical or intravenous administration to a mouse. *Cancer Gene Ther* 6, 367-372.

Wu, Q., Esuvaranathan, K. and Mahendran, R. (2004) Monitoring the response of orthotopic bladder tumors to granulocyte macrophage colony-stimulating factor therapy using the prostate-specific antigen gene as a reporter. *Clin Cancer Res* 10, 6977-6984.

Wu, Q., Mahendran, R. and Esuvaranathan, K. (2003) Nonviral cytokine gene therapy on an orthotopic bladder cancer model. *Clin Cancer Res* 9, 4522-4528.

Xu, H.J., Zhou, Y., Seigne, J., Perng, G.S., Mixon, M., Zhang, C., Li, J., Benedict, W.F. and Hu, S.X. (1996) Enhanced tumor suppressor gene therapy via replication-deficient adenovirus vectors expressing an N-terminal truncated retinoblastoma protein. *Cancer Res* 56, 2245-2249.

Yamashita, M., Rosser, C.J., Zhou, J.H., Zhang, X.Q., Connor, R.J., Engler, H., Maneval, D.C., Karashima, T., Czerniak, B.A., Dinney, C.P. and Benedict, W.F. (2002) Syn3 provides high levels of intravesical adenoviral-mediated gene transfer for gene therapy of genetically altered urothelium and superficial bladder cancer. *Cancer Gene Ther* 9, 687-691.

Yew, N.S., Zhao, H., Wu, I.H., Song, A., Tousignant, J.D., Przybylska, M. and Cheng, S.H. (2000) Reduced inflammatory response to plasmid DNA vectors by elimination and inhibition of immunostimulatory CpG motifs. *Mol Ther* 1, 255-262.

Yokoyama, H., Sasaki, K., Franks, M.E., Goins, W.F., Goss, J.R., de Groat, W.C., Glorioso, J.C., Chancellor, M.B. and Yoshimura, N. (2009) Gene therapy for bladder overactivity and nociception with herpes simplex virus vectors expressing preproenkephalin. *Hum Gene Ther* 20, 63-71.

Yoshimura, N., Kato, R., Chancellor, M.B., Nelson, J.B. and Glorioso, J.C. (2010) Gene therapy as future treatment of erectile dysfunction. *Expert Opin Biol Ther* 10, 1305-1314.

Zaharoff, D.A., Hoffman, B.S., Hooper, H.B., Benjamin, C.J., Jr., Khurana, K.K., Hance, K.W., Rogers, C.J., Pinto, P.A., Schlom, J. and Greiner, J.W. (2009) Intravesical immunotherapy of superficial bladder cancer with chitosan/interleukin-12. *Cancer Res* 69, 6192-6199.

Zang, Z., Mahendran, R., Wu, Q., Yong, T. and Esuvaranathan, K. (2004) Non-viral tumor necrosis factor-alpha gene transfer decreases the incidence of orthotopic bladder tumors. *Int J Mol Med* 14, 713-717.

Zhang, J., Ramesh, N., Chen, Y., Li, Y., Dilley, J., Working, P. and Yu, D.C. (2002) Identification of human uroplakin II promoter and its use in the construction of CG8840, a urothelium-specific adenovirus variant that eliminates established bladder tumors in combination with docetaxel. *Cancer Res* 62, 3743-3750.

Zhang, X., Atala, A. and Godbey, W.T. (2008) Expression-targeted gene therapy for the treatment of transitional cell carcinoma. *Cancer Gene Ther* 15, 543-552.

Zhang, X. and Godbey, W.T. (2010) Preclinical evaluation of a gene therapy treatment for transitional cell carcinoma. *Cancer Gene Ther*.

Zhang, Z., Shirakawa, T., Hinata, N., Matsumoto, A., Fujisawa, M., Okada, H., Kamidono, S., Matsuo, M. and Gotoh, A. (2003) Combination with CD/5-FC gene therapy enhances killing of human bladder-cancer cells by radiation. *J Gene Med* 5, 860-867.

Zhu, Z., Xing, S., Lin, C., Zhang, X., Fu, M., Liang, X., Zeng, F., Lu, G. and Wu, M. (2003) Bladder cancer therapy using combined proliferating cell nuclear antigen antisense oligonucleotides and recombinant adenovirus p53. *Chin Med J (Engl)* 116, 1860-1863.

15

Delivery Methods to Target RNAs in the Kidney

Csaba Révész and Péter Hamar
Semmelweis University, Budapest, Hungary

1. Introduction

Significant improvements have been made during the last 20 years in the therapy of renal diseases including the broadening of treatment options. Gene therapy is a potential modality for renal diseases for which we are yet unable to offer specific treatment. In spite of the revolutionary progress in the field of gene therapy, delivery to achieve safe clinical application remains one of the biggest challenges in biomedical research. In the present chapter we focus on nucleic acid (NA) therapy targeting messenger (mRNA) and micro (miRNA) RNA in the kidney.

2. RNA interference

RNA interference (RNAi), the sequence-specific post-transcriptional gene silencing mediated by small (19-25 nucleotide length) double-stranded RNAs (dsRNA), is of potential use as a therapeutic approach for the treatment of a variety of diseases (Dykxhoorn & Lieberman, 2006; Castanotto & Rossi, 2009). Small, non-coding RNA molecules such as microRNA (miRNA) and short interfering RNA (siRNA) are important regulators of gene expression, helping to control cellular metabolism, growth and differentiation, to maintain genome integrity, and to combat viruses and mobile genetic elements (C. Zhang, 2009; Moazed, 2009).

2.1 Biogenesis of small RNAs and mechanism of action

Following completion of the human genome project, a series of non-coding small RNAs have been discovered. Two main categories of small RNAs have been defined on the basis of their precursors. The cleavage of exogenous double-stranded RNA (dsRNA) precursors produced during viral infection or after artificial transfection generates siRNAs, whereas the processing of genome-encoded endogenous stem-loop RNA structures generates miRNAs.
Exogenous siRNAs and endogenous miRNAs are generated from dsRNA precursors that are produced in or introduced into cells (Siomi H. & Siomi M.C., 2009; Bartel, 2004).
During the mechanism of RNAi, double-stranded RNA is cleaved by an RNAseIII ribonuclease called Dicer into smaller fragments (21 to 23 nucleotides). The resulting fragments are then bound to an Argonaut family protein which functions as the core component of a protein-RNA complex called the RNA-induced silencing complex (RISC) or its nuclear form the RNA-induced transcriptional silencing complex (RITS). SiRNA/miRNA duplex is unwind by helicase, and the guide or antisense strand will then engage in selective degradation of the mRNA that is complementary to the guide strand.

As a post-transcriptional gene-silencing (PTGS) mechanism **exogenous siRNA** mediated RNAi causes degradation of the target mRNA and prevents protein synthesis (Rácz & Hamar, 2008). Physiologic function of RNAi is elimination of viral infections, as double stranded RNAs are often produced during the life cycle of viruses and are eliminated this way. However, siRNA mediated PTGS can be utilized therapeutically, by transfecting cells in vivo with siRNA complementary to a segment of a protein coding mRNA (Rácz & Hamar, 2006). The revolutionary aspect of siRNA therapy is that it acts on disease-associated key proteins by down regulating components of the pathway without permanent effects on the genome. Thus, siRNA treatment has the potential to prevent injury from occurring in addition to addressing existing injury.

Endogenous non-coding **miRNAs** are involved in post-transcriptional regulation of gene-expression. MiRNAs are generated from endogenous hairpin structured transcripts throughout the genome. MiRNA encoding genes are transcribed by RNA polymerase II (pol II) providing long precursor transcripts, known as primary miRNAs (pri-miRNAs). After transcription, Drosha RNase: a type III nuclear ribonuclease cleaves nucleotides from the pri-miRNA, processing it into shorter pre-miRNAs. Nuclear export factor Exportin-5 (Exp5/Xpo5) transports the pre-miRNA to the cytoplasm. Further cytoplasmic processing by Dicer (type III ribonuclease) cleaves pre-miRNA generating mature, double-stranded, 18-25 nucleotide-long miRNA. The guide strand is incorporated into RISC and remains stably associated with RISC, becoming the mature miRNA. The opposite (passenger) strand is disposed. The miRNA guides the RISC to the target mRNA with complementary sequence. In case of incompletely complementary sequences, translation of the target mRNA is silenced, and the mRNA is degraded by the RISC in case of fully complementary sequence. Unlike RNAi induced by siRNA, miRNA during regulation, cleavage of the mRNA occurs more seldom, only by complete match between the miRNA and the mRNA (Kaucsár et al., 2010).

MiRNAs and siRNAs control post-transcriptional gene expression by directing endonuclease cleavage of the target mRNA. This mechanism of action is referred to as slicer activity. For slicer activity fully complementary miRNA and target mRNA sequences are required. However, in some cases, few mismatches can be tolerated for cleavage. MiRNAs may also act a slicer-independent manner such as mRNA repression, or mRNA decapping (Valencia-Sanchez et al., 2006).

Regulatory miRNAs compose networks. This notion is supported by (i) the high number of non-coding RNAs which are functionally active and target signaling molecules, (ii) many genes encoding miRNAs are closely clustered in the genome and (iii) in some cases different miRNAs control a single mRNA target or vice versa a single miRNA may influence expression of multiple different target proteins. Human and murine kidney specific miRNA expression profiles have been reported and summarized (in Kaucsár et al., 2010).

2.1 Further small RNA types

A **non-coding RNA (ncRNA)** is a functional RNA molecule that is not translated into a protein. Non-coding RNAs include long known transfer RNA (tRNA) and ribosomal RNA (rRNA) involved in translation, as well as newly described RNAs involved in gene expression regulation such as:

- Small nuclear RNA (snRNA) - involved in mRNA splicing.
- Small nucleolar RNA (snoRNA) - direct the modification of ribosomal RNAs.

- Micro RNA (miRNA) and short interfering RNA (siRNA) - regulate gene expression.
- The P-element induced wimpy testis in Drosophila (piwi) (Saito et al., 2006) proteins regulate stem- and germ-line cell division (Cox et al., 2000). Piwi-interacting RNAs (piRNAs) isolated from mouse testes (Kim, 2006) are involved in defense of germ-line cells against parasitic DNA elements such as retrotransposons.

MiRNAs and siRNAs are about 20-25 nucleotides long. piRNAs have a broader average size ~24–31 nucleotides. siRNAs have been widely used in functional genomics and also have therapeutic potential.

3. Challenges in RNA-based therapy knocking down disease

Presently, therapeutic RNAi application faces three major obstacles:
i. *stability* of siRNA when administered in vivo,
ii. *delivery* across barriers in living organisms, and
iii. circumvention of *immune response*.

Efforts to improve the effect of RNAi-based nucleic acid (NA) therapy include,
i. *stabilization* of the nucleic acid against enzymatic degradation,
ii. enhancing *cellular uptake* of the nucleic acid, and
iii. limiting *immunoactivation* during in vivo application.

Stability of siRNA in vivo in biological milieu is one of the obstacles for therapeutic application. Numerous modifications are available, since chemically synthesized siRNAs became cheap and easy to synthesize. (For chemical modifications see 4.2.).

Delivery problems include rapid degradation of NAs and rapid renal clearance. Double stranded NAs have an advantageous resistant profile against nuclease degradation which can be further reduced by chemical modifications. Rapid renal clearance eliminates the therapeutically applied small NA from the circulation; however, this can be utilized as an advantage in targeting the kidney as tubular epithelial cells (TEC) may take up the NAs from the ultrafiltrate. Thus, TEC can be efficiently targeted this way (Molitoris et al., 2009).

Exogenously administered siRNAs may have undesired **side effects** (Rácz & Hamar, 2008). Such unwanted side-effects may include: unintended knockdown of partially complementary sequences may occur resulting in off-target silencing. Side effects induced by siRNAs have been shown to be concentration dependent. Off-target silencing is more likely to occur in case of high siRNA concentrations but sometimes may occur even in low siRNA concentration (Jackson et al, 2003). Moreover, high siRNA concentration can also induce gene activation of apoptosis and stress response (Semizarov et al., 2003) or can lead to non-selective translational shutdown (erre nem találtam hiv-t).

Immunological response is an other obstacle in therapeutic siRNA application. Toll-like receptors (TLRs) recognize pathogen-associated molecular patterns (PAMPs), such as bacterial wall endotoxins (LPS), viral dsRNA, and cytosine-guanine (CG) motifs. TLRs also recognize siRNA, and consequently TLR intracellular signaling pathways are activated leading to immune activation. Moreover, dsRNAs induce interferon response directly.

Delivery across barriers in living organisms, e.g. across biological membranes is a major issue for potential therapeutic application of siRNAs. Chemical modifications, complexation, conjugation with lipid bilayer-penetrating carriers assist this purpose. This chapter focuses on delivery issues of RNAi in order to influence pathological conditions in the kidney.

4. Delivery strategies

Delivery strategies to induce cellular uptake of the therapeutic nucleic acid include physical force or vector systems such as viral-, lipid- or complex- based delivery, or nanocarriers. From the initial applications with less possible clinical relevance, when NAs were addressed to renal cells with hydrodynamic high pressure injection systemically, a wide range of gene therapeutic viral and non-viral carriers have been applied already to target posttranscriptional events in different animal kidney disease models in vivo.

4.1 Physical approaches

One of the strategies for introducing NAs into cells and tissues is physical force. During these approaches hydrodynamic pressure is applied to force the NAs into tissue parenchyma and cells. The **hydrodynamic pressure** can be established systemically during the hydrodynamic procedure or locally during direct injections into the target organ.

Intrarenal, local delivery to the kidney can be achieved by different routes such as via the renal artery targeting glomeruli, via the renal vein targeting the tubulointerstitium, via the ureter into the renal pelvis and by subcapsular administration for intraparenchymal effects. Effects of the hydrodynamic pressure can be further enhanced by **temporary pore openings** in cell membranes by electroporation or sonoporation with ultrasound or micro-injection.

DY547-labeled non-target control siRNA or rhodamine-labeled p85α siRNA uptake followed by hydrodynamic or standard tail vein injection was noted in the kidney with consequent protein inhibition in case of p85α siRNA, but no signal was observed after intraperitonal or per rectum administration (Larson et al., 2007). Hydrodynamic administration resulted in a higher uptake in the kidney as well as in other target organs in contrast to standard intravenous injection (Larson et al., 2007).

In a mouse model of renal ischemia-reperfusion, Fas siRNA pretreatment hydrodynamically through the tail vein and/or injected locally into renal vein protected NMRI mice from renal ischemia-reperfusion injury (Hamar et al., 2004). Sufficient downregulation of the FAS apoptosis receptor substantially reduced functional deterioration of the kidney manifesting in significant survival advantage. Similar good results were achieved by silencing apoptosis cascade elements (Zheng et al., 2008) or the central inflammatory signaling element: nuclear factor kappa-b (NFkB) (Feng et al., 2009).

Apoptosis antagonizing transcription factor (AATF), a regulator of apoptotic pathways, was targeted in an *in vitro* model of kidney ischemia-reperfusion injury. In human kidney proximal tubule HK-2 cells and in primary renal tubule epithelial cells RNA interference-mediated silencing of AATF heightened whereas overexpression of transgenic AATF ameliorated superoxide accumulation and apoptotic cell death following hypoxia (Xie & Guo, 2006).

Gremlin siRNA plasmid suspended in 2 ml of the TransIT-EE Hydrodynamic buffer delivered weekly by hydrodynamic tail vein injection reversed diabetic nephropathy in streptozotocin-induced diabetic, uninephrectomized mice. Furthermore, high glucose induced collagen IV and MMP-2 activity was inhibited by lipofectamin transfection of the same gremlin construct in cultured mouse mesangial cells (Q. Zhang et al., 2010). Gremlin is highly expressed in kidney with diabetic nephropathy, mainly observed in areas of tubulointerstitial fibrosis, and its mRNA level correlates with the degree of the fibrosis.

4.2 Chemical modifications

Spontaneous uptake of siRNA by cells without additional carrier is reportedly less efficient when compared to strategies employing transfection reagents that complex or encapsulate siRNA. *Chemical modification* and bioconjugation with vehicles can drastically improve the stability and cellular uptake, allowing improvements in selectivity and reduced toxicity. While phosphodiester oligonucleotides are unstable in the biological milieu, several chemical modifications have been applied to enhance stability.

Before RNAi was discovered antisense oligonucleotides were used for experimental nucleic acid sequence specific inhibition of protein synthesis. Main differences between siRNA used in RNAi and previously popular antisense oligonucleotides (ASOs) is, that ASOs are single stranded and thus, much more sensitive to extracellular nuclease degradation, whereas siRNAs are more resistant due to their double stranded structure (Paroo & Corey, 2004).

First generation of chemically modified oligonucleotides was phosphorothioate RNA, later 2′ sugar modifications (2′-O-methyl and 2′-O-methoxy-ethyl-RNAs) were introduced (Monia, 1997). The hydrophilic character and anionic backbone of siRNAs reduces their uptake by the cells. While siRNA duplexes are relatively more stable in serum than single stranded siRNA, they easily undergo degradation by nucleases in vivo. This, with their limited capability to cross cellular lipid bilayers, represents a significant barrier to the therapeutic development of siRNA. A variety of chemical modifications have been tested to enhance effectiveness of oligonucleotide intracellular delivery, including chemical modifications to sugars (2′-sugar), backbones, or nucleobases. Conjugation to membrane penetrating vehicles has been also demonstrated to enhance stability, prevent triggering of an immune response, control pharmacokinetic profiles and reduce nonspecific effects. However, some of these modifications may affect biological activity (Rácz & Hamar, 2006, 2008).

4.3 Viral vectors

Besides chemical modifications *vector systems* have been used widely to protect and deliver NAs in vitro and in vivo. Gold standards of gene delivery are *viral vectors*. Several kinds of viral vectors have been used already in delivery applications into the kidney. Strategies employed in previous gene therapy applications can be readily adapted for use in RNAi. Viral vector containing expression cassettes coding for shRNA precursors, as an alternative to siRNA administration have been successfully used in the kidney employing plasmid DNA (pDNA) vectors. Few studies describe renal shRNA delivery with viral vectors such as, replication-deficient *adenoviral* delivery in rat cortical tubules, glomeruli or tubular epithelium of the outer medulla or *lentiviral* retrograde ureteral infusion to tubular epithelial cells in mice. Intraparenchymal delivery of lentivirus particularly induced transgene expression in the cortical and corticomedullary area of the kidney with lower expression in the medullary part. In a rat renal transplantation model, perfusion of the donor kidney with lentiviral vector induced significant target gene silencing. Transplantation offers an ex-vivo window enabling significant reduction of possible systemic side-effects of NA therapy. From a safety perspective, the use of lentiviral vectors may lead to unwanted insertion of the construct in vital gene regions.

Recombinant *adenoviruses and adeno-associated viruses (AVs, AAVs)* are capable of transducing cells with high efficiency. However, adenoviral vectors have been reported to be immunogenic. In mice, intraparenchymal or intrapelvic delivery of recombinant AAV induced transgene expression by epithelium of the tubules or mainly in the medulla, respectively. Despite recent concerns, recombinant AAVs are attractive vectors as they appear to be safe and capable of long-term gene expression. Although efficient delivery vehicles, adenoviruses are strong stimulators of innate and adaptive immune responses. This may cause toxicity and limit repeated administration. To modify tropism and reduce immune responses, recent studies have used surface modified or helper-dependent 'gutless' vectors. Helper dependent and chemically modified vectors may have an improved safety profile that could be better suited to clinical application.

Adeno-associated (AAV) virus-2 vector was used for inhibiting mineralocorticoid receptor (MR) by MR-shRNA expressing AAV. AAV MR-shRNA reduced MR expression in the kidney and prevented blood pressure increase, albuminuria, and renal failure in cold-induced hypertension in Sprague–Dawley rats (Wang et al., 2006).

Anti-luciferase siRNA-expressing piGENE hU6-stem21 pDNA was co-injected hydrodynamically with pGL3 firefly luciferase-expressing pDNA via tail vein in ddY mice in a dose- and time-dependence study of vector-based in vivo RNAi (Kobayashi et al., 2004). Authors investigated silencing efficiency in liver, kidney, lung and muscle. Viral vector mediated RNA silencing of the transgene 1 day after intravenous injection was almost as efficient in the kidney as in the liver.

Hemagglutination virus of Japan–envelope vector was used in uninephrectomized streptozotocin-induced diabetic mice to target mammalian translocase of inner mitochondrial membrane 44 (TIM44) (Y. Zhang et al., 2006). TIM44, a membrane anchor of mitochondrial heat-shock protein 70 (mtHsp70) to TIM23 complex is upregulated in diabetic mouse kidneys and is held responsible for superoxide production. RNAi to TIM44 reduced proteinuria, renal hypertrophy, renal cell proliferation and apoptosis, and suppressed superoxide production.

4.4 Non-viral carriers

Applying *non-viral* vehicles constitute promising alternatives to the use of viral vectors. Delivery of siRNA, especially with cationic preparations and biodegradable components have much better safety profiles than their viral counterparts, though their transfection efficiency is generally lower. The positive charge facilitates complex formation with NAs and endocytosis of the complex. The complex between the cationic carrier (lipids, polymers, peptides, nanoparticles) and the anionic NA is formed by electrostatic interaction.

4.4.1 Lipid-based delivery

Various lipid-based delivery systems have been developed for in vivo application of siRNA, including liposomes, micelles, emulsions, and solid lipid nanoparticles. Application of liposome-mediated gene carriers retrospects a long path from the seventies. Complexes between cationic lipid and DNA are named **lipoplexes**. Due to the high complexity of the self-assembly process, little is known about the mechanisms of formation. Multicomponent lipoplexes, incorporating three to six lipid species, have emerged as promising delivery candidates, with 10 to 100 times higher efficiency than binary complexes usually applied for gene delivery (Caracciolo et al., 2005, 2009). Our understanding about the bio-distribution of RNA-liposome complex is rather scarce; however, it is known to depend on the colloidal properties of the complex as well as their interaction with blood components. Surface charge is a main issue in half-life and destination of the complex. While lipoplexes with a strong anionic charge are usually absorbed by scavenger cells, resulting in a rapid elimination from the blood, a strongly positive surface favors the accumulation in the liver (Y.-C. Tseng et al, 2009).

Liposome-based transfection reagents have been successfully employed for *in vivo* siRNA delivery to the kidney, such as

cationic lipids

- N-[1-(2,3-Dioleoyloxy)propyl]-N,N,N-trimethylammonium methylsulfate (DOTAP)
- (3β-[N-(N′,N′-dimethylaminoethane)-carbamoyl])-cholesterol (DC-Chol)

or **neutral helper lipids**

- 1,2-dioleoyl-*sn*-glycero-3-phosphatid-ylcholine (DOPC),
- dioleoylphosphatidylethanolamine (DOPE).

Protection of nucleic acids with encapsulation into the liposome makes these lipid delivery strategies attractive for gene transfer. However, composition and surface charge pattern are important issues in organ targeting and potential immune recognition and response.

Lipoproteins have also been tested as lipid-based transfection reagents. Efficient and selective siRNA conjugation to bile acids and long-chain fatty acids, or cholesterol, depends on interactions with lipoprotein particles, lipoprotein receptors and transmembrane proteins (Wolfrum et al., 2007). High-density lipoprotein (HDL) directs siRNA delivery into the liver, gut, kidney and steroidogenic organs, whereas low-density lipoprotein (LDL) targets siRNA primarily to the liver. In a delivery study of lipoprotein-siRNA complexes it has been ascertained that ^{32}P-cholesterol-siRNA bound to HDL or albumin but not to LDL resulted in an accumulation in the kidney, while with LDL the main target organ was the liver.

Examples of successful lipid based siRNA delivery in renal pathologies

Intravenous RNAi-mediated inhibition of p53 delivered by **lipofectamin** transfection agent minimized renal injury in a hypoperfusion/ischemia and a cisplatin model of kidney damage in rats. P53 siRNA minimized renal p53 protein increase after ischemia-reperfusion injury. Proximal tubule cells were protected against ischemic and cisplatin-induced acute injury by chemically modified, 2′O-methylated p53 siRNA (Molitoris et al., 2009). Following i.v. injection, rapid glomerular filtration with subsequent proximal tubule brush border binding and endocytosis by proximal tubule cells were observed. The minimal labeling in the vasculature indicated rapid renal clearance.

Renal injury and diabetic nephropathy were ameliorated by **cholesterol-tagged** 12/15-lipoxygenase (12/15-LO) targeting siRNAs in streptozotocin-induced mouse model of type 1 diabetes (Yuan et al., 2008). Lipoxygenases (LO) are a family of non-heme iron-containing enzymes that insert molecular oxygen into polyunsaturated fatty acids. The 12/15-LO is involved in mesangial cell growth and extracellular matrix protein expression during glomerulosclerosis. Cholesterol conjugation was applied to enhance renal siRNA uptake. Significant reduction of 12/15-LO mRNA level was observed in murine mesangial cells *in vitro* and the examined tissues in vivo (spleen, kidney, liver, and heart), indicating broad tissue biodistribution of the siRNAs. Glomerular hypertrophy and mesangial matrix expansion were reduced.

Breast adenocarcinoma (MDA-MB-231) cells in vitro and in female SCID mice in vivo were treated with cationic liposome loaded with COX-2 siRNA (Mikhaylova et al., 2009). COX-2 is often upregulated in cancer. **DOTAP/DOPE** (DD) and DOTAP/DOPE/DOPE-PEG2000 (DDP) lipid mixtures were used for producing lipoplexes. For imaging purposes liposomes were loaded with different contrast agents. Incubation of DDP lipoplexes for extended periods demonstrated siRNA-dependent, sequence-specific downregulation of COX-2 protein expression in breast cancer cells. Also, tumor-bearing female SCID mice treated with DDP-COX-2 lipoplexes DY-647 labeled localization of COX-2 siRNA was observed in the tumor, lung and liver shortly after injection. In contrast, the fluorescence intensity in the kidney was lower, however, second highest signal of detectable fluorescence was observed in the kidneys 24h post injection.

Physical approaches (such as hydrodynamic in vivo delivery) are often combined with adaptation of different carriers. DY547- and rhodamine-labeled, chemically modified siRNAs mixed with DOTAP effectively appeared in the kidney after hydrodynamic and standard iv. injection, while i.p. and rectal administration were unsuccessful even with DOTAP liposomal transfection reagent (Larson et al., 2007).

RLIP76 multifunctional transporter, which is frequently over-expressed in malignant cells has been chosen as a target for kidney cancer in a study that compare anti-RLIP76 IgG, RLIP76 siRNA, or RLIP76 antisense oligodeoxynucleotide in Caki-2 kidney cancer xenograft bearing Hsd: athymic nude *nu/nu* mice (Singhal et al., 2009). Treatment with RLIP76 antibody, siRNA, or antisense caused regression of established Caki-2 kidney cancer xenografts. Messenger RNA targeting was performed with Quiagen's lipid-based **TransMessenger** transfection reagent. Caki-2 cells express RLIP76 3-fold compared to normal human kidney mesangial cells. The tumor-bearing animals were alive 4-times longer due to the RLIP76 antibody, RLIP76 siRNA, or RLIP76 antisense treatment. Administration of RLIP76 antibody, siRNA, or antisense caused regression of established Caki-2 kidney cancer xenografts.

4.4.2 Polymer-based delivery

Polymer-based delivery systems have been extensively used for plasmid DNA and more recently for siRNA. As with lipid-based delivery systems, polymeric delivery of siRNA usually involves a cationic moiety as a core component. Cationic polymers are generally classified into synthetic and natural polymers. **Synthetic** polymers include branched or linear *poly-(etilene-imine) (PEI)*, *poly-(L-lysine) (PLL)*, and *cyclodextrin*-based polycations. **Natural** cationic polymers include *chitosan, atelocollagen*, and cationic *polypeptides*. Cationic polymers (**polyplexes** if complexed with DNA) are key players of non-viral transfer systems due to their exclusive physicochemical properties (Kimura et al., 2001). Most important characteristics of non-viral carriers are charge ratio, which define their ability to carry NAs in therapeutically sufficient quantities (Almofti et al., 2003). An extensive research in polymer therapeutics led to new generations of polymers improving safety, biocompatibility, and efficiency. One novel approach aims at glomerular protein knockdown using **poly-(ethylene-glycol)-poly-(L-lysine) (PEG-PLL)** copolymer-based nanocarriers while avoiding size-selective restraints of the glomerular filter (Shimizu et al., 2010). These polymer nanocarriers have enhanced delivery and retention in the kidney compared to naked siRNA following intraperitoneal administration, more specifically to cells of the glomerulus. Furthermore, the applied PLL carrier proved superior with respect to glomerular targeting when compared to a viral delivery of siRNA. Notably, PEI-siRNA complexes displayed lower renal targeting compared to naked siRNA, however, naked siRNA taken up in the kidney was mostly degraded, whereas renal accumulation of PEI-siRNA resulted in a significantly higher proportion of intact siRNA (Malek et al., 2009).

In vivo pharmacokinetics, tissue distribution and adverse effects studies of PEG-PLL copolymer delivered siRNAs in mice revealed that PEI complexation substantially increased tissue uptake compared to naked siRNA (Malek et al., 2009). Application of naked siRNAs with almost no uptake of intact siRNA molecules was observed in the kidney, while PEI complexation led to a significant increase in levels of intact siRNAs. PEI (–PEG) complex uptake proved to be composition dependent.

In an other application of PEG-PLL glomerulonephritis was ameliorated by MAPK1 siRNA in lupus nephritis mouse model (Shimizu et al., 2010). PEG-PLL complexed siRNA transfected glomeruli successfully, unlike the naked siRNA. MAPK1 mRNA expression in isolated glomeruli was significantly suppressed in mice treated with the MAPK1 siRNA PEG-PLL complexes, whereas control or HVJ-E viral vector mediated siRNA had no effect on protein expression.

Based on a conception that **hyaluronic acid** (HA) plays an important role on receptor-mediated endocytosis, the effect of HA modification of siRNA/PEI complex has been investigated in B16F1 melanoma tumor-bearing mice (Jiang et al., 2008). The hyaluronic acid conjugated complex exhibited higher gene silencing efficiency in B16F1 murine melanoma cells with HA receptors than the siRNA/PEI complex alone. According to an *in vivo* biodistribution study, siRNA/PEI-HA complex accumulated mainly in tissues with HA receptors such as liver, kidney, and tumor. Anti-VEGF siRNA/PEI-HA complex was used successfully as target specific antiangiogenic therapeutics in the tissues with HA receptors, such as liver cancer and kidney cancer. Intratumoral injection of anti-VEGF siRNA/PEI-HA complex resulted in an effective inhibition of tumor growth by the HA receptor mediated endocytosis to tumor cells in mice.

Cationized gelatin delivered plasmid DNA expressing TGF-β type II receptor (TGF-βRII) complexed by siRNA prevented interstitial renal fibrosis (Kushibiki et al., 2005) in unilateral ureteral obstruction (UUO) model mice.

4.4.3 Aptamers

Aptamers (<lat.> aptus: fit), like antibodies are molecules that bind tightly to their specific molecular targets. Unlike antibodies aptamers can be synthesized and selected with pure chemical methods, and their production does not involve living systems. Target binding by aptamers is achieved by their 3 dimensional structure.

RNA oligonucleotide aptamers recognize their target specifically on the basis of their unique 3-dimensional structures. Application of aptamers as carriers is based on the specific interaction between the aptamer and its cellular membrane receptor. As aptamers bind their molecular targets like antibodies, internalization of the aptamer enables the cellular uptake via receptor-mediated endocytosis, thereby increasing local concentration of carried drugs in the targeted cells.

Spiegelmer aptamers are l-enantiomers, which are immunologically inert, and are not degraded by nucleases. Ccl2 antagonistic, PEGylated spiegelmer mNOX-E36 aptamer ameliorated diabetic nephropathy in mice (Ninichuk et al., 2008). mNOX-E36-3'PEG reduced the number of glomerular macrophages, significantly improved the glomerular filtration rate, reduced renal Ccl2 mRNA and protein expression, and thus protected from diffuse glomerulosclerosis.

Spiegelmer NOX-F37 aptamer targeting vasopressin-dependent activation of V_{1a} and V_2 receptors effectively neutralized vasopressin (AVP) and increased diuresis in healthy rats (Purschke et al., 2006).

4.4.4 Nanoparticles

Various types of *nanoparticles* are used in biomedical research. Few experiments have been already completed for kidney targeting.

- *Nanocrystals* are crystalline structures of aggregated molecules, mostly known as *quantum dots* and are used for biological imaging, semiconductors of material research and chemical engineering.
- *Nanotubes* are self-assembling sheets of atoms (often carbon atoms) arranged in tubes.
- *Fullerenes* are similar to carbon nanotubes in that their molecular framework is entirely composed of an extensive π-conjugated carbon skeleton.
- *Dendrimers* are unique molecular architectures having well defined structures with inner cavities to bind biomolecules that make them appropriate for gene delivery.

Quantum dots (Qdot) were applied for bioimaging purposes in the study, where uptake of siRNA/PEI complexes was enhanced with hyaluronic acid (HA) conjugation (referred earlier in 4.4.2, Jiang et al., 2008).

Nanofibrous scaffold mediated RNAi was applied successfully silencing GAPDH in human embryonic kidney 293 cells (HEK 293) (Cao et al., 2010). **Polycaprolactone** (PCL) nanofiber encapsulated GAPDH siRNA, and the released intact siRNA from scaffold resulted in successful transfection of HEK293 cells.

So far no attempt has been documented for *fullerene-* or *dendrimer-based* RNAi in the kidney, however several gene delivery studies of dendriplexes or fullerenes carrying DNA to other organs were published (Tomalia et al., 2007; Shcharbin et al., 2010; Zhong et al., 2008; Maeda-Mamiya et al., 2010).

Polyamidoamine (PAMAM) dendrimers bound EGFP-C2 marker gene and delivered it to many organs after intravenous injection that resulted in high expression in liver, kidney, lung, and spleen (Zhong et al., 2008).

Human embryonic kidney cells (HEK293), mouse embryonic cells (NIH/3T3), SV40 transformed monkey kidney fibroblasts (COS-7) and human epithelioid cervical carcinoma cells (HeLa) were efficiently transfected with **dendriplexes** carrying pDNA encoding firefly luciferase, beta-galactosidase or green fluorescent protein (Shcharbin et al., 2010).

To investigate a *fullerene* as nanocarrier, **tetra(piperazino)fullerene epoxide** (TPFE) conjugated Insulin 2 gene coding pDNA was administered to mice (Maeda-Mamiya et al., 2009). Plasmid insertion was more efficient when delivered with fullerene than when delivered with Lipofectin in kidney, liver and spleen. Application of TPFE fullerene carrier did not elevate blood urea nitrogen (BUN), whereas plasmid carried with Lipofectin increased BUN level that indicated a mild kidney toxicity.

5. Conclusion

Nucleic acid therapies reviewed in the present chapter are aimed at silencing messenger RNA. Recent advances in delivery systems may soon advance NA therapy from science fiction to science and medicine, thus enabling therapy of presently uncurable diseases of the kidney such as cancer, or fibrosis.

Delivery method	Carrier	Target RNA	Disease	Model	Functional assays	Author
Hydrodynamic / Lipid	TransIT In Vivo Gene Delivery System, DOTAP	p85α	Acute renal injury	Ischemia-reperfusion	Uptake, biodistribution	Larson et al., 2007
Hydrodynamic / Lipid	Lipofectamine 2000	Fas	Acute renal injury	Ischemia-reperfusion	Blood urea nitrogen, Fas Immunohisto-chemistry, apoptosis, histological scoring	Hamar et al., 2004
Hydrodynamic	n.a.	Apoptosis cascade elements	Acute renal injury	Ischemia-reperfusion	n.a.	Zheng et al., 2008
Hydrodynamic	n.a.	Nuclear factor kappa-b (NFkB)	Acute renal injury	Ischemia-reperfusion	n.a.	Feng et al., 2009
Hydrodynamic /Viral	Lipofectamine 2000	Apoptosis antagonizing transcription factor (AATF)	Acute renal injury	Ischemia-reperfusion	Apoptosis, oxidative stress, caspase activation, membrane lipid peroxidation	Xie & Guo, 2006
Hydrodynamic	pBAsi mU6 Neo/ TransIT-EE Hydrodynam ic Delivery System	Gremlin	Diabetic nephro-pathy	Streptozotozin -induced diabetes	Proteinuria, serum creatinine, glomerular and tubular diameter, collagen type IV/BMP7 expression	Q. Zhang et al., 2010
Viral/Lipid	pSUPER vector/ Lipofectamin e	TGF-β type II receptor	Interstitial renal fibrosis	Unilateral urethral obstruction	α-SMA expression, collagen content,	Kushibiki et al., 2005
Viral	Adeno-associated virus-2	Mineral corticoid receptor	Hyper-tension caused renal damage	Cold-induced hypertension	blood pressure, serum albumin, serum urea nitrogen, serum creatinine, kidney weight, urinary sodium	Wang et al., 2006
Hydrodynamic /Viral	pU6 vector	Luciferase	n.a.	n.a.	uptake	Kobayashi et al., 2004
Lipid	Lipoproteins, albumin	apoB1, apoM	n.a.	n.a.	Uptake, binding affinity to lipoproteins and albumin	Wolfrum et al., 2007
Lipid	Lipofectamin e2000	p53	Acute renal injury	Ischemic and cisplatin-induced acute injury	Histological scoring, apoptosis	Molitoris et al., 2009

Delivery method	Carrier	Target RNA	Disease	Model	Functional assays	Author
Lipid	DOTAP/DOPE, DOTAP/DOPE/ DOPE-PEG2000	COX-2	Breast adeno-carcinoma	MDA-MB-231 breast cancer xenograft-bearing mouse	Cell viability, uptake	Mikhaylova et al., 2009
Lipid	Cholesterol	12/15-lipoxygenase	Diabetic nephro-pathy	Streptozotocin -induced diabetes	Albuminuria, urinary creatinine, histology, type I and IV collagen, TGF-β, fibronectin, plasminogen activator inhibitor 1	Yuan et al., 2008
Lipid	Lipofectamine 2000	Mitochondrial membrane 44 (TIM44)	Diabetic nephro-pathy	Streptozotocin -induced diabetes	Cell proliferation and apoptosis, histology, ROS, mitochondrial import of Mn-SOD and glutathione peroxidase, cellular membrane polarization	Y. Zhang et al., 2006
Hydrodynamic / Lipid	Proteolipo-some	RLIP76	Renal carcinoma	Caki-2 kidney cancer xenograft-bearing mouse	uptake	Singhal et al., 2009
Polymer	PEGylated PEI	Luciferase pGL3	n.a.	n.a.	Uptake, biodistribution, erythrocyte aggregation	Malek et al., 2009
Polymer	PEGylated poly-L-lysine	MAPK1	Lupus glomerulo-nephritis	Glomerulo-nephritis	Proteinuria, glomerulosclerosis, TGF- β, , fibronectin, plasminogen activator inhibitor 1	Shimizu et al., 2010
Polymer/Nano particle	Hyaluronic acid/ Quantum dot/ PEI	VEGF	Kidney cancer/ melanoma	B16F1 melanoma tumor-bearing mouse	Biodistribution, citotoxicity, tumor volume, endocytosis	Jiang et al., 2008
Polymer/Nano particle	PEGylated polycapro-lactone nanofiber	GAPDH	n.a.	n.a.	cell viability, uptake	Cao et al, 2010
Aptamer	Spiegelmer mNOX-E36	CC chemokine ligand 2	Glomerulo sclerosis	Uninephrecto-mized mouse	urinary albumin, urinary creatinine, histopathology, glomerular filtration rate, macrophage count, serum Ccl2, Mac-2+, Ki-67+	Ninichuk et al., 2008

Delivery method	Carrier	Target RNA	Disease	Model	Functional assays	Author
Aptamer	Aptamer NOX-F37	vasopressin (AVP)	Congestive heart failure	n.a.	Binding affinity to D-AVP, Inhibition of AVP Signaling, Urine osmolality and sodium concentration,	Purschke et al., 2006
Aptamer	Aptamer A1, A2, and A3	glutamate receptor subunit 1(GluR1)	n.a.	Human embryonic kidney 293	binding	Liu et al., 2009

Table 1. Application of RNA interference in kidney disease models.

6. References

Almofti, M.R., Harashima, H., Shinohara, Y., Almofti, A., Baba, Y., Kiwada, H. (2003). Cationic liposome-mediated gene delivery: biophysical study and mechanism of internalization. *Arch Biochem Biophys,* (Feb 2003), Vol. 410, No. 2, pp. (246-253), ISSN 0003-9861

Bartel, D.P. (2004). MicroRNAs: Genomics, biogenesis, mechanism, and function. *Cell,* (Jan 2004), Vol. 116, No. 2, pp. (281-297), ISSN 0092-8674

Cao, H., Jiang, X., Chai, C. & Chew, S.Y. RNA interference by nanofiber-based siRNA delivery system. (2010). *J Controlled Release,* (Jun 2010), Vol. 144, No. 2, pp. (203-212), ISSN 0168-3659

Caracciolo, G., Pozzi, D., Amenitsch, H. & Caminiti, R. (2005). Multicomponent cationic lipid-DNA complex formation: Role of lipid mixing. *Langmuir,* (Dec 2005), Vol. 21, No. 25, pp. (11582-11587), ISSN 0743-7463

Caracciolo, G., Caminiti, R., Digman, M.A., Gratton, E. & Sanchez, S. (2009). Efficient escape from endosomes determines the superior efficiency of multicomponent lipoplexes. *J Physical Chem. B,* (Apr 2009), Vol. 113, No. 15, pp. (1995-4997), ISSN 1089-5647

Castanotto, D. & Rossi, J.J. (2009). The promises and pitfalls of RNA-interference-based therapeutics. *Nature,* (Jan 2009), Vol. 457, No. 7228, pp. (426-433), ISSN 0028-0836

Cox, D.N., Chao, A. & Lin, H. (2000). piwi encodes a nucleoplasmic factor whose activity modulates the number and division rate of germ line stem cells. *Development,* (Feb 2000), Vol. 127, No. 3, pp. (503-514), ISSN 1011-6370

Feng, B., Chen, G., Zheng, X., Sun, H., Zhang, X., Zhang, Z.-X., Xiang, Y., Ichim, T.E., Garcia, B., Luke, P., Jevnikar, A.M. & Min, W.-P. (2009). Small Interfering RNA Targeting RelB Protects Against Renal Ischemia-reperfusion Injury. *Transplantation,* (May 2009), Vol. 87, No. 9, pp. (1283–1289), ISSN 0041-1337

Gao, K. & Huang, L. (2009). Nonviral methods for siRNA delivery. *Molecular Pharmaceutics,* (May-Jun 2009), Vol. 6. No. 3, pp. (651-658), ISSN 1543-8384

Hamar, P., Song, E., Kökény, G., Chen, A., Ouyang, N. & Lieberman, J. (2004). Small interfering RNA targeting Fas protects mice against renal ischemia-reperfusion injury. *Proc Natl Acad Sci,* (Oct 2004), Vol. 101, No. 41, pp. (14883-14888), ISSN 0027-8424

Jackson, A.L., Bartz, S.R., Schelter, J., Kobayashi, S.V., Burchard, J., Mao, M., Li, B., Cavet, G. & Linsley, P,S. Expression profiling reveals off-target gene regulation by RNAi. *Nat Biotechnol,* (Jun 2003), Vol. 21, No. 6, pp. (635-637), ISSN 1087-0156

Jiang, G., Park, K., Kim, J., Kim, K.S. & Hahn, S.K. (2008). Target specific intracellular delivery of siRNA/PEI-HA complex by receptor mediated endocytosis. *Molecular Pharmaceutics,* (May-Jun 2009), Vol. 6, No. 3, pp. (727-737), ISSN 1543-8384

Juliano, R., Alam, R., Dixit, V. & Ming, X. (2008). Mechanisms and strategies for effective delivery of antisense and siRNA oligonucleotides. *Nucleic Acids Res,* (Jul 2008), Vol. 36, No. 12, pp. (4158-4171). ISSN 0305-1048

Juliano, R., Bauman, J., Kang, H. & Ming, X. (2009). Biological barriers to therapy with antisense and siRNA oligonucleotides. *Molecular Pharmaceutics,* (May-Jun 2009), Vol. 6, No. 3, pp. (686-695), ISSN 1543-8384

Kaucsár, T., Rácz, Zs. & Hamar, P. (2010). Post-transcriptional gene-expression regulation by micro RNA (miRNA) network in renal disease. *Adv Drug Deliv Rev,* (Nov 2010), Vol. 62, No. 14, pp. (1390-1401), ISSN 0169-409X

Kim, S., Garg, H., Joshi, A. & Manjunath, N. (2009). Strategies for targeted nonviral delivery of siRNAs in vivo. *Trends in Molecular Medicine,* (Nov 2009), Vol. 15, No. 11, pp. (491-500), ISSN 1471-4914

Kim, V.N. (2006). Small RNAs just got bigger: Piwi-interacting RNAs (piRNAs) in mammalian testes. *Genes Dev,* (Aug 2006), (Aug 2006), Vol. 20, No. 15, pp. (1993-1997), ISSN 0890-9369

Kimura T, Yamaoka T, Iwase R, Murakami A. (2001) Structure/function relationship in the polyplexes containing cationic polypeptides for gene delivery. *Nucleic Acids Res,* (2001) *Suppl.,* No . 1, pp (203-204), ISSN 0305-1048

Kobayashi, N., Matsui, Y., Kawase, A., Hirata, K., Miyagishi, M., Taira, K., Nishikawa, M. & Takakura, Y. (2004). Vector-Based in Vivo RNA Interference: Dose- and Time-Dependent Suppression of Transgene Expression. *Journal of Pharmacology and Experimental Therapeutics,* (Feb 2004), Vol. 308, No. 2, pp. (688-693), ISSN 0022-3565

Kushibikia, T., Nagata-Nakajimab, N., Sugaib, M., Shimizub, A. & Tabata, Y. (2005). Delivery of plasmid DNA expressing small interference RNA for TGF-b type II receptor by cationized gelatin to prevent interstitial renal fibrosis. *J Controlled Release,* (Jul 2005), Vol. 105, No. 3, pp. (318-331), ISSN 0168-3659

Larson, S.D., Jackson, L.N., Chen, A., Rychahou, P.G. & Evers, B.M. (2007). Effectiveness of siRNA uptake in target tissues by various delivery methods. *Surgery,* (Aug 2007), Vol. 142, No. 2, pp. (262-269), ISSN 0263-9319

Malek, A., Merkel, O., Fink, L., Czubayko, F., Kissel, T. & Aigner, A. (2009). In vivo pharmacokinetics, tissue distribution and underlying mechanisms of various PEI(-PEG)/siRNA complexes. *Toxicology and Applied Pharmacology,* (Apr 2009), Vol. 236, No. 1, pp. (97-108), ISSN 0041-008X

Marques, JT. & Williams, BR. (2005). Activation of the mammalian immune system by siRNAs. Nat Biotechnol, (Nov 2005), Vol. 23, No. 11, pp. (1399-1405), ISSN 1087-0156

Mikhaylova, M., Stasinopoulos, I., Kato, Y., Artemov, D. & Bhujwalla, ZM. (2011). Imaging of cationic multifunctional liposome-mediated delivery of COX-2 siRNA. *Cancer Gene Therapy,* (Mar 2011), Vol. 16, No. 3, pp. (217-226), ISSN 0929-1903

Moazed, D. (2009). Small RNAs in transcriptional gene silencing and genome defense. *Nature,* (Jan 2009), Vol. 457, No. 7228, pp. (413-420), ISSN 0028-0836

Molitoris, B.A., Dagher, P.C., Sandoval, R.M., Campos, S.B., Ashush, H., Fridman, E., Brafman, A., Faerman, A., Atkinson, S.J., Thompson, J.D., Kalinski, H., Skaliter, R., Erlich, S. & Feinstein, E. (2009). siRNA Targeted to p53 attenuates ischemic and cisplatin-induced acute kidney injury. *J Am Soc Nephrol,* (Aug 2009), Vol. 20, No. 8, pp. (1754-1764), ISSN 1046-6673

Monia, B.P. (1997). First- and second-generation antisense oligonucleotide inhibitors targeted against human c-raf kinase. *Ciba Found Symp.* Vol. 209, pp. (107-119), ISSN 0300-5208

Ninichuk, V., Clauss, S., Kulkarni, O., Schmid, H., Segerer, S Radomska, E., Eulberg, D., Buchner, K., Selve, N., Klussmann, S. & Anders, H.-J. (2008). Late onset of Ccl2 blockade with the Spiegelmer mNOX-E36-3'PEG prevents glomerulosclerosis and improves glomerular filtration rate in db/db mice. *Am J Pathol,* (Mar 2008), Vol. 172, No. 3, pp. (628-637), ISSN 0002-9440

Purschke, W.G., Eulberg, D., Buchner, K., Vonhoff, S. & Klussmann, S. (2006). An L-RNA-based aquaretic agent that inhibits vasopressin in vivo. *Proc Natl Acad Sci,* (Mar 2006), Vol. 103, No. 13, pp. (5173-5178), ISSN 0027-8424

Paroo, Z. & Corey, D.R. (2004). Challenges for RNAi in vivo. *Trends Biotech,* Vol. 22, No. 8, pp. (390-394), ISSN 0167-9430

Rácz, Zs. & Hamar, P. (2006). Can siRNA technology provide the tools for gene therapy of the future? *Curr Med Chem,* (Aug 2006), Vol. 13, No 19, pp. (2299-2307), ISSN 0929-8673

Rácz, Zs. & Hamar, P. (2008). RNA interference in research and therapy of renal diseases. *Contr Nephrol,* Vol. 159, pp. (78-95), ISSN 0302-5144

Saito, K., Nishida, K.M., Mori, T., Kawamura, Y., Miyoshi, K., Nagami, T., Siomi, H. & Siomi, M.C. (2006). Specific association of Piwi with rasiRNAs derived from retrotransposon and heterochromatic regions in the Drosophila genome. *Genes Dev,* (Aug 2006), Vol. 20, No. 16, pp. (2214-2222), ISSN 0890-9369

Semizarov, D., Frost, L., Sarthy, A., Kroeger, P., Halbert, D.N. & Fesik, S.W. Specificity of short interfering RNA determined through gene expression signatures. *Proc Natl Acad Sci,* (May 2003), Vol. 100, No. 11, pp. (6347-6352), ISSN 0027-8424

Shcharbin, D., Pedziwiatr, E., Blasiak, J. & Bryszewska. M. (2010). How to study dendriplexes II: Transfection and cytotoxicity. *J Control Release,* (Jan 2010), Vol. 141, No. 2, pp. (110-127), ISSN 0168-3659

Shimizu, H., Hori, Y., Kaname, S., Yamada, K., Nishiyama, N., Matsumoto, S., Miyata, K., Oba, M., Yamada, A., Kataoka, K. & Fujita, T. (2010). siRNA-Based Therapy Ameliorates Glomerulonephritis. *J Am Soc Nephrology,* (Apr 2010), Vol. 21, No. 4, pp. (622-633), ISSN 1046-6673

Singhal, S.S., Singhal, J., Yadav, S., Sahu, M., Awasthi, Y.C. & Awasthi, S.A. (2009). RLIP76: A Target for Kidney Cancer Therapy. *Cancer Res,* (May 2009), Vol. 69, No. 10, pp. (4244-4251), ISSN 0008-5472

Siomi, H. & Siomi, M.C. (2009). On the road to reading the RNA-interference code. *Nature,* (Jan 2009), Vol. 457, No. 7228, pp. (396-404), ISSN 0028-0836

Song, E., Lee, S.K., Wang, J., Ince, N., Ouyang, N., Min, J., Chen, J., Shankar, P. & Lieberman, J. (2003). RNA interference targeting Fas protects mice from fulminant hepatitis. *Nature Medicine,* (Feb 2003), Vol. 9, No. 3, pp. (347-351), ISSN 1078-8956

Tseng, Y.-C., Mozumdar, S. & Huang, L. (2009). Lipid-based systemic delivery of siRNA. *Adv Drug Deliv Rev,* (Jul 2009), Vol. 61, No. 9, pp. (721-731), ISSN 0169-409X

Tuschl, T., Zamore, P.D., Lehmann, R., Bartel, D.P. & Sharp, P.A. (1999). Targeted mRNA degradation by double-stranded RNA in vitro. *Genes Dev,* (Dec 1999), Vol. 13, No. 24, pp. (3191-3197), ISSN 0890-9369

Valencia-Sanchez, M.A., Liu, J., Hannon, G.J. & Parker, R. (2006). Control of translation and mRNA degradation by miRNAs and siRNAs. *Genes Dev,* (Mar 2006), Vol. 20, No. 5, pp. (515-524), ISSN 0890-9369

Wang, X., Skelley, L., Cade, R. & Sun, Z. (2006). AAV delivery of mineralocorticoid receptor shRNA prevents progression of cold-induced hypertension and attenuates renal damage. *Gene Therapy,* (Jul 2006), Vol. 13, No. 14, pp. (1097-1103), ISSN 0969-7128

Wolfrum, C., Shi, S., Jayaprakash, K.N., Jayaraman, M., Wang, G., Pandey, R.K., Rajeev, K.G., Nakayama, T., Charrise, K., Ndungo, E.M., Zimmermann, T., Koteliansky, V., Manoharan, M. & Stoffel, M. (2007). Mechanisms and optimization of in vivo delivery of lipophilic siRNAs. *Nature Biotechnology,* (Sep 2007), Vol. 25, No. 10, pp. (1149-1157), ISSN 1087-0156

Xie, J. & Guo, Q. (2006). Apoptosis antagonizing transcription factor protects renal tubule cells against oxidative damage and apoptosis induced by ischemia-reperfusion. *J Am Soc Nephrol,* (Dec 2006), Vol. *17, No. 12, pp. (3336–3346),* ISSN 1046-6673

Yuan, H., Lanting, L., Xu, Z.-G., Li, S.-L., Swiderski, P., Putta, S., Jonnalagadda, M., Kato, M. & Natarajan, R. (2008). Effects of cholesterol-tagged small interfering RNAs targeting 12/15-lipoxygenase on parameters of diabetic nephropathy in a mouse model of type 1 diabetes. *Am J Physiol Renal Physiol,* (Jun 2008), Vol. 295, pp. (F605-F617), ISSN 0363-6127.

Zhang, C. (2009). Novel functions for small RNA molecules. *Curr Opin Mol Ther,* (Dec 2009), Vol. 11, No. 6, pp. (641-651), ISSN 1464-8431

Zhang, Q., Shi, Y., Wada, J., Malakauskas, SM., Liu, M., Ren, Y., Du, C., Duan, H., Li, Y., Li, Y. & Zhang, Y. (2010). In vivo delivery of Gremlin siRNA plasmid reveals therapeutic potential against diabetic nephropathy by recovering bone morphogenetic protein-7. *PloS ONE,* (Jul 2010), Vol. 5, No. 7, e11709, pp. (1-13), ISSN 1932-6203

Zhang, Y., Wada, J., Hashimoto, I., Eguchi, J., Yasuhara, A., Kanwar, Y.S., Shikata, K. & Makino, H. (2006). Therapeutic approach for diabetic nephropathy using gene delivery of translocase of inner mitochondrial membrane 44 by reducing mitochondrial superoxide production. *J Am Soc Nephrol,* (Apr 2006), Vol. 17, No. 4, pp. (1090–1101), ISSN 1046-6673

Zheng, X., Zhang, X., Feng, B., Sun, H., Suzuki, M., Ichim, T., Kubo, N., Wong, A., Min, L.R., Budohn, M.E., Garcia, B., Jevnikar, A.M. & Min, W.P. (2008). Gene Silencing of Complement C5a Receptor Using siRNA for Preventing Ischemia/Reperfusion Injury. *Am J Pathol,* (Oct 2008), Vol. 173, No. 4, pp. (973–980), ISSN 0002-9440

Zhong, H., He, Z.G., Li, Z., Li, G.Y., Shen, S.R. & Li. X.L. (2008). Studies on polyamidoamine dendrimers as efficient gene delivery vector. *J Biomater Appl,* (May 2008), Vol. 22, No. 6, pp. (527-544), ISSN 0885-3282

16

Therapeutic Potential of Gene Transfer to Testis; Myth or Reality?

Yoshiyuki Kojima, Kentaro Mizuno, Yukihiro Umemoto, Shoichi Sasaki, Yutaro Hayashi and Kenjiro Kohri
Department of Nephro-urology, Nagoya City University Graduate School of Medical Sciences, Nagoya, Japan

1. Introduction

Although there have been many reports about gene transfer to testicules, the original purpose is to develop more effective and simple methods to obtain transgenic animals than the most widely used method, which is the direct microinjection of foreign DNA into pronuclei of fertilized eggs. In the future, however, this technique has the potential to be the most useful approach for the treatment of testicular disorders such as male infertility and testicular cancer. In addition to whether gene transfer to testis is technically possible, the issues of social acceptance, ethics and safety must be addressed before it could become a clinical option. Germ cell gene therapy is rejected on the grounds that gene transfer to normal germ cells would be possible to affect future generations without precise understanding of the mechanism and control of gene expression. Therefore, at present, we should not make exceptions to the standing ethical rules in future clinical application of gene transfer to normal germ cells and consider appropriate gene therapy that avoids gene transfer to normal germ cells. On the other hand, the basic common consensus throughout the world is that gene transfer to somatic cells and cancer cells can be applied to treat wide range of disorders. Up to now, there has been no report about clinical application of gene transfer to testis. In this chapter, we discuss the current understanding of gene transfer to testes in animals, and the future possibility of clinical application of this technique for human testicular disorders.

2. Normal function and anatomy of testis

The testis has two primary functions: the production of sperm (spermatogenesis), which ensures the survival of our species, and the secretion of steroid hormones (steroidogenesis), which is necessary for male sexual differentiation, male secondary sexual functions, including behavior and spermatogenesis. Three main cells, germ cells (spermatogenic cells) and the somatic cells such as Sertoli cells and Leydig cells play a significant role in maintaining these testicular functions. Germ cells in the testis are composed of spermatogonia, spermatocytes and spermatids. Spermatogenesis can be divided into several processes, including the proliferation and differentiation of spermatogonia, which are stem cells, meiosis of spermatocytes, and their morphological changes to spermatids. Sertoli and

Leydig cells support germ cell development, maturation and release into the seminiferous tubule lumen. The cell to cell crosstalk involves an intricate network of paracrine-autocrine systems that support endocrine input to modulate cell function (Saunders, 2003).

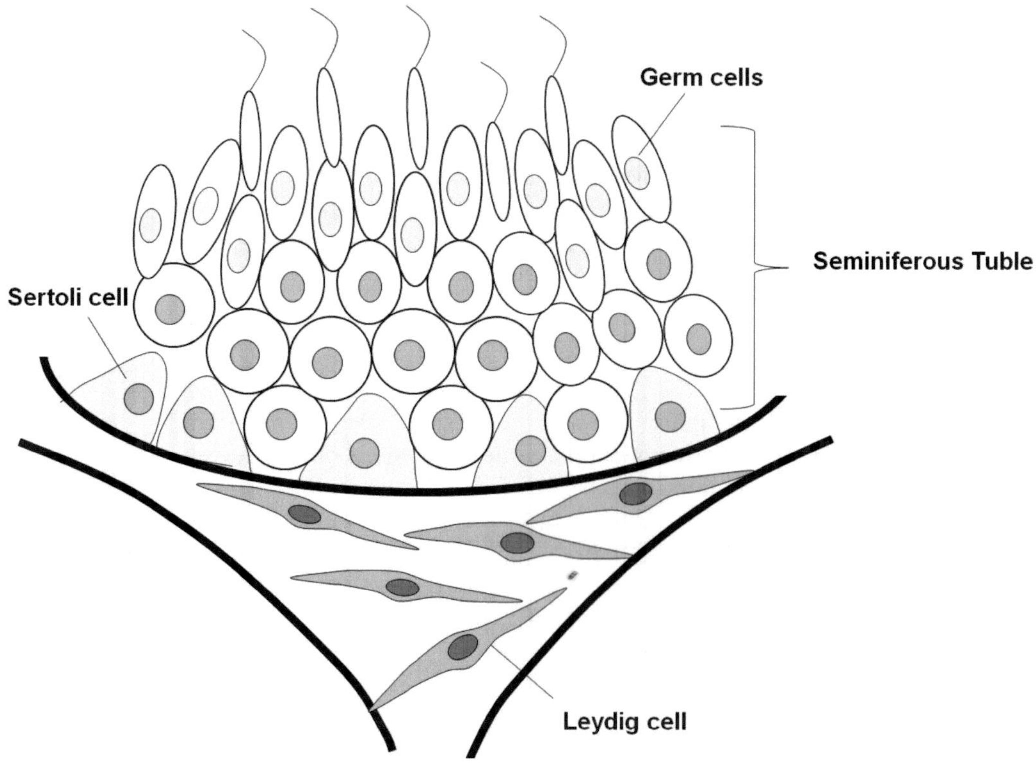

Fig. 1. Drawing of testis demonstrating relationships of seminiferous tubules and interstitium.

3. Possible methods of gene transfer to testis-animal studes

3.1 *In vivo* gene transfer

Establishment of the efficient methods of gene transfer to testis is important to apply for clinical use in the future. In animal studies, two methods, intratesticular injection and intratubular injection, can be used to perform gene transfer to the testis depending on the target cells. If the target cells are Leydig cells, intratesticular injection may be better, whereas if they are germ cells or Sertoli cells, intratubular injection may be preferable (Kojima, 2008a). These same basic methods will be used for humans.

3.1.1 Intratesticular injection

Intratesticular injection is a simpler method. DNA solution is injected directly into the testis through the scrotal skin using a needle and a disposable syringe. This technique allows the spread of DNA throughout the entire interstitial space of the testis, but not in the seminiferous tublues.

3.1.2 Intratubular injection

For intratubular injection, two injection techniques are available, antegrade injection and retrograde injection. The testis is pulled out and exposed under a dissecting microscope in both techniques. Injection of DNA containing Trypan blue dye is useful way to monitor the accuracy of the testis injection.

3.1.2.1 Antegrade injection

For the antegrade injection, a small incision is made in the tunica, and then DNA solution is directly injected into the seminiferous tubules using an injection glass micropipette. Injection is usually made at several sites in the testis (Kojima, 2003).

3.1.2.2 Retrograde injection

For the retrograde injection, the injection glass micropipette is inserted into the rete testis via the efferent duct to allow direct injection into the seminiferous tubules. (Kurokawa, 2005). This technique enables the more thorough spread of exogenous DNA throughout the entire seminiferous tubule.

3.2 *Ex vivo* gene transfer

The testicular cell and tissue transplantation system with gene transfer is sometimes a useful procedure for gene transfer to the testis to produce transgenic animals. In this system, transduced donor testicular cells populations are transplanted by efferent duct injection into recipient animals (Nagano, 2001; Orwig, 2002) or transduced donor testicular tissues are transplanted directly into the testis.

4. Vectors

Generally, there are two main types of gene delivery vectors: non-viral and viral. Although several researchers have attempted gene transfer into animal testis using these vectors to produce transgenic animals, the choice of vector is one of the most important issues when applying for clinical trials of gene therapy for male infertility. Since these vectors have their own characteristics, they should be clarified before being used for testis-mediated gene transfer *in vivo* (Table 1). If a suitable vector could be developed, gene therapy could be considered safer than ICSI (Lamb, 2008).

4.1 Non-viral vector

It has been shown that non-viral vectors have several advantages over viral ones, as they are simple and cheap manufacture, no insert-size limitation, low immunogenicity and, as a result, a good safety profile. On the other hand, the disadvantages are the short duration of expression, inefficient transfection and difficulty in targeting transfection (Navarro, 2008). These techniques are so uncontrollable and unpredictable that they will not be appropriate for use in clinical trials in the short term, although some may be useful to produce transgenic animals. To apply for clinical use in the future, significant modification will be required.

4.1.1 Naked DNA

Sperm cells have the capacity to capture foreign DNA (Brackett, 1971). Several reports have demonstrated that sperm-mediated gene transfer *in vitro*, which is based on the intrinsic

			Transgene Expression cells			
		Expression periods	Germ cell	sperm	Sertoli cell	Leydig cell
Non-viral vector	Naked DNA	NA	NA	+	NA	NA
	Liposome	< 1 week	-	+	-	-
	Electroporation	1-2 months	+	+	+	+
Viral Vector	Adenovirus	>2months	-	-	+	+
	Retrovirus	NA	+	NA	-	NA
	Lentivirus	> 6months	-	-	+	NA
	Baculovirus	NA	-	-	+	+

NA: not assessment

Table 1. Characteristics of vectors in testicular gene transfer system *in vivo*.

ability of sperm cells to bind and internalize exogenous DNA and to transfer it into the egg at fertilization, has succeeded in generating transgenic animals (Lavitrano, 1989, 1992, 1997, 2006; Francolini, 1993; Zani M, 1995).
On the other hand, Huguet E et al. (1998) analyzed the uptake of exogenous DNA by mouse and rat spermatozoa using *in vivo* methods. DNA was injected into the vas deferens, and spermatozoa were recovered 6 hr later. Uptake of exogenous DNA occurred in 60–70% of spermatozoa after *in vivo* DNA injection into the proximal region of the vas deferens (Huguet, 1998). These male mice injected with exogenous DNA encoding green fluorescent protein (GFP) were mated with normal estrus females, and 7.5% newborns were found positive by PCR for exogenous DNA. In these positive animals, some tissues showed GFP expression (Huguet, 2000).

4.1.2 Liposome

Cationic lipids interact with negatively charged nucleic acid molecules forming complexes in which the nucleic acid is coated by lipids (Felgner, 1987). The positive outer surface of the complex can associate with the negatively charged cell membrane, allowing the internalization of nucleic acid. In this technique, DNA is mixed with cationic lipid just before the addition of this complex to the testis. Several researchers have reported testis-mediated gene transfer using this method. As early as 3–4 days after microinjection of the exogenous gene mixed with cationic lipids into the seminiferous tubules, gene expression was observed within both immature and differentiated germ cells. By 40 days post-injection, the gene expression was restricted to the most immature germ cells in the basal portion of the seminiferous tubules (Celebi, 2002). Although transgene was transmitted to morula, blastocyst and mid-gestational fetuses, the ratio of animals carrying the exogenous gene decreased as they developed. Over 80% of morula-stage embryos expressed the exogenous gene, but only some postpartum progeny were foreign-DNA-positive with a high incidence of mosaicism (Yonezawa, 2001). Repeated injection with linearized plasmid DNA containing the *β-galactosidase* gene encapsulated with cationic liposome into the testis of adult mice via the scrotum resulted in the transmission of exogenous DNA sequences to blastocysts through fertilization (Ogawa, 1995). Sato et al. (1999, 2002) also attempted to transfect testicular spermatozoa with plasmid DNA by direct injection into testes to obtain transgenic animals. When injected males were mated with superovulated females 2 and 3 days after injection, more than 50% gene transmission was achieved in mid-gestational fetuses, and overt gene expression was not found in these fetuses. They suggested that plasmid DNA introduced into a testis is rapidly transported to the epididymis and then incorporated by epididymal spermatozoa.

4.1.3 Electroporation

Electroporation is a widely used technique for enhancing the efficiency of DNA delivery into cells. Application of electric pulses after local injection of DNA temporarily opens cell membranes and facilitates DNA uptake (De Vry, 2010). Electroporation provides more sperm cells to increase DNA uptake than unelectroporated spermatozoa (Gagné, 1991; Horan, 1992).

As a possible alternative and more effective method for generating transgenic mice, several researchers have attempted testis-mediated gene transfer using an *in vivo* electroporation method. After injection of exogenous DNA into the testis, the testes are held between a tweezer-type electrode, and square electric pulses are applied several times at 20–50 volts (Muramatsu, 1996, 1997; Yamazaki, 1998, 2000; Umemoto, 2002, 2005). Expression of the exogenous gene was clearly observed in germ cells of seminiferous tubules 48 hours after transfecting the mouse testis by *in vivo* electroporation (Muramatsu, 1997). Stable gene expression in spermatogenic cells using electroporation would be facilitated by *retroviral integrase* gene co-transfection (Ryoki, 2001). We also directly injected DNA, which was constructed as a cytomegalovirus enhancer/chicken β-actin promoter connected with the β-*galactosidase* gene (Umemoto, 2002, 2005), into mouse testes using a square-wave electroporator, and investigated the efficiency of gene transfer. The β-galactosidase activity was detected in germ cells and Sertoli cells in seminiferous tubules and in Leydig cells for 4 weeks (Umemoto, 2002, 2005); however, although electroporation is a simple and convenient technique for gene transfer to germ cells in the testis, the gene expression was deemed transient and uncontrollable (Umemoto, 2005). Another problem of electroporation is that the electric pulses themselves could result in testicular damage. In our previous reports, the Johnsen scores were significantly decreased and apoptotic cells were significantly increased in the testis several weeks after *in vivo* electroporation (Umemoto, 2002, 2005; Kojima, 2005). These results suggest that spermatogenic damage caused by electroporation itself could be important problems for clinical application.

Yomogida et al. (2002) investigated the rescue of spermatogenesis in Sl^{17H}/Sl^{17H} mutant mice, which are infertile because of an altered stem cell factor (SCF), by gene transfer using electroporation. Dobashi et al. (2005) showed that the transfer of erythropoietin to rat testes by *in vivo* electroporation might reduce the risk of germ cell loss caused by surgically induced cryptorchidism. To define the transcriptional regulatory elements of the *OAZt* gene promoter, *in vivo* DNA transfer to mouse testes was performed using electroporation (Ike, 2004). RNA interference (RNAi) technology has become a novel tool for silencing gene expression in cells or organisms, and has also been used to develop new therapeutics for certain diseases. RNAi against endogenous *Dmc1*, which encodes a DNA recombinase that is expressed and functionally required in spermatocytes, was introduced into mouse testis by electroporation and led to the same phenotypes observed in null mutant mice (Shoji, 2005). Thus, an *in vivo* RNAi system using electroporation may provide a rapid means for assessing the physiological role of the spermatogenetic gene.

4.2 Viral vector

Viral vectors provide the most efficient transfection. Their main disadvantages concern limitations on the size of inserted DNA, difficulty of manufacture and possible immunogenicity (Navarro, 2008).

4.2.1 Adenoviral vector

Adenoviruses are the most commonly used gene-delivery vectors due to the efficiency of their *in vivo* gene transfer. This opinion is based upon their natural ability to infect a broad array of both dividing and terminally differentiated, nondividing cell types, their capacity to deliver large amounts of DNA, and the ease at which this vector platform can be mass produced (Appledorn, 2008). Furthermore, adenovirus vector remain the gene transfer vector of choice for numerous human clinical trials, as more clinical trials utilize Ad-based vectors than any other vector currently available.

Several researchers have attempted to perform adenovirus-mediated gene transfer to animal testis *in vivo* (Blanchard & Boekelheide 1997; Kojima, 2003, 2008b; Takehashi, 2007). Intratesticular injection of adenoviral vector resulted in strong transgene expression in interstitial cells, including Leydig cells from seminiferous tubules (Kojima, 2003, Blanchard & Boekelheide, 1997). By contrast, intratubular injection resulted in transgene expression along the seminiferous tubules, in which strong expression was observed in Sertoli cells. No transgene expression was detected in germ cells by either method (Kojima, 2003, Blanchard & Boekelheide 1997).

Gene expression patterns by adenovirus-mediated gene transfer to the testis are particularly interesting and important from the viewpoint of gene therapy for male infertility in the future. Since it is not impossible to introduce a foreign gene precisely at specific chromosomal loci, abnormal sperm could be formed if a foreign gene is introduced into germ cells in the testis. This would increase the rate of offspring with anomalies; however, when an adenovirus vector is used, such problems can be avoided because of its biological characteristic of not introducing genes into germ cells in the testis. Fetuses and offspring produced by mating with males for several days after adenovirus-mediated gene transfer to the testis were normal and the number of neonates was not significantly different from that in the control group. None of the fetuses or offspring showed any abnormalities, and the transgene was not detected by RT-PCR and histochemical study (Kojima, 2003, 2008b). These results demonstrate that the risk of germline transmission following adenovirus-mediated gene transfer to the testis is extremely low (Kojima, 2008b).

There are two problems concerning transfection with the adenoviral vector, i.e., cytotoxicity as a general biological characteristic and the immune response (Yang, 1994, 1995; Amin, 1995); however, although apoptosis was detected in some spermatocytes and a slight immune response was observed for a short period, it was temporary. The testis did not become highly atrophic, severe deterioration of the tubules was not detected, sperm motility was not lowered and sperm abnormalities were not observed (Kojima, 2003); therefore, transfection by adenoviral vector was not considered to have any adverse effects on spermatogenic function overall. Adenovirus-mediated gene transfer to the testis has several advantages and can be exploited for the treatment of male infertility in the future; however, to achieve a better therapeutic effect in the future, the different strategies of adenoviral improvement should be combined.

Some studies have reported the effect of gene transfer to an animal model testis on spermatogenesis using an adenoviral vector *in vivo*. Transfer of the tumor suppressor protein *p53* gene to rat seminiferous tubules by adenoviral vector using the retrograde technique impaired spermatogenesis (Fujisawa, 2001). On the other hand, adenovirus-mediated *hepatocyte growth factor (HGF)* gene transfer into the testis in cryptorchidism rats inhibited germ cell apoptosis and restored spermatogenesis (Goda, 2004). To explore the therapeutic usefulness of the *HST-1/FGF-4* gene, which could be an important factor for spermatogenesis, in impaired spermatogenesis, adenovirus carrying the *HST-1/FGF-4* gene was administered into the testis of mice after adriamycin treatment, and *HST-1/FGF-4* gene transfer had a protective effect on experimentally induced testicular toxicity (Yamamoto, 2002).

4.2.2 Retroviral vector

Retroviral vectors based upon simple gammaretroviruses, complex lentiviruses, or potentially nonpathogenic spumaviruses represent relatively well-characterized tools that are widely used for stable gene transfer (Baum, 2006; Bushman 2007). They transfect by integrating the transgene into the target cell chromosome, but transgene expression ceases within days to weeks and tends to be shorter than adenovirus vectors. Unlike many other types of vectors currently being developed for gene therapy, retroviral vectors are able to genetically modify cells stably without perturbing cell growth (Kim, 2000). In the testis injected with retroviral vector into seminiferous tubules via rete testes, no cells with gene expression could be found (Ikawa, 2002); however, other researchers reported that retroviral vector was a powerful tool to transfer exogenous genes into the germ cell line and spermatogonia *in vitro* (Danno, 1999; De Miguel, 2003). Microinjection of a retroviral vector expressing the *β-galactosidase* gene into immature seminiferous tubules resulted in the direct transduction of spermatogonial stem cells, and the animals produced transgenic offspring after mating with females (Kanatsu-Shinohara, 2004).

4.2.3 Lentiviral vector

Lentviral vector are being increasingly used in basic and applied research. Human gene therapy clinical trials are currently underway using lentiviral vectors in a wide range of human diseases (Escors & Breckpot 2010). The capacity to efficiently transduce non-dividing cells, shuttle large genetic payloads, and maintain stable long-term transgene expression are attributes that have brought lentiviral vectors to the forefront of gene delivery vehicles for research and therapeutic applications in a clinical setting (Cockrell & Kafri, 2007). Testes transduced with lentiviral vector expressed the trangene without impairing spermatogenesis. Expression patterns were characteristic of Sertoli cells and gene expression was observed over a period of 6 months (Ikawa, 2002). Although spermatogenesis can be restored in *Sl/Sl^d* mutant mice by transducing Sertoli cells with lentiviral vectors generating a functional *c-kit* ligand, KL2, an insufficient number of spermatozoa for IVF were collected. Sperm collected from recipient testes were able to produce normal pups after intracytoplasmic sperm injection. None of the offspring carried the transgene, suggesting the inability of lentiviral vectors to infect spermatogenic cells *in vivo* (Ikawa, 2002).

4.2.4 Baculoviral vector

Since the discovery that baculoviruses can efficiently transduce mammalian cells, baculoviruses have been extensively studied as potential vectors for both *in vitro* and *in vivo* gene therapy (Hu, 2008). Baculovirus-mediated gene transfer is simple to perform, reproducible, and demonstrates no overt cell toxicity, and is particularly useful for repetitive or moderately high-throughput procedures, such as cell-based assays, or for situations where transfection procedures are inadequate (Merrihew, 2004; Kost, 2005). Baculovirus-mediated gene transfer to the testis via intratubular injection resulted in the gene expression in Sertoli cells but not in spermatocytes or sperm (Tani, 2003]. Park et al. (2009) demonstrated that intra-tunica albuguineal injection of GFP-baculovirus into the mouse testis resulted in a high level of GFP expression in the interstitial tissues. In addition, intra-tunica albuguineal injection of a modified baculovirus that encoded recombinant rat insulin-like growth factor binding protein (IGFBP)-5 resulted in an increase in IGFBP-5 in testis and semen.

5. Future prospects of gene therapy for male infertility

5.1 Abnormal sperm production and male infertility

Normal fertility is defined as achieving a pregnancy within one year by regular coital exposure. On the other hand, infertility is defined as the inability to conceive after one year of unprotected intercourse, which affects approximately 15% of couples trying to conceive in western countries. Worldwide more than 70 million couples suffer from infertility (Ombelet, 2008). It is generally reported that in approximately 30% of cases, infertility is mainly due to a male factor, and 70 to 90% of male infertility arises from impaired spermatogenesis with the clinical presentation of abnormal sperm production, such as oligozoospermia and azoospermia (Greenberg, 1978). The presented cases of male infertility include varicocele, cryptorchidism, obstruction of spermatic ducts, and endocrine disorders; however, most cases continue to be labeled with the diagnosis of "idiopathic infertility" or given descriptive diagnoses that do not provide a cause for their defect, although basic research helps to define the associated genes and the mechanisms responsible for the development, function and regulation of spermatogenesis (Matzuk & Lamb, 2008).

5.2 Present therapeutic options of male infertility and its limitation

Evolving therapies have allowed the use of sperm from men with compromised spermatogenesis, obstructive azoospermia, and sperm functional deficiency, enabling these men to procreate when unable to do so naturally (Oates, 2008). Assisted reproductive technology (ART) is the most appropriate management if a natural pregnancy fails to occur, and this is increasingly used in the treatment of both male and female infertility. Recently, severe male infertility, such as azoospermia, has been treated successfully by intracytoplasmic sperm injection (ICSI) (Palemo, 1992, 1996). Sperm can be obtained by microepididymal sperm aspiration (MESA), percutaneous sperm aspiration (PESA), and testicular sperm extraction (TESE) from patients with male infertility. ICSI involves the injection of a single sperm directly into the cytoplasm of a mature egg (oocyte) using a glass needle (pipette). ICSI guarantees high fertilization rates and could also theoretically lead to higher implantation rates. Fertilization rates were in the range of 60–90% and the delivery rate per retrieval was 38.5% in the first 560 couples (Palermo, 1996). Although ICSI allows otherwise sterile couples to become parents, there is still only an incomplete picture of the risks associated with the usage of these ART to offspring (Staessen, 1999; Alukal & Lamb, 2008). Several data have indicated a higher risk of congenital malformation (Sutcliffe, 2001; Hansen M, 2002), chromosome aneuploidy (In't Veld P, 1995; Liebaers, 1995; Loft A, 1999), low birth weight (Schieve, 2002), and imprinting defects such as Angelman syndrome (Cox, 2002) for children conceived by ICSI than for children conceived naturally. Additionally, this technique is not a cure per se for male infertility patients. The empirical treatments used in the past for male infertility patients are probably ineffective, and no effective treatments have been proved to improve spermatogenesis in idiopathic male infertility despite major advances in ART; therefore, additional prospective treatments for male infertility patients are needed to achieve paternity potential.

5.3 Therapeutic potential of gene transfer to tesits for male infertility

Fertilization is better *in vivo* than *in vitro* for male infertility. Clinically, testicular gene therapy may be useful to treat male infertility in the future because it is possible to promote spermatogenesis in male infertility patients diagnosed with pathological hypospermatogenesis, maturation arrest or Sertoli cells only. Since testicular cells play a significant role in creating life and personality, it is very important to understand the safety issues and to control the expression of transferred genes (Kojima, 2006a). Numerous difficult hurdles remain to be overcome in the clinical application of gene transfer to testis under the present conditions.

5.3.1 Appropriate methods and vectors of future gene therapy for male infertility

The basic common consensus throughout the world is that somatic gene therapy can be applied to treat a wide range of disorders, including cancer and inherited disease (Smith, 2003). The ethical issues in somatic gene therapy are primarily concerned with the risk of this procedure, such as vector toxicity and oncogenesis. On the other hand, although germline gene therapy is theoretically possible, it is rejected on the grounds that it would be possible to affect future generations without precise understanding about the mechanism and control of gene expression [(Kojima, 2006a). At present, we should not make exceptions to the standing ethical rules in future gene therapy for male infertility and consider appropriate gene therapy that avoids gene transfer to germ cells.

Within the seminiferous epithelium of seminiferous tubules, spermatogenesis occurs on the surface of Sertoli cells. In other words, Sertoli cells directly support spermatogenesis. They are involved in metabolic exchange with germ cells, as well as in their nutrition and the secretion of tubular fluid into the luminal compartment and the exclusive targets of follicle-stimulating hormone (FSH), androgens and other hormones within the testis (Brehm & Steger, 2005). On the other hand, Leydig cells are the main source of the androgen hormone, testosterone, which is located in the interstitial space, outside the seminiferous tubules. This function is regulated by luteinizing hormone (LH), paracrine factors secreted by cells within the seminiferous tubules and autoregulatory factors.

Disruption of spermatogenesis, which results in male infertility, can therefore be caused by defects affecting the germ cells or Sertoli cells or sometimes Leydig cell dysfunction. Germ cells are appropriate target cells of gene transfer into the testis to generate transgenic animals, while Sertoli cells and Leydig cells may be appropriate target cells for the clinical application of male infertility treatment on the basis of ethical issues. Viewed from this point, adenoviral-, lentiviral- or baculoviral-mediated gene transfer may be effective for transfecting testicular somatic cells, Sertoli cells or Leydig cells, because they can not introduce exogenous genes into germ cells, and are applicable vectors for *in vivo* gene therapy for male infertility in the future (Kojima, 2008a). Adenoviral vectors may currently be the most appropriate candidate to use in future clinical application because there is sufficient information from clinical trials about several other diseases.

Intratubular injection (antegrade injection or retrograde injection) is a useful technique to introduce genes into Sertoli cells, while intratesticular injection may be useful for Leydig cells.

It is important to choose an appropriate vector for clinical use. The disadvantage of liposome and electroporation methods for clinical application was that they showed potential for gene expression in germ cells and strong adverse effects on spermatogenesis. On the other hand, adenovirus-mediated gene transfer may be a more effective and superior method for transfecting testicular cells among these three methods and may be more applicable for gene therapy for male infertility in the future (Kojima, 2005).

5.3.2 Candidate genes of future gene therapy for male infertility

Spermatogenesis is a complex program of differentiation that takes place within the testicular seminiferous tubules, which are composed of germ cells and somatic Sertoli cells (Brehm & Steger, 2005; Bergmann 2005). Two control mechanisms are involved in the regulation of spermatogenesis; hormone and genetics. Sertoli cells trigger germ cell development by not only mediating hormonal stimuli of FSH and androgen secreted by Leydig cells, but also numerous genes. Understanding the mechanisms by which genes and gene products are expressed or repressed in the testes enables the development of strategies to treat male infertility. A lot of candidate male fertility-associated genes have been revealed from knockout mice phenotypes (Cram, 2001, O'Bryan MK & de Kretser, 2006). It is important to perform detailed phenotypic analysis in order to extract the maximum amount of information from each model; however, despite the identification of an increasing number of candidate genes involved in spermatogenesis, the range of diagnostic genetic tests for male infertility remains extremely limited (Nuti & Krausz, 2008). Normal spermatogenesis and fertility are dependent upon paracrine or autocrine interactions between somatic cells (Sertoli and Leydig cells) and germ cells, and upon endocrine support from the pituitary gland (Saunders, 2003).

Several possible genes may be essential for Sertoli and Leydig cell function to support normal spermatogenesis. Testicular gene therapy for these cells as target cells may be useful to treat male infertility in the future, especially for those who have no spermatozoa in their testes at all, such as pathological maturation arrest or Sertoli cells only. From our viewpoint, Sertoli cells are more appropriate target cells, because they perform crucial functions that initiate, promote and maintain spermatogenesis directly in seminiferous tubules.

Disorders of testicular function may originate as a result of abnormal development or proliferation of Sertoli cells (Sharpe, 2003). Idiopathic male infertility, including pathologically maturation arrest and Sertoli cell-only syndrome, may result in abnormal Sertoli cell function, which disrupts the normal progression of spermatogenesis [Kojima et al. 2006c].

Marker genes of maturity and immaturity of Sertoli cells include anti-Müllerian hormone, vimentin, connexin 26, connexin 43, aromatase, cytokeratin-18, GATA1, laminin α5, M2A antigen, $p27^{kip1}$, inhibin α, sulphated glycoprotein 2, androgen receptor and WT-1 (Brehm &

Steger, 2005; Sharpe, 2003). In addition, alterations of transcription regulation in the testis may cause idiopathic male infertility. Transcription factors include CREB, Sox3, Pem (Rhox5) and DAX1, which are essential for spermatogenesis and are expressed not in germ cells but in Sertoli cells of seminiferous tubules (Hummler, 1994; Yu, 1998; Weiss, 2003; Maclean, 2005a,b; Kojima, 2006c). Clarifying the role of these factors in spermatogenesis may advance the clinical application of gene therapy for patients with male infertility.

On the other hand, Leydig cells may also be target cells of gene therapy. Hypotheses about the underlying mechanism of the depletion of germ cells in Klinefelter syndrome males, which is the most common sex chromosome abnormality and the most frequent genetic cause of male infertility, include Leydig cell insufficiency and disturbed apoptosis regulation of Leydig cells (Aksglaede, 2006). There is also evidence of Leydig cell impairment in a proportion of men treated with cytotoxic chemotherapy for malignant disease (Howell, 2001). Endocrine disruptors can disrupt not only spermatogenesis but also normal endocrine function of Leydig cells, acting directly on Leydig cells to diminish testosterone production by interfering with the expression of specific genes in the steroidogenic pathway (Skakkebaek, 2001). Marker genes, including P450(CYP) steroid hydroxylase, 3β-HSD [143], Androgen receptor [144], LHR [145], Ad4BP/SF-1 [134,146,147] are expressed in Leydig cells (Weiss, 1992, Morohashi, 1993, 1994; Luo, 1994; Xu, 2007; Kojima, 2006c,], which are implicated in steroidogenesis or spermatogenesis. They may also be candidate genes for gene therapy in the future.

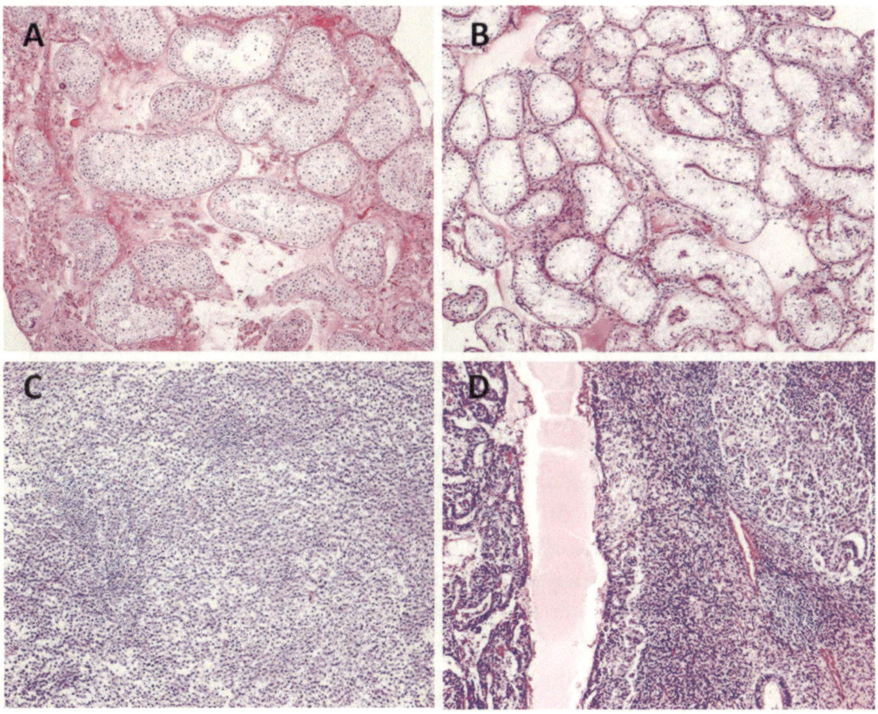

Fig. 2. Histological findings of normal spermatogenesis (A), male infertility, (Sertoli-cell only) (B) and testicular cancer; seminoma (C) and non-seminoma (embryonal carcinoma and teratoma) (D).

6. Future prospects of gene therapy for testicular cancer

6.1 Testicular cancer and germ cell tumor

Testicular cancer is the most frequent solid tumor in young male adults and a disease with elusive pathogenesis. Germ cell tumors (GCTs) represent 95% of all testicular cancers (Diamantopoulos, 2010). Testicular cancer represents the most curable solid tumor, with a 10-year survival rate of more than 95% (Travis, 2010). Especially, clinical stage I testicular cancer is highly curable. Since treatment for testicular cancer directly affects gonadal tissues, fertility rate after treatment for testicular cancer is reduced.

GCTs are divided into two broad group, seminnoma and non-seminoma. Seminoma retains the morphology of spermatogonial GCs. On the other hand, non-seminoma display embryonal and extra-embryonal differentiation patterns which include primitive zygotic (embryonal carcinoma), embryonal-like somatically differentiated (teratoma), and embryonally differentiated (choriocarcinoma and yolk-sac tumor) phenotypes (Chaganti & Houldsworth 2000).

6.2 Present therapeutic options of testicular cancer and its limitation

Treatment strategy is chosen according to the patient stage and prognostic group stratification. The standard therapy is generally considered to be radical orchiectomy even for bilateral testis cancer; however, partial orchiectomy should be undertaken only in selected patients -men with bilateral testicular cancer or GCTs in a solitary testis-if the size and location of the mass are amenable to surgery. Partial orchiectomy provides potential benefits over radical surgery by reducing the need for androgen substitution, lessening psychological stress, and preserving fertility, with a durable cure rate. However, partial orchiectomy is not always appropriate according to tumor size. Although alternative strategies of organ preservation, such as radiotherapy and chemotherapy, might be appropriate treatment options in the future, the safety and efficacy of these procedures have not been demonstrated in larger and prospective studies with longer follow-up (Zuniga, 2010). Therefore, gene therapy may be one of the options for testicular cancer in the future.

6.3 Therapeutic potential of gene transfer to tesits for testicular cancer

Several preclinical studies have demonstrated that gene therapy produced antitumor effects, suggesting its feasibility in clinical settings. Actual trials of gene therapy for certain cancers have already been reported; however, to our knowledge, there is no report about gene therapy for GCTs, because of complexity of its pathogenesis. Therefore, which method or vector is useful for clinical application has remained unknown.

A lot of researchers have attempted to identify the candidate genes of GCTs. Cytogenetic and molecular genetic analysis of GCTs has yielded important data relevant to the understanding of the mechanism of GC transformation (Chaganti & Houldsworth, 2000). Virtually 100% of tumors show increased copy number of the short arm of chromosome 12 (12p), as one or more copies of isochoromosome of12p or as tandem duplications of 12p, *in situ* or transposed elsewhere in the genome. This observation enhanced our understanding of the underlying genetic etiology of the disease because of its invariant presence (Houldsworth, 2006). Because the entire 12p, comprising about 400 genes, is involved, this would suggest that at least two, if not more, physically distant loci are the targets of the abnormality. In this region, there are several candidates with functions consistent with roles in cell growth, including *CCND2, GLUT3, GAPDH, TPI1 NANOG, DPPA3* and *GDF3*. It is

clear that gain of 12p is multifunctional with respect to biologic processes affected, which in this unique tumor system are inextricably linked; transformation and maintenance of pluripotency (Houldsworth, 2006). Epigenetic approach can also provide new knowledge about pathogenesis of GCTs. Aberrant promoter hypermethylation has been reported for several genes (*PRSS21, MGMT, RASSF1A*) in GCTs, suggestive of roles in GC transformation (Houldsworth, 2006).
Stem cell research has provided new insights on pathogenesis of GCTs. Cancer stem cells may be target for cancer cells (Hombach-Klonisch, 2008). It is becoming increasingly evidence that cancer constitutes a group of diseases involving altered stem cell maturation/differentiation and the disturbance of regenerative process. Previous study showed a substantial overlap in the expression patterns of testicular embryonal carcinomas and embryonic stem (ES) cells. Several candidate genes including *Oct3/4, SOX2, CENPA* and *PODXL*, which may contribute to the maintenance of plutipotency, have recently been detected. They may also be candidate genes for gene therapy in the future

7. Conclusions

Our limited understanding of the complex regulatory mechanisms underlying normal spermatogenesis and pathogenesis of GCTs makes it difficult to identify specific target genes for gene therapy for male infertility and GCTs. Recent remarkable advance in molecular approaches have contributed to find candidate genes and provided new knowledge on molecular genetics of testicular disorders including male infertility and GCTs. Although more genetic information about the molecular basis of spermatogenesis, male infertility and GCTs will be needed to apply gene therapy for male infertility and GCTs patients, these information will lead to new strategies for the clinical management and gene therapy will provides great benefits for the patients with these testicular diseases in the near future.

8. References

Aksglaede L, Wikström AM, Rajpert-De Meyts E, Dunkel L, Skakkebaek NE, Juul A. (2006) Natural history of seminiferous tubule degeneration in Klinefelter syndrome.Hum Reprod Update 12:39-48.
Alukal JP, Lamb DJ. Intracytoplasmic sperm injection (ICSI)--what are the risks? (2008) Urol Clin North Am. 35:277-288.
Amin R, Wilmott R, Schwarz Y, Trapnell B, Stark J (1995) Replication-deficient adenovirus induces expression of interleukin-8 by airway epithelial cells *in vitro*. Hum Gene Ther. 6:145-153.
Appledorn DM, Seregin S, Amalfitano A. (2008) Adenovirus vectors for renal-targeted gene delivery. Contrib Nephrol. 159:47-62.
Baum C, Schambach A, Bohne J, Galla M. Retrovirus vectors: toward the plentivirus? (2006) Mol Ther 13:1050-1063.
Bergmann M (2005) Spermatogenesis--physiology and pathophysiology Urologe A. 44:1131-1132.
Blanchard KT, Boekelheide K (1997) Adenovirus-mediated gene transfer to rat testis *in vivo*.Biol Reprod 56:495-500.

Brackett BG, Baranska W, Sawicki W, Koprowski H. (1971) Uptake of heterologous genome by mammalian spermatozoa and its transfer to ova through fertilization.Proc Natl Acad Sci U S A 68:353-357.

Brehm R, Steger K. (2005) Regulation of Sertoli cell and germ cell differentation. Adv Anat Embryol Cell Biol 181:1-93.

Bushman FD (2007) Retroviral integration and human gene therapy. J Clin Invest 117:2083-2086.

Celebi C, Auvray P, Benvegnu T, Plusquellec D, Jégou B, Guillaudeux T (2002) Transient transmission of a transgene in mouse offspring following *in vivo* transfection of male germ cells. Mol Reprod Dev 62: 477-482.

Chaganti RS, Houldsworth J (2000) Genetics and biology of adult human male germ cell tumors. Cancer Res. 60:1475-82

Cockrell AS, Kafri T (2007) Gene delivery by lentivirus vectors. Mol Biotechnol. 36:184-204.

Cox GF, Burger J, Lip V Mau UA, Sperling K, Wu BL, Horsthemke B (2002) Intracytoplasmic sperm injection may increase the risk of imprinting defects. Am J Hum Genet 71:162–16

Cram DS, O'Bryan MK, de Kretser DM (2001) Male infertility genetics--the future. J Androl 22:738-746.

Danno S, Itoh K, Baum C (1999) Efficient gene transfer by hybrid retroviral vectors to murine spermatogenic cells. Hum Gene Ther 10:1819-1831.

De Miguel MP, Donovan PJ. Determinants of retroviral-mediated gene delivery to mouse spermatogonia. Biol Reprod 2003; 68:860-866.

De Vry J, Martínez-Martínez P, Losen M, Temel Y, Steckler T, Steinbusch HW, De Baets MH, Prickaerts J (2010) *In vivo* electroporation of the central nervous system: a non-viral approach for targeted gene delivery. Prog Neurobiol. 92:227-44.

Diamantopoulos N, Kortsaris A (2010). Testicular germ cell tumors. J BUON. 15:421-34.

Dobashi M, Goda K, Maruyama H, Fujisawa M (2005) Erythropoietin gene transfer into rat testes by *in vivo* electropo-ration may reduce the risk of germ cell loss caused by cryptorchidism. Asian J Androl 7:369-373.

Escors D, Breckpot K. Lentiviral vectors in gene therapy: their current status and future potential (2010). Arch Immunol Ther Exp (Warsz). 58(2):107-19.

Felgner PL, Gadek TR, Holm M (1987) Lipofection: a highly efficient, lipid-mediated DNA-transfection procedure. Proc Natl Acad Sci U S A 84:7413-7417.

Francolini M, Lavitrano M, Lamia CL (1993) Evidence for nuclear internalization of exogenous DNA into mammalian sperm cells. Mol Reprod Dev 34:133-139.

Fujisawa M, Shirakawa T, Fujioka H (2001) Adenovirus-mediated p53 gene transfer to rat testis impairs spermatogenesis. Arch Androl 46:223-231.

Gagné MB, Pothier F, Sirard MA (1991) Electroporation of bovine spermatozoa to carry foreign DNA in oocytes. Mol Reprod Dev 29:6-15.

Goda K, Fujisawa M, Shirakawa T (2004) Adenoviral-mediated HGF expression inhibits germ cell apoptosis in rats with cryptorchidism. J Gene Med 6:869-876.

Goldstein M, Tanrikut C (2006). Microsurgical management of male infertility. Nat Clin Pract Urol 3:381-391.

Greenberg SH, Lipshultz LI, Wein AJ (1978) Experience with 425 subfertile male patients. J Urol 119:507-510.

Hansen M, Kurinczuk JJ, Bower C, Webb S (2002) The risk of major birth defects after intracytoplasmic sperm injection and *in vitro* fertilization. N Engl J Med 346:725–730.

Hombach-Klonisch S, Paranjothy T, Wiechec E, Pocar P, Mustafa T, Seifert A, Zahl C, Gerlach KL, Biermann K, Steger K, Hoang-Vu C, Schulze-Osthoff K, Los M (2008) Cancer stem cells as targets for cancer therapy: selected cancers as examples. Arch Immunol Ther Exp (Warsz). 56:165-80.

Horan R, Powell R, Bird JM, Gannon F, Houghton JA (1992) Effects of electropermeabilization on the association of foreign DNA with pig sperm.Arch Androl 28:105-114.

Houldsworth J, Korkola JE, Bosl GJ, Chaganti RS (2006). Biology and genetics of adult male germ cell tumors. J Clin Oncol. 24:5512-8.

Howell SJ, Shalet SM (2001) Testicular function following chemotherapy. Hum Reprod Update. 7:363-369.

Hu YC (2008) Baculoviral vectors for gene delivery: a review. Curr Gene Ther. 8:54-65.

Huguet E, Esponda P (1998). Foreign DNA introduced into the vas deferens is gained by mammalian spermatozoa. Mol Reprod Dev 51:42–52.

Huguet E, Esponda P (2000) Generation of genetically modified mice by spermatozoa transfection *in vivo*: preliminary results.Mol Reprod Dev 56:243-7.

Hummler E, Cole TJ, Blendy JA (1994) Targeted mutation of the CREB gene: compensation within the CREB/ATF family of transcription factors. Proc Natl Acad Sci U S A 91:5647-5651.

Ikawa M, Tergaonkar V, Ogura A, Ogonuki N, Inoue K, Verma IM (2002) Restoration of spermatogenesis by lentiviral gene transfer: offspring from infertile mice. Proc Natl Acad Sci U S A 99:7524-7529.

Ike A, Ohta H, Onishi M, Iguchi N, Nishimune Y, Nozaki M (2004) Transient expression analysis of the mouse ornithine decarboxylase antizyme haploid-specific promoter using *in vivo* electroporation. FEBS Lett 559:159-164.

In't Veld P, Branderburg H, Verhoeff A, Dhont M, Los F (1995) Sex chromosomal anomalies and intracytoplasmic sperm injection. Lancet 346:773

Kanatsu-Shinohara M, Toyokuni S, Shinohara T (2004)Transgenic mice produced by retroviral transduction of male germ line stem cells *in vivo*. Biol Reprod 71:1202-1207.

Kim SH, Kim S, Robbins PD (2006) Retroviral vectors. Adv Virus Res. 2000;55:545-563.

Kim SY. Assessing and communicating the risks and benefits of gene transfer clinical trials. Curr Opin Mol Ther. 8:384-389.

Kojima Y, Sasaki S, Umemoto Y, Hashimoto Y, Hayashi Y, Kohri K. (2003) Effects of adenovirus mediated gene transfer to mouse testis *in vivo* on spermatogenesis and next generation. J Urol 170:2109-2114.

Kojima Y, Sasaki S, Umemoto Y, Hashimoto Y, Hayashi Y, Kohri K (2005) Comparison of characteristics of several vectors to testicular gene transfer system. J Urol 173 (Suppl):407-408.

Kojima Y., Sasaki S, Kohri K (2006a) Therapeutic options: Current research and future prospects for gene therapy in andrology. In: Eds Hargreave T, Comhaire F and Schill W-B. Andrology for clinician. Heiderberg, Springer; pp592-598.

Kojima Y, Sasaki S, Hayashi Y, Umemoto Y, Morohashi K, Kohri K (2006b). Role of transcription factors Ad4BP/SF-1 and DAX-1 in steroidogenesis and spermatogenesis in human testicular development and idiopathic azoospermia. Int J Urol 13:785-793.

Kojima Y, Kurokawa S, Mizuno K, Umemoto Y, Sasaki S, Hayashi Y, Kohri K (2008a) Gene transfer to sperm and testis: future prospects of gene therapy for male infertility. Curr Gene Ther. 8:121-34

Kojima Y, Hayashi Y, Kurokawa S, Mizuno K, Sasaki S, Kohri K (2008b) No evidence of germ-line transmission by adenovirus-mediated gene transfer to mouse testes. Fertil Steril. 89:1448-1454.

Kost TA, Condreay JP, Jarvis DL (2005) Baculovirus as versatile vectors for protein expression in insect and mammalian cells. Nat Biotechnol 23:567-575.

Kuhlmann KF, Gouma DJ, Wesseling JG (2008) Adenoviral gene therapy for pancreatic cancer: where do we stand? Dig Surg. 25:278-292

Kurokawa S, Kojima Y, Mizuno K, Nakane A, Hayashi Y, Kohri K (2005) Effect of epidermal growth factor on spermatogenesis in the cryptorchid rat. J Urol. 174:2415-2419.

Lamb DJ. Would gene therapy for the treatment of male infertility be safe? (2008) Nat Clin Pract Urol. 5:594-595.

Lavitrano M, Camaioni A, Fazio VM, Dolci S, Farace MG, Spadafora C (1989) Sperm cells as vectors for introducing foreign DNA into eggs: genetic transformation of mice. Cell 57:717-723.

Lavitrano M, French D, Zani M, Frati L, Spadafora C (1992) The interaction between exogenous DNA and sperm cells. Mol Reprod Dev 31:161-169.

Lavitrano M, Maione B, Forte E (1997) The interaction of sperm cells with exogenous DNA: a role of CD4 and major histocompatibility complex class II molecules. Exp Cell Res 233:56-62.

Lavitrano M, Busnelli M, Cerrito MG, Giovannoni R, Manzini S, Vargiolu A. (2006) Sperm-mediated gene transfer. Reprod Fertil Dev 18:19-23.

Liebaers I, Bonduelle M, Van Assche E, Devroey P, Van Steirteghem A (1995) Sex chromosome abnormalities after intracytoplasmic sperm injection. Lancet 346:1095

Loft A, Petersen K, Erb K Mikkelsen AL, Grinsted J, Hald F, Hindkjaer J, Nielsen KM, Lundstrom P, Gabrielsen A, Lenz S, Hornnes P, Ziebe S, Ejdrup HB, Lindhard A, Zhou Y, Nyboe Andersen A (1999) Danish cohort of 730 infants born after intracytoplasmic sperm injection (ICSI) 1994–1997. Hum Reprod 14:2143–2148

Luo X, Ikeda Y, Parker KL (1994) A cell-specific nuclear receptor is essential for adrenal and gonadal development and sexual differentiation. Cell 77: 1994;481-90.

Matzuk MM, Lamb DJ (2008) The biology of infertility: research advances and clinical challenges. Nat Med. 14:1197-1213.

Maclean JA 2nd, Wilkinson MF. Gene regulation in spermatogenesis (2005a) Curr Top Dev Biol 71:131-197.

Maclean JA 2nd, Chen MA, Wayne CM (2005b) Rhox: a new homeobox gene cluster. Cell 120:369-382.

Merrihew RV, Kost TA, Condreay JP (2004) Baculovirus-mediated gene delivery into mammalian cells.Methods. Mol Biol 246:355-365.

Morohashi K, Zanger UM, Honda S, Hara M, Waterman MR, Omura T (1993) Activation of CYP11A and CYP11B gene promoters by the steroidogenic cell-specific transcription factor, Ad4BP. Mol. Endocrinol 7: 1196-204.

Morohashi K, Omura T (1994) Ad4BP/SF-1, a transcription factor essential for the transcription of steroidogenic cytochrome P450 genes and for the establishment of the reproductive function. FASEB J 10: 1569-77.

Muramatsu T, Shibata O, Ohmori Y, Okumura J (1996) *In vivo* electroporation: A convenient method for gene transfer to testicular cells in mice. Anim Sci Technol 67:975-982.

Muramatsu T, Shibata O, Ryoki S, Ohmori Y, Okumura J (1997) Foreign gene expression in the mouse testis by localized *in vivo* gene transfer. Biochem Biophys Res Commun 233:45-49.

Nagano M, Brinster CJ, Orwig KE, Ryu BY, Avarbock MR, Brinster RL (2001) Transgenic mice produced by retroviral transduction of male germ-line stem cells.Proc Natl Acad Sci U S A 98:13090-13095.

Navarro J, Risco R, Toschi M, Schattman G (2008) Gene therapy and intracytoplasmatic sperm injection (ICSI) - a review. Placenta. 29:193-199.

Nuti F, Krausz C (2008) Gene polymorphisms/mutations relevant to abnormal spermatogenesis. Reprod Biomed Online. 2008;16:504-513

Oates RD. The genetic basis of male reproductive failure. Urol Clin North Am.35:257-70

O'Bryan MK, de Kretser D (2006) Mouse models for genes involved in impaired spermatogenesis. Int J Androl 29:76-89.

Ogawa S, Hayashi K, Tada N, Sato M, Kurihara T, Iwaya M (1995) Gene expression in blastocysts following direct injection of DNA into testis. J Reprod Dev 41: 379-382.

Ombelet W, Cooke I, Dyer S, Serour G, Devroey P (2008) Infertility and the provision of infertility medical services in developing countries. Hum Reprod Update. 14:605-621

Orwig KE, Avarbock MR, Brinster RL (2002) Retrovirus-mediated modification of male germline stem cells in rats.Biol Reprod 67:874-879.

Palermo G, Joris H, Devroey P, Van Steirteghem AC (1992) Pregnancies after intracytoplasmic injection of single spermatozoon into an oocyte. Lancet. 340:17-18.

Palermo GD, Cohen J, Rosenwaks Z (1996). Intracytoplasmic sperm injection: a powerful tool to overcome fertilization failure. Fertil Steril 65:899-908.

Park HJ, Lee WY, Kim JH, Kim JH, Jung HJ, Kim NH, Kim BK, Song H (2009) Interstitial tissue-specific gene expression in mouse testis by intra-tunica albuguineal injection of recombinant baculovirus. Asian J Androl. 1:342-50.

Ryoki S, Park H, Ohmori Y, Shoji-Tanaka A, Muramatsu T (2001) An integrase facilitates long-lasting foreign gene expression *in vivo* in mouse spermatogenic cells. J Biosci Bioeng 91:363-367.

Sato M, Gotoh K, Kimura M (1999) Sperm-mediated gene transfer by direct injection of foreign DNA into mouse testis. Transgenics 2:357–369.

Sato M, Ishikawa A, Kimura M (2002). Direct injection of foreign DNA into mouse testis as a possible *in vivo* gene transfer system via epididymal spermatozoa. Mol Reprod Dev 61:49-56.

Saunders PT (2003) Germ cell-somatic cell interactions during spermatogenesis. Reprod Suppl. 61:91-101.

Schieve LA, Meikle SF, Ferre C, Peterson HB, Jeng G, Wilcox LS (2002) Low and very low birth weight in infants conceived with use of assisted reproductive technology. N Engl J Med 346:731–737

Sharpe RM, McKinnell C, Kivlin C, Fisher JS (2003) Proliferation and functional maturation of Sertoli cells, and their relevance to disorders of testis function in adulthood. Reproduction 2003;125:769-784.

Shoji M, Chuma S, Yoshida K, Morita T, Nakatsuji N (2005) RNA interference during spermatogenesis in mice. Dev Biol 282:524-534.

Skakkebaek NE, Rajpert-De Meyts E, Main KM (2001) Testicular dysgenesis syndrome: an increasingly common developmental disorder with environmental aspects. Hum Reprod 16:972-978.

Smith KR. Gene therapy: theoretical and bioethical concepts (2003) Arch Med Res 34: 247-268.

Staessen C, Camus M, Clasen K, De Vos A, Van Steirteghem A (1999) Conventional in-vitro fertilization versus intracytoplasmic sperm injection in sibling oocytes from couples with tubal infertility and normozoospermic semen. Hum Reprod 14:2474-2479.

Sutcliffe AG, Taylor B, Saunders K, Thornton S, Lieberman BA, Grudzinskas JG (2001) Outcome in the second year of life after in-vitro fertilisation by intracytoplasmic sperm injection: a UK case-control study. Lancet 357:2080–2084

Takehashi M, Kanatsu-Shinohara M, Inoue K (2007) Adenovirus-mediated gene delivery into mouse spermatogonial stem cells.Proc Natl Acad Sci U S A 2007;104:2596-2601.

Tani H, Limn CK, Yap CC (2003) *In vitro* and *in vivo* gene delivery by recombinant baculoviruses. 2003; J Virol 77:9799-9808.

Travis LB, Beard C, Allan JM, Dahl AA, Feldman DR, Oldenburg J, Daugaard G, Kelly JL, Dolan ME, Hannigan R, Constine LS, Oeffinger KC, Okunieff P, Armstrong G, Wiljer D, Miller RC, Gietema JA, van Leeuwen FE, Williams JP, Nichols CR, Einhorn LH, Fossa SD (2010) Testicular cancer survivorship: research strategies and recommendations. J Natl Cancer Inst. 102:1114-30.

Umemoto Y, Sasaki S, Kojima Y (2002) *In vivo* gene transfer to mouse testis and the influence of mouse spermatogenesis. J Urol 2002;167 (Suppl): 322.

Umemoto Y, Sasaki S, Kojima Y (2005) Gene transfer to mouse testes by electroporation and its influence on spermatogenesis. J Androl . 2005;26:264-271.

Weichselbaum RR, Kufe D. Gene therapy of cancer. Lancet 1997;349:10-12.

Weiss J, Axelrod L, Whitcomb RW, Harris PE, Crowley WF, Jameson JL (1992) Hypogonadism caused by a single amino acid substitution in the beta subunit of luteinizing hormone. N Engl J Med 326:179-183.

Weiss J, Meeks JJ, Hurley L, Raverot G, Frassetto A, Jameson JL (2003) Sox3 is required for gonadal function, but not sex determination, in males and females. Mol Cell Biol 23:8084-8091.

Xu Q, Lin HY, Yeh SD (2007) Infertility with defective spermatogenesis and steroidogenesis in male mice lacking androgen receptor in Leydig cells. Endocrine 32:96-106.

Yamamoto H, Ochiya T, Tamamushi S (2002) HST-1/FGF-4 gene activation induces spermatogenesis and prevents adriamycin-induced testicular toxicity. Oncogene 21:899-908.

Yamazaki Y, Fujimoto H, Ando H, Ohyama T, Hirota Y, Noce T (1998) *In vivo* gene transfer to mouse spermatogenic cells by deoxyribonucleic acid injection into seminiferous tubules and subsequent electroporation. Biol Reprod 59:1439-1444.

Yamazaki Y, Yagi T, Ozaki T, Imoto K (2000) *In vivo* gene transfer to mouse spermatogenic cells using green fluorescent protein as a marker. J Exp Zool 286:212-218.

Yang Y, Nunes FA, Berencsi K, Furth EE, Gönczöl E, Wilson JM (1994) Cellular immuninty to viral antigen limits E1-deleted adenoviruses for gene therapy. Proc Natl Acad Sci USA 91: 4407-4411.

Yomogida K, Yagura Y, Nishimune Y (2002) Electroporated transgene-rescued spermatogenesis in infertile mutant mice with a sertoli cell defect.Biol Reprod 67:712-717.

Yonezawa T, Furuhata Y, Hirabayashi K, Suzuki M, Takahashi M, Nishihara M (2001) Detection of transgene in progeny at different developmental stages following testis-mediated gene transfer. Mol Reprod Dev 60:196-201.

Yu RN, Ito M, Saunders TL, Camper SA, Jameson JL (1998) Role of Ahch in gonadal development and gametogenesis. Nat Genet 20:353-357.

Zani M, Lavitrano M, French D, Lulli V, Maione B, Sperandio S, Spadafora C (1995) The mechanism of binding of exogenous DNA to sperm cells: factors controlling the DNA uptake. Exp Cell Res 217:57-64.

Zuniga A, Lawrentschuk N, Jewett MA (2010). Organ-sparing approaches for testicular masses. Nat Rev Urol. 2010;7:454-64.

17

Quality of Life of Patients with Hormone Refractory Prostate Cancer After Gene Therapy

Akinobu Gotoh[1], Shuji Terao[1] and Toshiro Shirakawa[2]
[1]*Laboratory of Cell and Gene Therapy, Institute for Advanced Medical Sciences, Hyogo College of Medicine, Nishinomiya,*
[2]*International Center for Medical Research and Treatment, Kobe University School of Medicine, Kobe,*
Japan

1. Introduction

Bone metastasis in cancer patients is observed with high clinical frequency and is associated not only with cancer pain but also with pathological fractures, restriction of daily activities, and other skeletal-related events (SRE). It is therefore an issue with a very decisive effect on subsequent quality of life (QOL) (Chow & Bottomley, 2009). The development of new therapies for bone metastasis in recent years has allowed progress from the use of narcotic formulations, typical of which are the conventional opioid drugs, to treatments focused on 'bone health' which apply a multidisciplinary approach combining use for instance of high-strength bisphosphonate preparations and radionuclide therapy (Satoh et al., 2009). In prostate cancer and breast cancer, which have very high incidence of bone metastasis, there are many cases where survival of a number of years can be expected even at the stage of the illness where this kind of metastasis is present, and the therapeutic strategy needs to take account of QOL.

Each year thousands of men are diagnosed with prostate cancer; it is estimated that about 192,280 men will be diagnosed with this disease in 2009 (American Cancer Society, 2008). In advanced disease, androgen-deprivation therapy remains the best treatment. After a median response of 12 to 24 months, patients develop progressive hormone-refractory prostate cancer (HRPC) (Carroll et al., 2002, Chodak et al., 2002). Therefore, the development of new therapies with a survival advantage and greater antitumor effects is necessary. Gene therapy is a good candidate among new therapies.

The phase I clinical trial of the combination therapy of osteocalcin promoter-driven herpes-simplex-virus thymidine kinase (Ad-OC-TK) and valacyclovir (VAL) for the treatment of HRPC has been conducted previously at the University of Virginia (Kubo et al., 2003). Between August 2003 and March 2006, a phase I/II dose-escalating clinical trial of intratumoral injections of Ad-OC-TK was performed on 6 patients with HRPC in order to assess the potential toxicity and therapeutic effects of this treatment at Kobe University Hospital (Hinata et al., 2006, Shirakawa et al., 2007). In clinical oncological trials, the therapeutic effects on the tumor volume and the serum levels of tumor markers are frequently used as the primary therapeutic indices. However, recently, the assessment of QOL has become an important therapeutic index. Since prostate cancer generally has a

protracted natural history, it is particularly important for patients with HRPC to receive therapies that preserve or improve QOL, delay the progression of disease caused by severe pain, and provide quality-adjusted clinical benefits (Ho et al., 2006).
Among the QOL assessment systems developed so far are the European Organization for Research and Treatment of Cancer (EORTC), Quality of Life Questionnaire-Core 30 (QLQ-C30) (Aaronson et al., 1993), Functional Assessment of Cancer Therapy scale-General (FACT-G) (Cella et al., 1993) and MOS Short-Form 36-Item Health Survey (SF-36) (Ware & Sherbourne, 1992) systems, which have been translated and tested for use in a wide range of languages. Modules for quality of life assessment in specific diseases have also been developed and applied clinically, for instance EORTC-QLQ-LC13 (Bergman et al., 1994) and FACT-L (Cella et al., 1995) for lung cancer, EORTC-QLQ-BR23 (Sprangers et al., 1996) and FACT-B (Brady et al., 1997) for breast cancer, and European Organization for Research and Treatment of Cancer Quality of Life Questionnaire's prostate cancer-specific module (EORTC QLQ-PR25) (da Silva et al., 1993) and FACT-P (Esper et al., 1997) for prostate cancer. However, no QOL module had so far been developed for bone metastasis patients. We designed a questionnaire, formulated with reference to the EORTC-QLQ- PR25 assessment system. This is the first study, the short-term QOL and bodily pain of patients with HRPC who were undergoing a clinical trial involving the direct administration of the combination of Ad-OC-TK gene therapy plus VAL intra-lesionally in men with metastatic prostate cancer was evaluated.

2. Patients and methods

2.1 Eligibility criteria

The eligibility criteria included the presence of metastatic or locally recurrent prostate cancer, histologically confirmed adenocarcinoma, and confirmed disease progression despite surgery, radiation, androgen blockage, and/or conventional chemotherapy. Patients who were receiving androgen deprivation therapy including anti-androgen therapy underwent an at least 4-week anti-androgen withdrawal period before enrollment to exclude possible effects of anti-androgen withdrawal syndrome (Scher and Kelly, 1993). Luteinizing hormone-releasing hormone(LH-RH) agonist was continued during the anti-androgen withdrawal period and throughout the study. Further, each patient included must have had a lesion measurable by an imaging examination, and a single selected lesion had to be amenable to intralesional injection of the therapeutic agent.

2.2 Vector and valacyclovir

The replication-deficient adenoviral vector belongs to subgenus C, serotype 5 (Ad5) with the HSV-tk gene under the control of a tumor-restrictive OC promoter in the area of the excised E1 region. Ad-OC-TK was constructed via homologous recombination vector, as described previously (Ko et al., 1996). The Good Manufacturing Practice (GMP)-grade adenoviral vector (Lusky, 2005) was manufactured and characterized extensively by Molecular Medicine Bioservices (Carlsbad, CA) before clinical application. The oral antiviral agent valacyclovir (Valtrex; GlaxoSmithKline, Tokyo, Japan) has been approved in Japan for several indications, including treatment for herpes zoster and genital herpes. We used the worldwide-approved valacyclovir dosage of 1 g, three times daily (Tyring et al., 2000) in our clinical trial.

2.3 Study design

Six patients were divided into the low-dose and high-dose viral vector group (3 patients at each dose level). Ad-OC-TK was injected directly into the localized recurrent tumor or the bone metastatic lesion under the guidance of transrectal ultrasonography (TRUS) or computed tomography (CT). Only one index lesion per patient was selected, typically that representing the largest metastasis, causing severe bone pain at the metastatic site, or preventing urination by local recurrent tumor. The doses used were 2.5×10^9 (low-dose group: 3 patients) and 2.5×10^{10} (high-dose group: 3 patients) plaque-forming units (PFU) on Day 1 and Day 8. The patients were given 1 g of VAL three times daily for 21 days.

2.4 Assessment of the short-term QOL and bodily pain

Since there was no questionnaire for assessing the short-term QOL in patients receiving gene therapy for HRPC, we created a questionnaire (Table 1) (Terao, 2009) was created based on the EORTC QLQ-PR25 which is widely used to assess QOL in patients of prostate cancer. The questionnaire comprised scores evaluating role limitations in work (2 items), physical or social functioning (4 items), interpersonal relationships (2 items), emotional functioning (3 items), and sleep/vitality (2 items) as well as the global health status (2 items). A higher median value obtained on the symptom scale indicated a higher number of symptoms or problems. All the patients answered the questionnaire by themselves on days 0 (pretreatment), 14 and 28. The patients indicated how true a statement had been for them over the past 14 days using a 4-point scale as follows: 0, not at all; 1, a little bit; 2, quite a bit; 3, very much. All items were assigned equal weightage. Further, all the patients scored themselves on a visual analogue scale (VAS) with regard to their bodily pain on day 0, 14 and 28 as follows: 0%, they did not experience any bodily pain; 100%, they experienced severe bodily pain (EuroQol, 1990).

Global health status
- How much influence in your health?
- How much influence in your life?

Role limitation of work
- How much influence in your home works such as clean, shopping and so on ?
- How much influence in the work and the daily activity out of home?

Role limitation of physical or social
- How much influence to move your body such as stroll, running, sports and so on?
- How much influence to use a bus, a car, train, an airplane and so on?
- How much influence in the relationship having to do with the world?
- How much influence to call or meet your friends?

Personal relationship
- How much influence in the relation with your companion and partner?
- How much influence in the life with the family?

Emotional
- Did you felt depress?
- Did you felt anxiety and became nervous?
- Did you became miserable?

Sleep /Vitality
- How much influence in the dormancy?
- Did you felt fatigue?

Table 1. Questionnaire. Answer questions from 0-3 (0: not at all; 1: a little bit; 2: quite a bit; 3: very much).

2.5 Correlation of the change of PSA with QOL and bodily pain

The correlation of serum prostate-specific antigen (PSA) levels with short-term total QOL scores and bodily pain was assessed by measuring the rate of change (%) of the serum PSA levels, the short-term total QOL scores, and bodily pain from day 0 to day 28; these values were expressed as ⊿PSA, ⊿QOL, and ⊿Pain, respectively (Terao et al., 2009).

2.6 Statistical analysis

The short-term QOL scores of patients (nonparametric data) were analyzed by Friedman one-way ANOVA. The Spearman test was used to analyze the correlation of ⊿PSA with ⊿QOL and ⊿Pain. $P < 0.05$ was considered to be statistically significant.

3. Results

3.1 Patient characteristics

The mean age of the patients was 68 years (range, 63–77 years). The mean pretreatment serum PSA level was 222.7 ng/mL (range, 46.6–455.5 ng/mL). Three patients (50%) had been diagnosed with poorly differentiated adenocarcinoma and the other 3 (50%) had been diagnosed with moderately differentiated adenocarcinoma. All the patients had multiple bone metastatic lesions. In addition, 2 patients (33.3 %) had locally recurrent lesions. Two patients (33.3%) had undergone radical prostatectomy in the past and all the patients had been treated with androgen-deprivation therapy.

3.2 Short-term QOL and bodily pain

All 6 patients answered the questionnaires on days 0, 14 and 28. Table 2 (Terao, 2009) shows the short-term QOL scores of role limitations in work, physical or social functioning, interpersonal relationships, emotional functioning and sleep/vitality along with a total score of all items as well as the global health status.).

Items	pretreatment	Day 14	Day 28
QOL score			
Global health status	6.0 (5 - 7)	5.5 (5 - 6)	5.0 (4 - 6)*
Role limitations in work	6.0 (5 - 6)	4.5 (5 - 6)	4.0 (4 - 6)**
Physical or social functioning	11.0 (9 - 12)	8.5 (8 - 10)*	8.0 (6 - 10)*
Interpersonal relationships	6.0 (4 - 6)	5.0 (3 - 6)*	4.0 (3 - 6)**
Emotional functioning	7.5 (7 - 9)	7.0 (5 - 7)	5.0 (5 - 7)**
Sleep /Vitality	5.0 (4 - 6)	4.5 (4 - 6)	4.0 (4 - 5)**
Total score	42.0 (35 - 54)	34.0 (31 - 39)	30.5 (27 - 37)**
Bodily pain (%)	52.5 (10 - 70)	35.0 (5 - 50)	25.0 (5 - 50)**

Data is expressed as median (range). *p<0.05, ** p<0.01

Table 2. Scores of QOL and percent of bodily pain.

As compared with day 0, the scores for the global health status ($P < 0.05$), interpersonal relationships ($P < 0.01$), emotional functioning ($P < 0.01$) and sleep/vitality ($P < 0.01$) were significantly improved on day 28. Moreover, significant improvements in the short-term QOL scores were demonstrated with respect to the role imitations in work (day 14, $P < 0.05$; day 28, $P < 0.05$) and physical or social functioning (day 14, $P < 0.05$; day 28, $P < 0.01$). As compared with day 0, the total score of all items was also significantly improved on day 28 ($P < 0.01$). Further, as compared with day 0, the bodily pain was significantly reduced on day 28 ($P < 0.01$).

3.3 Correlation of ⊿PSA with ⊿QOL and ⊿Pain

Figure 1 shows the changes in the serum PSA levels of all patients from a period of 8 weeks before (-8 w) to 4 weeks after (4 w) the initial vector injection. The correlation of the serum PSA levels with the short-term total QOL scores and bodily pain is shown in Figure 2(A) and Figure 2(B), respectively. A significant correlation was observed between ⊿PSA and ⊿QOL ($P < 0.05$); however, it was not observed between ⊿PSA and ⊿Pain (Terao, 2009).

4. Discussion

Bone metastasis is found in 70 to 85% of autopsy cases in malignant tumor patients, and the bone is a potential site of metastasis in all cancerous tumors (Tubiana-Hulin, 1991). In recent years, the use of third-generation bisphosphonates and the progress of multidisciplinary approaches combining radiotherapy, chemotherapy, and other treatments has led to improvement in SREs and prolongation of survival in advanced cancers (Saad et al., 2002), so that long-term survival can be expected in prostate cancer, breast cancer, multiple myeloma, and other conditions even at the stage where bone metastasis is present. In conjunction with this progress, a strategy and response focused on long-term quality of life is required beginning from the initial stage of treatment. This is now coming to be seen as an important item for assessment when developing novel therapies. The present study consisted of a quality of life assessment in prostate cancer patients following the novel treatment of gene therapy.

QOL instruments, including EORTC QLQ-PR25, have been applied in several therapeutic trials of prostate cancer (Ho et al., 2006, Cella et al., 2006, Canil et al., 2005). The items in these questionnaires include questions regarding urinary conditions, for example pollakiuria, dysuria, and macrohematuria. Further, these questionnaires are employed for patients of prostate cancer in various stages. In this study, however, patients who have undergone various treatments—including radical prostatectomy, androgen-deprivation therapy and/or conventional chemotherapy—prior to gene therapy were targeted. Further, in 4 patients, the lesions that were injected with the vector were bone metastatic lesions alone. This study aimed at assessing the effect of gene therapy on bodily pain because most patients suffered pain at the site of vector-injected lesion. Moreover, there have been no questionnaires that assess QOL in patients receiving gene therapy for HRPC. Taking the above into consideration, a questionnaire based on EORTC QLQ-PR25 questionnaire (Table 1) was created and bodily pain was assessed by using VAS (Tearo et al., 2009).

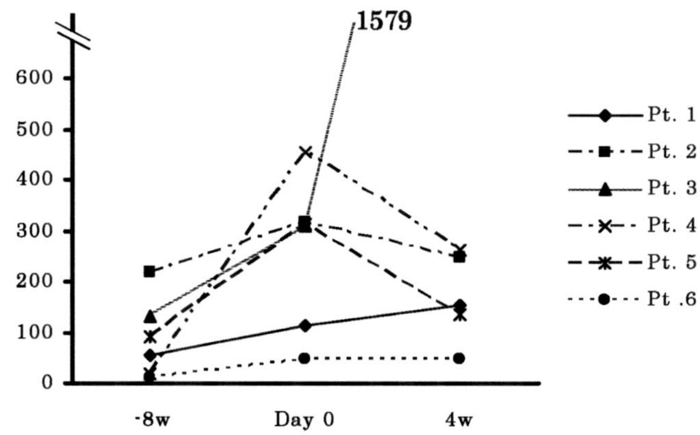

Fig. 1. The change of serum PSA level in all patients from before 8weeks (-8w) to after 4weeks (4w) of gene therapy.

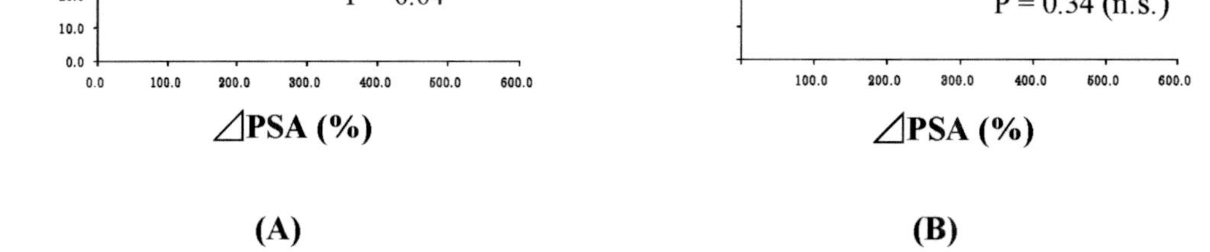

Fig. 2. (A) The correlation of PSA levels with short-term total QOL scores. (B) The correlation of PSA levels with bodily pain. Both were assessed by measuring the rate of change (%) of the serum PSA levels, the short-term total QOL scores, and bodily pain from day 0 to day 28; these values were expressed as ⊿PSA, ⊿QOL, and ⊿Pain, respectively.

Recently QOL is increasingly being recognized as a measure for assessing outcomes of therapeutic trials. Further, the assessment of the clinical effects of therapy on QOL is indispensable to the evaluation of therapeutic trials (Fayers & Bottomley, 2005). In several therapeutic trials for prostate cancer, the assessment of patients' QOL is incorporated as a therapeutic index. In this study, it was demonstrated that Ad-OC-TK plus VAL treatment significantly improved the short-term QOL scores and the total score using the modified questionnaire statistically correlated between ⊿PSA and ⊿QOL (Figure 2(A)). Therefore, although it will be necessary to compare the changes in QOL scores using the modified questionnaire to the changes in QOL scores using other typical questionnaires that are used for patients of HRPC, it is considered that the QOL of patients receiving Ad-OC-TK plus VAL treatment is worth assessing as a therapeutic index. Further, significant improvements in bodily pain were also observed. It is suggested that the clinical improvements may contribute to a significant improvement in bodily pain. Since the tumors of these patients displayed disease progression despite surgery, radiation, androgen-deprivation therapy and/or conventional chemotherapy, the serum PSA levels of all patients were very high prior to gene therapy. Following gene therapy, the serum PSA levels decreased in 2 patients, no change was observed in 1 patient and they were slightly increased in 2 patients (Figure 2(A)). Further, the induction of cell apoptosis in the vector-injected lesions of 5 patients examined by anti-ssDNA antibody staining on day 28 was also observed. However, a correlation between ⊿PSA and ⊿Pain was not demonstrated in spite of the clinical effects observed in the vector-injected lesion (Figure 2(B)). In this study, the Ad-OC-TK vector was injected directly into one single localized recurrent tumor or bone metastatic lesion despite of the fact that all the patients had multiple bone metastatic lesions. Especially in the case of patient 3, the pain in the non-vector injected lesions increased on day 28. This fact might be one reason that a correlation between ⊿PSA and ⊿Pain was not demonstrated (Terao et al., 2009).

Pain, which has been called the fifth vital sign, has come to be recognized as a crucial factor in assessing patient condition in the clinical environment. At the same time, however, pain is a subjective phenomenon, which makes it difficult to gain an accurate picture of a patient's pain. It will be important in future to perform diagnosis using more appropriate assessment methods. In the assessment of the efficacy of gene therapy as a novel cancer therapy, assessment methods emphasizing QOL are likely to receive important attention in the future. Since it has been found that the subjective sense of physical well-being in a large proportion of Japanese patients is centered not on the self but on external objects such as the family or the doctor, it would seem important to assess and select therapies with care, taking into account psychological aspects which patients find difficult to express for themselves, and basing the process on an assessment of the effect of each therapeutic method on the basic QOL.

5. Conclusion

It was demonstrated that Ad-OC-TK plus VAL gene therapy improved or preserved the short-term QOL and bodily pain of HRPC patients with metastatic or local recurrent tumors. These assessments may emerge as the new therapeutic indices of gene therapy for HRPC.

6. Acknowledgment

We thank all the patients for their participation in this study. This research was supported as a Japanese Research Project, Grant-in-aid for Scientific Research (A) : project 1420763.

7. References

Aaronson, N.K., Ahmedzai, S., & Bergman, B., et al. (1993). The European Organization for Research and Treatment of Cancer QLQ-C30; a quality-of-life instrument for use in international clinical trials in oncology. *J Natl Cancer Inst,* 85, 365-376.

American Cancer Society. (2008). Cancer Facts and Figures, 2008. Atlanta, GA, USA

Bergman, B., Aaronson, N.K. & Ahmedzai, S. (1994). The EORTC QLQ-LC13: a modular supplement to the EORTC Core Quality of Life Questionnaire (QLQ-C30) for use in lung cancer clinical trials. EORTC Study Group on Quality of Life. *Eur J Cancer,* 30A, 635-642.

Brady, M.J., Cella, D.F., & Mo, F. (1997). Reliability and validity of the Functional Assessment of Cancer Therapy-Breast quality-of-life instrument. *J Clin Oncol,* 15, 974-986.

Canil, C.M., Moore, M.J., & Seymour, L. et al. (2005). Randomized phase II study of two doses of gefitinib in hormone-refractory prostate cancer: a trial of the National Cancer Institute of Canada-Clinical Trials Group. J Clin Oncol. 23, 455–460.

Carroll, P.R., Kantoff, P.W., & Balk, S.P., et al. (2002). Second International Conference on Newer Approaches to Androgen Deprivation Therapy (ADT) in Prostate Cancer overview consensus statement—newer approaches to androgen deprivation therapy in prostate cancer. *Urology.* 60, 1–6.

Cella, D., Tulsky, D.S., & Gray, G., et al. (1993). The Functional Assessment of Cancer Therapy scale: development and validation of the general measure. *J Clin Oncol* 11, 570-579.

Cella, D., Bonomi, A.E., & Lloyd, S.R. (1995). Reliability and validity of the Functional Assessment of Cancer Therapy-Lung (FACT-L) quality of life instrument. *Lung Cancer,* 12, 199-220.

Cella, D., Petrylak, D., & Mulani, P., et al. (2006). Role of quality of life in men with metastatic hormone-refractory prostate cancer: how does atrasentan influence quality of life? *Eur Urol.* 49, 781–789.

Chodak, G.W., Keane, T., & Klotz, L., et al. (2002). Critical evaluation of hormonal therapy for carcinoma of the prostate. *Urology.* 60, 201–208.

Chow, E., & Bottomley, A. (2009). Understanding the EORTCQLQ-BM22, the module for patients with bone metastases. *Expert rev Pharmacoecon Outcomes Res,* 9, 461-465.

da Silva, F.C., Reis, E., Costa, T., & Denis, L., et al. (1993). Quality of life in patients with prostatic cancer. A feasibility study. The Members of Quality of Life Committee of the EORTC Genitourinary Group. *Cancer,* 71, 1138–1142.

Esper, P., Mo, F., & Chodak, G., et al. (1997). Measuring QOL in men with prostate cancer using the FACT-P instrument. *Urology,* 50, 920-928.

EuroQol. (1990). A new facility for the measurement of health-related quality of life. *The EuroQol Group. Health Policy,* 16, 199-208.

Fayers, P., & Bottomley, A. (2002). EORTC Quality of Life Group; Quality of Life Unit. Quality of life research within the EORTC-The EORTC QLQ-C30. European Organisation for Research and Treatment of Cancer. *Eur J Cancer,* 38, 125–133.

Hinata, N., Shirakawa, T., & Gotoh, A., et al. (2006). Progress report on phase I/II clinical trial of Ad-OC-TK plus VAL therapy for metastatic or locally recurrent prostate cancer: Initial experience at Kobe University. Int J Urol, 13, 834–837.

Ho, S., Wook, J., & Jong, J. (2006). Targeted-cryosurgical ablation of the prostate with androgen deprivation therapy: quality of life in high-risk prostate cancer patients. *Asian J Androl,* 8, 629–636.

Ko, S.C., Cheon, J., & Chung, L.K. (1996). Osteocalcin promoter-based toxic gene therapy for the treatment of osteosarcoma in experimental models. *Cancer Res,* 56, 4614-4619.

Kubo, H., Gardner, T.A., & Chung, L.W., et al.(2003). Phase I dose escalation clinical trial of adenovirus vector carrying osteocalcin promoter-driven herpes simplex virus thymidine kinase in localized and metastatic hormone-refractory prostate cancer. *Hum Gene Ther,* 14, 227–241.

Lusky, M. (2005) Good manufacturing practice production of adenoviral vectors for clinical trials. *Hum Gene Ther,* 16, 281-291.

Saad, F., Gleason, D.M., & Murray, R., et al. (2002). A randomized, placebo-controlled trial of zoledronic acid in patients with hormone-refractory metastatic prostate carcinoma. *J Natl Cancer Inst,* 94, 1458-1468.

Satoh, T., Kimura, M., & Matsumoto, K., et al. (2009). Single infusion of zoledronic acid to prevent androgen-deprivation therapy-induced bone loss in men with hormone-naïve prostate carcinoma. *Cancer,* 115, 3468-3474.

Scher, H.I., & Kelly, W.K. (1993). Flutamide withdrawal syndrome: Its impact on clinical trials in hormone-refractory prostate cancer. *J Clin Oncol,* 11, 1566-1572.

Shirakawa, T., Terao, S., & Gotoh, A., et al. (2007). Long-term outcome of phase I / II clinical trial of Ad-OC-TK/VAL gene therapy for hormone-refractory metastatic prostate cancer. Hum Gene Ther, 18, 1225-1232.

Sprangers, M.A., Groenvold, M., & Arraras, J.I. (1996). The European Organization for Research and Treatment of Cancer breast cancer-specific quality-of-life questionnaire module: first results from a three-country field study. *J Clin Oncol,* 14, 2756-2768.

Terao, S., Shirakawa, T., & Gotoh, A., et al. (2009). A pilot study of quality of life of patients with hormone-refractory prostate cancer after gene therapy. *Anticancer Res,* 29, 1533-1538.

Tubiana-Hulin, M. (1991). Incidence, prevalence and distribution of bone metastases. *Bone,* 12, S9-10.

Tyring, S.K., Beutiner, K.R., & Crooks, R.J., et al. (2000). Antiviral therapy for herpes zoster: Randomized, controlled clinical trial of valacyclovir and famciclovir therapy in immunocompetent patients 50 years and older. *Arch Fam Med,* 9, 863-869.

Ware, J.E. Jr, & Sherbourne, C.D. (1992). The MOS 36-item short-form health survey (SF-36). I. Conceptual framework and item selection. *Med Care,* 30, 473-483.

18

Fetal Gene Therapy

Christopher Porada and Graça Almeida-Porada
The Wake Forest Institute for Regenerative Medicine, Winston-Salem, North Carolina USA

1. Introduction

Gene therapy can be defined as the process by which a normal functional copy of a gene is transferred into the appropriate cells of an individual with the intent to correct a disease caused by a defect within the individual's own copy of the gene in question [1-3]. Gene therapy is still considered by many to be a relatively new therapeutic modality, having only developed over the last two decades. As such, it is still under intense experimental investigation to prove its therapeutic potential and safety before it can enter the clinic as a first line of treatment. Gene therapy promises to offer a precise means of permanently curing essentially any of the over 4000 currently known so-called monogenic diseases, which are caused by an error in only a single gene. These include, but are certainly not limited to, the hemophilias, lysosomal storage diseases like Gaucher's and Hurler's, hemoglobin disorders such as the thalassemias and sickle cell disease, diseases of immune function such as deficiencies in the shared γc receptor subunit or adenosine deaminase (ADA) deficiency, and cystic fibrosis. It is also anticipated that gene therapy will one day enable the treatment of a host of inherited or acquired disorders such as cancer, AIDS, and many others for which there is currently no cure [4-9].

2. Hemophilia a as an ideal target disease for correction with gene therapy

Among the monogenic disorders, the hemophilias, and hemophilia A in particular, represent ideal diseases to attempt to treat with gene therapy [10-13] because lifelong improvement or permanent cure is theoretically possible after only a single treatment. This is in contrast to current protein replacement-based therapies which, for hemophilia A, consist of frequent intravenous infusions of short-lived FVIII protein concentrates throughout the lifetime of the patient, without ever curing the underlying disease. The severity of hemophilia A is traditionally based on plasma levels of FVIII, with persons exhibiting less than 1% normal factor (<0.01 IU/mL) being considered to have severe hemophilia, persons with 1-5% normal factor moderately severe, and persons with 5%-40% of the normal FVIII levels mild [14-16]. Thus, even with the low levels of transduction that are routinely obtained with the current viral-based gene delivery systems, a marked clinical improvement would be anticipated in patients with hemophilia A, since even low levels of FVIII would likely convert most patients with severe hemophilia to either a moderate or mild phenotype, greatly improving their quality of life. Conversely, even supraphysiologic levels of FVIII as high as 150% of normal are predicted to be well tolerated, making the therapeutic window extremely wide [16]. In the past three decades, the remarkable progress in the understanding of the molecular basis of the disease, the identification and characterization of FVIII gene, structure, and biology has furthered the interest and feasibility of treating hemophilia A with gene therapy.

Based on the promise of lifelong cure following a single treatment and the encouraging preclinical results in murine and canine models, several clinical gene therapy trials in both hemophilia A and B have been undertaken. In each case, the treatment was well tolerated with the vectors and doses used. Despite the encouraging preliminary data from these studies [10, 13, 15-23], however, the plasma levels of FVIII achieved thus far have been insufficient to free the patients from the need of exogenous factor. In addition, expression of the FVIII transgene was often transient, and none of the trials exhibited a clear relationship between vector dose and resultant FVIII levels. Another major hurdle that has plagued the successful phenotypic correction of the hemophilias by factor replacement therapy is inhibitory antibody formation, which occurs in nearly 30% of patients with severe hemophilia A. The formation of these inhibitors greatly reduces the efficacy of subsequent FVIII infusions, and can ultimately lead to treatment failure, placing the patient at risk of life-threatening hemorrhage. Disappointingly, inhibitor formation has also observed when gene therapy has been used in an attempt to treat the hemophilias, since, as discussed in more detail below, the patient's immune system still "sees" the vector-encoded FVIII or FIX as foreign.

These clinical trials also raised the troubling possibility of inadvertent germline alteration when semen samples were found to be transiently positive for vector DNA [24, 25]. This is in contrast to prior studies conducted in experimental animals [26, 27], reinforcing the importance of the choice of animal model system employed when conducting pre-clinical studies, if one wishes to extrapolate results obtained in their model to what would likely happen in the clinic. The occurrence of insertional mutagenesis-mediated leukemogenesis in children who received murine retroviral vector-transduced hematopoietic cells as treatment for X-SCID [28-30] further supports the need to perform detailed analyses in a clinically predictive animal model prior to moving into human patients, since an adverse event of this nature was never observed in the decades of animal gene therapy experiments that led up to these clinical trials.

3. Animal models for testing gene therapy for hemophilia A

A number of animal models have been developed to evaluate new methods of not only treatment of coagulation disorders, but also the prevention and treatment of inhibitor formation. Dog models of hemophilia with congenital deficiency [31, 32] and mouse models obtained by gene targeting and knockout technology [33] are available to study FVIII function and gene therapy approaches for treating hemophilia A. Therapeutic benefit has been obtained in numerous studies using a variety of vector systems in the murine model [34-39], but phenotypic correction of hemophilia A in the dog has been much more difficult to achieve [40, 41], similar to findings in human patients, underscoring the value of large animal preclinical models for accurately predicting outcome in human patients. Transient hemophilic rabbit models induced by infusion of plasma containing inhibitors have been used to evaluate the effect of different bypass products to factor VIII [42], but this model, while valuable for inhibitor studies, does not accurately recapitulate the human disease, precluding its use for gene therapy studies.

3.1 Sheep as a preclinical model of hemophilia A

The ideal way to test gene therapy-based approaches to hemophilia A and evaluate long-term expression of clinically applicable FVIII-encoding gene therapy vectors would be to use an animal model that both closely resembles the disease process of HA and closely parallels normal human physiology. To this end, between 1979 and 1982, a number of male offspring of a single white alpine ewe at the Swiss Federal Institute of Technology all died several hours post-partum due to severe bleeding from the umbilical cord [43-45]. Daughters and granddaughters of this ewe also gave birth to lambs exhibiting the same pathology. Investigation of the affected animals showed extensive subcutaneous and intramuscular hematomas. Spontaneous hemarthroses were also frequent, leading to reduced locomotion and symptoms of pain in standing up, restricting nursing activity. Stronger injuries resulted in heavy bleeding and intensive pain. Laboratory tests showed increased PTT and FVIII levels (as assessed by aPTT) decreased to about 1% of that of the control animals. Replacement therapy with human FVIII (hFVIII) concentrate or fresh sheep plasma resulted in remission of disease and rapid clinical improvement.

Unfortunately, due to the expense and effort of maintaining these sheep, the Swiss investigators allowed the line to die out, saving only 6 straws of semen prior to allowing this valuable resource to pass into extinction. We recently used a variety of reproductive technologies to successfully re-establish this line of hemophilia A sheep and fully characterized both the clinical parameters and the precise molecular basis for their disease [46-51]. Importantly, chromogenic assays revealed undetectable FVIII activity in the circulation of these sheep, explaining their severe phenotype. In addition, we identified a frame-shift-induced premature stop codon as the molecular cause of the disease, just as occurs in a percentage of human patients with hemophilia A, making this line of sheep unique among animal hemophilia A models, since hemophilia A mice were generated through targeted gene deletion and the hemophilia A dog colonies exhibit a gene inversion.

In addition to the value of another large animal model of hemophilia A and the uniqueness of the mutation, sheep possess many characteristics that make them an ideal preclinical model for gene therapy, both postnatal and in utero. Firstly, sheep are fairly close in size to humans, weighing roughly 8lbs at birth and 150-200lbs as adults, likely obviating the need for scale-up of vector dose to move from experiments in sheep to human trials. In addition, the large size of the sheep, their long life span, and their relative ease of maintenance and breeding make it possible to conduct the long-term studies in large numbers of animals that are necessary to fully evaluate the efficacy and safety issues related to in utero gene therapy. Secondly, sheep share many important physiological and developmental characteristics with humans; for example, the pattern of fetal to adult hemoglobin switching, and the naturally occurring changes in the primary sites of hematopoiesis from yolk sac to fetal liver and finally to the bone marrow near the end of gestation. It is thus not surprising that fetal sheep have been used extensively in the study of mammalian fetal physiology, and results obtained with this model have been directly applicable to the understanding of human fetal growth and development. Thirdly, sheep are outbred, and thus represent a wide spectrum of genetic determinants of the immune response, as do humans. In addition, the development of the sheep immune system has been investigated in detail [52-58], making sheep well suited for studying the immunological aspects of gene therapy for HA. As the immune response to both the vector and the vector-encoded FVIII are likely to play a key role in FVIII inhibitor formation (or lack thereof), this represents an advantage not found in most other models, with the possible exception of the dog. For these reasons, we feel that the sheep are a particularly relevant model in which to examine fetal gene therapy in general and, in particular, for hemophilia A. An additional unique advantage to using sheep to study hemophilia A treatment is that in sheep, like human, a large percentage of the vWF is found within platelets rather than free in plasma. This is in contrast to dog (in which vWF circulates free in plasma [59, 60]), and may prove important given the vital role vWF plays in the stability/functionality of FVIII.

4. Rationale for performing gene therapy in utero

Importantly, many of the hurdles that have thus far prevented gene therapy from curing patients with hemophilia A, or many of the other diseases that have been investigated, could likely be circumvented by performing in utero gene therapy. At the present time, many of the diseases considered as candidates for gene therapy can be diagnosed relatively early in gestation, making it feasible to begin devising methods for performing gene therapy in utero rather than waiting until after birth. Methods for accessing both the sheep and the human fetus are well established and clinically viable. Indeed, fetal transfusions and in utero stem cell-based therapies have now been performed clinically by numerous investigators for decades, using a variety of protocols, in efforts to treat patients with a number of different diseases [61, 62]. While the stem cell trials have thus far only proven clinically successful in patients with immunodeficiencies, they have also demonstrated that accessing the early gestational human fetus multiple times poses minimal risks with modern imaging and ultrasound-guided delivery procedures[63]. Furthermore, it is important to note that experience and knowledge gained from studies performed in the fetal sheep model were used to design and perform the first curative human in utero transplantation for X-SCID [64], highlighting the value of the fetal sheep model for not only developing clinically viable methodology, but also for predicting clinical outcome. Using these established clinically applicable methodologies to perform gene therapy early in gestation would correct the disease prior to parturition, allowing the birth of a normal healthy baby who, ideally, would require no further treatments. Additionally, following prenatal diagnosis of disease, parents currently have only two options; pregnancy termination or birth of an affected child. In utero gene therapy would provide a much needed third option [65]. Although in vitro embryo screening and selection is a possible solution, this option is not widely available due to both its high cost and the lack of the required technology in developing countries. In utero gene therapy, in contrast, does not require any sophisticated equipment that would not already be in place for prenatal diagnosis. Indeed, several recent studies have now conclusively demonstrated the marked cost-effectiveness of prenatal screening for the hemophilias, even within developing third world countries [66-68].

Looking beyond the hemophilias, it is important to note that many of the diseases that could be treated with gene therapy exert a significant amount of irreversible damage to the patient prior to birth, during embryonic and fetal development. For example, irreversible neuronal damage is associated with inherited metabolic diseases such as Gaucher's, Lesch-Nyhan, and Tay Sachs. In these patients, post-natal gene therapy, while potentially capable of correcting the metabolic disorder, would be of only limited therapeutic benefit, since it could not reverse the damage which the gene defect had exerted during development. This is clearly in contrast to infants born with SCID or other genetic disorders, such as the hemophilias, who could theoretically be cured by postnatal gene therapy. Nevertheless, even in patients with diseases that can be cured postnatally, psychological and financial benefits exist to argue for performing correction in utero, since it would allow the birth of a healthy infant, who, ideally, would require no further treatments.

5. The fetus as a gene therapy recipient

In addition to the clinical and financial advantages of performing gene therapy prior to birth, numerous aspects of the fetus make it a more suitable gene therapy recipient than the adult. For example, due to their ability to integrate into the genome of the host cell, γ-retroviruses and lentiviruses have received a great deal of attention as gene delivery vectors, since transduction of a long-lived cell could provide lifelong therapy following a single administration. However, one of the main limiting factors to the successful application of these integrating vectors to in vivo gene therapy is the low level of initial transduction and the limited degree of expansion of transduced cells that occurs following gene therapy, since in the adult most cell populations in the body are relatively quiescent unless injury is used to induce cell cycling. In the case of hemophilia A, the primary site of FVIII synthesis under normal physiologic conditions is the liver [69]. Yet, in a mature animal, it is estimated that only 1 in 10,000 to 1 in 20,000 hepatocytes are actively cycling at any given time [70], making it very difficult to obtain meaningful levels of gene transfer unless the gene delivery system mediates extremely high efficiency transduction of quiescent cells, or injury such as partial hepatectomy is employed to induce cell division to enhance transduction and/or drive expansion of the limited numbers of transduced cells. In the fetus, the cells in all of the organs are actively cycling to support the continuous expansion that occurs throughout gestation. Thus, cells such as hepatocytes that are largely quiescent in the adult are far more mitotically active in the fetus. As such, these cells should be far more amenable to genetic correction with vectors requiring cell division. Furthermore, the active cycling of the cells in all of the organs to support the continuous expansion that occurs throughout gestation offers the possibility of achieving expansion of the gene-corrected cells during the remainder of gestation, such that transduction of even small numbers of target cells should lead to significant levels of gene-correction by birth.

6. Immunological advantages of in utero gene therapy

It is important to note that many patients suffer from the genetic diseases being targeted with gene therapy because they have never produced a single specific protein. As a result, their immune system has never "seen" this protein, and, following gene therapy, the cells of the immune system seek to eliminate any cells in the body that are expressing the very protein that could cure the patient of his/her disease. The low levels of gene delivery to the desired target cells and the immune response combine to yield very low levels of expression of the therapeutic protein, and even the small amounts that are produced are often only produced for a short time. In the case of hemophilia A, this cell-mediated immune response to the cells expressing the vector-encoded FVIII gene further complicates the already formidable challenge posed by the formation of inhibitory antibodies to the FVIII protein.

Remaining cognizant of the immune-aspects of hemophilia treatment, it is important to note that, in addition to the ability to target cells which are largely refractory to transduction in the adult, unique immunologic advantages also exist for performing gene therapy in utero. There is a window of time in early immunologic development, before thymic processing of mature lymphocytes, during which the fetus is largely tolerant of foreign antigens. Exposure to foreign antigens during this period often results in sustained tolerance, which can become permanent if the presence of the antigen is maintained [71]. When one considers that most individuals with a family history of hemophilia would likely go for early prenatal screening during pregnancy to ascertain whether the fetus was affected, it should be possible to perform in utero gene therapy relatively early in gestation. Given these unique immunological advantages presented by the early fetus, one can envision that in utero gene therapy would be an ideal approach for treating hemophilia A, since lifelong tolerance could be induced to FVIII. This would thus ensure that, even if in utero gene therapy was not curative, postnatal gene therapy or protein replacement could proceed safely without the risk of inhibitor formation.

7. Experimental in utero gene therapy studies

With the knowledge that performing gene therapy in utero would provide these advantages over existing post-natal approaches, we have spent the last decade and a half using the fetal sheep model to investigate whether it is possible to exploit the highly proliferative state and relative immuno-naïveté of the early gestational fetus to achieve significant levels of gene transfer by performing a single intraperitoneal injection of a γ-retroviral vector [72-82]. This approach to in utero gene therapy is safe and technically simple, involving only a single injection into the peritoneum of the fetus, and the injection can easily be given under ultrasound guidance, greatly increasing the clinical applicability of the approach. The straightforward nature of this approach enabled us to perform the gene transfer as early as 54 days of gestation (term: 145 days), improving the chances of achieving clinical benefit in diseases with early onset, and potentially allowing induction of immune tolerance to the vector-encoded gene.

8. Hematopoietic system

We focused our initial efforts on assessing whether this approach resulted in transduction of primitive hematopoietic stem/progenitor cells (HSC), since transduced HSC should provide a lifelong supply of gene-modified hematopoietic progeny, enabling long-term correction following a single in utero treatment. Based on the difficulty associated with transducing HSC in vitro without negatively affecting their in vivo engraftability/functionality [83], we reasoned that placing the vector directly in the fetus should conceivably expose all of the HSC present within the fetus to the vector while in their native microenvironment, potentially increasing the levels of gene transfer to the desired target cells. Indeed, in our initial studies, we observed levels of 2-3% gene-marked hematopoietic cells in the circulation [81, 82]. Furthermore, we found that by varying the age of the recipient at the time of gene transfer, we could markedly enhance the levels of hematopoietic cell transduction [75, 84].. If gene transfer was performed at only 54-57 days of gestation, gene-marking levels of 5-6% could be achieved in the peripheral blood, a level that could exert a beneficial effect in at least some genetic diseases. Importantly, these gene-marked hematopoietic cells persisted in these sheep over the course of 5 years of study [81, 82], transgene-positive CD34+ cells could be detected in the bone marrow of these animals several years post in utero gene transfer [85], and bone marrow cells isolated from these in utero gene transfer recipients successfully engrafted the hematopoietic system of secondary fetal sheep recipients upon re-transplantation. These three pieces of data provide compelling evidence that this approach enabled us to successfully insert genes into the stem cells of the hematopoietic system, suggesting this method could provide lifelong genetic correction.

9. Non-hematopoietic tissues

While transduction of clinically significant levels of HSC within these sheep following a single injection of vector into the peritoneal cavity hinted at the therapeutic potential of this simple approach to in utero gene therapy, the retroviral vectors we employed in these studies did not possess any type of targeting moiety which would restrict transduction to cells of the hematopoietic system. It was not surprising, therefore, when we examined other tissues of the recipients, to find that gene transfer was not limited to cells of the hematopoietic system, but had occurred in essentially all of the organs we examined, including numerous cell types within the liver, lung, and brain [79, 81, 82, 86]. Concomitantly, in utero gene transfer studies performed by other investigators in sheep, rodent, and non-human primate models employing a variety of viral-based gene delivery vectors produced similar results [78-81, 87-105], raising the exciting possibility that in utero gene therapy could potentially be used to treat not only hematologic disorders, but also numerous genetic disorders that affect tissues other than the hematopoietic system. For example, in the case of the hemophilias, this method could likely be used with success to delivering genes for the missing coagulation factors to the developing liver at levels that would covert patients with severe hemophilia to a moderate or even mild phenotype [79]. Moreover, tissue-specific expression is not necessary for factor VIII (the factor deficient in hemophilia A) or factor IX (the factor deficient in hemophilia B). Thus, the transfer of either of these genes into a wide range of tissues with ready access to the circulation, followed by long-term expression, would greatly enhance the therapeutic potential of this approach for treating/curing the hemophilias. Interestingly, although the incidence of hemophilia A is 7x's that of hemophilia B, the only studies that have explored the possibility of performing in utero gene therapy for the treatment of the hemophilias have been aimed at correcting hemophilia B (factor IX deficiency), and all but one group's studies [88, 99] have been performed in mice [87, 100, 101, 103-105], making it somewhat difficult to extrapolate the results to the human clinical setting.

Despite offering many advantages in the treatment of diseases such as the hemophilias, the widespread presence of gene-modified cells throughout the body also underscored the need to carefully examine the safety of this approach to in utero gene therapy, since expression of the transferred genetic material in all tissues may not always be desirable, and, in some cases, could in fact be deleterious, if the transgene in question requires tissue-specific expression. Based on our observations in the hematopoietic system, we first examined whether the developmental stage of the recipient might impact upon which tissues were modified following in utero gene therapy. Our initial results revealed that the liver, like the hematopoietic system, is more amenable to gene transfer at earlier stages of fetal development, leading us to believe that perhaps gene transfer was always most efficient if performed earlier in gestation. However, when we examined the lungs of these same recipients, we discovered that this belief was unfounded. In the lungs we observed exactly the opposite of what we had seen in the hematopoietic system and the liver, namely, that the levels of gene-marked cells were much higher if the transfer was performed later in gestation [79, 86]. These findings thus suggest that each tissue likely possesses its own unique developmental stage during which gene transfer is optimal. These findings also raised the intriguing possibility that it may be possible to choose, at least to some degree, which tissues will be modified following in utero gene transfer, by carefully selecting the age at which the transfer is performed.

10. Induction of immune tolerance following in utero gene transfer

As discussed previously, one of the major hurdles hindering treatment of the hemophilias by factor replacement therapy is the formation of inhibitory antibodies that can occur with repeated administration of these exogenous factors over time. While analyzing the tissues from the sheep that received in utero gene transfer, we noted that the thymus frequently exhibited transgene-positivity by PCR [81, 82]. Given the pivotal role of the thymus during the development of the fetal immune system's ability to distinguish self from non-self, we undertook studies to ascertain the immunologic significance of the presence of these transgene-positive cells within the thymus. In our first set of studies, [106] we demonstrated that in utero gene transfer successfully induced durable immune tolerance to the vector-encoded β-galactosidase. This tolerance induction appeared to involve both cellular and humoral mechanisms, since both antibody responses and cellular responses were blunted in these animals even several years after in utero gene transfer, providing strong evidence that IUGT induces immune tolerance to the protein product of the transgene. We next conducted studies to begin elucidating the mechanisms responsible for this observed tolerance and to assess whether the recipient gestational age had an impact upon transgene immunity/tolerance induction [107]. Immunohistochemistry revealed that thymic tissue is in fact transduced in the majority of animals following IUGT regardless of the age at which in utero gene transfer is performed. Importantly, however, we only observed transduction of thymic epithelial cells that are crucial for presentation of self-antigen during T cell thymic selection if gene transfer was performed prior to 72 days of gestation [term: 145 days], while after that point in gestation, predominantly CD45+ thymocytes were transduced. These analyses also revealed that, if in utero gene transfer is performed early in gestation, epithelial-like cells comprising the Hassall's corpuscles, as evidenced by their morphology, their CK-positivity, and their expression of thymic stromal lymphopoietin are also transduced. Flow cytometric analysis on the animals that received in utero gene transfer at varying gestational ages revealed that animals that received gene transfer early in gestation had significantly higher percentages of CD4+CD25+ Tregs within their periphery than did control animals or animals transduced later in gestation. These studies thus demonstrate that performing in utero gene transfer early in gestation takes advantage of multiple tolerogenic avenues present in the fetus, since it results in the transduction of both thymic epithelial cells, which may promote induction of central immune tolerance, and cells of Hassall's corpuscles, which can instruct dendritic cells to induce Tregs that can help maintain peripheral immune tolerance to the transgene products. These findings thus suggest that, even if not curative, in utero gene therapy would be ideal for a disease like hemophilia A, since lifelong tolerance could be induced to FVIII, thus overcoming the immune-related hurdles that currently hinder post-natal treatment of this disease. As discussed previously, however, in utero gene therapy studies to date have focused on hemophilia B [87, 88, 99-101, 103-105], rather than hemophilia A, which is intriguing, given the 7-fold higher incidence of hemophilia A, and the fact that patients with hemophilia A are more than 10x's as likely to develop inhibitory antibodies to the exogenous coagulation factor than patients with hemophilia B [108, 109]. While the choice to focus on hemophilia B is likely due to difficulties encountered in initial attempts to express FVIII as a transgene in the context of viral vectors [110], it nevertheless makes it unclear whether the ability to induce immune tolerance to marker gene products and FIX in utero will ultimately translate into the ability to induce tolerance to FVIII, given FVIII's apparent higher degree of immunogenicity.

11. Potential risk to fetal germline

While gene transfer to the vast majority of the fetal tissues would be desirable for correcting diseases, such as the hemophilias, that would benefit from widespread systemic release of a secreted transgene product, our analyses also revealed that the fetal reproductive tissues often contained the gene therapy vector sequences, raising the troubling possibility that the developing germline might have been modified as a result of in utero gene therapy. Since prior studies had demonstrated that both the embryonic germline [111-114] and isolated primordial germ cells (PGC) [115] can readily be infected with murine retroviral vectors and pass the vector genetic material to subsequent generations in a Mendelian fashion as part of the permanent genome, we used three approaches to examine this important issue in detail: 1) We performed immunohistochemical staining on tissue sections prepared from the in utero treated animals; 2) we performed genetic analysis on the sperm cells from the treated males; and 3) we performed breeding experiments in a limited number of animals [72, 80, 91, 116, 117]. These studies indicated that although the fetal ovaries appeared to be largely unaffected by this approach to in utero gene transfer, numerous cells within the developing fetal testes were in fact modified including interstitial cells, Sertoli cells, and small numbers of both immature germ cells within the forming sex cords and the resultant sperm cells. Importantly, however, gene-modified germ cells were only observed in 2 of the 6 animals examined in our studies, and, in these two animals, the incidence of germ cell modification was roughly 1 in 6250, a frequency that is well below the theoretical level of spontaneous mutation within the human genome [118]. This low frequency of modification coupled with observations that genetic alterations to the germ cells may produce deleterious effects, placing them at a disadvantage during fertilization suggest that the likelihood that any genetic alterations present would be passed to subsequent offspring would be extremely unlikely. In agreement with this supposition, we did not observe transfer of the vector sequences in any of the 10 offspring we studied, even when both the parents had received gene transfer in utero. This is clearly an issue that will need to be addressed in greater detail, nevertheless, prior to moving in utero gene therapy into clinical trials. This need for further investigation is underscored by the fact that, in other studies employing lentiviral vectors in non-human primates, the authors observed modification of the female germline, but no effect upon the male germ cells [90]. Thus, the issue of germline safety will likely have to be investigated in more than one preclinical model, and the specific vector being considered for clinical use will have to be employed, in order to obtain an accurate assessment of the risk posed by the procedure.

12. Conclusions

In conclusion, our findings in the sheep model and those of other groups exploring fetal gene delivery in sheep, mouse, and non-human primate substantial evidence now exists that in utero gene therapy possesses many advantages over postnatal gene therapy, both from a scientific standpoint and from a socioeconomic/psychological point of view, since it is one of the only therapies that could promise the birth of a normal healthy infant following prenatal diagnosis of disease. Importantly, in our in utero studies, none of the sheep that received murine MoLV-based vector preparations exhibited any type of pathology upon examination, even at time points of greater than 5 years post-transduction. Given the highly proliferative state of the fetus at the time of injection, the transduction of repopulating HSC, and the chance of insertional mutagenesis as a result of MoLV genomic integration, the lack of pathology within these animals is a finding of significance, and suggests that although not ideal, MoLV-based vectors may be relatively safe, at least in this context. Equally importantly, the risk to the fetus appears to be minimal, at least when administering the vector via the peritoneal cavity. Following in utero gene transfer, multiple tissues of the developing fetus were transduced and transgene expression persisted long-term (over 5 years), suggesting that this approach may one day be a viable therapeutic option for diseases affecting any of the major organ systems. Moreover, even if not curative, in utero gene therapy would be ideal for a disease like hemophilia A, since lifelong immunologic tolerance could be induced to FVIII, thus overcoming the immune-related hurdles that currently hinder post-natal treatment of this disease. Despite its great potential, however, it is important to realize that in utero gene therapy is still in the experimental stages and many issues need to be clarified before it can become a clinically viable treatment option for hemophilia A or any of the host of other monogenic diseases. Nevertheless, having recently re-established an extinct line of sheep with hemophilia A [43-45, 47-51] that accurately recapitulate the genetics and clinical symptoms of human patients with severe hemophilia A, we are now in an ideal position to apply our experience with in utero gene delivery and this clinically predictive large animal model to begin developing safe and effective approaches to treat hemophilia A with in utero gene therapy.

13. References

[1] Nathwani, A.C., R. Benjamin, A.W. Nienhuis, and A.M. Davidoff, *Current status and prospects for gene therapy.* Vox Sang, 2004. 87(2): p. 73-81.

[2] Nathwani, A.C., A.W. Nienhuis, and A.M. Davidoff, *Current status of gene therapy for hemophilia.* Curr Hematol Rep, 2003. 2(4): p. 319-27.

[3] Podsakoff, G.M., B.C. Engel, and D.B. Kohn, *Perspectives on gene therapy for immune deficiencies.* Biol Blood Marrow Transplant, 2005. 11(12): p. 972-6.

[4] Brenner, M.K. and F.V. Okur, *Overview of gene therapy clinical progress including cancer treatment with gene-modified T cells.* Hematology Am Soc Hematol Educ Program, 2009: p. 675-81.

[5] Ivanov, R., A. Hagenbeek, and S. Ebeling, *Towards immunogene therapy of hematological malignancies.* Exp Hematol, 2006. 34(3): p. 251-63.

[6] Pedersini, R., E. Vattemi, and P.P. Claudio, *Adenoviral gene therapy in high-grade malignant glioma.* Drug News Perspect. 23(6): p. 368-79.

[7] Rossi, J.J., C.H. June, and D.B. Kohn, *Genetic therapies against HIV.* Nat Biotechnol, 2007. 25(12): p. 1444-54.

[8] Sangro, B. and J. Prieto, *Gene therapy for liver cancer: clinical experience and future prospects.* Curr Opin Mol Ther. 12(5): p. 561-9.

[9] Touchefeu, Y., K.J. Harrington, J.P. Galmiche, and G. Vassaux, *Review article: gene therapy, recent developments and future prospects in gastrointestinal oncology.* Aliment Pharmacol Ther. 32(8): p. 953-68.

[10] Chuah, M.K., D. Collen, and T. VandenDriessche, *Clinical gene transfer studies for hemophilia A.* Semin Thromb Hemost, 2004. 30(2): p. 249-56.

[11] High, K.A., *Gene therapy: a 2001 perspective.* Haemophilia, 2001. 7 Suppl 1: p. 23-7.

[12] Pasi, K.J., *Gene therapy for haemophilia.* Br J Haematol, 2001. 115(4): p. 744-57.

[13] White, G.C., 2nd, *Gene therapy in hemophilia: clinical trials update.* Thromb Haemost, 2001. 86(1): p. 172-7.

[14] Agaliotis, D., *Hemophilia, Overview,* 2006.

[15] High, K.A., *Gene transfer as an approach to treating hemophilia.* Semin Thromb Hemost, 2003. 29(1): p. 107-20.

[16] Kay, M.A. and K. High, *Gene therapy for the hemophilias.* Proc Natl Acad Sci U S A, 1999. 96(18): p. 9973-5.

[17] Chuah, M.K., D. Collen, and T. Vandendriessche, *Preclinical and clinical gene therapy for haemophilia.* Haemophilia, 2004. 10 Suppl 4: p. 119-25.

[18] Graw, J., H.H. Brackmann, J. Oldenburg, R. Schneppenheim, M. Spannagl, and R. Schwaab, *Haemophilia A: from mutation analysis to new therapies.* Nat Rev Genet, 2005. 6(6): p. 488-501.

[19] Herzog, R.W. and V.R. Arruda, *Update on gene therapy for hereditary hematological disorders.* Expert Rev Cardiovasc Ther, 2003. 1(2): p. 215-32.

[20] Hough, C. and D. Lillicrap, *Gene therapy for hemophilia: an imperative to succeed.* J Thromb Haemost, 2005. 3(6): p. 1195-205.

[21] Nathwani, A.C., A.M. Davidoff, and E.G. Tuddenham, *Prospects for gene therapy of haemophilia.* Haemophilia, 2004. 10(4): p. 309-18.

[22] Roth, D.A., N.E. Tawa, Jr., J.M. O'Brien, D.A. Treco, and R.F. Selden, *Nonviral transfer of the gene encoding coagulation factor VIII in patients with severe hemophilia A.* N Engl J Med, 2001. 344(23): p. 1735-42.

[23] VandenDriessche, T., D. Collen, and M.K. Chuah, *Gene therapy for the hemophilias.* J Thromb Haemost, 2003. 1(7): p. 1550-8.

[24] Boyce, N., *Trial halted after gene shows up in semen.* Nature, 2001. 414(6865): p. 677.

[25] Marshall, E., *Gene therapy. Panel reviews risks of germ line changes.* Science, 2001. 294(5550): p. 2268-9.

[26] Arruda, V.R., P.A. Fields, R. Milner, L. Wainwright, M.P. De Miguel, P.J. Donovan, R.W. Herzog, T.C. Nichols, J.A. Biegel, M. Razavi, M. Dake, D. Huff, A.W. Flake, L. Couto, M.A. Kay, and K.A. High, *Lack of germline transmission of vector sequences following systemic administration of recombinant AAV-2 vector in males.* Mol Ther, 2001. 4(6): p. 586-92.

[27] Roehl, H.H., M.E. Leibbrandt, J.S. Greengard, E. Kamantigue, W.G. Glass, M. Giedlin, K. Boekelheide, D.E. Johnson, D.J. Jolly, and N.C. Sajjadi, *Analysis of testes and semen from rabbits treated by intravenous injection with a retroviral vector encoding the human factor VIII gene: no evidence of germ line transduction.* Hum Gene Ther, 2000. 11(18): p. 2529-40.

[28] Hacein-Bey-Abina, S., C. Von Kalle, M. Schmidt, M.P. McCormack, N. Wulffraat, P. Leboulch, A. Lim, C.S. Osborne, R. Pawliuk, E. Morillon, R. Sorensen, A. Forster, P. Fraser, J.I. Cohen, G. de Saint Basile, I. Alexander, U. Wintergerst, T. Frebourg, A.

Aurias, D. Stoppa-Lyonnet, S. Romana, I. Radford-Weiss, F. Gross, F. Valensi, E. Delabesse, E. Macintyre, F. Sigaux, J. Soulier, L.E. Leiva, M. Wissler, C. Prinz, T.H. Rabbitts, F. Le Deist, A. Fischer, and M. Cavazzana-Calvo, *LMO2-associated clonal T cell proliferation in two patients after gene therapy for SCID-X1*. Science, 2003. 302(5644): p. 415-9.

[29] Howe, S.J., M.R. Mansour, K. Schwarzwaelder, C. Bartholomae, M. Hubank, H. Kempski, M.H. Brugman, K. Pike-Overzet, S.J. Chatters, D. de Ridder, K.C. Gilmour, S. Adams, S.I. Thornhill, K.L. Parsley, F.J. Staal, R.E. Gale, D.C. Linch, J. Bayford, L. Brown, M. Quaye, C. Kinnon, P. Ancliff, D.K. Webb, M. Schmidt, C. von Kalle, H.B. Gaspar, and A.J. Thrasher, *Insertional mutagenesis combined with acquired somatic mutations causes leukemogenesis following gene therapy of SCID-X1 patients*. J Clin Invest, 2008. 118(9): p. 3143-50.

[30] Thrasher, A.J., H.B. Gaspar, C. Baum, U. Modlich, A. Schambach, F. Candotti, M. Otsu, B. Sorrentino, L. Scobie, E. Cameron, K. Blyth, J. Neil, S.H. Abina, M. Cavazzana-Calvo, and A. Fischer, *Gene therapy: X-SCID transgene leukaemogenicity*. Nature, 2006. 443(7109): p. E5-6; discussion E6-7.

[31] Hough, C., S. Kamisue, C. Cameron, C. Notley, S. Tinlin, A. Giles, and D. Lillicrap, *Aberrant splicing and premature termination of transcription of the FVIII gene as a cause of severe canine hemophilia A: similarities with the intron 22 inversion mutation in human hemophilia*. Thromb Haemost, 2002. 87(4): p. 659-65.

[32] Lozier, J.N., A. Dutra, E. Pak, N. Zhou, Z. Zheng, T.C. Nichols, D.A. Bellinger, M. Read, and R.A. Morgan, *The Chapel Hill hemophilia A dog colony exhibits a factor VIII gene inversion*. Proc Natl Acad Sci U S A, 2002. 99(20): p. 12991-6.

[33] Bi, L., A.M. Lawler, S.E. Antonarakis, K.A. High, J.D. Gearhart, and H.H. Kazazian, Jr., *Targeted disruption of the mouse factor VIII gene produces a model of haemophilia A*. Nat Genet, 1995. 10(1): p. 119-21.

[34] Gallo-Penn, A.M., P.S. Shirley, J.L. Andrews, D.B. Kayda, A.M. Pinkstaff, M. Kaloss, S. Tinlin, C. Cameron, C. Notley, C. Hough, D. Lillicrap, M. Kaleko, and S. Connelly, *In vivo evaluation of an adenoviral vector encoding canine factor VIII: high-level, sustained expression in hemophiliac mice*. Hum Gene Ther, 1999. 10(11): p. 1791-802.

[35] Garcia-Martin, C., M.K. Chuah, A. Van Damme, K.E. Robinson, B. Vanzieleghem, J.M. Saint-Remy, D. Gallardo, F.A. Ofosu, T. Vandendriessche, and G. Hortelano, *Therapeutic levels of human factor VIII in mice implanted with encapsulated cells: potential for gene therapy of haemophilia A*. J Gene Med, 2002. 4(2): p. 215-23.

[36] Moayeri, M., T.S. Hawley, and R.G. Hawley, *Correction of murine hemophilia A by hematopoietic stem cell gene therapy*. Mol Ther, 2005. 12(6): p. 1034-42.

[37] Moayeri, M., A. Ramezani, R.A. Morgan, T.S. Hawley, and R.G. Hawley, *Sustained phenotypic correction of hemophilia a mice following oncoretroviral-mediated expression of a bioengineered human factor VIII gene in long-term hematopoietic repopulating cells*. Mol Ther, 2004. 10(5): p. 892-902.

[38] Reddy, P.S., K. Sakhuja, S. Ganesh, L. Yang, D. Kayda, T. Brann, S. Pattison, D. Golightly, N. Idamakanti, A. Pinkstaff, M. Kaloss, C. Barjot, J.S. Chamberlain, M. Kaleko, and S. Connelly, *Sustained human factor VIII expression in hemophilia A mice following systemic delivery of a gutless adenoviral vector*. Mol Ther, 2002. 5(1): p. 63-73.

[39] Sarkar, R., R. Tetreault, G. Gao, L. Wang, P. Bell, R. Chandler, J.M. Wilson, and H.H. Kazazian, Jr., *Total correction of hemophilia A mice with canine FVIII using an AAV 8 serotype*. Blood, 2004. 103(4): p. 1253-60.

[40] Gallo-Penn, A.M., P.S. Shirley, J.L. Andrews, S. Tinlin, S. Webster, C. Cameron, C. Hough, C. Notley, D. Lillicrap, M. Kaleko, and S. Connelly, *Systemic delivery of an adenoviral vector encoding canine factor VIII results in short-term phenotypic correction, inhibitor development, and biphasic liver toxicity in hemophilia A dogs.* Blood, 2001. 97(1): p. 107-13.

[41] Scallan, C.D., D. Lillicrap, H. Jiang, X. Qian, S.L. Patarroyo-White, A.E. Parker, T. Liu, J. Vargas, D. Nagy, S.K. Powell, J.F. Wright, P.V. Turner, S.J. Tinlin, S.E. Webster, A. McClelland, and L.B. Couto, *Sustained phenotypic correction of canine hemophilia A using an adeno-associated viral vector.* Blood, 2003. 102(6): p. 2031-7.

[42] Turecek, P.L., H. Gritsch, G. Richter, W. Auer, L. Pichler, and H.P. Schwarz, *Assessment of bleeding for the evaluation of therapeutic preparations in small animal models of antibody-induced hemophilia and von Willebrand disease.* Thromb Haemost, 1997. 77(3): p. 591-9.

[43] Neuenschwander, S., L. Kissling-Albrecht, J. Heiniger, W. Backfisch, G. Stranzinger, and V. Pliska, *Inherited defect of blood clotting factor VIII (haemophilia A) in sheep.* Thromb Haemost, 1992. 68(5): p. 618-20.

[44] Backfisch, W., S. Neuenschwander, U. Giger, G. Stranzinger, and V. Pliska, *Carrier detection of ovine hemophilia A using an RFLP marker, and mapping of the factor VIII gene on the ovine X-chromosome.* J Hered, 1994. 85(6): p. 474-8.

[45] Neuenschwander, S. and V. Pliska, *Factor VIII in blood plasma of haemophilic sheep: analysis of clotting time-plasma dilution curves.* Haemostasis, 1994. 24(1): p. 27-35.

[46] Bormann C., L.C., Menges S., Hanna C., Foxworth G., Shin T., Westhusin M., Pliska V., Stranzinger G., Joerg H., Glimp H., Millsap L., Porada C., Almeida-Porada G., Kraemer D., *Reestablishment of an Extinct Strain of Sheep From a Limited Supply of Frozen Semen.* Reproduction, Fertility and Development 2005. 18(2): p. 201-202.

[47] Almeida-Porada, G., Desai, J., Long, C., Westhusin, M., Pliska, V., Stranzinger, G., Joerg, H., Thain, D., Glimp, H., Kraemer, D., Porada, C.D. , *Re-establishment and characterization of an extinct line of sheep with a spontaneous bleeding disorder that closely recapitulates human hemophilia A.* Blood, 2007. 110(11): p. 347a.

[48] Sanada, C., Wood, J.A., Liu, W., Lozier, J.N., Almeida-Porada, G., Porada, C.D., *A Frame Shift-Induced Stop Codon Causes Hemophilia A in Sheep.* . Blood, 2008. 112: p. Abstract #3378.

[49] Porada, C.D., C. Sanada, C.R. Long, J.A. Wood, J. Desai, N. Frederick, L. Millsap, C. Bormann, S.L. Menges, C. Hanna, G. Flores-Foxworth, T. Shin, M.E. Westhusin, W. Liu, H. Glimp, E.D. Zanjani, J.N. Lozier, V. Pliska, G. Stranzinger, H. Joerg, D.C. Kraemer, and G. Almeida-Porada, *Clinical and molecular characterization of a re-established line of sheep exhibiting hemophilia A.* J Thromb Haemost, 2010. 8(2): p. 276-85.

[50] Bormann, C., Long, C., Menges, S., Hanna, C., Foxworth, G., Westhusin, M., Pliska, V., Stranzinger, G., Glimp, H., Millsap, L., Porada, C., Almeida-Porada, G., Kraemer, D. , *Reestablishment of an extinct strain of sheep utilizing assisted reproductive technologies.* . Reproduction Fertility and Development 2007. 21(1): p. 153.

[51] Bormann C., L.C., Menges S., Hanna C., Foxworth G., Shin T., Westhusin M., Pliska V., Stranzinger G., Joerg H., Glimp H., Millsap L., Porada C., Almeida-Porada G., Kraemer D., *Reestablishment of an Extinct Strain of Sheep From a Limited Supply of Frozen Semen.* Reproduction, Fertility and Development 2006. 18(1): p. 201.

[52] Maddox, J.F., C.R. Mackay, and M.R. Brandon, *Ontogeny of ovine lymphocytes. I. An immunohistological study on the development of T lymphocytes in the sheep embryo and fetal thymus.* Immunology, 1987. 62(1): p. 97-105.

[53] Maddox, J.F., C.R. Mackay, and M.R. Brandon, *Ontogeny of ovine lymphocytes. III. An immunohistological study on the development of T lymphocytes in sheep fetal lymph nodes.* Immunology, 1987. 62(1): p. 113-8.

[54] Maddox, J.F., C.R. Mackay, and M.R. Brandon, *Ontogeny of ovine lymphocytes. II. An immunohistological study on the development of T lymphocytes in the sheep fetal spleen.* Immunology, 1987. 62(1): p. 107-12.

[55] Osburn, B.I., *The ontogeny of the ruminant immune system and its significance in the understanding of maternal-fetal-neonatal relationships.* Adv Exp Med Biol, 1981. 137: p. 91-103.

[56] Sawyer, M., J. Moe, and B.I. Osburn, *Ontogeny of immunity and leukocytes in the ovine fetus and elevation of immunoglobulins related to congenital infection.* Am J Vet Res, 1978. 39(4): p. 643-8.

[57] Silverstein, A.M., C.J. Parshall, Jr., and J.W. Uhr, *Immunologic maturation in utero: kinetics of the primary antibody response in the fetal lamb.* Science, 1966. 154(757): p. 1675-7.

[58] Tuboly, S., R. Glavits, and M. Bucsek, *Stages in the development of the ovine immune system.* Zentralbl Veterinarmed B, 1984. 31(2): p. 81-95.

[59] McCarroll, D.R., D.C. Waters, K.R. Steidley, R. Clift, and T.P. McDonald, *Canine platelet von Willebrand factor: quantification and multimeric analysis.* Exp Hematol, 1988. 16(11): p. 929-37.

[60] Parker, M.T., M.A. Turrentine, and G.S. Johnson, *von Willebrand factor in lysates of washed canine platelets.* Am J Vet Res, 1991. 52(1): p. 119-25.

[61] Flake, A.W. and E.D. Zanjani, *In utero hematopoietic stem cell transplantation: ontogenic opportunities and biologic barriers.* Blood, 1999. 94(7): p. 2179-91.

[62] Troeger, C., D. Surbek, A. Schoberlein, S. Schatt, L. Dudler, S. Hahn, and W. Holzgreve, *In utero haematopoietic stem cell transplantation. Experiences in mice, sheep and humans.* Swiss Med Wkly, 2006. 136(31-32): p. 498-503.

[63] Merianos, D., T. Heaton, and A.W. Flake, *In utero hematopoietic stem cell transplantation: progress toward clinical application.* Biol Blood Marrow Transplant, 2008. 14(7): p. 729-40.

[64] Flake, A.W., M.G. Roncarolo, J.M. Puck, G. Almeida-Porada, M.I. Evans, M.P. Johnson, E.M. Abella, D.D. Harrison, and E.D. Zanjani, *Treatment of X-linked severe combined immunodeficiency by in utero transplantation of paternal bone marrow.* N Engl J Med, 1996. 335(24): p. 1806-10.

[65] Coutelle, C., M. Themis, S.N. Waddington, S.M. Buckley, L.G. Gregory, M.S. Nivsarkar, A.L. David, D. Peebles, B. Weisz, and C. Rodeck, *Gene therapy progress and prospects: fetal gene therapy--first proofs of concept--some adverse effects.* Gene Ther, 2005. 12(22): p. 1601-7.

[66] Klein, I., H. Andrikovics, A. Bors, L. Nemes, A. Tordai, and A. Varadi, *A haemophilia A and B molecular genetic diagnostic programme in Hungary: a highly informative and cost-effective strategy.* Haemophilia, 2001. 7(3): p. 306-12.

[67] Peyvandi, F., *Carrier detection and prenatal diagnosis of hemophilia in developing countries.* Semin Thromb Hemost, 2005. 31(5): p. 544-54.

[68] Sasanakul, W., A. Chuansumrit, S. Ajjimakorn, S. Krasaesub, N. Sirachainan, S. Chotsupakarn, P. Kadegasem, and S. Rurgkhum, *Cost-effectiveness in establishing hemophilia carrier detection and prenatal diagnosis services in a developing country with limited health resources.* Southeast Asian J Trop Med Public Health, 2003. 34(4): p. 891-8.

[69] Hollestelle, M.J., T. Thinnes, K. Crain, A. Stiko, J.K. Kruijt, T.J. van Berkel, D.J. Loskutoff, and J.A. van Mourik, *Tissue distribution of factor VIII gene expression in vivo--a closer look.* Thromb Haemost, 2001. 86(3): p. 855-61.

[70] Fausto, N.a.W., E.M., *The Liver: Biology and Pathobiology*, ed. A.M. Arias, Boyer, J.L., Fausto, N., Jacoby, W.B., Scachter, D., and Shafritz, D.A.1994, New York: Raven. 1059-1084.

[71] Billingham, R.E., L. Brent, and P.B. Medawar, *Quantitative studies on tissue transplantation immunity. II. The origin, strength and duration of actively and adoptively acquired immunity.* Proc R Soc Lond B Biol Sci, 1954. 143(910): p. 58-80.

[72] Park P, Z.E., Porada CD. , *Risks to the germline following in utero gene transfer.* . Molecular Therapy, 2003. 7((5)): p. S137.

[73] Park P.J., A.-P.G., Glimp H.A., Zanjani E.D., Porada C.D. , *Germline cells may be at risk following direct injection gene therapy in utero.* Blood 2003. 102((11)): p. 874a.

[74] Park P.J., T.J., Almeida-Porada G., Zanjani E.D., Porada C.D. , *Male germline cells appear to be at risk following direct injection gene transfer in utero.* . Molecular Therapy 2004. 9 ((Suppl. 1)): p. S403.

[75] Porada C.D., A.-P.M.G., Torabi A., Zanjani E.D. , *In utero transduction of hematopoietic cells is enhanced at early gestational ages.* Blood, 2001. 98((Part 1)): p. 214a.

[76] Porada C.D., A.-P.M.G., Park P., Zanjani E.D. , *In utero transduction of lung and liver: gestational age determines gene transfer efficiency.* . Blood 2001. 98 ((Part 1)): p. 215a.

[77] Porada C.D., P.P., Torabi A., Almeida-Porada G., Zanjani E.D. , *Gestational age determines gene transfer efficiency to hematopoietic cells, lung and liver following in utero retroviral-mediated gene transfer.* . Molecular Therapy, 2002. American Society of Gene Therapy, Annual Meeting, Boston, MA .

[78] Porada, C.D., P. Park, G. Almeida-Porada, and E.D. Zanjani, *The sheep model of in utero gene therapy.* Fetal Diagn Ther, 2004. 19(1): p. 23-30.

[79] Porada, C.D., P.J. Park, G. Almeida-Porada, W. Liu, F. Ozturk, H.A. Glimp, and E.D. Zanjani, *Gestational age of recipient determines pattern and level of transgene expression following in utero retroviral gene transfer.* Mol Ther, 2005. 11(2): p. 284-93.

[80] Porada, C.D., P.J. Park, J. Tellez, F. Ozturk, H.A. Glimp, G. Almeida-Porada, and E.D. Zanjani, *Male germ-line cells are at risk following direct-injection retroviral-mediated gene transfer in utero.* Mol Ther, 2005. 12(4): p. 754-62.

[81] Porada, C.D., N. Tran, M. Eglitis, R.C. Moen, L. Troutman, A.W. Flake, Y. Zhao, W.F. Anderson, and E.D. Zanjani, *In utero gene therapy: transfer and long-term expression of the bacterial neo(r) gene in sheep after direct injection of retroviral vectors into preimmune fetuses.* Hum Gene Ther, 1998. 9(11): p. 1571-85.

[82] Tran, N.D., C.D. Porada, Y. Zhao, G. Almeida-Porada, W.F. Anderson, and E.D. Zanjani, *In utero transfer and expression of exogenous genes in sheep.* Exp Hematol, 2000. 28(1): p. 17-30.

[83] Peters, S.O., E.L. Kittler, H.S. Ramshaw, and P.J. Quesenberry, *Ex vivo expansion of murine marrow cells with interleukin-3 (IL-3), IL-6, IL-11, and stem cell factor leads to impaired engraftment in irradiated hosts.* Blood, 1996. 87(1): p. 30-7.

[84] Porada C.D., P.P., Torabi A., Almeida-Porada G., Zanjani E.D. , *Gestational age determines gene transfer efficiency to hematopoietic cells, lung and liver following in utero retroviral-mediated gene transfer.* . Molecular Therapy, 2002. American Society of Gene Therapy, Annual Meeting, Boston, MA
[85] Porada, C.D., D.D. Harrison-Findik, C. Sanada, V. Valiente, D. Thain, P.J. Simmons, G. Almeida-Porada, and E.D. Zanjani, *Development and characterization of a novel CD34 monoclonal antibody that identifies sheep hematopoietic stem/progenitor cells.* Exp Hematol, 2008. 36(12): p. 1739-49.
[86] Porada C.D., A.-P.M.G., Park P., Zanjani E.D. , *In utero transduction of lung and liver: gestational age determines gene transfer efficiency.* . Blood, 2001. 98 ((Part 1)): p. 215a.
[87] Chen, X.G., H.Z. Zhu, J.L. Gong, F. Li, and J.L. Xue, *Efficient delivery of human clotting factor IX after injection of lentiviral vectors in utero.* Acta Pharmacol Sin, 2004. 25(6): p. 789-93.
[88] David, A., T. Cook, S. Waddington, D. Peebles, M. Nivsarkar, H. Knapton, M. Miah, T. Dahse, D. Noakes, H. Schneider, C. Rodeck, C. Coutelle, and M. Themis, *Ultrasound-guided percutaneous delivery of adenoviral vectors encoding the beta-galactosidase and human factor IX genes to early gestation fetal sheep in utero.* Hum Gene Ther, 2003. 14(4): p. 353-64.
[89] Jimenez, D.F., C.I. Lee, C.E. O'Shea, D.B. Kohn, and A.F. Tarantal, *HIV-1-derived lentiviral vectors and fetal route of administration on transgene biodistribution and expression in rhesus monkeys.* Gene Ther, 2005. 12(10): p. 821-30.
[90] Lee, C.C., D.F. Jimenez, D.B. Kohn, and A.F. Tarantal, *Fetal gene transfer using lentiviral vectors and the potential for germ cell transduction in rhesus monkeys (Macaca mulatta).* Hum Gene Ther, 2005. 16(4): p. 417-25.
[91] Park, P.J., E. Colletti, F. Ozturk, J.A. Wood, J. Tellez, G. Almeida-Porada, and C. Porada, *Factors determining the risk of inadvertent retroviral transduction of male germ cells after in utero gene transfer in sheep.* Hum Gene Ther, 2009. 20(3): p. 201-15.
[92] Porada, C.D., N.D. Tran, G. Almeida-Porada, H.A. Glimp, J.S. Pixley, Y. Zhao, W.F. Anderson, and E.D. Zanjani, *Transduction of long-term-engrafting human hematopoietic stem cells by retroviral vectors.* Hum Gene Ther, 2002. 13(7): p. 867-79.
[93] Tarantal, A.F., V.K. Han, K.C. Cochrum, A. Mok, M. daSilva, and D.G. Matsell, *Fetal rhesus monkey model of obstructive renal dysplasia.* Kidney Int, 2001. 59(2): p. 446-56.
[94] Tarantal, A.F. and C.C. Lee, *Long-term luciferase expression monitored by bioluminescence imaging after adeno-associated virus-mediated fetal gene delivery in rhesus monkeys (Macaca mulatta).* Hum Gene Ther. 21(2): p. 143-8.
[95] Tarantal, A.F., C.C. Lee, D.F. Jimenez, and S.R. Cherry, *Fetal gene transfer using lentiviral vectors: in vivo detection of gene expression by microPET and optical imaging in fetal and infant monkeys.* Hum Gene Ther, 2006. 17(12): p. 1254-61.
[96] Tarantal, A.F., C.I. Lee, J.E. Ekert, R. McDonald, D.B. Kohn, C.G. Plopper, S.S. Case, and B.A. Bunnell, *Lentiviral vector gene transfer into fetal rhesus monkeys (Macaca mulatta): lung-targeting approaches.* Mol Ther, 2001. 4(6): p. 614-21.
[97] Tarantal, A.F., R.J. McDonald, D.F. Jimenez, C.C. Lee, C.E. O'Shea, A.C. Leapley, R.H. Won, C.G. Plopper, C. Lutzko, and D.B. Kohn, *Intrapulmonary and intramyocardial gene transfer in rhesus monkeys (Macaca mulatta): safety and efficiency of HIV-1-derived lentiviral vectors for fetal gene delivery.* Mol Ther, 2005. 12(1): p. 87-98.

[98] Tarantal, A.F., J.P. O'Rourke, S.S. Case, G.C. Newbound, J. Li, C.I. Lee, C.R. Baskin, D.B. Kohn, and B.A. Bunnell, *Rhesus monkey model for fetal gene transfer: studies with retroviral- based vector systems.* Mol Ther, 2001. 3(2): p. 128-38.

[99] Themis, M., H. Schneider, T. Kiserud, T. Cook, S. Adebakin, S. Jezzard, S. Forbes, M. Hanson, A. Pavirani, C. Rodeck, and C. Coutelle, *Successful expression of beta-galactosidase and factor IX transgenes in fetal and neonatal sheep after ultrasound-guided percutaneous adenovirus vector administration into the umbilical vein.* Gene Ther, 1999. 6(7): p. 1239-48.

[100] Waddington, S.N., S.M. Buckley, M. Nivsarkar, S. Jezzard, H. Schneider, T. Dahse, G. Kemball-Cook, M. Miah, N. Tucker, M.J. Dallman, M. Themis, and C. Coutelle, *In utero gene transfer of human factor IX to fetal mice can induce postnatal tolerance of the exogenous clotting factor.* Blood, 2003. 101(4): p. 1359-66.

[101] Waddington, S.N., M.S. Nivsarkar, A.R. Mistry, S.M. Buckley, G. Kemball-Cook, K.L. Mosley, K. Mitrophanous, P. Radcliffe, M.V. Holder, M. Brittan, A. Georgiadis, F. Al-Allaf, B.W. Bigger, L.G. Gregory, H.T. Cook, R.R. Ali, A. Thrasher, E.G. Tuddenham, M. Themis, and C. Coutelle, *Permanent phenotypic correction of hemophilia B in immunocompetent mice by prenatal gene therapy.* Blood, 2004. 104(9): p. 2714-21.

[102] Lipshutz, G.S., L. Flebbe-Rehwaldt, and K.M. Gaensler, *Reexpression following readministration of an adenoviral vector in adult mice after initial in utero adenoviral administration.* Mol Ther, 2000. 2(4): p. 374-80.

[103] Lipshutz, G.S., R. Sarkar, L. Flebbe-Rehwaldt, H. Kazazian, and K.M. Gaensler, *Short-term correction of factor VIII deficiency in a murine model of hemophilia A after delivery of adenovirus murine factor VIII in utero.* Proc Natl Acad Sci U S A, 1999. 96(23): p. 13324-9.

[104] Schneider, H., S. Adebakin, M. Themis, T. Cook, A.M. Douar, A. Pavirani, and C. Coutelle, *Therapeutic plasma concentrations of human factor IX in mice after gene delivery into the amniotic cavity: a model for the prenatal treatment of haemophilia B.* J Gene Med, 1999. 1(6): p. 424-32.

[105] Schneider, H., C. Muhle, A.M. Douar, S. Waddington, Q.J. Jiang, K. von der Mark, C. Coutelle, and W. Rascher, *Sustained delivery of therapeutic concentrations of human clotting factor IX--a comparison of adenoviral and AAV vectors administered in utero.* J Gene Med, 2002. 4(1): p. 46-53.

[106] Tran, N.D., C.D. Porada, G. Almeida-Porada, H.A. Glimp, W.F. Anderson, and E.D. Zanjani, *Induction of stable prenatal tolerance to beta-galactosidase by in utero gene transfer into preimmune sheep fetuses.* Blood, 2001. 97(11): p. 3417-23.

[107] Colletti, E., S. Lindstedt, P. Park, G. Almeida-Porada, and C. Porada, *Early Fetal Gene Delivery Utilizes both Central and Peripheral Mechanisms of Tolerance Induction.* Experimental Hematology, 2008. 36(7): p. 816-22.

[108] Chitlur, M., I. Warrier, M. Rajpurkar, and J.M. Lusher, *Inhibitors in factor IX deficiency a report of the ISTH-SSC international FIX inhibitor registry (1997-2006).* Haemophilia, 2009. 15(5): p. 1027-31.

[109] Ehrenforth, S., W. Kreuz, I. Scharrer, R. Linde, M. Funk, T. Gungor, B. Krackhardt, and B. Kornhuber, *Incidence of development of factor VIII and factor IX inhibitors in haemophiliacs.* Lancet, 1992. 339(8793): p. 594-8.

[110] Ponder, K.P., *Hemophilia gene therapy: a Holy Grail found.* Mol Ther. 19(3): p. 427-8.

[111] Doehmer, J., M. Breindl, K. Willecke, and R. Jaenisch, *Genetic transmission of Moloney leukemia virus: mapping of the chromosomal integration site.* Haematol Blood Transfus, 1979. 23: p. 561-8.
[112] Jaenisch, R., *Germ line integration and Mendelian transmission of the exogenous Moloney leukemia virus.* Proc Natl Acad Sci U S A, 1976. 73(4): p. 1260-4.
[113] Jahner, D., K. Haase, R. Mulligan, and R. Jaenisch, *Insertion of the bacterial gpt gene into the germ line of mice by retroviral infection.* Proc Natl Acad Sci U S A, 1985. 82(20): p. 6927-31.
[114] Soriano, P. and R. Jaenisch, *Retroviruses as probes for mammalian development: allocation of cells to the somatic and germ cell lineages.* Cell, 1986. 46(1): p. 19-29.
[115] Allioli, N., J.L. Thomas, Y. Chebloune, V.M. Nigon, G. Verdier, and C. Legras, *Use of retroviral vectors to introduce and express the beta-galactosidase marker gene in cultured chicken primordial germ cells.* Dev Biol, 1994. 165(1): p. 30-7.
[116] Park P.J., A.-P.G., Glimp H.A., Zanjani E.D., Porada C.D. , *Germline cells may be at risk following direct injection gene therapy in utero.* Blood, 2003. 102((11)): p. 874a.
[117] Park P.J., T.J., Almeida-Porada G., Zanjani E.D., Porada C.D. , *Male germline cells appear to be at risk following direct injection gene transfer in utero.* . Molecular Therapy, 2004. 9 ((Suppl. 1)): p. S403.
[118] Kazazian, H.H., Jr., *An estimated frequency of endogenous insertional mutations in humans.* Nat Genet, 1999. 22(2): p. 130.

Part 4

Gene Therapy in Other Diseases

19

Genetic Addiction Risk Score (GARS): Testing For Polygenetic Predisposition and Risk to Reward Deficiency Syndrome (RDS)

Kenneth Blum[1,2,3,4,7] et al.*

[1]*Departement of Psychiatry and McKnight Brain Institute, University of Florida, Gainesville*
[2]*Dominion Diagnostics Laboratory, North Kingstown, Rhode Island,*
[3]*Department of Nutrigenomics, LifeGen, Inc. San Diego, California,*
[4]*Department of Holistic Medicine, G & G Holistic Addiction Treatment Center, North Miami Beach, Florida,*
[7]*Department of clinical Neurology, Path Foundation NY, New York, New York USA*

1. Introduction

Dopamine is a neurotransmitter in the brain, which controls feelings of wellbeing. This sense of wellbeing results from the interaction of dopamine and neurotransmitters such as serotonin, the opioids, and other brain chemicals. Low serotonin levels are associated with depression. High levels of the opioids (the brain's opium) are also associated with a sense of wellbeing. (Blum et al., 2010).

Dopamine has been called the "anti-stress" and/or "pleasure" molecule. When released into the synapse, dopamine stimulates a number of receptors (D1 - D5), which results in increased feelings of wellbeing and stress reduction (Kreek and Koob, 2007). The mesocorticolimbic dopaminergic pathway plays an important role in mediating reinforcement of natural rewards such as food and sex, as well as unnatural rewards such as drugs of abuse (Bruijnzeel et al., 2007). Natural rewards include satisfaction of physiological drives (e.g. hunger and reproduction) and unnatural rewards are learned and involve satisfaction of acquired pleasures such as hedonic sensations derived from alcohol and other drugs, as well as from gambling and other risk-taking behaviors. (Olsen, 2011).

---

*Frank Fornari[2], B.William Downs[3], Roger L. Waite[3], [4]John Giordano[4], Andrew Smolen[5], Yijun Lui[1], Jai Tain[6], Neil Majmundar[7] and Eric R. Braverman[7,8]

1 *Departement of Psychiatry and McKnight Brain Institute, University of Florida, Gainesville, USA*
2 *Dominion Diagnostics Laboratory, North Kingstown, Rhode Island, USA*
3 *Department of Nutrigenomics, LifeGen, Inc. San Diego, California, USA*
4 *Department of Holistic Medicine, G & G Holistic Addiction Treatment Center, North Miami Beach, Florida, USA*
5 *Institute for Behavioral Genetics, University of Colorado, Boulder, Colorado, USA*
6 *Medical Image Processing Group, Institute of Automation, Chinese Academy of Sciences, Beijing, CHINA & Life Sciences Research Center, School of Life Sciences and Technology, Xidian University, Xi'an, Shaanx, CHINA*
7 *Department of clinical Neurology, Path Foundation NY, New York, New York. USA*
8 *Department of Neurological Surgery, Weill-Cornell College of Medicine, New York, New York*

The DRD2 gene is responsible for the synthesis of dopamine D2 receptors (Grady et al., 1989). Further depending on the genotype (allelic form A1 versus A2), the DRD2 gene dictates the number of these receptors at post-junctional sites (Blum et al., 1990; Noble et al. 1991). A low number of D2 receptors leads to hypodopaminergic function. When there is a paucity of dopamine receptors, the person is more prone to seek any substance or behavior that stimulates the dopaminergic system (Conrad et al., 2010). The D2 receptor has been associated with pleasure, and the DRD2 gene has been referred to as a reward gene (Heber & Carpenter, 2011).

Although the DRD2 gene, and especially the Taq1 A1 allele, has been most associated with neuropsychiatric disorders in general and in alcoholism in particular, it is likely involved in other addictions (e.g., carbohydrate). It may also be involved in co-morbid antisocial personality disorder symptoms, especially in children and adults with attention deficit hyperactivity disorder (ADHD), or Tourettes Syndrome, and high novelty seeking behaviors (Noble, 2003).

Reward Deficiency Syndrome was first defined in 1996 as a putative predictor of impulsive and addictive behaviors (Blum et al., 1996). Herein, "Reward Deficiency Syndrome" or "RDS" refers to a group of related addictive behaviors. Dopamine is a major component in the mechanisms related to RDS and brain function. Specifically, RDS involves dopamine resistance, a form of sensory deprivation of the brain's reward or pleasure mechanisms (Bowirrat & Oscar-Berman, 2005). The syndrome can be manifested in relatively mild or severe forms that follow as a consequence of an individual's biochemical inability to derive reward from ordinary, everyday activities. The DRD2 A1 genetic variant is also associated with a spectrum of impulsive, compulsive, and addictive behaviors (Gardner, 2011). RDS or anti-reward pathways unite these disorders and explain how certain genetic anomalies give rise to complex aberrant behavior.

In discussing RDS, specific reference is made to an insensitivity and inefficiency in the brain's reward system. There may be a common neurocircuitry, neuroanatomy, and neurobiology for multiple addictions and for a number of psychiatric disorders. Due to specific genetic antecedents and environmental influences, a deficiency of for example, the D2 receptors may predispose individuals to a high risk for multiple addictive, impulsive, and compulsive behaviors. It is well known that alcohol and other drugs of abuse, as well as most positive reinforcements (e.g., sex, food, gambling, aggressive thrills, etc.), cause activation and neuronal release of brain dopamine, which can decrease negative feelings and satisfy abnormal cravings for substances such as alcohol, cocaine, heroin, and nicotine, which, among others, are linked to low dopamine function (Blum et al., 2008).

In individuals possessing an abnormality in the DRD2 gene, the brain lacks enough dopamine receptor sites to achieve adequate dopamine sensitivity and function from the "normal" dopamine produced in the Reward Center of the brain. Carriers of the A1 DRD2 gene variant may have unhealthy appetites, abuse cocaine, indulge in overeating (which can lead to obesity) or, on the other extreme, be anorexic and/or suffer greater consequences of chronic stress (Bau et al., 2000). In these individuals, their addictive brains lead to generalized craving behavior. In essence, they seek substances including alcohol, opiates, cocaine, nicotine, and/or glucose (all substances known to cause preferential release of dopamine at the Nucleus accumbens (NAc)) to activate dopaminergic pathways in order to offset their low D2 receptors, which are caused by the dopamine D2 receptor gene Taq1 A1 allele antecedents (Sullivan et al., 2011). However, evidence is emerging that anterior cingulate cortex rather than the NAc may be involved in operant effort-based decision making (Walton et al., 2009). In addition, the DRD2 A1 polymorphism is also associated with abnormally aggressive behavior, which also stimulates the brain's use of dopamine (Chen et al., 2005).

2. Candidate genes and predisposition to reward dependence behaviors

RDS is linked to flawed dopamine metabolism, and especially to low D2 receptor density. Moreover, RDS results from a dysfunction in the mesolimbic system of the brain, which directly links abnormal craving behavior with a defect in the Dopamine D2 Receptor Gene (DRD2) as well as other dopaminergic genes (D1, D3, D4, and D5, DATA1, MAO, COMT), including many genes associated with the brain reward function (Pinto & Ansseau, 2009), as listed in Table 1, below.

REWARD -DEPENDENCE- PATH WAY	CANDIDATE GENES
Signal Transduction	ADCY7
Signal Transduction	AVPR1A
Signal Transduction	AVPR1B
Signal Transduction	CDK5R1
Signal Transduction	CREB1
Signal Transduction	CSNKLE
Signal Transduction	FEV
Signal Transduction	FDS
Signal Transduction	FOSL1
Signal Transduction	FOSL2
Signal Transduction	GSK3B
Signal Transduction	JUN
Signal Transduction	MAPK1
Signal Transduction	MAPK3
Signal Transduction	MAPK14
Signal Transduction	MPD2
Signal Transduction	MGFB
Signal Transduction	NTRK2
Signal Transduction	NTSR1
Signal Transduction	NTSR2
Signal Transduction	PPP1R1B
Signal Transduction	PRKCE
Serotonin	HTRIA
Serotonin	HTRIB
Serotonin	HTR2A
Serotonin	HTR2C
Serotonin	HTR3A
Serotonin	HTR3B
Serotonin	MAOA
Serotonin	MAOB

REWARD -DEPENDENCE- PATH WAY	CANDIDATE GENES
Serotonin	SLC64A
Serotonin	TPH1
Serotonin	TPH2
Opioid	OPRMI
Opioid	OPRKI
Opioid	PDYN
Opioid	PMOC
Opioid	PRD1
Opioid	OPRL1
Opioid	PENK
Opioid	PNOC
GABA	GABRA2
GABA	GABRA3
GABA	GABRA4
GABA	GABRA6
GABA	GABRB1
GABA	GABRB2
GABA	GABRB3
GABA	GABRD
GABA	GABRE
GABA	GABRG2
GABA	GABRG3
GABA	GABRQ
GABA	SLC6A7
GABA	SL6A11
GABA	SLC32A1
GABA	GAD1
GABA	GAD2
GABA	DB1
Dopamine	COMT
Dopamine	DDC
Dopamine	DRD1
Dopamine	DRD2
Dopamine	DRD3
Dopamine	DRD4
Dopamine	DRD5
Dopamine	SLC18A2
Dopamine	SLC6A3
Dopamine	TH
Cannabinoid	CNR1

REWARD -DEPENDENCE- PATH WAY	CANDIDATE GENES
Cannabinoid	FAAH
Cholinergic	CHRMI
Cholinergic	CHRM2
Cholinergic	CHRM3
Cholinergic	CHRM5
Cholinergic	CHRNA4
Cholinergic	CHRNB2
Adrenergic	ADRA1A
Adrenergic	ADRA2B
Adrenergic	ADRB2
Adrenergic	SLC6A2
Adrenergic	DRA2A
Adrenergic	DRA2C
Adrenergic	ARRB2
Adrenergic	DBH
Glycine	GLRA1
Glycine	GLRA2
Glycine	GLRB
Glycine	GPHN
NDMA	GR1K1
NDMA	GRINI
NDMA	GRIN2A
NDMA	GRIN2B
NDMA	GRIN2C
NDMA	GRM1
Stress	CRH
Stress	CRHEP
Stress	CRHR1
Stress	CRHR2
Stress	GAL
Stress	NPY
Stress	NPY1R
Stress	NPY2R
Stress	NPY5R
Drug Metabolizing	ALDH1
Drug Metabolizing	ALDH2
Drug Metabolizing	CAT

REWARD -DEPENDENCE- PATHWAY	CANDIDATE GENES
Drug Metabolizing	CYPZE1
Drug Metabolizing	ADH1A
Drug Metabolizing	ADH1B
Drug Metabolizing	ADH1C
Drug Metabolizing	ADH4
Drug Metabolizing	ADH5
Drug Metabolizing	ADH6
Drug Metabolizing	ADH6
Drug Metabolizing	ADH7
Others	BDNF
Others	CART
Others	CCK
Others	CCKAR
Others	CLOCK
Others	HCRT
Others	LEP
Others	NR3C1
Others	SLC29A1
Others	TAC

Table 1. Genes involved in various Reward Dependence Pathways.

The genesis of all behavior, be it "normal" (socially acceptable) or "abnormal" (socially unacceptable), derives from an individual's genetic makeup at birth. This genetic predisposition, due to multiple gene combinations and polymorphisms, is expressed differently based on numerous environmental factors including family, friends, educational and socioeconomic status, environmental contaminant exposure, and the availability of psychoactive drugs, including food. The core of predisposition to these behaviors is a set of genes interacting with the environment , which promote a feeling of wellbeing via neurotransmitter interaction at the "reward center" of the brain (located in the meso-limbic system), leading to normal dopamine release (Kendler et al 2011).

Subjects afflicted with RDS carry polymorphic genes in dopaminergic pathways that result in hypo-dopominergic function caused by a reduced number of dopamine D2 receptors, reduced synthesis of dopamine (by dopamine beta –hydroxylase), reduced net release of pre-synaptic dopamine (from, e.g., the dopamine D1 receptor), increased synaptic clearance due to a high number of dopamine transporter sites (dopamine transporter), and low D2 receptor densities (dopamine D2 receptor), making such people more vulnerable to addictive behaviors (Comings and Blum, 2000). The RDS concept involves shared genes and their mRNA expressions and behavioral tendencies, including dependence on alcohol, psycho-stimulants, marijuana, nicotine (smoking), and opiates, altered opiate receptor function, carbohydrate issues (e.g., sugar-binging), obesity, pathological gambling, sex addiction, premeditated aggression, stress, pathological aggression, and certain personality disorders, including novelty-seeking and sex addiction. The common theme across all of these substances and behaviors is that they induce pre-synaptic dopamine release (Dreyer,

2010). Spectrum disorders such as ADHD, Tourettes Syndrome, and Autism are also included due to dopamine dysregulation. As well as other rare mutations (Sundaram et al., 2010) have been associated with Tourettes and Autism. One example includes the association with Neuroligin 4 (NLGN4) is a member of a cell adhesion protein family that appears to play a role in the maturation and function of neuronal synapses (Lawson-Yuen et al., 2008).

3. Neurogenetics of reward deficiency syndrome (RDS)

Since the discovery of the double helix, explorations of brain function in terms of both physiology and behavioral traits have resulted in a plethora of studies linking these activities to neurotransmitter functions having a genetic basis. The mechanisms underlining gene expression and the potential impairments due to polygenic inheritance -- and as such, predisposition to addiction and self-destructive behaviors -- have been studied. Our studies have shown that the prevalence of the DRD2 A1 allele in Cocaine dependent (CD) subjects (n = 53) was 50.9%. It was significantly higher than either the 16.0% prevalence ($P < 10(-4)$) in non-substance abusing controls (n = 100) or the 30.9% prevalence ($P < 10(-2)$) in population controls (n = 265) wherein substance abusers were not excluded. Logistic regression analysis of CD subjects identified potent routes of cocaine use and the interaction of early deviant behaviors and parental alcoholism as significant risk factors associated with the DRD2 A1 allele. The cumulative number of these risk factors in CD subjects was positively and significantly ($P < 10^{-3}$) related to DRD2 A1 allelic prevalence. The data showing a strong association of the minor alleles (A1 and B1) of the DRD2 with CD indicates that a gene, located on the q22-q23 region of chromosome 11, confers susceptibility to this drug disorder (Noble et al.,1993)

Over half a century of dedicated and rigorous scientific research on the mesolimbic system, has provided insight into the addictive brain and the neurogenetic mechanisms involved in man's quest for happiness (Blum et al., 2009). In brief, the site of the brain where one experiences feelings of wellbeing is the mesolimbic system. This part of the brain has been termed the "reward center". Chemical messages including serotonin, enkephalins, GABA, and dopamine (DA) work in concert to provide a net release of DA at the nucleus accumbens (NAc), a region in the mesolimbic system. It is well known that genes control the synthesis, vesicular storage, metabolism, receptor formation, and neurotransmitter catabolism. The polymorphic versions of these genes have certain variations that could lead to an impairment of the neurochemical events involved in the neuronal release of DA. The cascade of these neuronal events has been termed "Brain Reward Cascade". See Figure 1. A breakdown of this cascade ultimately leads to a dysregulation and dysfunction of DA. Since DA has been established as the "pleasure molecule" and the "anti-stress molecule," any reduction in its function could lead to reward deficiency and resultant aberrant substance seeking behavior and a lack of wellness (Blum & Kozlowski, 1989).

It is well -known that humans are biologically predisposed to drink, eat, reproduce, and desire pleasurable experiences (Tindell et al. , 2006, Peciña et al., 2006). Impairment in the mechanisms involved in these natural processes lead to multiple impulsive, compulsive, and addictive behaviors governed by genetic polymorphisms. While there are a plethora of genetic variations at the level of mesolimbic activity, polymorphisms of the serotonergic-2A receptor (5-HTT2a), serotonergic transporter (5HTTLPR), dopamine D2 receptor (DRD2), dopamine D4 receptor (DRD4), dopamine transporter (DAT1), and Catechol-o-methyl–

transferase (COMT), and monoamine-oxidase (MOA) genes, as well as other genes, predispose individuals to excessive cravings and resultant aberrant behaviors.

As stated earlier, an umbrella term to describe the common genetic antecedents of multiple impulsive, compulsive, and addictive behaviors is RDS. Individuals possessing a paucity of serotonergic and/or dopaminergic receptors and an increased rate of synaptic DA catabolism, due to high catabolic genotype of the COMT gene, or high MOA activity are predisposed to self-medicating with any substance or behavior that will activate DA release including alcohol, opiates, psychostimulants, nicotine, glucose, gambling, sex, and even excessive internet gaming, among others. Use of most drugs of abuse, including alcohol, is associated with release of dopamine in the mesocorticolimbic system or "reward pathway" of the brain (Di Chiara, 1995). Activation of this dopaminergic system induces feelings of reward and pleasure. However, reduced activity of the dopamine system (hypodopaminergic functioning) can trigger drug-seeking behavior. Variant alleles can induce hypodopaminergic functioning through reduced dopamine receptor density, blunted response to dopamine, or enhanced dopamine catabolism in the reward pathway. Cessation of chronic drug use induces a hypodopaminergic state that prompts drug-seeking behavior in an attempt to address the withdrawal-induced state (Berridge, 2009).

Acute utilization of these substances can induce a feeling of wellbeing. But, unfortunately sustained and prolonged abuse leads to a toxic pseudo feeling of well being resulting in tolerance and disease or discomfort. Thus, low DA receptors due to carrying the DRD2 A1 allelic genotype results in excessive cravings and consequential behavior, whereas normal or high DA receptors results in low craving induced behavior. In terms of preventing substance abuse, or excessive glucose craving, one goal is to induce a proliferation of DA D2 receptors in genetically prone individuals. Experiments in vitro have shown that constant stimulation of the DA receptor system via a known D2 agonist in low doses results in significant proliferation of D2 receptors in spite of genetic antecedents. In essence (Boundry et al., 1996) D2 receptor stimulation signals negative feedback mechanisms in the mesolimbic system to induce mRNA expression causing proliferation of D2 receptors. This molecular finding serves as the basis to naturally induce DA release to also cause the same induction of D2-directed mRNA and thus proliferation of D2 receptors in the human. This proliferation of D2 receptors in turn, will induce the attenuation of craving behavior. In fact this has been proven with work showing DNA-directed over-expression (a form of gene therapy) of the DRD2 receptors and significant reduction in both alcohol and cocaine craving-induced behavior in animals (Filtz et al.,1994). These observations are the basis for the development of a functional hypothesis of drug-seeking and drug use. The hypothesis is that the presence of a hypodopaminergic state, regardless of the source, is a primary cause of drug-seeking behavior. Thus, genetic polymorphisms that induce hypodopaminergic functioning may be the causal mechanism of a genetic predisposition to chronic drug use and relapse. Finally, utilizing the long term dopaminergic activation approach will ultimately lead to a common safe and effective modality to treat RDS behaviors including Substance Use Disorders (SUD), Attention Deficit Hyperactivity Disorder (ADHD), and obesity among other reward deficient aberrant behaviors (Rothman & Glowa, 1995; Peng et al., 2010).

Support for the impulsive nature of individuals possessing dopaminergic gene variants is derived from a number of important studies illustrating the genetic risk for drug-seeking behaviors based on association and linkage studies implicating these alleles as risk antecedents having impact in the mesocorticolimbic system (see Figure 1).

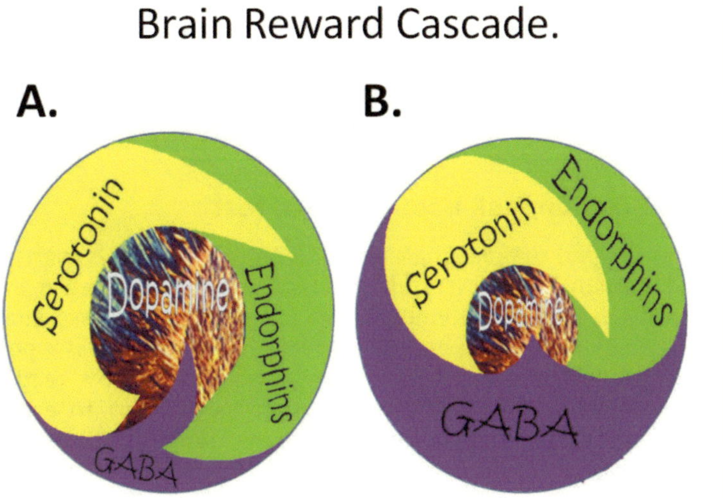

Fig. 1. Schematic of Brain reward Cascade Normal and abnormal representation. (A) represents the normal physiologic state of the neurotransmitter interaction at the mesolimbic region of the brain. Briefly, serotonin in the hypothalamus stimulates neuronal projections of methionine enkephalin in the hypothalamus that, in turn, inhibits the release of GABA in the substania nigra, thereby allowing for the normal amount of Dopamine to be released at the Nucleus Accumbens (NAc; reward site of the brain). (B) Represents hypodopaminergic function of the mesolimbic region of the brain. The hypodopaminergic state is due to gene polymorphisms as well as environmental elements, including both stress and neurotoxicity from aberrant abuse of psychoactive drugs (*i.e. alcohol, heroin, cocaine etc).* Genetic variables include serotonergic genes (serotonergic receptors [5HT2a]; serotonin transporter 5HTlPR); endorphinergic genes (the mu OPRM1 gene; proenkephalin (PENK); PENK polymorphic 3' UTR dinucleotide (CA) repeats}; GABergic genes (GABRB3); and dopaminergic genes (including ANKKI Taq A; DRD2 C957T, DRD4 7R, COMT Val/met substitution, MAO-A uVNTR, and SLC6A3 9 or 10R). Any of these genetic and or environmental impairments could result in reduced release of dopamine and or reduced number of dopaminergic receptors. Taken from Blum et al IIOAB 1(2) 2010.

In doing association studies that require a representative control sample for a single RDS psychiatric diagnosis or for potential subsets of RDS, one limitation relates to controls poorly screened for multiple RDS behaviors and other related psychiatric disorders (Neiswanger et al.,1995). Missing behaviors that are part of the RDS subset may be the reason for spurious results when genotyping for single subsets of RDS behaviors. For example, in our unpublished study, an individual may not drink alcohol or use drugs but may have other RDS behaviors such as overeating or intensive video-gaming. In support of this, a very strong association of the dopamine D2 receptor A1 allele (100%) was found in one family (Family A) studied over five generations. In addition, every individual in another family, Family B, also had at least one dopaminergic high risk allele (100%) (48% carried the DRD2 A1 allele). Moreover, in Family B only three adult individuals exhibited no addictive behavior. When compared to results in which 55 RDS subjects carried the

DRD2 A1 allele at a frequency of 78.2% and the results of a study in which 597 severe alcoholics carried the A1 allele at a frequency of 49.3%, there was a significant difference between these two groups ($X^2=16.9$, $p<0.001$). This demonstrated that the A1 allele's prevalence increases with multiple RDS behaviors. The results from these experiments show that multifaceted non-specific RDS behaviors should be considered as the true "reward" phenotype (endophenotype) instead of a single subset RDS behavior such as alcoholism.

4. The Genetic Addiction Risk Score (GARS) test

Very few behaviors depend upon a single gene. Complexes of genes (polygenic) drive most of heredity-based human actions, and RDS is no exception (Greven et al., 2011). For example, DRD2 and DAT1 gene polymorphisms are significantly associated with reward-dependent traits such as cocaine dependence (Brousse et al., 2010). As a polygenic disorder involving multiple genes and many polymorphisms, RDS likely requires a threshold number of RDS-associated polymorphisms in order to manifest in a particular subject. Unaffected individuals in the population carry some of these alleles. For example, the dopamine D2 receptor gene A1 allele is present in about one-third of unscreened Americans (Noble, 2003).

The GARS test has direct implications for both the diagnosis and targeted treatment of RDS behaviors by analyzing the association of dopaminergic genetic polymorphisms. Without being bound to a particular theory, in keeping with the concept of common neurogenetic mechanisms we believe that RDS is a basic phenotype covering many reward behaviors and psychiatric disorders, including spectrum disorders (Blum & Gold, 2011). The test provides for the first time a polygenic diagnosis of RDS predisposition. Such tests can be used, for example, to determine stratified genetic risk of patients with addictive behaviors upon their entry into a treatment facility, as information about an individual's genetic predisposition to RDS based on the analysis of a number of RDS-associated alleles will be very useful.

4.1 RDS-associated SNPs

RDS-associated SNPs can be identified by any suitable method, including DNA sequencing of patients diagnosed with one or more RDS behaviors. After validation, newly identified RDS-associated SNPs can be used in the test. As will be appreciated, once identified and validated, the presence, if any, of one or more RDS-associated SNPs in the nucleic acids derived from a biological sample taken from a patient can be determined using any suitable now known or later-developed assay, including those that rely on site-specific hybridization, restriction enzyme analysis, or DNA sequencing. Table 2 below, lists a number of particularly preferred RDS- associated SNPs, whereby, the detection of which can be used for the GARS test.

GENE	SNP
DRD2	CTGGACGTCCAGCTGGGCGCCTGCCT[C/T]GACCAGCACTTTGAGG ATGGCTGTG
	AGGAACTCCTTGGCCTAGCCCACCCT[G/T]CTGCCTTCTGACGGCCC TGCAATGT
	CTGCTTCCCACCTCCCTGCCCAGGCC[A/G]GCCAGCCTCACCCTTGC GAACCGTG
	GTCACTATTATGGTTTTTATTACTAT[G/T]GCTCTTTTTGAGGAATTG GGAAATT

GENE	SNP
	CTGACTCTCCCCGACCCGTCCCACCA[C/T]GGTCTCCACAGCACTCC CGACAGCC
	CCACCAGCTGACTCTCCCCGACCCGT[C/G]CCACCACGGTCTCCAC AGCACTCCC
	ACCCATCTCACTGGCCCCTCCCTTTC[A/C]CCCTCTGAAGACTCCTG CAAACACC
	TTTTGCTGAGTGACCTTAGGCAAGTT[G/T]CTTACCTTCTATGAGCCT GTTTCCT
	TGTGATGAATGGGTGCCAAATACACA[A/G]ATACAGAATCTAAGA AAACACATGG
	CTAGAGGAAGTGATGTTCAACAGACA[A/G]ACAACTGAAGGATGT GTAGGAATTA
	TGGAAGTCATGTGCTTTGTATGAAAC[A/G]CCTTGGAATGCTGATA AGTTTAATT
	GTCTAAAGCAAATGGAACCTTTAGGG[A/G]GAGAGATTTGTGTTTG CTGTGTCCC
	GAGGGGACTGGGGTCAGGCCTCATTC[A/G]GGTTCCCTAGAGTGGA AAGGATTGG
	GTATCAGACAGATCTAGGCTCAAATA[A/C]CAGCTTCAGTTCTCAC CACCTGTGT
	CCTGAGTGCACAGGATGCTGGAGCCT[C/T]CCAGTTTCTCTGGCTTT CATCTCGT
	AATCCCCCAACCCCTCCTACCCGTT[- /C]CAGGCCGGGGATCGCCGAGGAGGTA
	GAGGACCCAGCCTGCAATCACAGCTT[A/G]TTACTCTGGGTGTGGG TGGGAGCGC
5HT2A	GCTCAATGGTTGCTCTAGGAAAGCAG[C/T]ATTCTGAAGAGGCTTC TAAAGACAA
	CTGTGAACTCAGGAGCAAGTGCACAC[A/G]TTGCTTATCACTTACC AGAAGCATT
	CTCTGGTTTTAAGCAAGTCATTTAAT[- /C/T]GGAGTTTTTTTCTCCCATAAAATG
	AAATGGTCCTACCATCTATCCAGATA[C/T]ACAGCTTAAAAACTTA GGAGTCTCT
	TGCTATTTGTAATGCTGCTTATTAGA[G/T]ACATCGCTGATCCTCCTG TCAACTC
	ATGAACCAAATTGCATGAGCTCTATT[A/G]TGTGCCCCTCTTGTAAT ATAAAAAT
	CAGGCAGAATTTCCACAAATGAAATG[C/G]AAATTCAGATATATAT CTCTTAATC
	TCACTCATAACTGAAGATCATTTCAC[C/T]TTTGAATGAGAATTTGT CTCTGAAG
	TGGGCAGAGGAGGGGAAGGGTCACTG[C/T]ACTCAGGGACAAGAG AAGGGGTGGG
	ATCAGTGTGGTCACTTCACTGCTTGC[C/G]AAGGATTCCATCTAATT CTGAGGAA
	AGGCTCTACAGTAATGACTTTAACTC[C/T]GGAGAAGCTAACACTT CTGATGCAT
	TATGTCCTCGGAGTGCTGTGAGTGTC[C/T]GGCACTTCCATCCAAAG CCAACAGT
ANKK1	GGAGGGGGGTCTTGCCCTCAGCCTCA[C/T]GCAGGTTGGGGTCAGC CTGACGGGA

GENE	SNP
	GGAGGGGGGTCTTGCCCTCAGCCTCA[C/T]GCAGGTTGGGGTCAGCCTGACGGGA
	CCTGCAAGCTGTCGCTGCGCCAGCCC[A/G]GGGAGGTGAGTGTGTGGGCTGGGCA
	ACTTTGCAGCCCAGAATGGGGATGAC[C/G]GCACTGCGCGCCTGCTCCTGGACCA
OPRK1	AATTTCCCAAAAACTACAGTTTTTTT[-/T]TCTTAGCATGCTATTCAGGTAAACA
	TTTGCTAGGTAAGGTTCAGCACCCAT[C/T]TGCTGTGGCCTTCCTATGAAACGTA
	ATGACTAGTCGTGGAGATGTCTTCGT[A/C]CAGTTCTTCGGGAAGAGAGGAGTTC
	GAAAACACAAGTGTGATCAAATGCCA[C/T]GGACCCACAGGAAGCTGGTGGCTCT
	AAGAAATTGTCTGCATATAAACAAAT[A/G]CATCACATTTCCACAAAAGACTTTG
	TGAGAGCTAATGTTTCAAAGAAACTT[G/T]AAATTCCCAAGATTAAAATTATTGT
	CCCAGTAAGTGAATTAAATACTTTCA[C/T]AGACACTCTCCATCTAGTAGAACAA
	TGATAGGCACTGGTTCTACAGTGAGA[C/T]ATATCTCTCCTAAGTCTGGTGACAA
	ACAGTGGCACGATCTCGGCTCACTGC[A/C]ACCTCCACCTCCCGGGTTTAAGTGA
	TTACCTGGCTAACAGTTTTCTATCTC[C/T]CACACGAGCCTGGTGGGAGGCAGTG
	AGCTCTTGTTATCTTACCATTCCCAC[A/G]TTGATTCTCATTTTTATCCCTCTCC
	TCAAGATAGCTAATTGAGAACAAGCA[C/T]GAGACTCCACTCCTGGTCCCCAAGC
	CCATTTTCTTTTCTTCTTTGCTTGTC[G/T]TTTTTTTCTGTTTGTTTTTCTTTTC
	AGAAAATAACTTTTGCTAGATTCACC[A/G]TTGGTTATAGACCTGCATGATCTAA
	GTGATGTTACCAGCCTGAGGGAAGGA[A/G]GGTTCACAGCCTGATATGTTGGTGA
	AGTTAGCTCTGGTCAAGGCTAAAAAT[C/G]AATGAGCAAAATGGCAGTATTAACA
	AATTTTATTAGATTAAACAATTTTTA[A/G]CAGACCTCATGCTTGTTGGAGATAA
	GGTCCAGGGTACACAACCAAGCAGCC[A/T]TGCTCTAGAGCCCAGCAAGACAGGG
	ACTGAAGAATAATCATGCTTAACTCA[A/G]GAGAAATGCTCCACCAGACGGGCTG
	GCACATTTACTGTTTTGTCTAACCTG[C/T]CTAGCCATTTCAGTCAAGCTGATTG
	GCAATCAGAAAGAAATTCAGTTATTA[C/T]AGTATATGCAAGTCACACTGCAAGC
	AATGAAACACAAATCATAATCTCTGA[A/G]GCAAATAAGAATGGAAGGACTCCTG
	TTTAGGGCAAGTCAGAAAGTCCAAAA[A/G]TGCCTCAGATATTCTGTGTGAGTGA
	AAAAACTGGGCCTGAGCTCAGATGAA[C/T]TGGAGAACTGAACTTTGGCTTAGAA

GENE	SNP
	GAGTCATCAGCTCCCAAGGTTTTCTG[C/T]ATGGCTCTGTTTTTATGA TTTCTGT
	GTGTGTACTGCAGTCTGGTCCCATCG[C/T]ATTGCCTTGTGGGATTT GGGAGTAG
COMT	GCTCCTACGGTCCCTCAGGCTTGGAG[A/G]GTCACTTTAAACAATA AAAAGCAAC
	TGTGGTTACTTTCTGGAGAGAGCATG[C/T]GGCATGCAGGAGCTGG AGGGGGGGT
	AAAAGTTACGCTTAATAATGAATGTT[G/T]CAGCACTTTCTTCTCTT CAGGTATT
	CTGTGAGGCACTGAGGATGCCCTCAC[A/G]CGTGCATCTGCATGTG GCGTGCATG
	CTGGTTTGTGTATGTTCTTGGTAAAC[C/T]AGCCCTTGGTCTTACACA TCATTTC
	GCTTCCCTGTTCTCTTCTGCTCTGTC[C/T]TCTGGTGCCCTGAGGCTG GCCTCCA
	GGCATTTCTGAACCTTGCCCCTCTGC[A/G]AACACAAGGGGGCGAT GGTGGCACT
	ATAAGTAACTGTCGAGAAGATTCTCA[C/T]AGGAGACCACGTGGGT TGCCTGAAG
SLC6A3	AATGTCCTCAGCTGGTTCTTCCCCCA[A/G]TGCCCTGATCCTGGGCT CACATGTG
	GAGACGAAGACCCCAGGAAGTCATCC[C/T]GCAATGGGAGAGACA CGAACAAACC
	AAAATCAAGTAATGATTGATTTGTAG[A/G]AGTTTGAGTGAGGCAT CGGATCCCC
	ACCGTGCCCAGCCCTGTGTGGGCATC[A/G]GAGGTGGTTCCCTCTG GTCCTGTCG
	GTCCAGGCCCCAGGAGCTGCCGCAGC[A/G]GGCAGTGGAAGGAAG GCACGTTCAG
	CAGCTTCCCCTCCCAACACAGAGGCG[A/C]GGCCCAAGTGCAGGA CTCACAACGG
	AAGACACAGTGACGGTATACTCATGA[C/T]GGAATATGATTCGGCC TTAAAACAA
	AAGGCGAAGCCGGCGATGGTACGTAC[A/G]TTGGTGACGCAGAAC AGGGACAGGA
	GCCATCGCCACGCTCCCTCTGTCCTC[A/G]GCCTGGGCCGTGGTCTT CTTCATCA
	TGCTTCCTGCTACCAGCAGGCAGACT[C/T]GGATGGAGGTGGAGGG GACGAGAGT
	CACGGTAAAAATACAAGGACAGTGTG[A/T]GCAGCAGAATGGCCA GGCAGACCAC
	AGGGTTATTAGGATGCTGTGGTCATG[C/T]CGTGTGTGGATGAGTCC ATGCTGTT
	GCCAGGCAGGGGCTGGTGGAGGTGCA[C/G]GGCCTGGAGGAACAC AGAGCCCAGC
	AGGAGAGGACGTTTGCGCGATTCTCC[C/G]CAGATCCAGTGTTTCC CGTCAGCCA
	GGCTCGTGGCCCTGCGGGCGGATCTT[G/T]GGAAGAGCTTGTTCAC ACTCACCTA
	TCGAGGCAGGGCCACCGGGGACGTCC[A/G]AGAACATTGGTGATC CCTTCCCAGG
	AATGCAGGCGTGGGACAAGGCAGCTC[C/T]GAGTCCTGCTCAATGG TTTTGTGAC

GENE	SNP
	GAGCTCATCCTTGTCAAGGAGCAGAA[C/T]GGAGTGCAGCTCACCAGCTCCACCC
	GTGGGGAGGGGTGCAGGGGAAGGAGG[A/G]GCAAACCAGAGTGTCTGTCTTGAGG
	AAACACGCTGCTGCTGGATCCAAATG[A/C]CAGAAGTCGCCCTGGCTGGGGCGGT
	CTGCGCGCTGGTGCTCTGGGCAGGGC[G/T]GGGAGGCCGGGCGAGGACTCGCCAG
	GGAGCCAGGACGCGAGGGCGACCCCG[A/T]CGGCGGGAGGGCGGGGCGGGGCGGA
HTR3B	CCTTTACAGCCTTTACCTAAGGCAGT[A/G]CTCTTGCTGACATTCAGGACACTAA
	TTTGGCCTTCTCTCTTGGGCCAAGGA[A/G]TTTCTGCTCTATTGCATGTTCTCAT
	GAGAGCTCCTTGGAGATGGAATAGGC[C/T]CCAAGGTTAGCCTGTAATTGCCTCC
	CCTTAGCACCTGTGTGTCTATCATTC[C/T]GGGCAGGAAAACTTGCACAATTAAA
PPARG	AAACTCTGGGAGATTCTCCTATTGAC[C/G]CAGAAAGCGATTCCTTCACTGATAC
	AGGATTTTCTTACATTTAAAGCAGAA[C/T]GACACTACTGATACACAAAAGTAAA
	GAGAAATCTTCGGAGGGCTCACCAGC[A/G]TCACAAGTAGGTAGACCAGAAGAGG
	GTTTACAGACCTTGTCAGAGTTGGTA[C/G]TAATTCCAGAATATAATCATTTCAA
	TGGTTGACACAGAGATGCCATTCTGG[C/G]CCACCAACTTTGGGATCAGCTCCGT
	GATTTATTTAAATCATCTCTAATTCT[C/T]ACAACTCCGAAAAGATAAGAAAACA
	AGGATTTTCTTACATTTAAAGCAGAA[C/T]GACACTACTGATACACAAAAGTAAA
	GTTGGGGATCCAGTTGGCCTCATTCT[A/G]AGCTGGCTGTGGATTCACAGAAGAA
	AAGATACGGGGGAGGAAATTCACTGG[A/G]TTTTACAATATATTTTTCAAGGCAA
	GAGAAATCTTCGGAGGGCTCACCAGC[A/G]TCACAAGTAGGTAGACCAGAAGAGG
ChREBP	GACAAAAAGCAATTGAGGTCCAGGAG[C/G]TGCCGCCCACCCGGCTCCTCCTCTG
FTO	GCTGTCAGCACCTGGTACAAATACCA[A/G]GATAGGGTTTTTGGGGCCACATTTT
	GCATGCCAGTTGCCCACTGTGGCAAT[A/C]AATATCTGAGCCTGTGGTTTTTGCC
	AGGTTCCTTGCGACTGCTGTGAATTT[A/T]GTGATGCACTTGGATAGTCTCTGTT
	GATGACAACATGCAAACTTTATGGCC[A/G]GAAACCAAAGAGTCAGGCAAAATAT
	AAAAGAAAGTAAACATATTTAAGGTC[A/G]TAAATAAGGCCATGTCTAATAGTGA
	AGGAATGTTCTGATGGCTTGGCCCAG[G/T]TGGTGACTGTGCAGATAGACTGAAG
	TCAGCACCCAAGGGACCATCAAAGAG[A/G]CTGTTGTGGAGAGGGAATCCGAAGG

GENE	SNP
	TGGAGTGTTTTTCCTTCACCTTTTCC[A/G]GTCTCTGGGTTGCATCGC CAGACTG
	TGTCTAGCCCTGTGGGTTTACATTAG[A/T]TAGGGTAGGTTATTGCT GCAACGTA
	CTATCCAGGATGGCTCTAAAGGGACT[C/T]CGCTATAGGTTGGGGC TATGATAGA
	GCTTATATTCAAAGCTCCAGGTAAAT[A/G]TAAGATGTTGCTATAAT TACCTAAG
	GGTAGGCAGGTGGATCTGAAATCTCA[C/T]ATAGTACCAAGACACG TGACTAGGA
	TTGATTCTTATACTTTTTTGTTTAGT[C/T]GTTGAAATATGTTGTTTTG GTTGAA
	AATTAGGAAGATTTGAGTAGCTAAAA[A/G]TTCCAAGAGTGGAAT AATAGTTTA
	TTTGGTGCACTCCCAATTTACTCTAA[A/T]CTTCTACGGGCTTCCTTG GAGAAAC
	GACCTGAAAATAGGTGAGCTGTCAAG[G/T]TGTTGGCAGGGAGAG GCTCCTCTGG
	TGGTTCACTGCATATTCCCAGTAATT[C/G]GAACAATGCCTGACATG AAGTAGAC
	TTAGAATGTCTGAATTATTATTCTAG[A/G]TTCCTTGCGACTGCTGTG AATTTG
	TTGATTTCGGTAGTCATAACACCACC[C/T]TGGAAGGCACCCTAGA TAGAGGTCA
	TTCATTCTACCTGTCTTTAGTATCAT[A/G]GGGGTAGTTACCTCAGC GGGGGTAG
	TTGCTCAAGGTCACACAGTAACCTTA[A/G]GTAGGCAGGATAAGCT CTGGTTCTG
	TATGATGGTTAGGTTAGGTTGCAAGT[C/T]TTGGAATATATGCAGAG GAATAACT
	TTATAAACCTCTAAAATAGTTACTAA[A/G]TAAGTTATTCTTTTAGG TATTTTTC
	TTTTATTTCCGCAATCACTCCCTAAT[C/G]TTTATTTCTTTTTTGCTTC GCATCA
	TAGCATTTTTCTGGAGCGTAATTTCA[C/T]AATGTGAATCAGAAGTC TTAATAGT
	GAGCACAGGTGGAGAGAAAGGGGAGT[A/G]AGAGAAGCAAAGAA GAAAAGCCTTT
	TAGGGACACAAAAAGGGACATACTAC[A/G]TGAATTACTAATATCT AAGAAAATA
	ATGAATTACTAATATCTAAGAAAATA[C/T]GATACATTTGAGAACT TAGATGAAG
	GAAATGTGGTGTAGACGTGACCCAGG[A/G]GGAAATGAGTTTTGTT GGACAGATT
	CTACATCTCCTACTTAGCCGAGGTCT[C/T]TTCACTCTCTGGGCAAG TCTCCTCA
	ACACGGCTGAAGAGTCAGGAGTGGGA[C/T]GAAAAATACACTTCA TTTGTAGGTG
	GCACATTTATGCCTTTTATATGCCAC[A/G]TACACACGAAAACTccat atattct
	AGAGTGAATAAAATTATTTCTAAATT[C/T]ATGCTTCATACCGTGTG TAATTTAG
	TGTTGCAACAGAGATGATGGCAGTTT[C/T]GGCCACGGTGTAAGAA GCAGAGGTG

GENE	SNP
	ACATCTGCCTTCCCAGAGAAAGGAAA[A/G]TCAATGTTTAAAGTCT ATTTAAAAA
TNF Alpha	GGGAAGCAAAGGAGAAGCTGAGAAGA[C/T]GAAGGAAAAGTCAG GGTCTGGAGGG
	GGAGGCAATAGGTTTTGAGGGGCATG[A/G]GGACGGGGTTCAGCC TCCAGGGTCC
	TGGCCCAGAAGACCCCCCTCGGAATC[A/G]GAGCAGGGAGGATGG GGAGTGTGAG
	TCTTTCTGCATCCCCGTCTTTCTCCA[C/T]GTTTTTTCTCTCCATCCC TCCCTA
	GTTGAATGCCTGGAAGGTGAATACAC[A/G]GATGAATGGAGAGAG AAAACCAGAC
MANEA	CATTTTACAATAGATAAATGCTTGTG[C/T]TACCTAAAGCACTTAGC ACACAGTT
Leptin OB	GCTCTGGGAATGTCTATCCTATGCAA[C/T]GGAGATAAGGACTGAG ATACGCCCT
	ATGCAATGGAGATAAGGACTGAGATA[C/T]GCCCTGGTCTCCTGCA GTACCCTCA
	GGAGCCCCGTAGGAATCGCAGCGCCA[A/G]CGGTTGCAAGGTAAG GCCCCGGCGC
	AAGTTCCTGACCTCTGAATGAGAGGG[A/G]CTGTGTAAGGCCAATG CCTGGGAGG
	AATAAAAATAAATGTTCTTCCTTGCA[A/T]TGAAGTTAAATATGTAA ATTCTCAA
	ACTTAGGTATTAGAGGGTGGCCATTA[C/T]TTGAGAGTGACTATGA CCACAGTTA
	TGGGTGAATGTGTTATGCTCTCTCCC[A/G]CCACCATGTCTTTATAC CCCCTGAT
	CTCCCAGTGGGTGGGAGAGAAAGGAC[A/G]TAAGGAAGCAAGTGG TAAAGGCCCT
PEMT	ATCCCTTCACCAGAGTGATTTCCTCG[A/C]GGCAGGTGCCTGGGGT AGCCACTGG
	GGACTGCCTGGTTGTGCTTCGGACCC[A/G]GAGGCAGACAGAGGA GGCCTTTGAA
MAO-A	CCCACTAGGCAAGCCTCCTAAAAGCA[A/G]TATGGTTGTAGATCAC TGGAAAATA
	GTAAACATGCAAACTGAAACATTAGC[A/G]CCCATTTATTCAGCAT CTTAGAAGA
	GAGTGAAGGCCAGGTACAGAGGAAAT[A/G]AAGCATTCCAAATAA TGCCAGGTAA
	CCAAAGTTAACTTGTGAACCCTTCTA[A/G]TAAACTGCTCCAAGAT ATGACAAAA
	GTTTGCCATGGATGAACCACCAGGAT[A/G]GTGGGGGAGACAGAA AAGGTTGATG
	GGAAAATTCCCCTTCCCCTAAGACAT[C/T]CACCCTTCTGGTTTGGG TAATTCCT
	GCAGAGAGAAACCAGTTAATTCAGCG[G/T]CTTCCAATGGAGCTG TCATTAAGT
	GTGCATGATGTATTACAAGGAGGCC[G/T]TCTGGAAGAAGAAGGGT AGGCTGCT
	AGAGAAGGAAGTGGTGTCCCCACAAA[G/T]GAATTGCTAAGGAGT TCCACAGCCT
	AAGAGAAAACAAAGCTGAAATGCTGC[A/G]AGTCAATAATATCGT TGCTTTAACA

GENE	SNP
	TTTGACAACTATTTCTAGAATTTGCA[C/T]TGAACTCTGCTTTTCCTT TTAAATT
	GGTCTCGGGAAGGTGACCGAGAAAGA[C/T]ATCTGGGTACAAGAA CCTGAATCAA
CRH	CTGTCCCACAACATGGGGTCTTACAG[C/T]TCTTTGATGTATCCCCC CACAGGGG
	GCCTCTGGGGTCACCAGGTACATCTT[C/T]GATCTTGGCCACACTGG AGAGTCAA
	TTTCTAAACACAGAGGACTGGTGTTG[C/T]GTTATGCAAAGAAAAA TGCTTCTTA
	AAGACACTCAGGTGCAGGGACCCTCT[A/C]CATTTTTGCCCAGCAG CAGCCATGC
	AGGGCCAGGAACCATGAACCAGCGCG[G/T]GTGGGGGCAGCCTCT TCAGGCCTGG
	GGCACACCAGTCCTTTTGAGCCCCAG[C/T]GTCCCCAGGTTAATAA CCTAGAATT
	TGAACACGGAGGCCACACAAGAGTGG[A/G]TTCCAAGTGAAGGAG TGACCAACTC
	TCCTTTCCTGGGATCACAGAGGGAAG[C/T]GCGGGGGAGCCTAGAG AGCACCACA
	TACAGGTGAAGGAAAGTGATTCTTTC[C/T]CCGTTAACTTTGTTTCA CGCCAGAT
	CCCCCAACCAGAGATGATGATGGGGG[A/G]CAGGGGAGGCACCAA ACCCTGGGCC
	AGCAGCATACCCCTAGGGACCTAGGA[A/G]CAGGGAGGGAGAGA GGCAGCCCTGG
	CAGCTGGCACTGACAGCCTGGGGGGG[- /C/G]CGCTCTCCCCCTGCAGCCGTGCAGG
	GAGCACAAGAAGGCCAGCCCACTGGG[C/G]CCTGGGGCTGCCCTC GGCAACCGTG
	CTGCTTCCCACCAATCAGCACAGCTC[A/C]TGCCTGGGGCTGGGAC ACACTCCCG
ADIPOQ	ATCAGAATGTGTGGCTTGCAAGAACC[A/G]GCTCAGATCCTGCCCT TCAAAAACA
	GTTCTACTGCTATTAGCTCTGCCCGG[G/T]CATGACCAGGAAACCA CGACTCAAG
STS	GATGACAAGCCAGGCAGGGAGGAATG[A/G]ACCTGGATTCCTGGT GAAGGACGTG
VDR	GTCAGCGATTCTTAATATAAGAAAAA[A/G]TGGTGAAATGTGTTTA GAGTGTGCT
	CCTGGGGTGCAGGACGCCGCGCTGAT[C/T]GAGGCCATCCAGGACC GCCTGTCCA
	GTTCCTGGGGCCACAGACAGGCCTGC[A/G]CATTCCCAATACTCAG GCTCTGCTC
	CATAAGACCTACGACCCCACCTACTC[C/T]GACTTCTGCCAGTTCCG GCCTCCAG
	TGGCCTGCTTGCTGTTCTTACAGGGA[C/T]GGAGGCAATGGCGGCC AGCACTTCC
	TGTGGGGGTGGGCCAGCCCAGCTTAG[A/G]TTATCTTGGCTCATTGT CCACTAGT
DBI	TCTGTCCTCAGGCCAGGGCTTCGCTG[A/C]AGCCCCGGCCACTCCCT AGTGCCTG
	TACGAACTCACTGTAAAACTCACCTT[C/T]GCCATAAGACCTTCTTC AACTAAGT

GENE	SNP
	ACAGAGTTTACGAACTCACTGTAAAA[C/T]TCACCTTCGCCATAAG ACCTTCTTC
	GGAGAGAAAACAAAGTCAATGGGGCA[C/T]GTGTGGGAAACCAGC CTGACCTGTG
	TTACAGGGACTTCCAAGGAAGATGCC[A/G]TGAAAGCTTACATCAA CAAAGTAGA
GABRA6	TTGGGAAAGGAGAGTCTGAAGGGACA[A/G]TGCATGGTCGGAGAG CAGTGACAAT
	AAATTGGAAATCTGTAACGCAGCTTC[C/T]GTAAGCATGTGTGGGC AAAAAAGCA
	TTCTTTCCATCTGGCACCTATTTATT[C/G]ACTATTTATGCATTCGTT GAATTAT
	CTCTTTCACCATTGACAAATATTTAT[G/T]GACGACTTACTTTCTATG TAAGGTC
GABRB3	CGTTCAGTTTAGTAAGCAAAGGCTTC[C/T]TGGCTTCTCTGGTGATG GGGTTTGT
	AGCTTACCATTTAAGTAGAACTGTTT[A/G]AGATGCTGGACATTCTA ATACAATC
	CCAAATCTGAAATTTACTTGTCACTT[C/T]AGAGTTGTCTTTGAACG GAAAGATT
	TCTGTTGAGTGATAATCTTTCTCGCA[A/G]ATAACTCACAATATTTA AAAATTGT
	AAGAACTCTTCCATGATTGAAATGGT[A/C]GCACATGGAATAACAT CGATAAGTT
	ACAGCAGGTTGGAGCACAGGGCCTAA[A/G]TGGGAGGCCAGGGAG GTGGGCAGAG
	ATTGCTGATTTTCAGGCAAACTATGT[A/T]ACATGGCTTTCAATGGG TGCTTGGC
MTHFR	GAAGCAGTTAGTTCTGACACCAACAA[A/G]TGGTGATAAGAGGTTG ATAGCCTAG
	GTGGGGGGAGGAGCTGACCAGTGAAG[A/C]AAGTGTCTTTGAAGT CTTTGTTCTT
	CTTGAAGGAGAAGGTGTCTGCGGGAG[C/T]CGATTTCATCATCACG CAGCTTTTC
	AGATGTTCCACCCCGGGCCTGGACCC[C/T]GAGCGGCATGAGA
MLXIPL	GACAAAAAGCAATTGAGGTCCAGGAG[C/G]TGCCGCCCACCCGGC TCCTCCTCTG
	CAGGTAACTGACCCTTCACACATTTA[C/T]GGTGCCCATCTGACATT CATAGCAT
VEGF	GCGCGCGGGCGTGCGAGCAGCGAAAG[C/G]GACAGGGGCAAAGT GAGTGACCTGC
	AGACATGTCCCATTTGTGGGAACTGT[A/G]ACCCTTCCTGTGTGAGC TGGAGGCA
	AGACATGTCCCATTTGTGGGAACTGT[A/G]ACCCTTCCTGTGTGAGC TGGAGGCA
	ACATCCTGAGGTGTGTTCTCTTGGGC[C/T]TGGCAGGCATGGAGAG CTCTGGTTC
	AGCATTCCCGGGCGGGTGACCCAGCA[C/T]GGTCCCTCTTGGAATT GGATTCGCC
	ATCCTCTTCCTGCTCCCCTTCCTGGG[A/G]TGCAGCCTAAAAGGACC TATGTCCT

Table 2. RDS-associated SNPs.

4.2 Testing parameters and assay requirements: a note on methodology

A common class of experiments, known as a multiplexed assay or multiplexed biochemical experiment, comprises of reacting a sample known or suspected to contain one more target analyte species with a set of "probe" molecules. Multiplexing allows two or more, often many more (e.g., 10, 50, 100, 1,000 or more), target analyte species to be probed simultaneously (i.e., in parallel). Genome Wide scans have now been used to identify gene clusters in alcohol and drug addiction (Agrawal et al., 2010). For example, in a gene expression assay, each species of target analyte, usually a nucleic acid (i.e., DNA or RNA) of known nucleotide sequence but whose presence in a particular sample is suspected but is not known with certainty, can be detected using a short probe nucleic acid (e.g., a synthetically produced oligonucleotide) having a nucleotide sequence at least a portion of which is sufficiently complementary to the target sequence in the particular target analyte to allow stable hybridization under the various assay conditions used (including hybridization and stringent washing conditions) so that probe/target hybrids can later be detected using a desired detection scheme. As those in the art appreciate, such assays can involve those wherein target analyte species are labeled (or not) with a detectable label or wherein the various target analyte-specific probe species are labeled (directly or indirectly) with any suitable label that can be detected by the detector used with the particular assay format (e.g., bead-based formats, gene arrays, etc.). Labels include fluorescent molecules.

For example, in many known DNA/genomic bead-based multiplex assays, each probe species includes a DNA molecule of a predetermined nucleotide sequence and length attached to an encoded or otherwise identifiable bead or particle. When a labeled "target" analyte (in this case, a detectably labeled (e.g., fluorescently labeled) DNA molecule containing a target nucleotide sequence) is mixed with the probes, segments of the labeled target analyte selectively bind to complementary segments of the DNA sequence of one of the bead-bound probe species. The probes are then spatially separated and examined for fluorescence. The beads that fluoresce indicate that molecules of the target analyte have attached or hybridized to complementary probe molecules on that bead. The DNA sequence of the target analyte can then be determined, as the complementary nucleotide sequence of the particular probe species hybridized to the labeled target is known, and identification of the encoded bead indicates which probe species was bound to that bead. In addition, in such assays the level of fluorescence is indicative of how many of the target molecules hybridized (or attached) to the probe molecules for a given bead. As is known, similar bead-based assays may be performed with any set of known and unknown molecules, analytes, or ligands.

In such bead-based assays, the bead-bound probes are allowed to mix with samples that may contain the target analytes without any specific spatial position; as such, such assays are commonly called "random bead assays". In addition, because the bead-bound probes are free to move (usually in a liquid medium), the probe molecules and target analytes have a better opportunity to interact than in other assay techniques, such as in a conventional planar microarray assay format.

There are many bead/substrate types that can be used for tagging or otherwise uniquely identifying individual beads with attached probes. Known methods include using polystyrene latex spheres that are colored or fluorescently labeled. Other methods include using small plastic particles with a conventional bar code applied, or a small container having a solid support material and a radio-frequency (RF) tag. Still other bead-based approaches involve vary small encoded beads, particles, or substrates capable of providing a large number of unique codes (e.g., greater than 1 million codes) are known.

In multiplex assays designed to simultaneously examine 2-25 or so different target analyte species, other assay formats can be adapted for use in the GARS test. Indeed, any format suited for analysis of multiple genes, either simultaneously in one or more parallel reactions or in different reactions carried out in series or at different times, can readily be adapted for use.

5. Brief description of risk alleles in a number of reward genes

5.1 Dopamine D2 receptor gene (DRD2)

The dopamine D2 receptor gene (DRD2) first associated with severe alcoholism is the most widely studied gene in psychiatric genetics (Blum et a l., 1990). The *Taq*1 A is a single nucleotide polymorphism (SNP rs: 1800497) originally thought to be located in the 3'-untranslated region of the DRD2 but has since been shown to be located within exon 8 of an adjacent gene, the ankyrin repeat and kinase domain containing 1 (ANKK1). Importantly, while there may be distinct differences in function, the mis-location of the *Taq*1 A allele may be attributable to the ANKKI and the DRD2 being on the same haplotype or the ANKKI being involved in reward processing through a signal transduction pathway (Neville et al.,2004). The ANKKI and the DRD2 gene polymorphisms may have distinct, different actions with regard to brain function (Huang et al, 2009). Presence of the $A1^+$ genotype (A1/A1, A1/A2) compared to the A^- genotype (A2/A2) is associated with reduced receptor density. (Noble et al, 1991; Montag et al., 2010; Jönsson et al., 1999). This reduction causes hypodopaminergic functioning in the dopamine reward pathway. Other DRD2 polymorphisms such as the C (57T, A SNP (rs: 6277) at exon 7 also associates with a number of RDS behaviors including drug use (Duan et al., 2003). Compared to the T^- genotype (C/C), the T^+ genotype (T/T, T/C) is associated with reduced translation of DRD2 mRNA and diminished DRD2 mRNA, leading to reduced DRD2 density and a predisposition to alcohol dependence (Hirvonen et al.,2004) The *Taq*1 A allele is a predictive risk allele in families (Hill et al., 2008).

More recently, the DRD2 haplotypes I-C-G-A2 and I-C-A-A1 have been found to occur with a higher frequency in alcoholics [P=0.026, odds ratio (OR): 1.340; P=0.010, OR: 1.521, respectively]. The rare haplotype I-C-A-A2 occurred less often in alcoholics (P=0.010, OR: 0.507), and was also less often transmitted from parents to their affected children (1 vs. 7). Among the subgroups, I-C-G-A2 and I-C-A-A1 had a higher frequency in Cloninger 1 alcoholics (P=0.083 and 0.001, OR: 1.917, respectively) and in alcoholics with a positive family history (P=0.031, OR: 1.478; P=0.073, respectively). Cloninger 2 alcoholics had a higher frequency of the rare haplotype D-T-A-A2 (P<0.001, OR: 4.614) always compared with controls. In patients with positive family history, haplotype I-C-A-A2 (P=0.004, OR: 0.209) and in Cloninger 1 alcoholics, haplotype I-T-A-A1 (P=0.045 OR: 0.460) was less often present, confirming that haplotypes, which are supposed to induce a low DRD2 expression, are associated with alcohol dependence. Furthermore, supposedly high-expressing haplotypes weakened or neutralized the action of low-expressing haplotypes (Kraschewski et al 2009).

5.2 D4 dopamine receptor (DRD4)

There is evidence that the length of the D4 dopamine receptor (DRD4) exon 3 variable number of tandem repeats (VNTR) affects DRD4 functioning by modulating the expression and efficiency of maturation of the receptor. (Schoots & Van Tol 2003). The 7 repeat (7R) VNTR requires significantly higher amounts of dopamine to produce a response of the same magnitude as other size VNTRs (Oak et al., 2000). This reduced sensitivity or "dopamine resistance" leads to hypodopaminergic functioning. Thus 7R VNTR has been associated with substance-seeking behavior (McGeary et al., 2007). Survival analysis has revealed that by 25 years of age 76% of subjects with a DRD4 7-repeat allele have significantly more persistent ADHD compared with 66% of subjects without the risk allele. In contrast, there were no significant associations between the course of ADHD and the DAT1 10-repeat allele (P=0.94) and 5HTTLPR long allele, suggesting that the DRD4 7-repeat allele is associated with a more persistent course of ADHD (Biederman et al., 2009). This is consistent with the finding of the presence of the 7R DAT genotype in the heroin addict. Moreover, in a study evaluating the role of dopamine D4 receptor (DRD4) exon 3 polymorphisms (48 bp VNTR) in the pathogenesis of alcoholism, significant differences in the short alleles (2-5 VNTR) frequencies were found between controls and patients with a history of delirium tremors and/or alcohol seizures (p = 0.043) (Grzywacz et al., 2009). A trend was also observed in the higher frequency of short alleles amongst individuals with an early age of onset of alcoholism (p = 0.063). These results indicate that inherited short variants of DRD4 alleles (3R) may play a role in pathogenesis of alcohol dependence and carriers of the 4R may have a protective effect for alcoholism risk behaviors. It is of further note that the DRD4 7-repeat allele is significantly over-represented in the opioid-dependent cohort and confers a relative risk of 2.46 (Kotler et al., 1997).

5.3 Dopamine transporter gene (DAT1)

The dopamine transporter protein regulates dopamine -mediated neurotransmission by rapidly accumulating dopamine that has been released into the synapse (Vandenbergh, 1998). The dopamine transporter gene (SLC6A3 or DAT1) is localized to chromosome 5p15.3. Moreover, there is a VNTR polymorphism within the 3′ non-coding region of DAT1 (Michelhaugh et al., 2001). There are two important alleles that may independently increase risk for RDS behaviors. The 9 repeat (9R) VNTR has been shown to influence gene expression and to augment transcription of the dopamine transporter protein, resulting in an enhanced clearance of synaptic dopamine, yielding reduced levels of dopamine to activate postsynaptic neurons. Presence of the 9R VNTR has also been linked to Substance Use Disorder (SUD) (Guindalini et al., 2006). Moreover, in terms of RDS behaviors, tandem repeats of the dopamine transporter gene (DAT) have been associated with high risk for ADHD in children and in adults alike (Vandenbergh et al., 2002; Cook et al., 1995). The 10-repeat allele is significant for hyperactivity-impulsivity (HI) symptoms (Lee et al., 2007).

5.4 Catechol-O-methyltransferase (COMT)

The catechol-O-methyltransferase (COMT) is an enzyme involved in the metabolism of dopamine, adrenaline and noradrenaline. The Val158Met polymorphism of the COMT gene has been previously associated with a variability of the COMT activity, and alcoholism. Serý (2006) found a relationship between the Val158Met polymorphism of the COMT gene and alcoholism in male subjects. Serý (2006) found the significant difference between male alcoholics and male controls in allele and genotype frequencies (p<0,007; and p<0, 04 respectively. Interestingly in one of the subjects genotyped herein, who battles with heroin as an addiction while carrying the DRD2 A1 allele also carried the low enzyme COMT activity genotype (A/A). This is agreement with the work of Cao *et al.* (2003) who did not find an association with the high G/G and heroin addiction. No differences in genotype and allele frequencies of 108 val/met polymorphism of COMT gene were observed between heroin-dependent subjects and normal controls (genotype-wise: chi-square=1.67, P=0.43; allele-wise: chi-square=1.23, P=0.27). No differences in genotype and allele frequencies of 900 Ins C/Del C polymorphism of COMT gene were observed between heroin-dependent subjects and normal controls (genotype-wise: chi-square=3.73, P=0.16; allele-wise: chi-square=0.76, P=0.38). While there is still some controversy regarding the COMT association with heroin addiction it was also interesting that the A allele of the val/met polymorphisms (-287 A/G) found by Cao *et al.* (2003) was found to be much higher in heroin addicts than controls. Faster metabolism results in reduced dopamine availability at the synapse, which reduces postsynaptic activation, inducing hypodopaminergic functioning. Generally Vanderbergh et al. (1997) and Wang et al. (2001) support an association with the Val allele and SUD but others do not (Samochowise et al. 2006).

5.5 Monoamine – Oxidase A

Monoamine oxidase-A (MAOA) is a mitochondrial enzyme that degrades the neurotransmitters serotonin, norepinephrine, and dopamine. This system is involved with both psychological and physical functioning. The gene that encodes MAOA is found on the X chromosome and contains a polymorphism (MAOA-uVNTR) located 1.2 kb upstream of the MAOA coding sequences (Shih, 1991). In this polymorphism, consisting of a 30-base pair repeated sequence, six allele variants containing either 2-, 3-, 3.5-, 4-, 5-, or 6-repeat copies have been identified (Zhu & Shih, 1997). Functional studies indicate that certain alleles may confer lower transcriptional efficiency than others. The 3-repeat variant conveys lower efficiency, whereas 3.5- and 4-repeat alleles result in higher efficiency (Brummett et al., 2007). The 3- and 4-repeat alleles are the most common, and to date there is less consensus regarding the transcriptional efficiency of the other less commonly occurring alleles (e.g., 2-, 5-, and 6-repeat). The primary role of MAOA in regulating monoamine turnover, and hence ultimately influencing levels of norepinephrine, dopamine, and serotonin, indicates that its gene is a highly plausible candidate for affecting individual differences in the manifestation of psychological traits and psychiatric disorders (Shih et al., 1999). For example, recent evidence indicates that the MAOA gene may be associated with depression (Brummett et al., 2008) and stress (Lee et al., 2009). However, evidence regarding whether higher or lower MAOA gene transcriptional efficiency is positively associated with psychological pathology as been mixed. The low-activity 3-repeat allele of the MAOA-uVNTR polymorphism has been positively related to symptoms of antisocial personality (Ponce et al., 2009) and cluster B personality disorders. Other studies, however, suggest that alleles associated with higher transcriptional efficiency are related to unhealthy psychological characteristics such as trait aggressiveness and impulsivity. High MAO activity and low levels of dopamine are 2 important factors in the development of alcohol dependence. MAO is an important enzyme associated with the metabolism of biogenic amines. Therefore, Huang *et al.* (2007) investigated whether the association between the dopamine D2 receptor (DRD2) gene and alcoholism is affected by different polymorphisms of the MAO type A (MAOA) gene. The genetic variant of the DRD2 gene was only associated with the anxiety, depression (ANX/DEP) ALC phenotype, and the genetic variant of the MAOA gene was associated with ALC. Subjects carrying the MAOA 3-repeat allele and genotype A1/A1 of the DRD2 were 3.48 times (95% confidence interval = 1.47-8.25) more likely to be ANX/DEP ALC than the subjects carrying the MAOA 3-repeat allele and DRD2 A2/A2 genotype. The MAOA gene may modify the association between the DRD2 gene and ANX/DEP ALC phenotype.

Overall, Vanyukov et al (2004) suggested that, although not definitive, variants in MAOA account for a small portion of the variance of SUD risk, possibly mediated by liability to early onset behavioral problems (Vanyukov et al., 2004).

5.6 Serotonin transporter gene

The human serotonin (5-hydroxytryptamine) transporter, encoded by the SLC6A4 gene on chromosome 17q11.1-q12, is the cellular reuptake site for serotonin and a site of action for several drugs with central nervous system effects, including both therapeutic agents (e.g. antidepressants) and drugs of abuse (e.g. cocaine). It is known that the serotonin transporter plays an important role in the metabolic cycle of a broad range of antidepressants, antipsychotics, anxiolytics, antiemetics, and anti-migraine drugs. Salz *et al.* (2009) found an excess of -1438G and 5-HTTLPR L carriers in alcoholic patients in comparison to the heroin dependent group [OR (95% CI)=1.98 (1.13-3.45) and 1.92 (1.07-3.44), respectively]. The A-1438G and 5-HTTLPR polymorphisms also interacted in distinguishing alcohol from heroin dependent patients (df) =10.21 (4), p=0.037). The association of -1438A/G with alcohol dependence was especially pronounced in the presence of 5-HTTLPR S/S, less evident with 5-HTTLPR L/S and not present with 5-HTTLPR.

5.7 Gamma-aminobutyric acid (GABA) receptor genes

Gamma-aminobutyric acid (GABA) receptor genes have also received some attention as candidates for drug use disorders. One reason for this is that the dopamine and GABA systems are functionally interrelated (White, 1996). Research suggests that dopamine neurons projecting from the anterior ventral tegmental area to the NAc are tonically inhibited by GABA through its actions at the GABAA receptor (Ikemoto, Kohl, & McBride, 1997). Moreover, it has been shown that alcohol (Theile, Morikawa, Gonzales, & Morrisett, 2008) or opioid (Johnson & North, 1992) enhancement of GABAergic (through GABAA receptor) transmission inhibits the release of dopamine in the mesocorticolimbic system. Thus, a hyperactive GABA system, by inhibiting dopamine release, could also lead to hypodopaminergic functioning. Because of this, GABA genes are of interest in the search for causes of drug use disorders. A dinucleotide repeat (DNR) polymorphism of the GABA receptor β3 subunit gene (GABRB3) results in either the presence of the 181-bp G1 or 11 other repeats designated as non-G1 (NG1). Research indicates that the NG1 is more prevalent in children of alcoholics (COAs; Namkoong, Cheon, Kim, Jun, & Lee, 2008). Presence of the NG1 has been associated with alcohol dependence (Noble et al., 1998; Song et al., 2003). In addition, other GABA receptor genes have also been associated with this disorder (Edenberg et al., 2004).

6. Multiplex analysis and GARS

There is a need to classify patients at genetic risk for drug seeking behavior prior to or upon entry to residential and or non-residential chemical dependency programs. Instead of continuing to evaluate single gene associations to predict future drug abuse, it seems parsimonious to evaluate multiple genes involved in the brain reward cascade and hypodopaminergic antecedents. As described in this example, such methods employ RDS-associated gene panels to stratify or classify patients entering a treatment facility as having low, moderate, or high genetic predictive risk based on a number of now known and/or later discovered RDS risk alleles. Our laboratory developed a Genetic Addiction Risk Score (GARS) for this purpose. This example describes genetic studies for seven RDS-associated alleles for six candidate genes in a patient population (n=26) of recovering poly-drug abusers (Blum et al., 2010).

To determine RDS risk severity for each of these 26 patients, the percentage of prevalence of the risk alleles was calculated and a severity score based on the percentage of these alleles present in a given patient was developed. Subjects carry the following risk alleles: DRD2=A1; SLC6A3 (DAT) =10R; DRD4=3R or 7R; 5HTTIRP = L or $L_{A;}$ MAO= 3R; and COMT=G. As depicted in Tables 5 and 6, below, Low Severity (LS) = 1-36%, Moderate Severity (MS) =37-50%, and High Severity (HS) = 51-100%, scores were assigned. Two distinct ethnic populations among the 26 patients were studied. Group 1 consisted of 16 male Caucasian psycho-stimulant addicts and Group 2 consisted of 10 Chinese heroin-addicted males. Based on this analysis, the 16 Caucasian 100% of subjects had at least one risk allele (see tables 5 and 6). Therefore, using this approach it was found that 81% of the patients were at moderate to high risk for addictive behavior. Of particular interest was the discovery that 56% of the subjects carried the DRD2 A1 allele (9/16).

Out of the nine Chinese heroin addicts (Group 2), it was found that 11% (1) were HS, 56% (5) were MS, and 33% (3) were LS. These scores were then converted to a fraction and represented as GARS, whereby the average GARS was found to be: 0.28 Low Severity; 0.43 moderate severity; and 0.54 high severity, respectively. Therefore, using GARS it was discovered that 67% of the Group 2 patients were at moderate to high risk for addictive behavior. As with Group 1, 56% of the Group 2 subjects carried the DRD2 A1 allele (5/9). Statistical analysis revealed that the two groups did not differ in terms of overall severity (67% vs. 81%) in these two distinct populations. Combining these two independent study populations reveals that subjects entering a residential treatment facility for poly-drug abuse carry at least one risk allele (100%). Moreover, 74% of the combined 25 subjects who were genotyped by SNP analysis had a moderate-to-high GARS.

The 16 patients of Group 1 were interviewed and evaluated for chemical dependence using a standard battery of diagnostic tests and questionnaires. The tests included the following: a drug history questionnaire; a physical assessment, urine drug tests; a breathalyzer; complete CBC blood test; and a symptom severity questionnaire. The patients were determined to be substance dependent according to Diagnostic and Statistical Manual (DSM-IV) criteria. All patients were residential in-patients enrolled in 30-90 day chemical dependence rehabilitation programs at either of two treatment centers in the U.S.

Table 3 shows the demographics of the 16 patients, including gender, race, age, and length of abstinence. The median age was 29.5 ± 8.8 SD years. The population breakdown was as follows: 87.5 % Caucasian and 12.5% Hispanic. The average number of months abstinent for the entire population was 9.5 ±23.3. There were 3 pure cocaine-only addicts; 4 cocaine crack addicts; and 9 cocaine plus other drugs of abuse (alcohol, opiates and marijuana).

Table 4 includes genotype data from a functional MRI (fMRI) study in China evaluating involving 10 heroin-addicted Chinese males with a median age of 33 ± 7.6 SD years. Diagnosis of heroin dependence was also determined in this group using DSM-1 V criteria and other behavioral instruments. The average number of months abstinent for the entire population was 16 ± 7.9.

	Median ±st.dev.	**(min, max)**	***N (total = 16)***
Age	29.5 ±8.80	(19, 48)	16
Clean time (months)	9.5 ±23.33	(2, 101)	16
Race = Caucasian			14
Race = Hispanic			2
Sex = Male			16
Primary Substance = Cocaine only			3
Primary Substance = Crack cocaine			4
Primary Substance = Cocaine + Other*			9

Table 3. Demographics of all Caucasian subjects combined.

	Median ±st.dev.	**(min, max)**	***N (total = 10)***
Age	33 ± 7.57	(20, 44)	10
Clean time (months)	16 ± 7.91	(1, 24)	10
Race = Chinese			10
Sex = Male			10
Primary Substance = Heroin only			10
Primary Substance = Heroin + other			0

*One sample was eliminated because genotyping could not be performed. Source Blum et al 2010.

Table 4. Demographics of all Chinese subjects combined*.

6.1 Genotyping

Genotyping (Blum et al., 2010) was performed as follows. Each patient was also genotyped for the following gene polymorphisms: MAOA-VNTR, 5HTTLPR, SLC6A3, DRD4, ANKKI, DRD2 TaqIA (rs1800497), and the COMT val^{158}met SNP (rs4680). Genotypes were scored independently by two investigators.

The dopamine transporter (DAT1, locus symbol SLC6A3, which maps to 5p15.3, contains a 40 base-pair Variable Number Tandem Repeat (VNTR) element consisting of 3-11 copies in the 3' untranslated region (UTR) of the gene.

The dopamine D4 receptor (DRD4), which maps to 11p15.5, contains a 48 bp VNTR polymorphism in the third exon, which consists of 2-11 repeats.

Monoamine Oxidase A upstream VNTR (MAOA-uVNTR). The MAOA gene, which maps to Xp11.3-11.4, contains a 30 bp VNTR in the 5′ regulatory region of the gene that has been shown to affect expression. A genotype by environment interaction has been reported for this polymorphism.

Serotonin Transporter-Linked Polymorphic region (5HTTLPR). The serotonin transporter (5HTT, Locus Symbol SLC6A4), which maps to 17q11.1-17q12, contains a 43 bp insertion/deletion (ins/del) polymorphism in the 5′ regulatory region of the gene. A SNP (rs25531, A/G) in the Long form of 5HTTLPR has functional significance: The more common L_A allele is associated with the reported higher basal activity, whereas the less common L_G allele has transcriptional activity no greater than the S. The SNP rs25531 is assayed by incubating the full length PCR product with the restriction endonuclease MspI.

For all of the above VNTR and ins/del polymorphisms, PCR reactions contained approximately 20 ng of DNA, 10% DMSO, 1.8 mM MgCl2, 200 μM deoxynucleotides, with 7′-deaza-2′-deoxyGTP substituted for one half of the dGTP, 400 nM of appropriate forward and reverse amplification primers, and 1 unit of AmpliTaq Gold® polymerase, in a total volume of 20 µl. Amplification was performed using touchdown PCR. After amplification, an aliquot of PCR product was combined with loading buffer containing size standard (Genescan 1200 Liz) and analyzed with an ABI PRISM® 3130 Genetic Analyzer.

DRD2 TaqIA (rs1800497). The gene encoding the dopamine D2 receptor maps to 11q23, and contains a polymorphic TaqI restriction endonuclease site located within exon of the adjacent ANKKI gene that was originally thought to be located in the 3' untranslated region of the gene. The A1 allele has been reported to reduce the amount of receptor protein. This SNP was assayed using a Taqman (5'Nuclease) assay.

COMT val^{158}met SNP (rs4680). The gene encoding COMT maps to 22q11.21, and codes for both the membrane-bound and soluble forms of the enzyme that metabolizes dopamine to 3-methoxy-4-hydroxyphenylethylamine. An A→G mutation results in a valine to methionine substitution at codons 158/108, respectively. This amino acid substitution has been associated with a four-fold reduction in enzymatic activity. The COMT SNP was assayed with a Taqman method.

6.2 Genetic Addiction Risk Score (GARS)

In terms of genotyping data it has been determined that when multiple RDS-associated genes are analyzed, such as the genes for serotonergic- 2A receptor (5-HTT2a), serotonergic transportor (5HTTLPR), (dopamine D2 receptor (DRD2), Dopamine D4 receptor (DRD4), Dopamine transporter (DAT1), Catechol-o-methyl -transferase (COMT), and monoamine-oxidase (MOA), 100% of all subjects carried at least one risk allele. To our knowledge this is the first reported attempt to stratify or classify addiction risk by incorporating an algorithm formulation that combines genotyping results for a number of RDS-associated risk alleles by pre-assigning an allele as a risk allele having predictive value for drug use. Previously, Blum et al (1996) using Bayesian statistics it was shown that the DRD2 A1 allele had a predictive value of 74.4% for all Reward Deficiency Syndrome (RDS). Here, the subjects studied in this investigation had multiple drug abuse relapses and presented to in-patient residential treatment programs.

Sub	MAOAuVNTR	5HTTLPR	5HTTLPR	SLC6A3	DRD4	DRD2	COMT	Any risk allele	SEVERITY* GARS
1	3R	S/L	S/LG	9R/10R	4R/4R	A1/A2	G/G	POSITIVE	0.46–MS
2	3R	S/L	S/LA	10R/10R	4R/7R	A2/A2	G/G	POSITIVE	0.62 -HS
3	3R	L/L	LA /LG	9R/9R	3R/4R	A1/A2	A/G	POSITIVE	0.57-HS
4	4R	S/L	S/LA	10R/10R	3R/7R	A2/A2	G/G	POSITIVE	0.46-MS
5	4R	L/L	LA/LA	10R/10R	4R/7R	A2/A2	A/G	POSITIVE	0.62 -HS
6	3R	S/S	S/S	9R/10R	4R/7R	A2/A2	A/G	POSITIVE	0.30 -LS
7	4R	S/L	S/LG	10R/10R	4R/4R	A1/A1	A/A	POSITIVE	0.38 -MS
8	4R	S/L	S/LA	9R/10R	3R/4R	A2/A2	A/A	POSITIVE	0.23-LS
9	3R	L/L	LA//LA	9R/9R	4R/7R	A2/A2	A/G	POSITIVE	0.54-HS
10	4R	L/L	LA/LA	9R/10R	4R/4R	A2/A2	G/G	POSITIVE	0.54 -HS
11	3R	S/L	S/ LA	9R/10R	4R/4R	A1/A2	G/G	POSITIVE	0.54-HS
12	4R	L/L	LA/LA	9R/10R	4R/4R	A1/A2	A/G	POSITIVE	0.54-HS
13	4R	S/L	S/ LA	10R/10R	4R/4R	A1/A2	A/G	POSITIVE	0.46 -MS
14	4R	S/S	S/S	9R/10R	4R/4R	A1/A2	G/G	POSITIVE	0.30-LS
15	3R	L/L	LA / LA	10R/10R	4R/4R	A1/A2	A/G	POSITIVE	0.69 -HS
16	4R	S/L	S/LA	10R/10R	4R/7R	A1/A2	A/A	POSITIVE	0.46-MS

Table 5. Group 1 genotyping data for each Caucasian patient. Data taken from Blum *et al.* 2010.

The finding that 75% of these individuals have moderate-to-high GARS, whereas only 25% had low GARS, indicates that pre-screening patients prior enrolling in a treatment program could be beneficial. Clinically, this will be important for understanding expectations of future success and the need for intensive treatment involving genomic solutions coupled with medical therapies, including bio-holistic therapies. It will also reduce quilt and denial of the entering patient.

Subject	MAOAuVNTR	5HTTLPR	5HTTLPR	SLC6A3	DRD4	*DRD2*	*COMT*	Any risk allele	SEVERITY* GARS
1	4R	S/L	S/LA	10R/10R	4R/4R	A2/A2	A/A	POSITIVE	0.30-LS
2	3R	S/S	S/S	10R/10R	2R/4R	A1/A2	GAG	POSITIVE	0.38-MS
3	4R	S/S	S/S	10R/10R	3R/4R	A1/A2	G/G	POSITIVE	0.46-MS
4	3R	S/S	S/S	10R/10R	4R/6R	A2/A2	G/G	POSITIVE	0.38-MS
5	4R	S/S	S/S	10R/10R	4R/4R	A1/A2	A/G	POSITIVE	0.30-LS
6	3R	L/L	S/ LG	10R/10R	4R/4R	A1/A2	ND	POSITIVE	0.45 -MS
7	4R	L/L	LA/LG	10R/10R	4R/4R	A1/A2	A/G	POSITIVE	0.54 -HS
8	4R	S/S	S/S	10R/10R	4R/5R	A2/A2	A/G	POSITIVE	0.23-LS
9	3R	S/L	S/LA	10R/10R	2R/4R	A2/A2	A/G	POSITIVE	0.46-MS

Table 6. Group 2 genotyping data for each Chinese patient. Data taken from Blum et al 2010.

The GARS study supports the understanding that identifying hypodopaminergic genotypes may be the best predictor of adult and adolescent drug abuse or other SUD behavior. These results are also consistent with a number of functional MRI studies that show that the hypodopaminergic DRD2 A1 genotype leads to blunted responses that can could lead to aberrant drug and/or food seeking behavior (Stice et al., 2008), while the hyperdopaminergic A2 genotype serves as a protective factor against the development of drug disorders (Volkow et al 2006).

A further strength of this study is that only male subjects were used. Males with hypodopaminegic functioning are more likely to abuse drugs that stimulate the mesocorticolimbic system than those with normal dopaminergic functioning. In contrast, females living in a negative environment are at increased risk (possibly not due to their genotypes) for using more drugs and even more types of drug that increase their risk for SUD.

Another strength of this study is that it is in agreement with the work of Conner *et al.* [2010] confirming the importance of the cumulative effect of multiple genotypes coding for hypodopaminergic functioning, regardless of their genomic location, as a predictive method of drug use in males. Moreover, it extends the current literature, by suggesting for the first time a simple method using genetic testing to classify risk behavior in male patients seeking in-patient residential treatment (see table 7).

6.3 A representative RDS gene panel

Table 7, describes a RDS-associated gene/polymorphism panel that can be used in accordance with the potential development of the GARS test.

Gene	Significance	Comment
ALDH2	$P = 5 X 10^{-37}$	With alcoholism and alcohol-induced medical diseases
ADH1B	$P = 2 X 10^{-21}$	With alcoholism and alcohol-induced medical diseases
ADH1C	$P = 4 X 10^{-33}$	With alcoholism and alcohol-induced medical diseases
DRD2	$P = 1 X 10^{-8}$	With alcohol and drug abuse
DRD4	$P = 1 X 10^{-2}$	With alcohol and drug abuse
SLC6A4	$P = 2 X 10^{-3}$	With alcohol , heroin, cocaine, methamphetamine dependence
HTRIB	$P = 5 X 10^{-1}$	With alcohol and drug abuse
HTRI2A	$P = 5 X 10^{-1}$	With alcohol and drug abuse
TPH	$P = 2 X 10^{-3}$	With alcohol and drug abuse
MAOA	$P = 9 X 10^{-5}$	With alcohol and drug abuse
OPRD1	$P = 5 X 10^{-1}$	With alcohol and drug abuse
GABRG2	$P = 5 X 10^{-4}$	With alcohol and drug abuse
GABRA2	$P = 7 X 10^{-4}$	With alcohol and drug abuse
GABRA6	$P = 6 X 10^{-4}$	With alcohol and drug abuse
COMT*	$P = 5 X 10^{-1}$	With alcohol and drug abuse in Asians
DAT1	$P = 5 X 10^{-1}$	With alcohol and drug abuse in Asians
CNR1	$P = 5 X 10^{-1}$	With alcohol and drug abuse
CYP2E1*	$P = 7 X 10^{-2}$	With alcohol LIVER DISEASE

Table 7. An RDS gene panel. Chen et al. Journal of Psychoactive drugs. June 2011.

7. Conclusion

The need to genetically test individuals, especially at entry into a residential or even non-residential chemical dependency program, has long been recognized. In the GARS study, a high percentage (75%) of subjects were found to carry a moderate to high GARS, and 100% of individuals tested possessed at least one of the RDS risk alleles tested. It is of some interest that in the Group 2 population only rare DRD4 alleles such as 2R, 5R, and 6R were found. This study supports our understanding that hypodopaminergic state is due to gene polymorphisms, as well as environmental elements including both stress and neurotoxicity from aberrant abuse of psychoactive drugs (e.g., alcohol, heroin, cocaine etc). This study demonstrates that useful genetic variables include serotonergic genes (e.g., serotonergic receptors [5HT2a], serotonin transporter 5HTlPR, etc.), endorphinergic genes (e.g., mu OPRM1 gene, proenkephalin (PENK) [PENK polymorphic 3' UTR dinucleotide (CA) repeats]), and dopaminergic genes (e.g., ANKKI Taq A; DRD2 C957T, DRD4 7R, COMT Val/met substation, MAO-A uVNTR, and SLC3 9 or 10R). Future studies could add other genes (e.g., GABARB3) and D3 dopamine receptor.

Any of these genetic and/or environmental impairments could result in reduced release of dopamine and or reduced number of dopaminergic receptors. The use of GARS will have prevention and treatment benefits in those patients afflicted with genetic antecedents to RDS-seeking behaviors.

8. Conflict of interest

Kenneth Blum, B.William Downs. and Roger Waite owns stock in LifeGen, Inc. the world wide distributors of the GARS test based on US and foreign patents. Frank Fornari is an consultant and owns interest in Dominion Diagnostics Lab the commercial developers of the GARS test. John Giordano is a LifeGen, Inc. partner.

9. References

Agrawal, A.; Lynskey, M.T.; Todorov, A.A.; Schrage, A.J.; Littlefield, A.K.; Grant, J.D.; Zhu, Q.; Nelson, E.C.; Madden, P.A.; Bucholz, K.K.; Sher, K.J. & Heath, A.C. (2010). A Candidate Gene Association Study of Alcohol Consumption in Young Women*. *Alcohol Clin Exp Res*, (published online ahead of print December 8 2010)

Bau, C.H.; Almeida, S. & Hutz, M.H. (2000). The TaqI A1 allele of the dopamine D2 receptor gene and alcoholism in Brazil: association and interaction with stress and harm avoidance on severity prediction. *Am J Med Genet*, Vol.96, No.3, (June 2000), pp. 302-206, ISSN 1552-4833

Berridge, K.C. (2009). 'Liking' and 'wanting' food rewards: brain substrates and roles in eating disorders. *Physiol Behav*, Vol.97, No.5, (July 2009), pp. 537-550, ISSN 0031-9384

Biederman, J.; Petty, C.R.; Ten Haagen, K.S.; Small, J.; Doyle, A.E.; Spencer, T.; Mick, E.; Monuteaux, M.C.; Smoller, J.W.; Faraone, S.V. (2009). Effect of candidate gene polymorphisms on the course of attention deficit hyperactivity disorder. *Psychiatry Res*, Vol.170, No.2-3, (December 2009), pp. 199-203, ISSN 0165-1781

Blum, K. & Gold, M.S. (2011). Neuro-chemical activation of brain reward meso-limbic circuitry is associated with relapse prevention and drug hunger: a hypothesis. *Med Hypotheses*, Vol.76, No.4, (April 2011), pp. 576-584, ISSN 0306-9877

Blum, K.; Giordano, J.; Morse, S.; Liu, Y.; Tan, J.; Bowirrat, A.; Smolen, A.; Waite, R.; Downs, W.; Madigan, M.; Kerner, M.; Fornari, F.; Stice, E.; Braverman, E.; Miller, D.; Bailey, J. (2010). Genetic Addiction Risk Score (GARS) Analysis: Exploratory Development of Polymorphic Risk Alleles in Poly-drug Addicted Males. *The IIOAB Journal*, Vol.1, No.2, (July 2010), pp. 1-14, ISSN 0976-3104

Blum, K.; Chen, T.J.H.; Chen, A.L.H.; Bowirrat, A.; Downs, B.W.; Waite, R.L.; Reinking, J.; Kerner, M.; Braverman, D.; DiNubile, N.; Rhoades, P.; Braverman, E.R.; Blum, S.H.; Oscar-Berman, M.; Paolomo, T.; Stice, E.; Gold, M.; Comings, D.E. & Savarimuthu, S. (2009) Genes and Happiness. *Gene Therapy and Mol Biol*, Vol.13, (June 2009)

Blum, K.; Chen, A.L.; Chen, T.J.; Braverman, E.R.; Reinking, J.; Blum, S.H.; Cassel, K.; Downs, B.W.; Waite, R.L.; Williams, L.; Prihoda, T.J.; Kerner, M.M.; Palomo, T.; Comings, D.E.; Tung, H.; Rhoades, P. & Oscar-Berman, M. (2008). Activation instead of blocking mesolimbic dopaminergic reward circuitry is a preferred modality in the long term treatment of reward deficiency syndrome (RDS): a commentary. *Theor Biol Med Model*, Vol.12, No.5, (November 2008), pp. 24, ISSN 1742-4682

Blum, K.; Sheridan, P.J.; Wood, R.C.; Braverman, E.R.; Chen, T.J.; Cull, J.G. & Comings, D.E. (1996). The D2 dopamine receptor gene as a determinant of reward deficiency syndrome. *J R Soc Med*, Vol.89. No.7, (July 1996), pp. 396-400, ISSN 0141-0768

Blum, K.; Noble, E.P.; Sheridan, P.J.; Montgomery, A.; Ritchie, T.; Jagadeeswaran, P.; Nogami, H.; Briggs, A.H. & Cohn, J.B. (1990). Allelic association of human dopamine D2 receptor gene in alcoholism. *JAMA*, Vol.263, No.15, (April 1990), pp. 2055-2060, ISBN 0098-7484

Boundy, V.A.; Lu, L. & Molinoff, P.B. (1996). Differential coupling of rat D2 dopamine receptor isoforms expressed in Spodoptera frugiperda insect cells. *J Pharmacol Exp Ther*, Vol.276, No.2, (February 1996), pp. 784-794, ISSN 0022-3565

Bowirrat, A. & Oscar-Berman, M. (2005). Relationship between dopaminergic neurotransmission, alcoholism, and Reward Deficiency syndrome. *Am J Med Genet B Neuropsychiatr Genet*, Vol.132B, No.1, (January 2005), pp. 29-37, ISSN 1552-4841Brousse, G.; Vorspan, F.; Ksouda, K.; Bloch, V.; Peoc'h, K.; Laplanche, J.L.; Mouly, S.;

Schmidt, J.; Llorca, P.M. & Lepine, J.P. (2010). Could the inter-individual variability in cocaine-induced psychotic effects influence the development of cocaine addiction? Towards a new pharmacogenetic approach to addictions. *Med Hypotheses*, Vol.75, No.6, (December 2010), pp. 600-604, ISSN 0306-9877

Bruijnzeel, A.W.; Repetto, M. & Gold, M.S. (2004). Neurobiological mechanisms in addictive and psychiatric disorders. *Psychiatr Clin North Am*, Vol.27, No.4, (December 2004), pp.661-674, ISSN 0193-953X

Brummett, B.H.; Boyle, S.H.; Siegler, I.C.; Kuhn, C.M.; Surwit, R.S.; Garrett, M.E.; Collins, A.; Ashley-Koch, A.; Williams, R.B. (2008). HPA axis function in male caregivers: effect of the monoamine oxidase-A gene promoter (MAOA-uVNTR). *Biol Psychol*, Vol.79, No.2, (October 2008), pp. 250-255, ISSN 0301-0511

Brummett, B.H.; Krystal, A.D.; Siegler, I.C.; Kuhn, C.; Surwit, R.S.; Züchner, S.; Ashley-Koch, A.; Barefoot, J.C.; Williams, R.B. (2007). Associations of a regulatory polymorphism of monoamine oxidase-A gene promoter (MAOA-uVNTR) with symptoms of depression and sleep quality. *Psychosom Med*, Vol.69, No.5, (June 2007), pp. 396-401, ISSN 0033-3174

Cao, L.; Li, T.; Liu, X. (2003). Association study of heroin dependence and catechol-O-methyltransferase gene. *Zhonghua Yi Xue Yi Chuan Xue Za Zhi*, Vol.20, No.2, (April 2003), pp. 127-130, ISSN 1003-9406

Chen, T.J.H.; Blum, K.; Chen, A.L.C.; Bowirrat, A.; Downs, W.B.; Madigan, M.A.; Waite, R.L.; Bailey, J.A.; Kerner, M.; Yeldani, Majmundar, N.; Giordano, J.; Morse, S.; Miler, D.; Fornari, F.; Braverman, E.R. Neurogenetics and clinical evidence for the putative activation of the brain reward circuitry by amino-acid precursor-catabolic enzyme inhibition therapeutic agent (a Neuroadaptagen): Proposing an addiction candidate gene panel map. *Journal Of Psychoactive Drugs* (in press) 2011.

Chen, T.J.; Blum, K.; Mathews, D.; Fisher, L.; Schnautz, N.; Braverman, E.R.; Schoolfield, J.; Downs, B.W. & Comings, D.E. (2005). Are dopaminergic genes involved in a predisposition to pathological aggression? Hypothesizing the importance of "super normal controls" in psychiatricgenetic research of complex behavioral disorders. *Med Hypotheses*, Vol.65, No.4, (2005), pp. 703-707, ISSN 0306-9877

Comings, D.E. & Blum, K. (2000). Reward deficiency syndrome: genetic aspects of behavioral disorders. *Prog Brain Res*, Vol.126, (2000), pp. 325-341, ISSN 0079-6123

Conner, B.T.; Hellemann, G.S.; Ritchie, T.L.; Noble, E.P. (2010). Genetic, personality, and environmental predictors of drug use in adolescents. *J Subst Abuse Treat*, Vol.38, No.2, (March 2010), pp. 178-190, ISSN 0740-5472

Conrad, K.L.; Ford, K.; Marinelli, M. & Wolf M.E. (2010). Dopamine receptor expression and distribution dynamically change in the rat nucleus accumbens after withdrawal from cocaine self-administration. *Neuroscience*, Vol.169, No.1, (August 2010), pp. 182-194, ISSN 0306-4522

Cook, E.H. Jr.; Stein, M.A.; Krasowski, M.D.; Cox, N.J.; Olkon, D.M.; Kieffer, J.E.; Leventhal, B.L. (1995). Association of attention-deficit disorder and the dopamine transporter gene. *Am J Hum Genet*, Vol.56, No.4, (April 1995), pp. 993-998, ISSN 0002-9297

Di Chiara, G. (1995). The role of dopamine in drug abuse viewed from the perspective of its role in motivation. *Drug Alcohol Depend*, Vol.38, No.2, (May 1995), pp. 95–137, ISSN 0376-8716

Dreyer, J.L. (2010). New insights into the roles of microRNAs in drug addiction and neuroplasticity. *Genome Med*, Vol.2, No.12, (December 2010), pp. 92, ISSN 1794-994X

Duan, J.; Wainwright, M.S.; Comeron, J.M.; Saitou, N.; Sanders, A.R.; Gelernter, J. & Gejman, P.V. (2003). Synonymous mutations in the human dopamine receptor D2 (DRD2) affect mRNA stability and synthesis of the receptor. *Hum Mol Genet*, Vol.12, No.3, (February 2003), pp. 205-216, ISSN 0964-6906

Edenberg, H. J.; Dick, D.M.; Xuei, X.; Tian, H.; Almasy, L.; Bauer, L.O.; Crowe, R.R.; Goate, A.; Hesselbrock, V.; Jones, K.; Kwon, J.; Li, T.K.; Nurnberger, J. I. Jr.; O'Connor, S. J.; Reich, T.; Rice, J.; Schuckit, M.A.; Porjesz, B.; Foroud, T.; Begleiter, H. (2004). Variations in GABRA2 encoding the alpha 2 subunit of the GABA (A) receptor, are associated with alcohol dependence and with brain oscillations. *American Journal of Human Genetics*, Vol.74, No.4, (April 2004), pp. 705−714, ISSN 0002-9297

Edwards, S. & Koob, G.F. (2010). Neurobiology of dysregulated motivational systems in drug addiction. *Future Neurol*, Vol.5, No.3, (May 2010), pp. 393-401, ISSN 1479-6708

Filtz, T.M.; Guan, W.; Artymyshyn, R.P.; Facheco, M.; Ford, C. & Molinoff, P.B. (1994). Mechanisms of up-regulation of D2L dopamine receptors by agonists and antagonists in transfected HEK-293 cells. *J Pharmacol Exp Ther*, Vol.274, No.3, (December 1994), pp. 1574-1582, ISSN 0022-3565

Gardner, E.L. (2011). Addiction and brain reward and antireward pathways. *Adv Psychosom Med*, Vol.30, (published online ahead of print April 19 2011), pp. 22-60, ISSN 0065-3268

Grandy, D.K.; Litt, M.; Allenm, L.; Bunzow, J.R.; Marchionni, M.; Makam, H.; Reed, L.; Magenis, R.E. & Civelli, O. (1989). The human dopamine D2 receptor gene is located on chromosome 11 at q22-q23 and identifies a TaqI RFLP. *Am J Hum Genet*, Vol.45, No.5, (November 1989), pp. 778-785, ISBN 0002-9297

Greven, C.U.; Rijsdijk, F.V. & Plomin, R. (2011). A twin study of ADHD symptoms in early adolescence: hyperactivity-impulsivity and inattentiveness show substantial genetic overlap but also genetic specificity. *J Abnorm Child Psychol*, Vol.39, No.2, (February 2011), pp. 265-275, ISSN 0091-0627

Grzywacz, A.; Kucharska-Mazur, J.; Samochowiec, J. (2009). Association studies of dopamine D4 receptor gene exon 3 in patients with alcohol dependence. *Psychiatr Pol*, Vol.42, No.3, (May-June 2009), pp. 453-461, ISSN 0033-2674

Guindalini, C.; Howard, M.; Haddley, K.; Laranjeira, R.; Collier, D.; Ammar, N.; Craig, I.; O'Gara, C.; Bubb, V.J.; Greenwood, T.; Kelsoe, J.; Asherson, P.; Murray, R.M.; Castelo, A.; Quinn, J.P.; Vallada, H.; Breen, G. (2006). A dopamine transporter gene functional variant associated with cocaine abuse in a Brazilian sample. *Proc Natl Acad Sci U S A*, Vol.103, No.12, (March 2006), pp. 4552-4557, ISSN 0027-8424

Heber, D. & Carpenter, C.L. (2011). Addictive Genes and the Relationship to Obesity and Inflammation. *Mol Neurobiol*, (published online ahead of print April 19 2011)

Hill, S.Y.; Hoffman, E.K.; Zezza, N.; Thalamuthu, A.; Weeks, D.E.; Matthews, A.G.; Mukhopadhyay, I. (2008). Dopaminergic mutations: within-family association and linkage in multiplex alcohol dependence families. *Am J Med Genet B Neuropsychiatr Genet*, Vol.147B, No.4, (June 2008), pp. 517-526, ISSN 1552-4841

Hirvonen, M.; Laakso, A.; Någren, K.; Rinne, J.O.; Pohjalainen, T.; Hietala, J. (2004). C957T polymorphism of the dopamine D2 receptor (DRD2) gene affects striatal DRD2 availability in vivo. *Mol Psychiatry*, Vol.9, No.12, (December 2004), pp. 1060-1061, ISSN 1359-4184

Huang, W.; Payne, T.J.; Ma, J.Z.; Beuten, J.; Dupont, R.T.; Inohara, N. & Li, M.D. (2008) Significant association of ANKK1 and detection of a functional polymorphism with nicotine dependence in an African-American sample. *Neuropsychopharmacology*, Vol.34, No.2, (January 2009), pp. 319-330, ISSN 0893-133X

Huang, S.Y.; Lin, W.W.; Wan, F.J.; Chang, A.J.; Ko, H.C.; Wang, T.J.; Wu, P.L.; Lu, R.B. (2007). Monoamine oxidase-A polymorphisms might modify the association between the dopamine D2 receptor gene and alcohol dependence. *J Psychiatry Neurosci*, Vol.32, No.3, (May 2007), pp. 185-192, ISSN 1180-4882

Ikemoto, S., Kohl, R. R., & McBride, W. J. (1997). GABA (A) receptor blockage in the ventral tegmental area increases extracellular levels of dopamine in the nucleus accumbens of rats. *Journal of Neurochemistry*, Vol.69, No.1, (July 1997), pp. 137–143, ISSN 0022-3042

Johnson, S. W.; North, R. A. (1992). Opioids excite dopamine neurons by hyperpolarization of local interneurons. *Journal of Neuroscience*, Vol.12, No.2, (February 1992), pp. 483–488, ISSN 0270-6474

Jönsson, E.G.; Nöthen, M.M.; Grünhage, F.; Farde, L.; Nakashima, Y.; Propping, P. & Sedvall, G.C. (1999). Polymorphisms in the dopamine D2 receptor gene and their relationships to striatal dopamine receptor density of healthy volunteers. *Mol Psychiatry*, Vol.4, No.3, (May 1999), pp. 290-296, ISSN 1359-4184

Kendler, K.S.; Aggen, S.H.; Knudsen, G.P.; Røysamb, E.; Neale, M.C. & Reichborn-Kjennerud, T. (2010). The structure of genetic and environmental risk factors for syndromal and subsyndromal common DSM-IV axis I and all axis II disorders. *Am J Psychiatry*, Vol.168, No.1, (January 2011), pp. 29-39, ISSN 002-953X

Koob, G. & Kreek, M.J. (2007). Stress, dysregulation of drug reward pathways, and the transition to drug dependence. *Am J Psychiatry*, Vol.164, No.8, (August 2007), pp. 1149-1159, ISSN 0002-953X

Kotler, M.; Cohen, H.; Segman, R.; Gritsenko, I.; Nemanov, L.; Lerer, B.; Kramer, I.; Zer-Zion, M.; Kletz, I.; Ebstein, R.P. (1997). Excess dopamine D4 receptor (D4DR) exon III seven repeat allele in opioid-dependent subjects. *Mol Psychiatry*, Vol.2, No.3, (May 1997), pp. 251-254, ISSN 1359-4184

Kraschewski, A.; Reese, J.; Anghelescu, I.; Winterer, G.; Schmidt, L.G.; Gallinat, J.; Finckh, U.; Rommelspacher, H.; Wernicke, C. (2009). Association of the dopamine D2 receptor gene with alcohol dependence: haplotypes and subgroups of alcoholics as key factors for understanding receptor function. *Pharmacogenet Genomics*, Vol.19, No.7, (July 2009), pp. 513-527, ISSN 1744-6872

Lawson-Yuen, A.; Saldivar, J.S.; Sommer, S. & Picker, J. (2008). Familial deletion within NLGN4 associated with autism and Tourette syndrome. *Eur J Hum Genet*, Vol.16, No.5, (May 2008), pp. 614-618, ISSN 1018-4813

Lee S.Y.; Hahn, C.Y.; Lee, J.F.; Huang, S.Y.; Chen, S.L.; Kuo, P.H.; Lee, I.H.; Yeh, T.L.; Yang, Y.K.; Chen, S.H.; Ko, H.C.; Lu, R.B. (2010). MAOA Interacts With the ALDH2 Gene in Anxiety-Depression Alcohol Dependence. *Alcohol Clin Exp Res*, Vol.34, No.7, (July 2010), pp. 1212-1218, ISSN 0145-6008

Lee, S.Y.; Hahn, C.Y.; Lee, J.F.; Chen, S.L.; Chen, S.H.; Yeh, T.L.; Kuo, P.H.; Lee, I.H.; Yang, Y.K.; Huang, S.Y.; Ko, H.C.; Lu, R.B. (2009). MAOA-uVNTR polymorphism may modify the protective effect of ALDH2 gene against alcohol dependence in antisocial personality disorder. *Alcohol Clin Exp Res*, Vol.33, No.6, (June 2009), pp. 985-990, ISSN 0145-6008

Lee, S.S.; Lahey, B.B.; Waldman, I.; Van Hulle, C.A.; Rathouz, P.; Pelham, W.E.; Loney, J.; Cook, E.H. (2007). Association of dopamine transporter genotype with disruptive behavior disorders in an eight-year longitudinal study of children and adolescents. *Am J Med Genet Neuropsychiatr Genet*, Vol.144B, No.3, (April 2007), pp. 310-317, ISSN 1552-4841

Lusher, J.M.; Chandler, C.; Ball, D. (2001). Dopamine D4 receptor gene (DRD4) is associated with Novelty Seeking (NS) and substance abuse: the saga continues. *Mol Psychiatry*, Vol.6, No.5, (September 2001), pp.497-499, ISSN 1359-4184

McGeary, J.E.; Esposito-Smythers, C.; Spirito, A.; Monti, P.M. (2006). Associations of the dopamine D4 receptor gene VNTR polymorphism with drug use in adolescent psychiatric inpatients. *Pharmacol Biochem Behav*, Vol.86, No.2, (February 2007), pp. 401-406, ISSN 0091-3057

Michelhaugh, S.K.; Fiskerstrand, C.; Lovejoy, E.; Bannon, M.J.; Quinn, J.P. (2001). The dopamine transporter gene (SLC6A3) variable number of tandem repeats domain enhances transcription in dopamine neurons. *J Neurochem*, Vol.79, No.5, (December 2001), pp. 1033-1038, ISSN 0022-3042

Montag, C.; Markett, S.; Basten, U.; Stelzel, C.; Fiebach, C.; Canli, T. & Reuter, M. Epistasis of the DRD2/ANKK1 Taq Ia and the BDNF Val66Met polymorphism impacts novelty seeking and harm avoidance. *Neuropsychopharmacology*, Vol.35, No.9, (August 2010), pp. 1860-1867. ISSN 0893-199X

Namkoong, K.; Cheon, K. A.; Kim, J. W.; Jun, J. Y.; Lee, J. L. (2008). Association study of dopamine D2, D4 receptor gene, GABAA receptor β subunit gene, serotonin transporter gene polymorphism with children of alcoholics in Korea: A preliminary study. *Alcohol*, Vol.42, No.2, (March 2008), pp. 77−81, ISSN 1535-7414

Neiswanger, K.; Kaplan, B.B. & Hill, S.Y. (1995). What can the DRD2/alcoholism story teach us about association studies in psychiatric genetics? *Am J Med Genet*, Vol.60, No.4, (August 1995), pp. 272-275, ISSN 0148-7299

Neville, M.J.; Johnstone, E.C. & Walton, R.T. (2004). Identification and characterization of ANKK1: a novel kinase gene closely linked to DRD2 on chromosome band 11q23.1. *Hum Mutat*, Vol.23, No.6, (June 2004), pp. 540-545, ISSN 1059-7794

Noble, E.P. (2003). D2 dopamine receptor gene in psychiatric and neurologic disorders and its phenotypes. *Am J Med Genet B Neuropsychiatr Genet*, Vol.116B, No.1, (January 2003), pp. 103-125, ISSN 1552-4841

Noble, E. P.; Zhang, X.; Ritchie, T.; Lawford, B. R.; Grosser, S. C.; Young, R.M.; Sparkes, R. S. (1998). D2 dopamine receptor and GABA (A) receptor β3 subunit genes and alcoholism. *Psychiatry Research*, Vol.81, No.2, (November 1998), pp. 133−147, ISSN 0165-1781

Noble, E.P.; Blum, K.; Khalsa, M.E.; Ritchie, T.; Montgomery, A.; Wood, R.C.; Fitch, R.J. & Ozkaragoz, T. (1993). Allelic association of the D2 dopamine receptor gene with cocaine dependence. *Drug Alcohol Depend*, Vol.33, No.3, (October 1993), pp. 271-285, ISSN 0376-8716

Noble, E.P.; Blum, K.; Ritchie, T.; Montgomery, A. & Sheridan, P.J. (1991). Allelic association of the D2 dopamine receptor gene with receptor-binding characteristics in alcoholism. *Arch Gen Psychiatry*, Vol.48, No.7, (July 1991), pp. 648-654, ISSN 0003-990X

Oak, J.N.; Oldenhof, J.; Van Tol, H.H. (2000). The dopamine D (4) receptor: one decade of research. *Eur J Pharmacol*, Vol.405, No.1-3, (September 2004), pp. 303-327, ISSN 0014-2999

Olsen, C.M. (2011). Natural rewards, neuroplasticity, and non-drug addictions. *Neuropharmacology*, (published online ahead of print April 1 2011)

Peciña, S.; Smith, K.S. & Berridge, K.C. (2006). Hedonic hot spots in the brain. *Neuroscientist*, Vol.12, No.6, (December 2009), pp. 500-511, ISSN 1073-8584

Peng, X.Q.; Xi, Z.X.; Li, X.; Spiller, K.; Li, J.; Chun, L.; Wu, K.M.; Froimowitz, M. & Gardner, E.L. (2010). Is slow-onset long-acting monoamine transport blockade to cocaine as methadone is to heroin? Implication for anti-addiction medications. *Neuropsychopharmacology*, Vol.35, No.13, (December 2010), pp. 2564-2578, ISSN 0893-133X

Pinto, E. & Ansseau, M. (2009). Genetic factors of alcohol dependence. *Encephale*, Vol.35, No.5, (October 2009), pp. 461-469, ISSN 0013-7006

Ponce G, Pérez-González R, Aragüés M, Palomo T, Rodríguez-Jiménez R, Jiménez-Arriero MA, Hoenicka J. (2009). The ANKK1 kinase gene and psychiatric disorders. *i.* Jul;16(1):50-9

Rothman, R.B. & Glowa, J.R. (1995). A review of the effects of dopaminergic agents on humans, animals, and drug-seeking behavior, and its implications for medication development. Mol Neurobiol, Vol.11, No.1-3, (August-December 1995), pp. 1–19, ISSN 0893-7648

Saiz, P.A.; Garcia-Portilla, M.P.; Florez, G.; Arango, C.; Corcoran, P.; Morales, B.; Bascaran, M.T.; Alvarez, C.; San Narciso, G.; Carreño, E.; Alvarez, V.; Coto, E.; Bobes, J. (2009). Differential role of serotonergic polymorphisms in alcohol and heroin dependence. *Prog Neuropsychopharmacol Biol Psychiatry*, Vol.33, No.4, (June 2009), pp. 695-700, ISSN 0278-5846

Samochowiec, J.; Kucharska-Mazur, J.; Grzywacz, A.; Jabłoński, M.; Rommelspacher, H.; Samochowiec, A., Sznabowicz, M.; Horodnicki, J.; Sagan, L.; Pełka-Wysiecka J.

(2006). Family-based and case-control study of DRD2, DAT, 5HTT, COMT genes polymorphisms in alcohol dependence. *Neurosci Lett*, Vol.410, No.1, (December 2006), pp. 1-5, ISSN 0304-3940

Schoots, O.; Van Tol, H.H. (2003). The human dopamine D4 receptor repeat sequences modulate expression. *Pharmacogenomics J*, Vol.3, No. 6, (2003), pp. 343-348, ISSN 1470-269X

Serý, O.; Didden, W.; Mikes, V.; Pitelová, R.; Znojil, V.; Zvolský, P. (2006). The association between high-activity COMT allele and alcoholism. *Neuro Endocrinol Lett*, Vol.27, No.1-2, (February-April 2006), pp. 231-235, ISSN 0172-780X

Shih, J.C.; Chen, K. and Ridd, M.J. (1999). Monoamine Oxidase: From Genes to Behavior. *Annu Rev Neurosci*, Vol.22, (1999), pp.197–217, ISSN 0147-006X

Shih, J.C. (1991). Molecular basis of human MAO A and B. *Neuropsychopharmacology*, Vol.4, No.1, (January 1991), pp.1-7, ISSN 0893-133X

Song, J.; Koller, D. L.; Foroud, T.; Carr, K.; Zhao, J.; Rice, J.; Nurnberger, J. I. Jr.; Begleiter, H.; Porjesz, B.; Smith, T. L.; Schuckit, M. A.; Edenberg, H. J. (2003). Association of GABA (A) receptors and alcohol dependence and the effects of genetic imprinting. *American Journal of Medical Genetics Part B, Neuropsychiatric Genetics*, Vol.117B, No.1, (February 2003), pp. 39–45, ISSN 1552-4841

Stice, E.; Spoor, S.; Bohon, C. & Small, D.M. (2008). Relation between obesity and blunted striatal response to food is moderated by TaqIA A1 allele. *Science*, Vol.322, No.5900, (October 2008), pp.449-452, ISSN 0036-8075

Sullivan, J.M.; Risacher, S.L.; Normandin, M.D.; Yoder, K.K.; Froehlich, J.C. & Morris, E.D. (2011). Imaging of alcohol-induced dopamine release in rats: Preliminary findings with [(11) C] raclopride PET. *Synapse*, (published online ahead of print February 9 2011)

Sundaram, S.K.; Huq, A.M.; Wilson, B.J. & Chugani, H.T. (2010). Tourette syndrome is associated with recurrent exonic copy number variants. *Neurology*, Vol.74, No.20, (May 2010), pp. 1583-1590, ISSN 0028-3878

Theile, J. W.; Morikawa, H.; Gonzales, R. A.; Morrisett, R. A. (2008). Ethanol enhances GABAergic transmission onto dopamine neurons in the ventral tegmental area of the rat. *Alcohol: Clinical & Experimental Research*, Vol.32, No.6, (June 2008), pp. 1040–1048, ISSN 0145-6008

Tindell, A.J.; Smith, K.S.; Peciña, S.; Berridge, K.C. & Aldridge, J.W. (2006). Ventral pallidum firing codes hedonic reward: when a bad taste turns good. *J Neurophysiol*, Vol.96, No.5, (November 2006), pp. 2399-2409, ISSN 0022-3077

Vandenbergh, D.J.; Bennett, C.J.; Grant, M.D.; Strasser, A.A.; O'Connor, R.; Stauffer, R.L.; Vogler, G.P.; Kozlowski, L.T. (2002). Smoking status and the human dopamine transporter variable number of tandem repeats (VNTR) polymorphism: failure to replicate and finding that never-smokers may be different. *Nicotine Tob Res*, Vol.4, No.3, (August 2002), pp. 333-340, ISSN 1462-2203

Vandenbergh, D.J. (1998). Molecular cloning of neurotransmitter transporter genes: beyond coding region of cDNA. *Methods Enzymol*, Vol.296, (1998), pp. 498-514, ISSN 0076-6879

Vandenbergh, D.J.; Rodriguez, L.A.; Miller, I.T.; Uhl, G.R.; Lachman, H.M. (1997). High-activity catechol-O-methyltransferase allele is more prevalent in polysubstance abusers. *Am J Med Genet*, Vol.74, No.4, (July 1997), pp. 439-442, ISSN 1552-4825

Vanyukov, M.M.; Maher, B.S.; Devlin, B.; Tarter, R.E.; Kirillova, G.P.; Yu, L.M.; Ferrell, R.E. (2004). Haplotypes of the monoamine oxidase genes and the risk for substance use disorders. *Am J Med Genet B Neuropsychiatr Genet*, Vol.125B, No.1, (February 2004), pp.120-125, ISSN 1552-4841

Volkow, N.D.; Wang, G.J.; Begleiter, H.; Porjesz, B.; Fowler, J.S.; Telang, F.; Wong, C.; Ma, Y.; Logan, J.; Goldstein, R.; Alexoff, D.; Thanos, P.K. (2006). High levels of dopamine D2 receptors in unaffected members of alcoholic families: possible protective factors. *Arch Gen Psychiatry*, Vol.63, No.9, (September 2006), pp. 999-1008, ISSN 0003-990X

Walton, M.E.; Grovesm J.; Jennings, K.A.; Croxson, P.L.; Sharp, T.; Rushworth, M.F. & Bannerman, D.M. (2009). Comparing the role of the anterior cingulate cortex and 6-hydroxydopamine nucleus accumbens lesions on operant effort-based decision making. *Eur J Neurosci*, Vol.29, No.8, (April 2009), pp. 1678-1691, ISSN 0953-816X

Wang, T.; Franke, P.; Neidt, H.; Cichon, S.; Knapp, M.; Lichtermann, D.; Maier, W.; Propping, P.; Nöthen, M.M. (2001). Association study of the low-activity allele of catechol-O-methyltransferase and alcoholism using a family-based approach. *Mol Psychiatry*, Vol.6, No.1, (January 2001), pp.109-111, ISSN 1359-4184

White, F. J. (1996). Synaptic regulation of mesocorticolimbic dopamine neurons. *Annual Review of Neuroscience*, Vol.19, (1996), pp. 405–436, ISSN 0147-006X

Zhu, Q.S.; Shih, J.C. (1997). An extensive repeat structure down-regulates human monoamine oxidase A promoter activity independent of an initiator-like sequence. *J Neurochem*, Vol.69, No.4, (October 1997), pp.1368-1373, ISSN 0022-3042

Ponce G, Pérez-González R, Aragüés M, Palomo T, Rodríguez-Jiménez R, Jiménez-Arriero MA, Hoenicka J. The ANKK1 kinase gene and psychiatric disorders.; Neurotox Res. 2009 Jul;16(1):50-9.

20

Current and Future Biological Treatments in Inflammatory Bowel Disease

Jesus K. Yamamoto-Furusho
Inflammatory Bowel Disease Clinic, Department of Gastroenterology, Instituto Nacional de Ciencias Médicas y Nutrición; Vasco de Quiroga 15, Tlalpan México

1. Introduction

The biologic approach to IBD therapy has developed in recent years as a result of a better understanding of specific immunopathological processes in intestinal inflammation.
Advances in the development of biologic drugs were the result of two major findings, in basic research: 1) The ability to dissect immunopathologies in the intestinal mucosa up to the level of single molecules. The best example of such progress is the generation of sophisticated experimental models of inflammatory bowel disease such as knock-out and transgenic mice in which experimental colitis is exacerbated or ameliorated because of the lack or over expression of a single gene. Treatment strategies to decrease/neutralize or increase the concentration or effect of the protein encoded by that gene can be performed. 2) Advances in biotechnology now enable the insertion of genes into viral vectors so that targeted delivery of cytokines is possible, antisense oligonucleotide can be designed to hybridize with target RNA's thus the expression of specific molecules can be decreased, commercial amounts of growth factors generated and humanized antibodies creating less immunogenicity can be engineered.
There are several categories of treatments that are relevant to IBD such as 1) Anti-Tumoral Necrosis Factor alfa (TNF-α) antibodies; 2) Selective adhesion blockade; 3) Recombinant cytokines; 4) Growth factors; 5) Immunostimulation; 6) Nucleic acid based therapies; 7) Gene therapy; 8) Autologous bone-marrow transplantation; 9) Helminths, 10) Apheresis.

2. Anti-tnf alpha therapies

TNF-α mediates multiple proinflammatory signals that play a central role in the pathogenesis of IBD, including neutrophil recruitment to local sites of inflammation, activation of both coagulation and fibrinolysis, and induction of granuloma formation. Increased numbers of TNF-α producing cells are present in intestinal biopsy specimens from IBD patients, more frequently in Crohn's disease tissues than ulcerative colitis [1].

2.1 INFLIXIMAB

Infliximab is a chimeric (75% human / 25% mouse) anti-TNFα monoclonal antibody; TNFα mediates multiple pro-inflammatory processes central to the pathogenesis of IBD.

Infliximab was demonstrated to be effective in both the induction and maintenance therapy for refractory luminal and fistulizing CD. In a randomized double-blind placebo controlled trial, 108 patients with moderate-to-severe CD which is resistant to conventional therapy, were treated with the single intravenous infusion of either placebo or infliximab at a dose of 5 mg/kg, 10 mg/kg or 20 mg/kg.
The rates of the clinical response at 4 week were 81% for infliximab 5 mg/kg, 50% for infliximab 10 mg/kg and 64% for infliximab 20 mg/kg, all of which were significantly higher than that for the placebo-treated group. The clinical remission rate at 4 week was also significantly higher in the infliximab-treated group than in the placebo-treated group (33% *vs* 4%) [2]. In a randomized, double-blind, placebo-controlled trial for the treatment of fistulizing disease, 94 CD patients with draining abdominal and perianal fistulas refractory to conventional therapy were treated with three intravenous infusions at week 0, 2 and 6 of either a placebo or infliximab at a dose of 5 mg/kg or 10 mg/kg. The response rates were significantly greater in the infliximab 5 mg/kg group (68%) and in the infliximab 10 mg/kg group (56%) than that in the placebo-treated group (26%). The rates of a complete closure of the fistulas were also significantly higher in the infliximab 5 mg/kg and 10 mg/kg group (55% and 38% respectively) compared with the placebo-treated group (13%) [3].
Rutgeerts et al. [4] who described the ACT 1 and 2 trials. These trials enrolled patients with moderate–severe UC refractory to aminosalicylates (ACT 1), corticosteroids, and/or immunosupressives (ACT 1 and 2). A total of 728 patients were randomized to receive a standard induction schedule of infliximab (5 or 10 mg/kg) or placebo at weeks 0, 2, and 6 followed by every 8 week "maintenance" dosing. Patients were followed for 54 weeks in ACT 1 and 30 weeks in ACT 2. Clinical responses after 8 weeks were reported in 69% and 64% of patients receiving infliximab 5 mg/kg in ACT 1 and 2, and in 61% and 69% of patients who received 10 mg/kg, compared to 37% and 29% of patients who received placebo. In both studies, patients who received infliximab were more likely to have a clinical response at week 30 and by week 54 in ACT 1, 45% and 44% of patients who had received 5 or 10 mg/kg infliximab "maintained" their clinical response compared with 20% of patients randomized to placebo.

2.2 ADALIMUMAB

Adalimumab is a subcutaneously administered IgG1 monoclonal antibody that binds with high specificity and affinity to human TNFα and consists of human-derived heavy and light chain variable regions and human IgG1 constant region. Adalimumab is now approved in the US and Europe for the treatment of CD.
The CLASSIC I trial randomized 299 moderate to severe CD patients naïve to anti-TNF therapy to one of three dose combinations administered at week 0 and 2 (160/80 mg, 80/40 mg, or 40/20 mg) or placebo. At week 4, 36% (P = 0.001), 24% (P = 0.06), and 18% (P = 0.36) in the adalimumab groups, respectively, were in clinical remission compared to 12% in the placebo group [5]. Fifty-five patients who were in remission at week 4 of CLASSIC were randomized to receive continued adalimumab 40 mg every other week, weekly or placebo for up to one year as part of the CLASSIC trial in which 74%, 83% and 44% of patients, respectively, maintained remission at week 56 [6]. Similar to the ACCENT study with infliximab, immunomodulator therapy again did not alter these results[7]. Finally, the CHARM trial (n = 854) examined adalimumab induction and maintenance efficacy in patients with moderate to severe active CD. An 80 mg dose at week 0 and 40 mg dose at

week 2 were administered to all patients, with 499 (58%) achieving clinical response and then randomized to placebo, adalimumab 40 mg every other week, or 40 mg weekly through week 56. Significantly higher rates of remission were seen in the adalimumab groups compared to placebo at both week 26 (40% and 47% *vs* 17%, $P < 0.001$) and week 56 (36% and 41% *vs* 12%, $P < 0.001$). The adalimumab groups also had significantly more steroid discontinuation and complete fistula closure. Safety data was comparable to other TNF therapy [8].

2.3 CERTOLIZUMAB

Certolizumab pegol or CDP870 (UCB; Smyrna, GA) is a monoclonal humanized anti-TNFα antibody Fab′ fragment linked chemically to polyethylene glycol (PEG). In contrast to infliximab and adalimumab the antibody fragment does not induce apoptosis [9]. Certolizumab has been evaluated in both induction and maintenance trials for CD [9,10]. In 92 patients with moderate to severe CD randomized to a single intravenous dose of 1.25, 5, 10 or 20 mg/kg of CDP870 or placebo, the primary endpoints of clinical response or remission after four weeks were not different between treatment groups and placebo, but the remission rate at week 2 was 47% in the 10 mg/kg group compared to 16% in the placebo group ($P = 0.041$) [10]. The PRECISE 1 study compared subcutaneous certolizumab (100, 200 or 400 mg) to placebo administered at week 0, 4, and 8 in 292 patients with moderate-severe CD. While all doses of certolizumab produced significant clinical benefit over placebo at week 2, 400 mg had the strongest effect at all time points, most markedly at week 10 (52.8% *vs* 30.1%, $P = 0.006$); however, no statistical significance in clinical response was seen at week 12, the primary endpoint. When re-analyzed according to stratification by C-reactive protein level (> 10 mg/L), the 400 mg group had a significantly better response at week 12 (53.1% *vs* 17.9%, $P = 0.005$) that was attributed to a lower placebo response rate than those patients with a CRP < 10. In the PRECISE 2 trial, patients who responded to a 400 mg induction dose at week 0 and 2 (428/668, 64%) were randomized to receive 400 mg certolizumab or placebo every 4 week for 26 week. Significantly more patients in the certolizumab arm achieved clinical response (62.8% *vs* 36.2%, $P < 0.001$) and remission (47.9% *vs* 28.6%, $P < 0.001$) at week 26 [11]. Safety and tolerability were similar to other anti-TNF agents, although patients treated with certolizumab had lower rates of autoantibody formation.

3. Selective adhesion blockade

Many adhesion molecules play an important role in trafficking leukocytes into the inflamed gut wall and they are up-regulated in both CD and UC. α4-integrins, predominantly expressed on lymphocytes, usually exist in combination with a β subunit and interact with adressins expressed on endothelium. α4β1-integrin binds to vascular cellular adhesion molecule 1 (VCAM-1) and α4β7-integrin binds to mucosal addressing cell adhesion molecule 1 (MAdCAM-1). The interaction between α4β7-integrin and MAdCAM-1 is important in mediating lymphocytes homing to the gut mucosa [12].

Leukocyte function-associated antigen 1 (LFA-1) expressed on leukocytes interacts with intercellular adhesion molecule 1 (ICAM-1), which is constitutively expressed at low levels on vascular endothelial cells and a subset of leukocytes, and they are up-regulated on many cell types in response to pro-inflammatory mediators [13].

3.1 NATALIZUMAB

Natalizumab, a humanized IgG4 anti-α4-integrin monoclonal antibody, inhibits both α4β7-integrin/MAdCAM-1 interaction and α4β1/VCAM-1 binding. It was already approved by Food Drug Administration (FDA) for use in patients with Crohn´s disease in 2007. The mechanism of action consists of natalizumab interrupted lymphocyte trafficking into the intestine [14]. In a large placebo-controlled randomized trial including 248 patients with moderate to severe CD, patients were treated twice at 4 week intervals with 3 or 6 mg/kg of natalizumab or placebo. A significantly higher number of patients achieved remission at week 6 only in the 3 mg/kg natalizumab group compared with the two infusions of placebo group (44% *vs* 27%) [15]. A larger phase 3 trial of ENACT-1 in 905 patients with moderate to severe CD treated with natalizumab and concurrent immunosuppressive therapies, prior anti-TNF-α therapy or elevated CRP levels showed a significant response rate compared with placebo-treated patients [16]. Three hundred and thirty-nine patients with CD who responded to natalizumab were followed by 12 months (ENACT-2), natalizumab demonstrated a significant superiority over the placebo in its ability to sustain both the response and remission at all consecutive time points over a 6 months period and enabled patients to be successfully withdrawn from steroids [17]. In an uncontrolled short term pilot study in 10 patients with active UC, a single 3 mg/kg intravenous infusion of natalizumab showed a short-term benefit [18]. Natalizumab is efficacious in multiple sclerosis (MS) as well [19,20]. Against these effects of natalizumab in IBD and MS, 3 patients receiving repeated treatment with natalizumab developed JC virus related progressive multifocal leukoencephalopathy (PML) [21-23]. PML, which almost invariably occurs in patients with AIDS or leukemia or in organ-transplant recipients, is a fatal opportunistic infection of the central nervous system caused by the reactivation of a clinically latent JC polyomavirus infection. Two patients with MS had been receiving the concomitant administration of interferon β-1a [21,22] and 1 patient with CD had been treated with natalizumab monotherapy [23].

3.2 MLN-02

MLN-02 is a humanized anti-α4β7-integrin blocks specifically the α4β7-integrin/MAdCAM-1 interaction. A randomized placebo-controlled trial in 185 patients with mild to moderately active UC treated with placebo, 0.5 mg/kg MLN-02 or 2.0 mg/kg MLN-02 intravenously on day 1 and 29 demonstrated that on day 57, 2.0 mg/kg MLN-02 showed significantly greater remission rates over the placebo (36.9% *vs* 20.7%) [24].

A randomized placebo-controlled trial in 181 patients with moderately active UC treated by two infusions with placebo, 0.5 mg/kg MLN-02, or 2.0 mg/kg MLN-02 intravenously demonstrated that on day 43 the remission rates were significantly higher in the actively treated groups (0.5 mg/kg: 33%, 2.0 mg/kg: 34%) than in the placebo-treated group (15%) [25]. MLN-02 appears to be a generally well-tolerated and effective therapy especially for active UC, but further trials are necessary to confirm these findings.

3.3 ALICAFORSEN (ISIS 2302)

ISIS 2302 is a 20 base phosphorothioate oligodeoxynucleotide designed to specifically hybridize to the 3′-untranslated region of the human ICAM-1 mRNA. Treatment of ISIS 2302 *in vitro* resulted in a highly specific reduction in ICAM-1 mRNA and, consequently, a marked decrease in ICAM-1 protein expression [26].

A pilot trial in patients with moderate CD (including 15 patients treated with 13 intravenous infusions of 0.5, 1.0 or 2.0 mg/kg ISIS 2302 *vs* 5 patients with placebo over 26 day) demonstrated a higher remission rate in ISIS 2302-treated group compared with the placebo-treated group on day 33 (47% *vs* 20%) [27, 28]. Another larger randomized placebo-controlled trial also failed to show any benefit of ISIS 2302 for active CD [29]. Two hundred and ninety-nine patients with moderately active, steroid-dependent CD received placebo or ISIS 2302 (2 mg/kg intravenously three times a week) for 2 or 4 week in month 1 and 3. There were no differences in the steroid-free remission rates at week 14 between the ISIS 2302-treated groups (2 week: 20.2%, 4 week: 21.2%) and the placebo-treated group (18.8%). This suggested that ISIS 2302 may be effective when given in adequate doses. In another study patients were infused with high dose ISIS 2302 (250 mg to 350 mg) intravenously three times a week for 4 week, showed a 41% remission rate [30]. A randomized placebo-controlled trial in 40 patients with mild to moderately active distal UC treated with 60 mL alicaforsen enema (0.1, 0.5, 2, or 4 mg/mL or placebo) once daily for 28 consecutive days showed a beneficial effect at the highest dose [31]. An open-label, uncontrolled study in 12 patients with chronic unremitting pouchitis treated with 240 mg alicaforsen enema nightly for 6 week demonstrated a significant improvement in the pouchitis disease activity index and an endoscopic mucosal appearance at week 6 [32].

4. Recombinant cytokines

MRA (Anti-IL-6 receptor antibody)

IL-6 is one of the major inflammatory cytokines. IL-6 can transduce signals into cells without IL-6 receptor expression when IL-6 binds to soluble IL-6 receptor. The expression of IL-6 and soluble IL-6 receptor increases in patients with active CD [33, 34]. A pilot randomized double blind placebo-controlled trial of a humanized anti-IL-6 receptor monoclonal antibody that included thirty-six patients were randomized biweekly to receive either a placebo, 8 mg/kg MRA or MRA/placebo alternately for 12 week. The clinical remission rate with biweekly MRA was significantly higher than with placebo (80% *vs* 31%) [35].

4.1 FONTOLIZUMAB (Anti-interferon-γ antibody)

Interferon-γ is a key cytokine that enhances the development of a Th1 immune response. Fontolizumab is a humanized monoclonal antibody directed against interferon-γ. A phase 2 study of fontolizumab at intravenous doses of 4 mg/kg or 10 mg/kg in 133 patients with moderate to severe active CD did not demonstrate efficacy at day 28. However, exploratory analyses based on 91 patients who received a second dose of fontolizumab at day 28 did demonstrate efficacy. This effect was most prominent in patients with elevated baseline concentrations of CRP [36]. An additional phase 2 study of fontolizumab at lower subcutaneous doses of 1.0 mg/kg or 4.0 mg/kg in 196 patients with active CD did not demonstrate efficacy at day 28 [37]. These results indicate that a single dose may not be sufficient to achieve a significant improvement. Further clinical studies of fontolizumab for the induction and maintenance of remission in patients with CD are required.

4.2 ANTI-IL2 Receptor (CD25) Antibodies

Daclizumab: IL-2 is a major T cell growth factor, which is secreted by activated T cells and acts via the high-affinity IL-2 receptor on T cells themselves to promote cell survival and proliferation. The IL-2 receptor α-chain (CD25) is a component of high-affinity IL-2 receptor

and it is expressed on activated T cells. Daclizumab is a humanized monoclonal antibody to CD25, which blocks the binding of IL-2 to the IL-2 receptor. An open label pilot study of daclizumab suggested that it was beneficial for patients with active UC [38]. However, a recent placebo-controlled phase 2 trial of daclizumab at intravenous doses of 1 mg/kg twice with a 4-week interval or 2 mg/kg every 2 week for a total of four doses in 159 patients with active UC failed to show any efficacy [39].
Basiliximab is a chimeric monoclonal antibody against CD25, which blocks the binding of IL-2 to the IL-2 receptor. Two uncontrolled pilot studies suggested that basiliximab in combination with steroids may be effective for steroid resistant UC [40, 41]. A large randomized controlled trial is required to confirm the therapeutic benefit of this antibody.

4.3 VISILIZUMAB

Visilizumab, an anti-CD3 monoclonal antibody is undergoing evaluation in severe UC. In an open-label phase I trial, 79% and 54% of steroid-refractory UC patients treated with 10 mcg/kg per day (n = 24) for two consecutive days experienced response and remission respectively at day 30, and 100% of those treated with 15 mcg/kg per day (n = 8) achieved both clinical response and remission [42]. Sixty-three percent of patients receiving the higher dose remained in remission at one year. Almost two-thirds of patients experienced symptoms of cytokine release syndrome 1-3 hr post-infusion, including nausea, chills, fever, headache and arthralgias [43].

5. Growth factors

Growth factors may restore the protective and reparative foundation of the colon, and therefore represent a possible therapeutic option for UC. Growth factors that have been identified as potentially beneficial in treating UC include transforming growth factor β (TGF-β), epidermal growth factor (EGF), keratinocyte growth factor-1 and 2 (KGF-1 or 2, also known as fibroblast growth factor 7 or 10). Repifermin is a truncated, purified KGF-2 expressed in *Escheria coli*, and induces the proliferation of intestinal and colonic mucosa and reduces intestinal ulcers and inflammation in animal models [44]. Intravenously administered repifermin (1-50 μg/kg) for five consecutive days did not yield different rates of clinical response or remission at week 4 compared to placebo in patients with active UC [44].
EGF is a mitogenic peptide produced by salivary and duodenal Brunner's glands, topical application is beneficial in wound healing and systemic EGF is useful in treating neonatal necrotizing enterocolitis [45]. An 83% remission rate was demonstrated in patients with mild to moderate left-sided UC (n = 24) randomized to daily EGF enemas for 2 week compared to 8% in the placebo group ($P < 0.001$); disease activity, endoscopic and histologic scores remained significantly better in the EGF group through 12 week [45]. It aids mucosal healing by stimulating local prostaglandin synthesis and epithelial cell regeneration *via* up-regulation of EGF and its receptor, neutrophil suppression, and decreased production of inflammatory cytokines stimulated by NSAIDs and/or *H pylori* [46]. A small open-label trial in which twice daily Rebamipide enemas were given to patients with UC proctitis for one month demonstrated significant clinical, endoscopic and histopathologic improvement [47].

6. Immunostimulation

The greatest evidence supporting the use of colony-stimulating factors in intestinal inflammation comes from studies conducted in patients with active Crohn's Disease (CD): sargramostim and filgrastim.

6.1 GM-CSF

Initial findings suggested that patients treated with sargramostim (GM-CSF) (Immunex Corporation, Seattle, WA, USA) in active CD had a high rate of clinical response and remission, with limited side effects [48]. This 8-week, open-label, dose-escalating study, was conduced on 15 patients with Crohn's Disease Activity Index (CDAI) greater than 220 but lower than 475. Among them, 80% achieved clinical response (decrease in CDAI >70 points) and 53% achieved remission (CDAI <150). The response rate was 75%, 85%, and 75% in the 4, 6, and 8 µg/kg per day dose groups. The only patient with fistula had complete clinical closure of a chronic recto-vaginal fistula. Treatment with sargramostim also improved quality of life.

Lastly, the Sargramostim in Crohn's Disease Study Group [49] conducted a multicenter, randomized, placebo-controlled trial, where 124 patients were included. Patients were randomly assigned in a 2:1 ratio to receive sargramostim (6 µg per kilogram of body weight) or placebo subcutaneously daily for 56 days. The primary end point was clinical response and other end points included changes in disease severity, quality of life, and adverse events.

The primary end point was not proven, this was achieved in 54% in the sargramostim group and 44% in the placebo group ($P = 0.28$), but a clinical response defined by a decrease from baseline of at least 100 points in the CDAI score was significantly higher in the sargramostim group than in the placebo group (48% vs 26%, $P = 0.01$), as well as the remission rate (40% vs 19%, $P = 0.01$). The improvement, including remission rates, was also superior in the sargramostim group thirty days after treatment. In patients in whom the validated Crohn's Disease Endoscopic Index of Severity was assessed, the median post-treatment scores were significantly lower in the sargramostim group, but the median decrease between the two groups was not. Draining fistulae was eliminated in 4 of 8 of patients in the treatment group and in 2 of 5 in the placebo group. Only 1 of 78 patients had detectable neutralizing antibodies at day 57, and no association was observed with adverse events. Treatment with GM-CSF may provide effective synergistic or single-agent treatment alternatives to immunosuppression for IBD [50], but evidence that supports its recommendation as treatment remains weak.

6.2 G-CSF

Dejaco *et al* [51] performed an open-label pilot study with filgrastim (Neupogen®, Amgen Inc, Thousand Oaks, CA, USA) in 5 CD patients with severe endoscopic postoperative recurrence, but with clinically inactive CD (CDAI <150). Patients received 300 µg of filgrastim subcutaneously, three times weekly for a total of 12 weeks, for the primary objective of evaluating safety and efficacy in this group of patients. Efficacy was evaluated by ileocolonoscopy, including histopathological examination according to Rutgeerts' rating for postoperative recurrence, which was performed before treatment and within 1 week after the end of treatment. Four patients had stricturing and one had penetrating behavior. Complete mucosal healing occurred in 2 patients after treatment (1 patient after 12 weeks of therapy and in 1 patient 9 months after treatment cessation), and all other patients had no response. In 1 patient closure of perianal fistulas was noted. This study suggested that despite the small number of patients filgrastim seems to be safe, well tolerated, and might provide efficacy in CD.

Korzenik et al [52] conducted a 12 week open-label trial with filgrastim (Neupogen®, Amgen Inc, Thousand Oaks, CA, USA) that offered preliminary evidence that is a safe and potentially effective therapy for the treatment of active CD and fistulous complications. Twenty CD patients with a CDAI >220 and ≤450 were enrolled. Primary end point was a decrease in the CDAI of >70 points and remission was considered to be a CDAI <150 points. All patients received filgrastim daily for 12 weeks at an initial dose of 300 μg subcutaneously. The absolute neutrophil count (ANC) was monitored weekly and was targeted between 25 and 35 × 10^9. The dose was adjusted downward by 100 μg if ANC exceeded this range, and after a subsequent reduction to 100 μg/day, the dose was lowered to 75 μg/day. Five patients (25%) achieved remission during the study, 11 (55%) demonstrated a decrease of at least 70 points, and 3 of 4 (75%) patients with fistulae had a positive response (defined as closure of more than 50% of fistulae). Among responders at week 12, 4 of 11 patients (36%) maintained response for additional 4 weeks after completion of therapy and the others had an increase in disease activity.

7. Nucleic acid based therapies

Nucleic acid based therapies have focused on the use of antisense phosphorothioate oligonucleotide to the p65 subunit of NF-κB and ICAM-1 antisense oligonucleotide (Alicaforsen, ISIS-2302). In a pilot study 11 steroid-refractory or resistant IBD patients were given a single dose of rectal antisense NF-κB p65 oligonucleotide. An improvement in clinical, endoscopic and histologic scores was seen at day 7 in 71% of the treatment group compared with 25% of the placebo group [53].

ISIS-2302 is a 20-base pair complementary nucleotide chain that hybridizes with ICAM-1 mRNA that is thus degraded by RNAse-H and the message and expression of ICAM-1 is therefore decreased. In patients treated with doses between 300-350 mg infused 3 times weekly for 4 weeks, it seemed to have higher benefit in those with active CD [54].

Immunostimulatory DNA sequences, ISS-DNA, also known as CpG DNA, are unmethylated CpG dinucleotides within consensus sequences present in bacterial and viral genomes. ISS-DNA and their synthetic analogues activate innate immunity *via* Toll-like receptor 9. ISS-ODN (Liposomal immunostimulatory DNA sequence) was shown to prevent and ameliorate the severity of colitis in animal models [55] and therefore may be effective also in the treatment of human IBD. Clinical trials to test their efficacy are underway.

8. Gene therapy

Gene therapy strategies using plasmid IL-10 vectors or an adenovirus IL-10 constructs seem to be a potent approach for the treatment of IBD. Barbara *et al* [56] reported that gene transfer was achieved by intraperitoneal injection of non-replicating human adenovirus bearing IL-10 gene, either 24 hr before or 1 hr after intrarectal administration of TNBS (trinitrobenzenesulfonic acid) in rats. IL-10 gene transfer prior to colitis improved colitis macroscopically and histologically.

9. Allogenic bone-marrow transplantation

Allogenic bone-marrow transplants in CD patients were noted to induce prolonged disease remission, providing evidence of the role of bone-marrow T cells in this disease.
The goal of autologous haematopoietic stem-cell transplantation (HSCT) is resetting T cell responses by eliminating all circulating T cells. A phase I study in 12 patients with refractory CD showed that 11 patients entered a sustained remission (CDAI <150). After a median follow-up of 18.5 months, only one patient has developed a recurrence of active CD, which occurred 15 month after HSCT [57].

10. Helminths

Helminthic colonization has been theorized to be protective against the development of IBD based both on epidemiologic and animal model data.
Another strategy for resetting the T-cell repertoire has been proposed based on the helminths. The immune system has evolved with the presence of these helminths, which functions to expand the T regulatory cell population, enhancing IL-10 production and shifting a T_H1 type process more towards T_H2 [58]. An RCT of *Trichiuris suis*, a pig worm, using 2 500 *Trichiuris suis* ova administered orally once every two weeks, in UC has shown a response of 44% of the treatment group *versus* 14% of receiving placebo group [59]. An open label study of 29 patients with active CD identified high rates of response (79.3%) and remission (72.4%).

11. Apheresis

Selective apheresis of leukocytes, including the targeted removal of monocytes, granulocytes, and lymphocytes is a growing area of research in the treatment of UC.
Review of leukocyte apheresis studies shows efficacy in inducing remission across various UC populations in small open trials [60], but the inherent process of apheresis makes controlled studies difficult to conduct. Two larger trials have demonstrated that leukocyte apheresis (n = 76) and granulocyte/monocyte apheresis (Adacolumn®) (n = 69) are equally or more effective than steroids in the induction of remission [61, 62], with fewer adverse events [61] and greater steroid-sparing effects [62]. In the only controlled trial to date, 19 patients with moderate to severe UC treated with five weekly sessions of either leukocyte sham apheresis (followed by every other week for 4 wk) or sham apheresis demonstrated that the leukocyte apheresis group had significantly greater clinical improvement (80%) than the sham group (33%)[63]. Maintenance of remission after apheresis has been equivocal: in one study of 71 patients with active UC treated with leukocyte apheresis, only 27% of those with an initial response (n = 53) maintained remission for more than six months; rapid response to treatment was the only factor correlated with long-term response in multivariate analysis [64]. In another study, however, 26 of 33 patients maintained remission at one year after 11 weekly sessions of granulocyte/monocyte apheresis [65]. Apheresis may be effective in other settings as well, including a small group of patients with toxic megacolon [66], acute pouchitis [67] and a patient with pyoderma gangrenosum [68].

12. Conclusion

Several biological agents are already approved and in evaluation for treatment of IBD patients who had no response to conventional treatment (5-ASA, steroids, immnunomodulators). These antibody-based therapies consisting of monoclonal antibodies directed against several cytokines (anti-TNFα, IL6, IL-2R, Interferon γ) and selective adhesion molecules (Natalizumab, MLN-02, Alicaforsen). In addition to the cytokine treatment as near- to middle-term additions to therapeutic options, therapies directed to receptors involved in T-cell activation such as Abatacept (CTLA4-Ig) targeting the recruitment of inflammatory cells will soon be important for the care of IBD patients unresponsive to other modalities. However, there are new potential therapies directed to enhance the innate immune system (Sargramostin, filgastrim) and miscellaneous such as nucleic acid based therapies (ISS-DNA), allogenic bone-marrow trasplants, helminths, apheresis and gene therapy.

13. References

[1] Breese EJ, Michie CA, Nicholls SW, et al. (1994) *Gastroenterology* 106:1455-1466.

[2] Targan SR, Hanauer SB, van Deventer SJ, Mayer L, Present DH, Braakman T, DeWoody KL, Schaible TF, Rutgeerts PJ. (1997) *N Engl J Med* 337: 1029-1035

[3] Present DH, Rutgeerts P, Targan S, Hanauer SB, Mayer L, van Hogezand RA, Podolsky DK, Sands BE, Braakman T, De-Woody KL, Schaible TF, van Deventer SJ. (1999) *N Engl J Med* 340: 1398-1405

[4] Rutgeerts P, Sandborn WJ, Feagan BG, et al. (2005) *N Engl J Med* 353:2462-2476.

[5] Hanauer SB, Sandborn WJ, Rutgeerts P, Fedorak RN, Lukas M, MacIntosh D, Panaccione R, Wolf D, Pollack P. (2006) *Gastroenterology* 130: 323-333.

[6] Rutgeerts PJ, Mellili LE, Li J, Pollack PF. (2006) *Gastroenterology* 130: A479

[7] Panaccione R, Hanauer SB, Fedorak R, Rutgeerts P, Sandborn WJ, Pollack P. (2006) *Gastroenterology* 130: A479

[8] Colombel JF, Sandborn WJ, Rutgeerts P, Enns R, Hanauer SB, Panaccione R, Schreiber S, Byczkowski D, Li J, Kent JD, Pollack PF. (2007) *Gastroenterology* 132: 52-65.

[9] Schreiber S, Rutgeerts P, Fedorak RN, Khaliq-Kareemi M, Kamm MA, Boivin M, Bernstein CN, Staun M, Thomsen OO, Innes A. (2005) *Gastroenterology* 129: 807-818

[10] Winter TA, Wright J, Ghosh S, Jahnsen J, Innes A, Round P. (2004) *Aliment Pharmacol Ther* 20: 1337-1346

[11] Sandborn WJ, CJ, Panes J, Scholmerich J, McColm JA, Schreiber S. (2006) *Am J Gastroenterol* 101: S454-S455

[12] Farstad IN, Halstensen TS, Kvale D, Fausa O, Brandtzaeg P. (1997) *Am J Pathol* 150: 187-199.

[13] To SS, Newman PM, Hyland VJ, Robinson BG, Schrieber L. (1996) *Arthritis Rheum* 1996; 39: 467-477

[14] Gordon FH, Lai CW, Hamilton MI, Allison MC, Srivastava ED, Fouweather MG, Donoghue S, Greenlees C, Subhani J, Amlot PL, Pounder RE. (2001) *Gastroenterology* 121: 268-274

[15] Ghosh S, Goldin E, Gordon FH, Malchow HA, Rask-Madsen J, Rutgeerts P, Vyhnalek P, Zadorova Z, Palmer T, Donoghue S. Natalizumab for active Crohn's disease. (2003) *N Engl J Med* 348: 24-32

[16] Rutgeerts P, Colombel J, Enns R, Feagan B, Hanauer S, Lawrance I, Panaccione R, Sanders M, Schreiber S, Targan S, Van Deventer S, Sandborn W. (2003) *Gut* 52: A239
[17] Sandborn W, Colombel JF, Enns R, Feagan B, Hanauer S, Lawrance I, Panaccione R, Sanders M, Schreiber S, Targan S, Van Deventer S, Rutgeerts P. (2004) *Gastroenterology* 127: A332
[18] Gordon FH, Hamilton MI, Donoghue S, Greenlees C, Palmer T, Rowley-Jones D, Dhillon AP, Amlot PL, Pounder RE. (2002) *Aliment Pharmacol Ther* 16: 699-705
[19] Miller DH, Khan OA, Sheremata WA, Blumhardt LD, Rice GP, Libonati MA, Willmer-Hulme AJ, Dalton CM, Miszkiel KA, O'Connor PW. (2003) *N Engl J Med* 348: 15-23
[20] Yednock TA, Cannon C, Fritz LC, Sanchez-Madrid F, Steinman L, Karin N. (1992) *Nature* 356: 63-66
[21] Kleinschmidt-DeMasters BK, Tyler KL. *N Engl JMed* 2005; 353: 369-374
[22] Langer-Gould A, Atlas SW, Green AJ, Bollen AW, Pelletier D. *N Engl J Med* 2005; 353: 375-381
[23] Van Assche G, Van Ranst M, Sciot R, Dubois B, Vermeire S, Noman M, Verbeeck J, Geboes K, Robberecht W, Rutgeerts P. (2005) *N Engl J Med* 353: 362-368
[24] Feagan BG, Greenberg G, Wild G, McDonald J, Fedorak R, Pare P, Kishimoto K, Gutierrez-Ramos JG, Krop J. (2003) *Gastroenterology* 124: A25-26
[25] Feagan B, Greenberg G, Wild G, McDonald J, Fedorak R, Pare P, Kishimoto K, Gutierrez-Ramos JG, Krop J, Vandervoort M. (2003) *Gastroenterology* 125: 606
[26] Bennett CF, Condon TP, Grimm S, Chan H, Chiang MY. (1994) *J Immunol* 152: 3530-3540.
[27] Yacyshyn BR, Bowen-Yacyshyn MB, Jewell L, Tami JA, Bennett CF, Kisner DL, Shanahan WR Jr. (1998). *Gastroenterology* 114: 1133-1142
[28] Schreiber S, Nikolaus S, Malchow H, Kruis W, Lochs H, Raedler A, Hahn EG, Krummenerl T, Steinmann G. (2001) *Gastroenterology* 120: 1339-1346
[29] Yacyshyn BR, Chey WY, Goff J, Salzberg B, Baerg R, Buchman AL, Tami J, Yu R, Gibiansky E, Shanahan WR. (2002) *Gut* 51: 30-36
[30] Yacyshyn BR, Barish C, Goff J, Dalke D, Gaspari M, Yu R, Tami J, Dorr FA, Sewell KL. (2002) *Aliment Pharmacol Ther* 16: 1761-1770
[31] van Deventer SJ, Tami JA, Wedel MK. (2004) *Gut* 53: 1646-1651.
[32] Miner P, Wedel M, Bane B, Bradley J. (2004) *Aliment Pharmacol Ther* 19: 281-286
[33] Hosokawa T, Kusugami K, Ina K, Ando T, Shinoda M, Imada A, Ohsuga M, Sakai T, Matsuura T, Ito K, Kaneshiro K. (1999) *J Gastroenterol Hepatol* 1999; 14: 987-996
[34] Ito H, Takazoe M, Fukuda Y, Hibi T, Kusugami K, Andoh A, Matsumoto T, Yamamura T, Azuma J, Nishimoto N, Yoshizaki K, Shimoyama T, Kishimoto T. (2004) *Gastroenterology* 2004; 126: 989-996.
[35] Hommes D, Mikhajlova T, Stoinov S, et al. (2004) *Gastroenterology* 127: A332
[36] Protein Design Labs reports progress on two humanized antibodies at International Organization of Inflammatory Bowel Disease. PDL Press release. March 2004. Available from: URL: http://www.pdl.com
[37] Van Assche G, Dalle I, Noman M, Aerden I, Swijsen C, Asnong K, Maes B, Ceuppens J, Geboes K, Rutgeerts P. (2003) *Am J Gastroenterol* 98: 369-376
[38] Protein Design Labs reports negative results in phase II clinical trial with daclizumab in ulcerative colitis. PDL Press release. May 2004. Available from: URL: http://www.pdl.com
[39] Creed TJ, Norman MR, Probert CS, Harvey RF, Shaw IS, Smithson J, Anderson J, Moorghen M, Gupta J, Shepherd NA, Dayan CM, Hearing SD. (2003) *Aliment Pharmacol Ther* 18: 65-75

[40] Creed T, Probert C, Dayan C, Hearing S. (2004) *Gastroenterology* 126: A75
[41] Creed TJ, Probert CS, Norman MN, Moorghen M, Shepherd NA, Hearing SD, Dayan CM. (2008) *Aliment Pharmacol Ther* 23: 1435-1442
[42] Plevy S, Regueiro M, et al.. (2004) *Gastroenterology* 126: A75
[43] Carpenter PA, Appelbaum FR, Corey L, Deeg HJ, Doney K, Gooley T, Krueger J, Martin P, Pavlovic S, Sanders J, Slattery J, Levitt D, Storb R, Woolfrey A, Anasetti C. (2002) *Blood* 99: 2712-2719
[44] Sandborn WJ, Sands BE, Wolf DC, Valentine JF, Safdi M, Katz S, Isaacs KL, Wruble LD, Katz J, Present DH, Loftus EV Jr, Graeme-Cook F, Odenheimer DJ, Hanauer SB. (2003) *Aliment Pharmacol Ther* 17: 1355-1364.
[45] Sinha A, Nightingale J, West KP, Berlanga-Acosta J, Playford RJ. (2003) *N Engl J Med* 349: 350-357
[46] Arakawa T, Kobayashi K, Yoshikawa T, Tarnawski A. (1998) *Dig Dis Sci* 43: 5S-13S
[47] Makiyama K, Takeshima F, Hamamoto T. (2005) *Dig Dis Sci* 50: 2323-2329
[48] Dieckgraefe BK, Korzenik JR. 2002. *Lancet,* 260:1478-80.
[49] Korzenik JR, Dieckgraefe BK, Valentine JF, et al. 2005. *N Engl J Med,* 352:2193-201.
[50] Dieckgraefe BK, Korzenik JR, Anant S. 2006. *Ann N Y Acad Sci,* 1072:300-6.
[51] Dejaco C, Lichtenberger C, Miehsler W, et al. 2003. *Digestion,* 68:63-70.
[52] Korzenik JR, Dieckgraefe BK. 2005. *Aliment Pharmacol Ther,* 21:391-400.
[53] Loftberg R, Neurath M, Ost A, Petterson S. *Gastroenterology* 122:A60
[54] Barish CF. (2005) 5: 1387-1391.
[55] Rachmilewitz D, Katakura K, Karmeli F, Hayashi T, Reinus C, Rudensky B, Akira S, Takeda K, Lee J, Takabayashi K, Raz E. (2004) *Gastroenterology* 126: 520-528.
[56] Barbara G, Xing Z, Hogaboam CM, Gauldie J, Collins SM. (2000) *Gut* 46: 344-349
[57] Oyama Y, Craig RM, Traynor AE, Quigley K, Statkute L, Halverson A, Brush M, Verda L, Kowalska B, Krosnjar N, Kletzel M, Whitington PF, Burt RK. (2005) *Gastroenterology* 128: 552-563
[58] Summers RW, Elliott DE, Urban JF Jr, Thompson RA, Weinstock JV. (2005) Gastroenterology 128: 825-32.
[59] Summers RW, Elliott DE, Qadir K, Urban JF Jr, Thompson R, Weinstock JV. (2005) *Gut* 54: 87-90.
[60] Katz S. (2005) *J Clin Gastroenterol* 39: 557-569
[61] Sawada K, Muto T, Shimoyama T, Satomi M, Sawada T, Nagawa H, Hiwatashi N, Asakura H, Hibi T. (2003) *Curr Pharm Des* 9: 307-321
[62] Hanai H, Watanabe F, Yamada M, Sato Y, Takeuchi K, Iida T, Tozawa K, Tanaka T, Maruyama Y, Matsushita I, Iwaoka Y, Kikuch K, Saniabadi AR. (2004) *Digestion* 70: 36-44
[63] Sawada K, Kusugami K, Suzuki Y, Bamba T, Munakata A, Hibi T, Shimoyama T. (2005) *Am J Gastroenterol* 100: 1362-1369
[64] Takemoto K, Kato J, Kuriyama M, Nawa T, Kurome M, Okada H, Sakaguchi K, Shiratori Y. (2007) *Dig Liver Dis* 2007; 39: 422-429
[65] Hanai H, Watanabe F, Takeuchi K, Iida T, Yamada M, Iwaoka Y, Saniabadi A, Matsushita I, Sato Y, Tozawa K, Arai H, Furuta T, Sugimoto K, Bjarnason I. (2003) *Clin Gastroenterol Hepatol* 1: 28-35
[66] Sawada K, Egashira A, Ohnishi K, Fukunaga K, Kusaka T, Shimoyama T. (2005) *Dig Dis Sci* 50: 767-773
[67] Sakuraba A, Sato T, Iwakami Y, Takada Y, Inoue N, Takaishi M, Ogata H, Iwao, Hibi T. (2006) *Gastroenterology* 130: A661
[68] Fujimoto E, Fujimoto N, Kuroda K, Tajima S. *Br J Dermatol* 2004; 151: 1090-1092

21

Gene Therapy for Alpha-1-Antitrypsin Deficiency Diseases

Parveen Salahuddin
Interdisciplinary Biotechnology Unit, A.M.U. Aligarh, India

1. Introduction

Alpha-1-antitrypsin (AAT) deficiency was first described in 1963 by Laurell and Eriksson (Laurell & Eriksson, 1963). They reported an absence of the alpha-1-band in electrophoresis. Alpha -1 -antitrypsin deficiency is one of the most common lethal hereditary disorder of Caucasians of European descent. Alpha -1- antitrypsin also known as α-1-proteinase inhibitor is an archetypal member of the serine proteinase inhibitors, "serpins". The function of alpha -1- antitrypsin is to protect the lower respiratory tract of lungs from proteolytic attack by neutrophil elastase (NE) (Carrell et al., 1982; Brantly et al., 1988). The low circulating levels of AAT expose the lungs to uncontrolled proteolytic attack and predispose the Z homozygous to early-onset panlobular emphysema (Brantly et al., 1988) and liver diseases (Sharp et al., 1969; Sveger, 1976; Eriksson et al., 1986). AAT is synthesized primarily by hepatocytes (Koj et al., 1978; Eriksson et al., 1978) and also by other cells such as monocytes, macrophages, breast carcinoma cells and cornea (Boskovic & Twing, 1998; Geboes et al., 1982; Perlmutter et al., 1985; Ray et al., 1977). In addition, there is a local production of AAT within the lungs by alveolar macrophages and epithelial cells. AAT is present in the plasma at concentrations of 190-280 mg/dl. AAT is a single chain glycoprotein of molecular weight 52kDa containing 394 amino acid residues with the active site residue methionine located at amino acid position 358. AAT also contains three oligosaccharide chains linked to Asn 46, Asn83 and Asn247 respectively. AAT is encoded at the PI locus on chromosome 14 (14q24.3-q32.1) (Cox, 1982, 1985; Schroeder et al., 1985). The PI locus is 12.2 kb in length with 4 coding exons (II, III, IV, and V), 3 noncoding exons (IA, IB, IC) and 6 introns; the region coding for the reactive site loop is located in exon V. AAT shows co-dominant pattern of inheritance (Eriksson, 1965). Accumulating evidence shows that AAT may also exhibit anti-inflammatory activities independent of its protease inhibitor function (Dabbagh et al., 2001; Jeannin et al., 1998; Ikari et al., 2001; Weiss et al., 1993; Bucurenci et al., 1992). For example AAT has been shown to stimulate fibroblast proliferation and procollagen synthesis (Dabbagh et al., 2001) and up-regulate human B cell differentiation into IgE-and IgG4-secreting cells (Jeannin et al., 1998). AAT also inhibits neutrophil superoxide production (Bucurenci et al., 1992), induces the release of macrophage derived interleukin-1 receptor antagonist (Churg et al., 2001) and reduces bacterial endotoxin and TNFα lethal effect *in vivo* (Jie et al., 2003; Libert et al., 1996). AAT also increases the expression of cytokine IL-10 (Janciauskiene et al., 2007). A novel finding indicates that AAT protects the insulin secreting β-cells of pancreas from apoptosis (Zhang et al.,2007).

AAT consists of three β sheets (A-C) , nine helices (A-I) and a mobile reactive site loop that presents the peptide sequence as a pseudosubstrate for target proteinase (Elliott et al., 1996a, 1998, 2000; Ryu et al., 1996; Kim et al., 2001). The active site, Met 358-Ser359, acts as a bait for neutrophil elastase (Johnson & Travis, 1978). After docking, the serine proteinase cleaves the P1-P1'(Met 358-Ser359) of AAT (Wilczynska et al., 1995) and the proteinase is then inactivated by mousetrap action that swings it from upper to lower pole of the inhibitor in association with the insertion of reactive site loop as an extra strand (s4A) in β-sheet A (Wilczynska et al., 1997; Stratikos & Gettins, 1997, 1998,1999; Huntington et al., 2000). This process is accompanied by loss of secondary structure in the serine proteinase and also dramatic rearrangements of the active site. Distortion around the active site of proteinase moves the loop containing the catalytic serine 6A° away from the catalytic histidine residue and thereby disrupts the oxyanion hole (Huntington et al., 2000). These effects results in the inhibition of deacylation reaction. However, after a very long period of time the inhibitory complex breaks down and the active proteinase is released from the complex (Plotnick et al., 2002).

AAT is a highly pleomorphic gene with approximately 125 single nucleotide polymorphisms (SNPs) (Wood & Stockley, 2007) in which a proportion of variants show altered AAT levels or function. These polymorphic variants occur due to amino acid substitutions/deletions which results in charge differences. Based on charge differences, these variants have been identified by isoelectric focusing in the pH range of 4.0-5.0. The most anodal variant is termed as "B" and the most cathodal variant as "Z" (Brantly, 1992; Cox, 2001). The normal variants migrate in the middle region in an isoelectric focusing; hence they are termed as "M". Although, approximately 50 normal AAT variants have been described (Boskovic & Twing, 1998) of these only four normal variants namely M1(Val213), M1(Ala213), M2 and M3 are relatively common with an allelic frequencies among Europeans of Northern European descent of greater than 95% (Kueppers & Christopherson , 1992; Dykes et al.,1984). The M1 (Val213) allele is the most common (allelic frequency 44%-49%) followed by M1 (Ala213) (20%-23%), M2 (14-19%) and M3 (10%-11%) (Kueppers & Christopherson, 1992; Dykes et al., 1984; Nukiwa et al., 1987a). The phylogenetic tree of four of these variants shows that M3 variant is an ancestral protein (Salahuddin, 2010). Variants may also be classified based upon their effect on AAT levels and function. These are normal, deficient, null (nil detectable) or dysfunctional. Deficient variants are susceptible to lungs or liver diseases, whilst null alleles show only lungs diseases. Dysfunctional alleles which while present at a detectable level do not function normally such as the F variant. The majority of clinical diseases of AAT occur due to deficiency and null alleles.

Since AAT molecule has a Met358 residue at its active site, therefore it is readily oxidized by cigarette smoke and thereby resulting in recruitment of inflammatory cells to the lungs. Oxidation of Met358 causes in decrease in association rate constant of AAT for NE by more than 1,000-fold (Travis, 1988).Therefore, cigarette smoking in Z homozygous patients renders an already poorly defended lungs completely defenseless. One unanswered question relating to the pathogenesis of the emphysema is variation in the extent of the disease in individuals matched by age, AAT serum levels, AAT phenotype, and smoking history. This possibly occurred due to variations in the genetic expression of the NE gene.

The Z variant is a more common deficiency variant in Northern Europe whereas S variant is more common in South-West Europe. In Z AAT deficiency variant there is a single base substitution (GAG →AAG) in the codon for residue 342. This causes in amino acid substitution of Glu342 by Lys342 (Jeppsson, 1976). In native state the Glu 342 forms salt bridge with Lys 290. This salt bridge maintains stable closure of β-sheet A. Mutation of Glu 342 to Lys342 disrupts the structure of β-sheet A. Thus, the β-sheet A undergoes expansion and easily accepts reactive site loop of neighbouring AAT molecule as β-strand and consequently polymers of Z AAT are formed. These polymers tangle in the endoplasmic reticulum of the liver to form inclusion bodies (Lomas et al., 1992; Skinner et al., 1998). The accumulated polymerized protein is retained in the periportal cells of the liver as diastase-resistant periodicacid/ schiff positive inclusions. The polymerized insoluble protein present in the endoplasmic reticulum of hepatocytes eventually causes neonatal hepatitis, juvenile cirrhosis and hepatocellular carcinoma (Geboes et al., 1982; Perlmutter et al., 1985; Ray et al., 1977). Owing to the polymerization in the ER of hepatocytes, the AAT is not secreted into the blood stream therefore the levels of circulating AAT in plasma decrease to <11 µM or <570 µg/ml and are unable to protect the lungs from proteolytic degradation. Thus, Z AAT homozygous is predisposed to develop early onset panlobular emphysema (Boskovic & Twing, 1998). Only a subset of patients with AAT deficiency experience liver disease. In these patients a cascade of aberrant signals are also triggered within the hepatocyte, most likely due to the result of an unfolded protein response. However, the downstream details remain unclear. The mode of polymerization seen in ZAAT also underlies the Mmalton (52Phe deleted) (Matsunaga et al., 1990) and Siiyama (Ser53Phe) variants of AAT (Seyama et al., 1991, 1995; Lomas et al., 1993).The S variant (Glu264Val) shows a slower rate of polymer formation because the structural changes in β -sheet A are not substantial (Elliott et al., 1996b; Mahadeva et al., 1999) resulting in a milder form of serum deficiency with no clinical consequences. If an individual has the genotype PiSZ, then their clinical phenotype for liver disease (Mahadeva et al., 1999) and lung disease in smokers (Turino et al., 1996) is intermediate between that of PiZ and PiS subjects. There are many null-allelic variants of AAT that are absent in plasma, and are termed as QO rather than Pi. In QOgranite falls genotype there is deletion of a single base pair that leads to the premature stop codon and unstable mRNA (Nukiwa et al., 1987b). Likewise there is deletion of 2 bp in exon IV in QOhong kong causing in a premature stop codon, and unstable mRNA hence a truncated protein (Sifers et al., 1988). Thus, both QO granite falls and QO hong kong show accumulation in the endoplasmic reticulum of the liver resulting in plasma deficiency. Similarly, an amino acid substitution at the active site (Met358Arg), in dysfunctional Pittsburgh AAT results in reduced neutrophil elastase inhibitory activity as well as inhibition of factor IXa, kallikrein and factor XIIf (Scott et al., 1986)

Gene therapy is a therapeutic strategy in which genetic material, in the form of cDNA /RNA is transferred to an individual to correct a hereditary disorder or to treat and/or prevent an acquired disease (Anderson, 1992; Miller,1992; Crystal,1992; Mulligan, 1993). Gene therapy depends upon vectors for carrying normal gene. These vectors integrate with host genome and all cells resulting from cell division of the host cell will contain the copy of the correct gene in place of the defective one. Gene therapy can be classified into three distinct classes: 1) gene addition also known as gene replacement, ii) gene reprogramming and iii) gene repair. Gene addition is currently the most popular technique which is clinically tested. Gene addition is used for curing diseases that occur due to loss-of-function mutations. This technique involves delivery of a corrected copy of the defective gene without removal of the endogenous mutated gene. Advantages of gene addition lie in its simplicity, whereas a disadvantage is lack of regulated gene expression in some cases. For a less complex diseases, gene replacement strategies are most suitable. However, for more complex diseases in which the gene product requires regulated gene expression, gene reprograming is more appropriate. The gene reprogramming approach involves inhibition of the expression of mutated gene by modification of messenger RNA (mRNA). Although, this approach also expresses an additional genetic material within cells, the net result is correction (or reprogramming) of endogenous mutant gene. This is in contrast to the expression of additional intact functional gene in gene addition technique. A disadvantage of this technique is inefficient nature of the reprogramming. The third approach namely, gene repair is a more developed technique than gene addition or reprogramming approaches. This technique in contrast to gene addition involves correction of mutant sequences at the genomic DNA level but is limited owing to its low efficiency. There are various types of viral and non-viral vectors. The examples of some viral vectors are retroviruses, adenoviruses and adeno-associated viruses (AAVs) and examples of non-viral vectors is liposomal vector and other means by which it is transported into the cell are naked DNA injection and gold-particle bombardment.

For the treatment of patients with AAT deficiency with impaired lungs function is weekly infusion of AAT protein derived from human plasma (Heresi & Stoller, 2008). However, this method has several disadvantages like high cost, inconvenient route of administration, risks of blood borne diseases and time-consuming nature of the therapy thus provide an impetus to develop alternative treatment modalities such as gene therapy. Indeed a phase I AAT gene therapy clinical trial has been approved at the University Of Florida College Of Medicine, Gainesville, Florida, USA. The trial involves intramuscular injection of AAT gene using a recombinant adeno-associated virus (rAAV) vector and thus provides stable plasma levels (Song et al., 2002). In view of above, in this chapter I have discussed about viral and non-viral vectors in gene therapy, their advantages and disadvantages and their applications in alpha-1-antitrypsin deficiency diseases.

2. Viral vectors for gene therapy

2.1 Retroviruses

Retroviruses (Retroviridae) are enveloped single stranded RNA viruses that have been widely used in gene transfer technique. The retrovirus is reverse transcribed from single-stranded RNA genome into a double stranded DNA, which can integrate into host chromosomes (Fields & Knipe, 1986). The retrovirus genome contains three open reading frames that encode for group specific antigens (gag) that codes for core and structural proteins of virus, similarly, polymerase (pol) codes for reverse transcriptase, protease and integrase, and envelope (env) codes for retroviral coat proteins. All of the retroviral genomes have packaging signal Ψ and *cis* acting sequences known as long terminal repeat (LTR) present at each ends. These LTR and neighboring sequences act *in cis* during viral gene expression, and packaging, retro-transcription and integration of the genome (Figure 1). The common example of retroviral vector is Moloney Murine Leukaemia Virus (Mo-MLV). This virus has varying cellular tropisms depending upon the receptor binding domain of envelope glycoprotein. Retroviral vectors upon binding to the host cell receptor undergo conformational changes within envelope glycoprotein leading to their fusion with the host cell membrane and thereby release capsid core into the cytoplasm. Once inside the cytoplasm the single stranded RNA genome is reverse transcribed into double stranded DNA proviral genome by an enzyme reverse transcriptase. The proviral genome subsequently forms a preintegration complex with the viral integrase and thereby it is transported to the nuclear membrane. The pre-integration complex enters the nucleus during mitosis as nuclear membrane is disrupted (Roe et al., 1993).

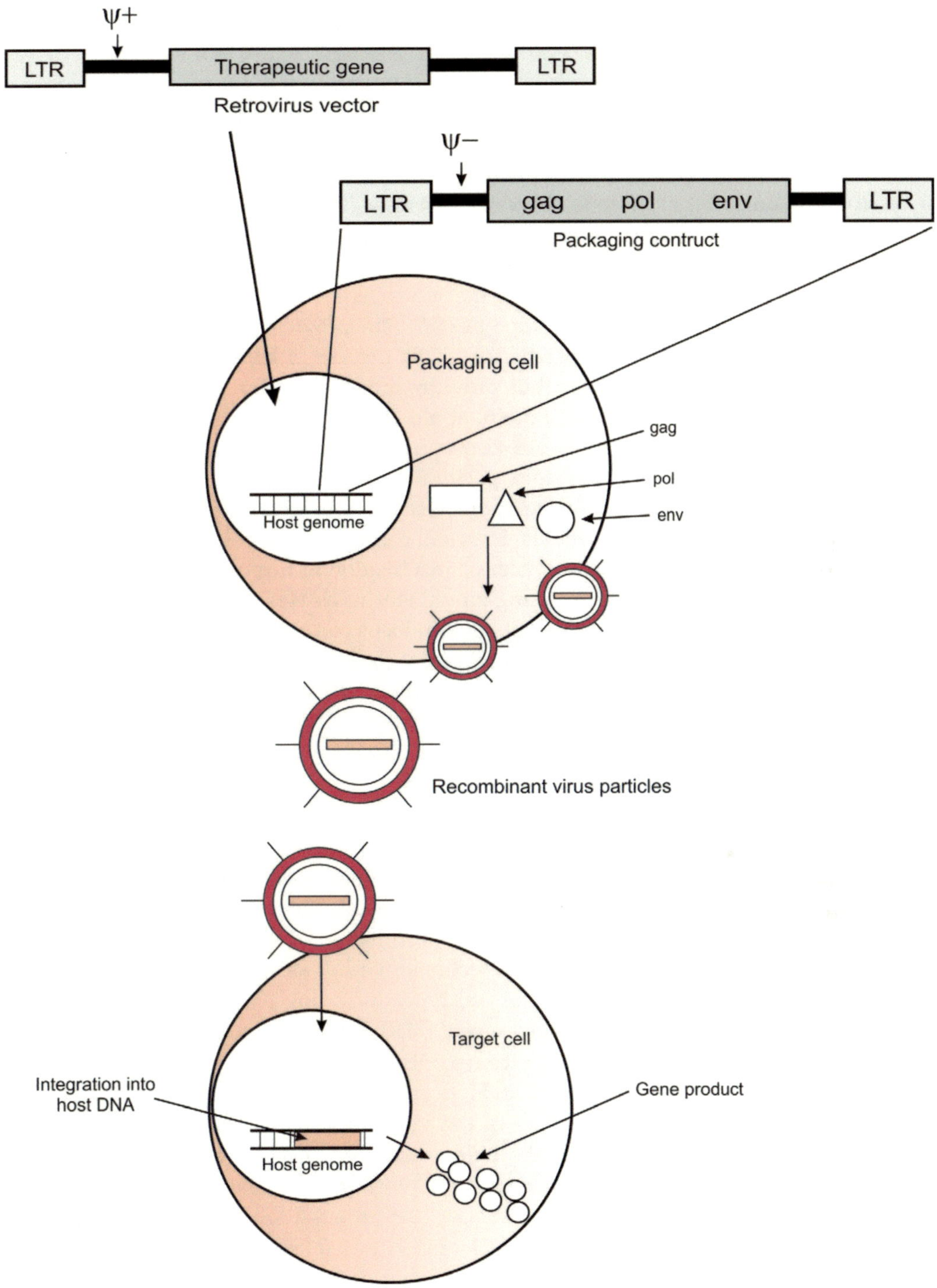

Fig. 1. Structure of retroviral and retroviral gene transfer and production. The *gag, pol* and *env* genes required for viral production are integrated into the packaging cells genome. The vector provides the viral packaging signal, commonly denoted Ψ, and a target gene

After entering the nucleus, the viral integrase randomly integrates the proviral genome into the host chromosomal genome and consequently the viral genes are expressed by host replication machinery. Retroviral vectors are created by removal of the operon like retroviral *gag, pol* and *env* genes. These genes are replaced by therapeutic gene of interest (Figure.1). Up to eight kb of exogenous DNA can be inserted and expressed in place of the viral gene. The LTRs and Ψ sequence are the only viral sequences that are present in vector, and thus this vector is insufficient to express the viral proteins. To express the viral proteins, it is necessary to supply the viral genes *gag, pol* and *env in trans* (Figure. 1). This can be achieved by creating packaging cell lines that express these genes. Removal of *gag, pol* and *env* genes *in vivo* reduce immune responses against the virus. The tropism of retroviruses can be modified by removing the native envelope protein and providing an alternative envelope glycoprotein *in trans* during virus production. This process is known as pseudotyping of virus. The pseudotyping of retrovirus thus provides broader tropism and enhanced stability upon concentration (Kang et al., 2002; Stein, et al., 2005; Wong et al., 2004). One problem encountered in gene therapy using retroviruses is that the integrase enzyme can insert genetic material of the virus at random position in the genome of the host. If genetic material is inserted in the middle of gene of the host cell, this gene will be disrupted causing insertional mutagenesis. If the gene is inserted during regulation of cell division, an uncontrolled division may occur like cancer or inactivation of tumour supressor gene. This problem has recently been solved by using zinc finger nucleases (Durai et al., 2005) or by including certain sequences such as the beta-globin locus control region to direct integration to specific chromosomal sites. Other disadvantages include limited insert capacity (8kb), low titer, their inactivation by human complement factor and their inability to transduce non-dividing cell. Their advantages are : ability to transduce dividing cell, inability to express viral proteins that could be immunogenic and their ability to achieve long term transgene expression.

2.2 Adenoviruses

Adenoviruses are medium-sized (90-100nm) non-enveloped icosahederal viruses composed of nucleocapsid and double-stranded linear DNA (Fields & Knipe, 1986). There are over 51 different serotypes in humans, which are responsible for 5-10% of upper respiratory infection in children and several types of infections in adult as well. They efficiently infect and express their genes in wide variety of cell types including dividing and non-dividing cell. The adenovirus has inverted terminal repeat (ITR) (Figure. 2) sequence at its both ends, and the gene transcript can be divided into two distinct phases: early genes (E) expressed before the onset of viral DNA replication and late genes (L) expressed after the onset of viral replication. One of the essential proteins in the viral replication process is the E1A gene product. The E1A is the first gene to be expressed after infection and has a keyrole as transactivator of all other adenoviral genes. Viral infection is mediated through binding of fiber knob protein of the virus to the primary Coxsackie-Adenovirus Receptors (CAR) (Bergelson et al., 1997) present on the cell surfaces. This is followed by interaction between the cell surface integrins alpha v beta 3 and alpha v beta 5 and virion penton base (Wickham et al., 1993). Consequently, the adenovirion is endocytosed through clathrin-coated pit into an endosome. After this the pH of endosome decreases leading to conformational changes in varion capsid proteins which culminate in the release of viral capsid into the cytoplasm.

The viral capsid translocates from cytoplasm to nucleus of cell where viral genome is released and undergoes replication and transcription as an extrachromosomal element (Figure 2). Adenoviruses infects a variety of quiescent and proliferating cells in different species and can mediate normal gene expression. The transgene expression is mostly transient due to host immune responses (Yang et al., 1996; Stein et al., 1998). The adenoviral vectors have been shown to give therapeutic levels of human alpha-1-antitrypsin (Kay et al., 1995).

First generation recombinant adenovirus vectors (rADs) are generally derived from the human adenovirus serotypes 2 and 5 and these vectors are rendered replication-defective through deletion of the E1-region. Large foreign DNA is inserted in place of E1 deleted region of adenoviral genome (Figure.2). These rADs are propagated in cell line expressing E1 segment (Figure 2). For insertion of larger transgenes, first generation rADs may also carry deletions in the E3 region (Bett et al. , 1994). Several such cell lines like HEK 293(Graham et al.,1977) and 911(Falloux et al., 1996) have been developed that are cable to propagating replication defective rADs vector.

Recently, new varieties of rADs vectors have been developed that are less immunogenic than first generation rADs vectors. These vectors lack or are defective in the E2, E3 or E4 regions and can be propagated in trans-complementing cell lines (Englehardt et al., 1994a, b; Yang et al .,1994; Brough et al., 1996).Additionally, there are vectors called gutless vectors that are devoid of all viral genes and contain only ITR and packaging signal of wild type virus. These gutless vectors can carry up to 35kb of foreign DNA (Kochanek et al., 1996; Parks et al., 1996; Schneider et al., 1998). In order to propagate, these gutless vectors need helper virus containing all genes for virus assembly *in trans* (Parks et al., 1996). Gutless adenoviruses have been shown to give rise to sustain transgene expression compared to first generation adenoviruses (Morsy et al., 1998).

2.3 Adeno-associated viruses

Adeno-associated Viruses (AAVs) belong to the family Parvoviridae. AAVs are small single-stranded DNA genome containing inverted terminal repeats (ITRs) at both ends of the DNA strands and contains two open reading frames (ORFs): rep and cap. The rep is composed of four overlapping genes encoding rep proteins required for the AAV life cycle and the cap contains overlapping nucleotide sequences of capsid proteins namely VP1, VP2 and VP3. These capsid proteins interact together to form a capsid of icosahederal symmetry. The ITRs are the only *cis* acting elements required for efficient encapsidation and integration of the viral genome into the genome of the host cells (Samulski et al., 1989). The wild-type AAV is non-pathogenic. AAVs infects broad host range. The AAVs genome integrates into specific locus on human chromosome 19 (Kotin & Berns, 1989). The AAV vectors can transduce both mitototic and post mitototic cells (Summerford & Samulski, 1998; Summerford et al., 1999). The AAV does not integrate into the genome rather it transduces cells and expresses the transgene as an episome. Disadvantages of AAV vector is that it is unable to replicate unless sequences are provided *in trans* by a helper virus such as adenovirus and HSV. Other disadvantage of this vector is limited packaging capacity for transgene (4.7 kb). These adenovirus (Schiedner et al., 1998; Morral, et al., 1998) and rAAV vectors have been shown to achieve stable levels of alpha-1-antitrypsin greater than 800 µg/ml.

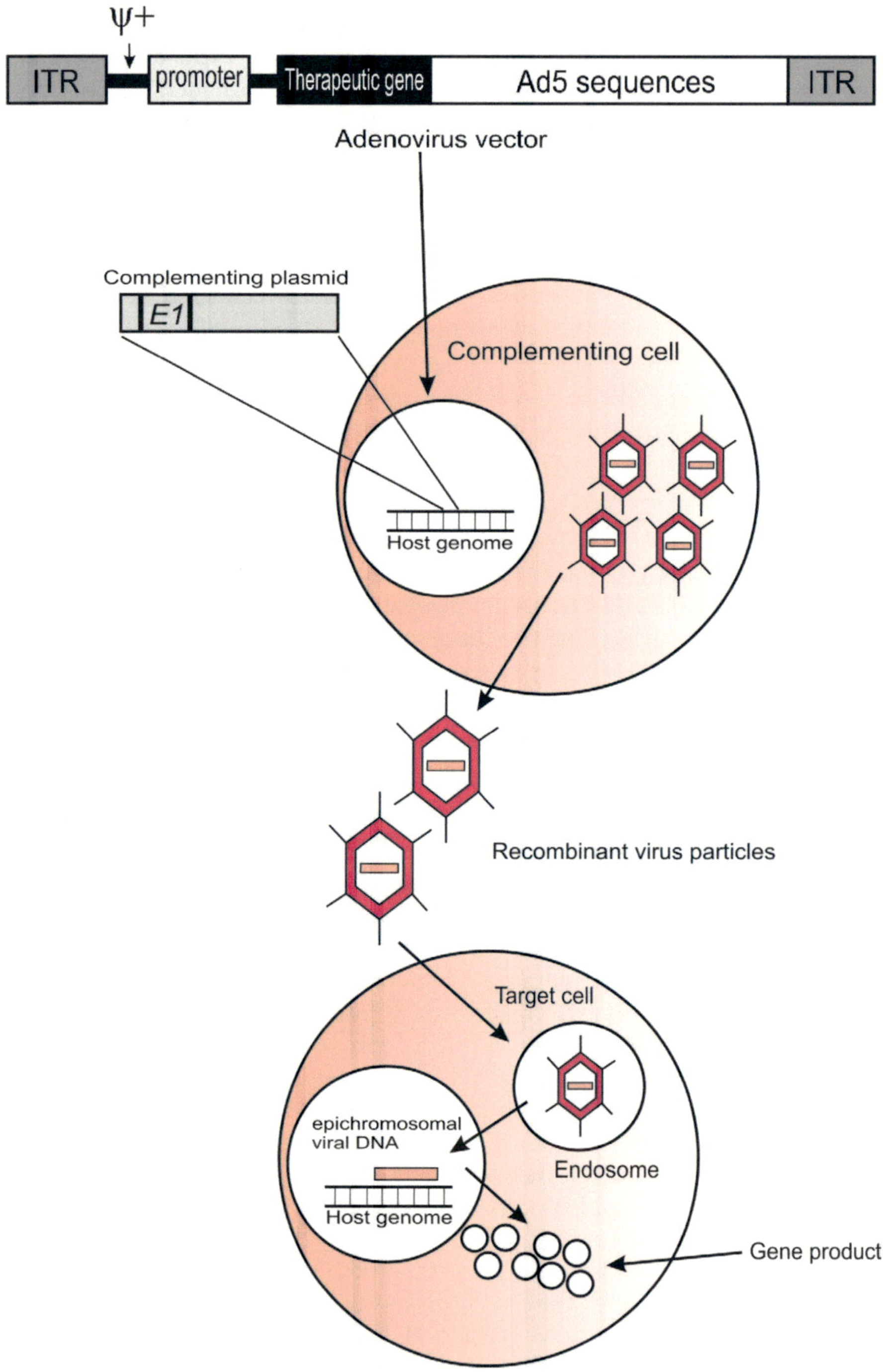

Fig. 2. Structure of adenoviral vector and principle of adenovirus production. Adenovirus vectors are based on serotypes 2 and 5. Therapeutic genes are placed into the deleted E1 region of the viral genome, driven by internal promoters. The function of E1 for production of viral particles is provided by the complementing cell line expressing E1.

3. Non-viral vectors for gene therapy

Non-viral vectors for gene delivery has several advantages over viral vectors. Viruses cause an immune response that can make repeated administrations ineffective. Non-viral vectors on the other hand do not elicit a specific immune response. Non-viral vectors do not randomly integrate DNA into the genomic DNA of the host. Nonviral vectors can also carry more DNA than viral vectors, allowing the delivery of larger genes. In addition, nonviral vectors are easier and less expensive to manufacture. Moreover, vector like plasmids are non-pathogenic and therefore they carry less risk to harm than most viral vectors. Disadvantage of using nonviral vectors for gene therapy are its low efficiency of transgene expression and short duration of expression. Non-viral vectors can be divided into two distinct categories: physical and chemical. Physical methods involve forcing the plasmid into cells through electroporation, sonoporation, or particle bombardment. Chemical methods employ lipids, polymers, or proteins that will complex with DNA, condensing it into particles and directing it to the cells. Many types of DNA deliveries have been proposed. They are i) naked DNA ii) cationic lipids iii) cationic polymers.

3.1 Naked DNA

Naked DNA (in the form of a plasmid) can be transferred by directly injecting into muscle cells (Wolff et al., 1990).Though, it is not very efficient, but can result in prolonged low level expression *in vivo*. The simplicity of this method and sustained expression has led to the development of DNA vaccines. Several approaches have been developed to enhance the efficiency of gene transfer *via* naked DNA including gene gun (Yang et al., 1990) and electroporation (Rols et al., 1998). These physical approaches allow DNA to directly penetrate cell membrane and bypass endosome/lysosome, thus avoiding enzymatic degradation. Further, it has been reported that intramuscular injection of plasmid DNA followed by electroporation results in an impressive level of gene expression (Rizzuto et al., 1999).

3.2 Cationic lipids

Gene transfer can be achieved either by direct intratissue injection of naked plasmid DNA or by intratracheal and intravenous injection which generally requires the use of a delivery vector or vehicle. Various types of synthetic vectors have been developed for gene transfer. Among these, cationic lipid- and polymer-based systems have been the most extensively studied. Cationic lipids are amphiphilic molecules consisting of hydrophilic and hydrophobic regions, i.e., a (charged) cationic (amine) headgroup, attached via a linker (for example glycerol) to a hydrophobic double hydrocarbon chain or a cholesterol derivative. Positively charge head group of cationic lipids and cationic polymers form complexes with negatively charged phosphate backbone of DNA through electrostatic interactions thereby it spontaneously form compact structures called lipoplexes. The cationic lipid-DNA complexes are protected from extracellular or intracellular nucleases. Furthermore, positive charges of lipolexes, tend to electrostatically interact with the negatively charged molecules of the cell membrane. This may facilitate their cellular uptake. Transfection efficiency of cationic lipids depend on the structure of cationic lipids (the geometric shape, the number of charged groups per molecules, the nature of lipid anchor, and linker bondages), the charge ratio used to form DNA–lipid complexes, the size of DNA, conformation of DNA and the properties of the colipid (Wasungu & Hoekstra, 2006). These colipids are mostly cholesterol and dioleoylphosphatidylethanolamine (DOPE). The role of these colipids in cationic liposome-mediated gene transfer depends upon the structure of cationic lipid. Some cationic lipids require DOPE for a normal level of transfection, while other cationic lipids like double fatty chains are capable of forming bilayer or micellar structures that do not depend upon helper lipid for transfection. Most cationic lipids are more or less toxic to cells, and inclusion of colipid DOPE reduce the charge ratio thereby reducing toxicity.

3.3 Cationic polymers

Cationic polymers have also been extensively used for gene transfer. When cationic polymers are mixed with DNA, they form nanosized complexes that are known as polyplexes. These polyplexes are more stable than lipoplexes. Among cationic polymers, PEI is most effective polymer used for transfection. PEI was first used in gene transfer in 1995 (Boussif et al., 1995). These PEI exist as either linear or branched polymer. PEI contains high content of amine groups most of which are nonprotonated at the physiological pH. These nonprotonated amines exert buffering effect, which effectively stop the acidification of the endosomal pH by neutralizing the protons that are pumped by membrane transporter, ATPase (Akinc et al., 2005; Yamashiro et al., 1983). This eventually leads to influx of chloride counter ions within the compartment and thereby osmotic pressure develops that causes the swelling and breakdown of the endosomal membrane. Transfection capacity and toxic nature of PEI depends on its molecular weight (MW), configuration, and the charge ratio of polymer to DNA used. Several studies have demonstrated that high molecular weight PEI (greater than 25,000 Da) is toxic and less efficient in transfection while polymers prepared from medium to low MW (5,000–25,000 Da) are less toxic and more efficient in transfection (Fischer et al., 1999). Besides this, branched PEI shows high toxicity and low transfection efficiency compared to polyplexes prepared from linear chain of PEI (Wightman et al., 2001).

4. Gene therapy applications in alpha-1 -antitrypsin deficiency diseases

The deficiency of AAT in plasma causes reduced protection against neutrophil elastase in lungs, this eventually leads to emphysema. A logical approach to treat this disease is to raise the levels of AAT in plasma to above 11μM (570–800 μg/mL; 57–80 mg/dL). One specific treatment for AAT deficiency available at present is augmentation therapy which involves administration of plasma purified AAT intravenously. According to Hubbard and Crystal (1990), approximately only 2-3% of the infused AAT actually reach the lungs. Therefore, alternative routes of administration, such as inhalation of nebulized AAT powder or aerosolized AAT solution (Hubbard et al., 1989; Hubbard & Crystal, 1990; Sandhaus, 2004; Taylor & Gumbleton, 2004), provided the protection against lungs diseases. However, for treating lungs and liver diseases alternative therapy namely gene therapy provides long term solution (Flotte, 2002; Stecenko & Brigham, 2003; Sandhaus, 2004). Several vectors containing cDNA of AAT have been constructed for treating AAT deficiency diseases. These vectors are retroviral (Kay et al., 1992), adenoviral (Jaffe et al., 1992; Rosenfeld et al., 1991; Morral et al., 1998; Schiedner et al., 1998; Kay et al., 1995) and adeno-associated viral (Lu et al., 2006; Song et al.,1998;2001) Besides this, AAT gene can also be transferred by liposomal vectors (Alino et al., 1994; Canonico et al., 1994), naked DNA injection and gold-particle bombardment (Qiu et al., 1996).

First clinical trial has demonstrated that AAT gene could be transferred in humans (Brigham et al., 2000). Patients with AAT deficiency received a single dose of non-viral cationic liposome and AAT complex into one nostril, while other nostril acts as a control. Protein was detected in nasal lavage fluid, with maximum levels on fifth day, which is approximately one third of the normal levels. This rise in AAT was not seen in fluid from the control nostril. Besides this, levels of the pro-inflammatory cytokine, IL-8, was decreased in the treated nostril. Surprisingly, when purified AAT protein was intravenously administered, the decrease in pro-inflammatory cytokine, IL-8, levels was not observed in normal nasal implying that different routes of administrationmay lead to variations in the production level of IL-8.

The retroviral vector containing cDNA of human AAT with constitutive promoter have also been used as a delivery system. After packaging into an infectious virus, the provirus was integrated into murine fibroblasts and it expressed and secreted human AAT. This AAT was found to be glycosylated, reacted normally with human NE, and had a normal half-life in plasma. When these cells were transplanted into the peritoneal cavity of nude mice, one month latter human AAT was present in plasma and most notably it was present in lung epithelial lining fluid (Garver et al., 1987).Thus, this vector has a potential to cure lungs disease associated with AAT deficiency. The disadvantage of retroviral vector system is that transgene expression is low. Therefore researchers have to resort to better vector systems like adenovirus and adeno-associated virus.

The adenoviral vectors containing human AAT cDNA have been delivered to different organs and cells. For example replication-deficient adenoviral vector containing an adenovirus major late promoter and a recombinant human AAT gene (Ad-AAT) was infected to epithelial cells of the cotton rat respiratory tract both *in vitro* and *in vivo* (Rosenfeld et al., 1991). Results *in vitro* demonstrated that human alpha-1-antitrypsin was synthesized as well as secreted. Whereas *in vivo* intratracheal administration of Ad-AAT to these rats, resulted in the synthesis and secretion of human AAT by lung tissue, and AAT was detected in the epithelial lining fluid for at least 1 week. This mode of administration of Ad-AAT has a potential to cure emphysema. Similarly, when replication defective adenovirus vector containing human AAT cDNA was transferred to human endothelial cells *in vitro* and in the lumen of intact human umbilical veins *ex vivo* (Lemarchand et al., 1992), the infection resulted in the expression of AAT transcripts and synthesis and secretion of AAT both in cell culture (0.3-0.6 μg) and in the vein perfusates (13 μg/ml). The therapeutic level of AAT was achieved in vein perfusate. In another study recombinant adenoviral vectors containing human alpha-1-antitrypsin cDNA under the transcriptional control of the phosphoglycerate kinase (PGK) or RSV-LTR promoters was constructed and transduced in mouse hepatocytes *in vivo* (Kay et al., 1995). The therapeutic serum level of human alpha-1-antitrypsin of up to 700 micrograms/ml was achieved *in vivo*. Thus, this vector has a capacity to cure liver and lungs diseases, but it cannot knock down the expression of misfolded Z AAT in liver. The adenoviruses are pathogenic in nature as well as immunogenic, therefore they have limited applications in treating AAT deficiency diseases.

Recombinant adeno-associated viral vectors have been most successful delivery system so far, as they are capable of achieving therapeutic levels of AAT (Lu et al., 2006; Song et al., 1998) and are less likely to induce an inflammatory response than adenoviral vectors. Studies have been conducted to examine delivery of rAAV-AAT vectors to muscle, lung, or liver (Song et al., 1998, 2001; Virella-Lowell et al., 2005; Liqun Wang et al., 2009). Although, maximum expression could be achieved by each delivery route, however the use of muscle injection has several advantages over other approaches , such as a more favorable profile of anti-capsid effector T-cell responses (Manno et al., 2006; Brantly et al., 2009) and a lower level of dissemination to distant sites (Manno et al., 2003; 2006). A phase I trial of intramuscular injection of a rAAV2-AAT vector has recently been completed but levels of gene expression were found to be very low and generally undetectable. Studies have shown that AAV1 capsid transduction and expression in muscle was substantially more efficient than AAV2 (Xiao et al., 1999; Chao et al., 2001; Gao et al., 2002; Rabinowitz et al., 2002; Hauck & Xiao, 2003). The phase I trial of a rAAV1-AAT vector has been initiated (Brantly et al., 2009.). There are several problem associated with rAAV: firstly scarcity of available AAV2 receptors on the apical surface of airway epithelium, secondly degradation of AAV in the cytoplasm, and thirdly lack of integration of rAAV has limited its efficacy in clinical trials. Several alternative AAV serotypes such as rAAV5, rAAV8, rAAV9, or AAV2 capsid mutants with specifically targeted ligands have been developed. These alternative capsids may bypass the binding and internalization barriers and achieve improved gene expression from a single administration. Among these tested rAAV serotypes, the rAAV8 was found to be more powerful gene therapy vector as it efficiently transduced many different tissues *in vivo* and transduced a high percentage of cells in the lung when delivered intratrachealy (Liqun Wang et al., 2009). It should be noted these approaches whilst potentially protecting the lungs and other tissues, will not influence the liver disease.

The Z AAT variant undergoes polymerization; therefore it accumulates in the ER of hepatocytes. Hence it is associated with liver disease; therefore gene therapy aiming at inhibiting the expression of the Z AAT gene in liver represents a promising therapeutic approach. A number of methods aimed at turning off production of the abnormal Z AAT protein are being considered. These include the use of and siRNA, ribozyme technology, gene repair, PNA and SDF. In a recent report, small-interfering RNAs (siRNAs) was designed to downregulate endogenous Z AAT within hepatocytes. Three different siRNA sequences were cloned into a recombinant adeno-associated virus (rAAV), either singly or as a trifunctional (3X) construct. Each of these vectors demonstrated activity independent of other. These studies showed a decrease in total human Z AAT when rAAV-3X-siRNA packaged into AAV8 capsids was used, thus removing ZAAT accumulation from liver. The rAAV8-3X-siRNA vector may hold promise as a potential therapy for patients with AAT liver disease (Cruz et al., 2007a). Similarly, ribozyme-mediated specific gene replacement also represents a novel mode of gene therapy that aims to treat the AAT deficiency by inhibiting the expression of the mutated gene and at the same time also replacing the defective gene with a normal AAT gene in the liver (Ozaki et al., 1999). Unfortunately, this approach has not been successful todate. A technology called gene repair has been developed which uses chimeric RNA/DNA oligonucleotides to "patch" a single gene mutation. RNA complementary to the area surrounding the point mutation is synthesised with a contiguous DNA oligonucleotide made of the corrected sequence. In model systems, chimeraplast constructs were capable of correcting targeted single site gene mutation (Cole-Strauss et al., 1999). Another mode of gene therapy utilizes second- as well as third-generation oligonucleotides based on a peptide nucleic acid (PNA). These PNA are analogs in which the phosphodiester backbone is replaced by repetitive units of the pseudo-peptide polymer N-(2-aminoethyl) glycine to which the purine and pyrimidine bases are attached by a methyl carbonyl linker (Pellestor & Paulasova, 2004). PNAs hybridize to complementary DNA or RNA in a sequence specific manner. These PNAs are more stable and form hybrid with DNA by displacing one strand of DNA thereby inhibiting gene transcription. Similarly, when these PNAs bind to RNA they act as an antisense (McLean et al., 2009). The potential of PNA in treating AAT deficiency diseases remains to be seen. Furthermore, small DNA fragments (SDFs) have been used for correcting the sequence of variant AAT. This strategy involves small fragment homologous replacement (SFHR) in which the sequences can be directly altered, inserted or deleted. These SDFs can directly convert the mutant sequence to a wild-type genotype, thereby restoring the normal phenotype. Indeed SDFs of normal M and Z AAT sequences were synthesized and transfected into peripheral blood monocytes of PiM subjects and PiZ subjects. The defective gene was corrected in Z AAT monocytes *in vitro* and consequently this treatment was associated with an increase in AAT secretion. This technology has potential to protect both lungs and liver (McLean et al., 2009; McNab et al., 2007). The rAAV2 vectors, such as those used in current clinical trials, appear to be incapable of stably transducing more than 5% of the hepatocyte population. Recently, AAV2 and pseudotyped vectors for serotypes 1, 5, and 8 carrying the human AAT transgene were injected into C57Bl/6 mice. Circulating hAAT level was found to be highest for AAV8 injected animals. Most notably, up to 40% of total liver cells stained positive for the transgene in AAV2/8 subjects. This suggests that different types of AAV use different cellular pathways for infection and AAV8 serotype is a powerful gene therapy vector (Conlon et al., 1982).

The transfection efficacy of several non-viral plasmid vectors containing the full genomic hAAT gene with its natural promoter (pTG7101) and others containing the cDNA of hAAT gene driven by cytomegalovirus immediate-early promoter or the 0.5 kb upstream of hAAT gene sequence has been studied by hydrodynamic tail-vein injection (20 mg/mouse) (Alino et al., 2003).These studies demonstrated that only pTG7101 plasmid results in expression of hAAT in plasma. Further, it was found that hAAT remains long-term stable in plasma, with therapeutic concentrations of hAAT (40.9 mg/ml). In addition, 4 months after transfection, the efficacy of transgenic expression (amount of RNA/DNA) in mouse liver was 50–80% that normally expressed by the mouse gene. Researchers have constructed non-viral plasmid vector which contained AAT gene and eukaryotic replication initiation sequences from Epstein–Barr virus, EBNA1 and from its family of binding sites. Using hydrodynamic injection approach, they found greater than 300 mg/ml of AAT in serum, and increased in serum AAT concentrations occurred for greater than nine months after a single dose of administration of the vector (Stoll et al., 2001). These studies demonstrated that naked plasmid DNA injection is a good technique for curing AAT diseases. Similarly, intravenous injection of linear DNA encoding the AAT gene driven by an RSV promoter into mice is reported to achieve 10–100 fold higher serum AAT concentrations than similar administration of circular DNA with expression persisting for at least 9 months (Chen et al., 2001). Thus, the linear form of the DNA may contribute to more excessive and prolonged *in vivo* expression than the circular DNA.

Studies have shown that lipoplex technology can deliver normal AAT gene to human respiratory epithelium *in vivo* (Brigham et al., 2000). This mode of therapy is safe, but their limitations are similar to those of other nonviral gene therapy. Despite of some progress, the lipid vectors are still inefficient in targeting the genes to distant tissues. Efforts are in way to improve these vectors which include modification of their surface to improve their biocompatibility with biological fluids and tissue specificity, and inclusion of active components that help to overcome the cellular barriers in transfection.

Adult stem cell-based gene therapy holds several unique advantages including avoidance of germline or other undesirable cell transductions. Moreover, stem cells have a capacity for both self-renewal indefinitely and differentiation, making them an ideal vehicle for permanent delivery of normal genes to those affected by loss-of-function genetic mutations. Research using stem cells have also shown some potential for treatment of AAT disease, though these approaches will require further development before clinical use. Since stem cells can differentiate into liver cells that are capable of expressing AAT (Zhou et al., 2007; Moriya et al., 2007; Saito et al., 2006), thus transplanting these cells into deficient patients might facilitate normal production of AAT. This approach however would not prevent accumulation of misfolded AAT in the liver, therefore it would not necessarily affect liver disease. Alternatively, an approach targeting the lung might be used, in this technique human embryonic stem cells are differentiated into alveolar epithelial type II cells (Wang et al., 2007). This alveolar type II cells capable of producing AAT could be transplanted to AAT deficient patients for producing AAT.

5. Future prospects

To further enhance this transduction of viral vectors researchers have developed a novel AAV vector that packages a double-stranded (ds) genome (Richard, 2011). These vectors bypass the rate limiting step of second-strand synthesis resulting in both increased and faster transgene expression. In liver, researchers have been able to demonstrate dsAAV 2 transduction is 90% whereas dsAAV 8 transduction is over 95% using a lower dose. Thus, it is evident that suppression of PiZZ gene expression along with the successful gene addition strategy should eliminate both liver and lungs diseases respectively. It should be noted that although AAV2 and AAV8 transduce the liver with high efficiency the overall tropism is broad and is not restricted to liver cells. Several steps including viral binding, endocytosis, trafficking and uncoating are required for cell specific transduction and research are on way to relate structure to function using a shuffled serotype capsid library (Richard, 2011). Thus, transduction by these alternative serotypes vectors could be restricted to liver cells. Additionally, to down-regulate Z-AAT researchers have also begun to examining innovative approach for long-term expression of therapeutic RNAs using the recombinant adeno-associated virus (rAAV) vector, including spliceosome-mediated RNA trans-splicing (SMaRT) (Cruz et al., 2007b). This technology has a potential to correct Z AAT mutation at the molecular level. Recent reports indicate that chemical chaperones, such as 4-phenylbutyric acid (4-PBA), can assist the proper folding of Z AAT (Burrows et al., 2000). This implies that transduction of rAAV-Hsp70 vectors construct into liver cells of animals and humans could increase the folding of mutant AAT in a native configuration and facilitate degradation of the misfolded protein (Flotte, 2011). Lastly, by analyzing all of the data of preclinical and clinical studies, more efficient vector systems could be designed in future to cure AAT deficiency diseases.

6. Conclusions

These viral and non-viral vectors showed advantages as well as disadvantages in curing AAT deficiency diseases. Among tested rAAV serotypes, the rAAV8 was found to be more powerful gene therapy vector for treating lungs and liver diseases. For liver diseases several approaches have been implemented like siRNA, ribozyme technology, gene repair, PNA and SDF. Their usefulness in clinical trials remain to be seen. The newly developed AAV vector that packages ds DNA looks promising for treating AAT deficiency diseases.

7. Acknowledgements

Author is thankful to DISC, Interdisciplinary Biotechnology Unit and Aligarh Muslim University for facilities.

8. References

Akinc, A.; Thomas, M.; Klibanov, A. M. & Langer, R.(2005). Exploring polyethylenimine-mediated DNA transfection and the proton sponge hypothesis. *The Journal of Gene Medicine,* Vol 7, No.5, pp.657-63, ISSN 1099-498X

Alino, S. F.; Crespo, J.; Bobadilla, M.; Lejarreta, M.; Blaya, C. & Crespo, A.(1994). Expression of human α -1-antitrypsin in mouse after in vivo gene transfer to hepatocytes by small liposomes. *Biochemical and Biophysical Research Communications,* Vol 204, No.3, pp. 1023–1030, ISSN 0006-291X

Alino, S. F.; Crespo, A. & Dasí, F. (2003).Long-term therapeutic levels of human alpha-1 antitrypsin in plasma after hydrodynamic injection of nonviral DNA. *Gene Therapy,* Vol 10, No. 19, pp. 1672-1679, ISSN 0969-7128

Anderson, W. F.(1992). Human gene therapy. *Science,* Vol 256, No.5058, pp. 808-813, ISSN 0036-8075

Bergelson, J. M.; Cunningham , J. A.; Droguett, G.; Kurt-Jones , E. A.; Krithivas, A.; Hong, J. S.; Horwitz, M. S.; Crowell, R. L. & Finberg, R. W. (1997). Isolation of common receptor for Coxsackie B viruses and Adenoviruses 2 and 5. *Science,* Vol 275, No. 5304, pp.1320-1323, ISSN 0036-8075

Bett, A. J.; Haddara, W.; Prevec, L. & Graham, F. L.(1994). An efficient and flexible system for construction of adenovirus vectors with insertions or deletions in early regions 1 and 3.*Proceeding of the National Academy of Science of the United State of America,* Vol 91, No.19, pp. 8802-8806, ISSN 0027-8424

Boskovic, G. & Twining, S. S. (1998). Local control of α 1-proteinase inhibitor levels: regulation of α 1-proteinase inhibitor in the human cornea by growth factors and cytokines. *Biochimica et Biophysica Acta,* Vol 1403, No. 1, pp. 37- 46. ISSN 0005-2736

Boussif, O.; Lezoualch, F.; Zanta, M. A.; Mergny, M. D.; Scherman, D.; Demeneix, B. & Behr, J. P. (1995). A versatile vector for gene and oligonucleotide transfer into cells in culture and in vivo:polyethylenimine. *Proceeding of the National Academy of Science of the United State of America,* Vol 92, No.16, pp.7297-7301, ISSN 0027-8424

Brantly, M.; Nukiwa, T. & Crystal, R.G. (1988). Molecular basis of α1- antitrypsin deficiency. *American Journal of Medicine,* Vol 84, No. 6A, pp.13-31, ISSN 0002-9343

Brantly, M. (1992). Diagnosis and treatment of αl-antitrypsin. *The Endocrinologist,* Vol 2, No. 1, pp. 33-39, ISSN 1051-2144

Brantly, M. L.; Chulay, J. D.; Wang, L.; Mueller, C.; Humphries, M.; Spencer, L.T.; Rouhani, F.; Conlon, T. J.; Calcedo, R.; Betts, M. R.; Spencer, C.; Byrne, B. J.; Wilson, J. M. & Flotte, T.R. (2009). Sustained transgene expression despite T lymphocyte responses in a clinical trial of rAAV1-AAT gene therapy. *Proceeding of the National Academy of Science of the United State of America,* Vol 106, No. 38. pp.16363-16368 ISSN 0027-8424

Brigham, K. L.; Lane, K. B.; Meyrick, B.; Stecenko, A. A.; Strack, S.; Cannon, D. R.; Caudill, M. & Canonico, A. E. (2000).Transfection of nasal mucosa with a normal alpha-1 antitrypsin (AAT) gene in AAT deficient subjects: comparison with protein therapy. *Human Gene Therapy,* Vol 11, No.7, pp. 1023–1032, ISSN 1043-0342

Brough, D. E.; Lizonova, A.; Hsu, C.; Kulesa, V. A. & Kovesdi, I.(1996.).A gene transfer vector-cell line system for complete functional complementation of adenovirus early regions E1 and E4. *The Journal of Virology,* Vol 70, No.9, pp. 6497-6501, ISSN 0022-538X

Bucurenci, N.; Blake, D. R.; Chidwick, K. & Winyard, P. G. (1992).Inhibitionof neutrophil superoxide production by human plasma α1-antitrypsin. *FEBS Letters,* Vol 300, No.1, pp.21-24, ISSN 0014-5793

Burrows, J. A.; Willis, L. K. & Perlmutter, D. H. (2000). Chemical chaperones mediate increased secretion of mutant α1-antitrypsin(α1-AT) Z: a potential pharmacological strategy for prevention of liver injury and emphysema in α1-AT deficiency. *Proceeding of the National Academy of Science of the United State of America,* Vol 97, No. 4, pp. 1796-1801, ISSN 0027-8424

Canonico, A. E.; Conary, J. T.; Meyrick, B.O. & Brigham, K.L.(1994).Aerosol and intravenous transfection of human □-1-antitrypsin gene to lungs of rabbits. *American Journal of Respiratory Cell and Molecular Biology,* Vol 10, No.1, pp. 24–29, ISSN 1044-1549

Carrell, R. W.; Jeppsson, J. O.; Laurell, C. B.; Brennan, S. O.; Owen, M. C.; Vaugham, I. & Boswell, D.R. (1982). Structure and variation of human α 1- antitrypsin. *Nature,* Vol 298, No. 5872, pp.329-334, ISSN 0028-08363

Chao, H.; Monahan, P. E.; Liu, Y.; Samulski, R. J. & Walsh, C. E. (2001). Sustained and complete phenotype correction of hemophilia B mice following intramuscular injection of AAV1 serotype vectors. *Molecular Therapy,* Vol 4, No.3, pp.217-222, ISSN 1525-0016

Chen, Z.Y.; Yant, S. R.; He, C.Y.; Meuse, L.; Shen, S. & Kay, M. A. (2001).Linear DNAs concatemerize in vivo and result in sustained transgene expression in mouse liver. *Molecular Therapy,* Vol 3, No.3, pp. 403-410, ISSN 1525-0016

Churg, A.; Dai, J.; Zay, K.; Karsan, A.; Hendricks, R.; Yee, C.; Martin, R.; Mac-Kenzie, R.; Xie, C.; Zhang, L.; Shapiro, S. & Wright, J. L. (2001). α-1-antitrypsin and a broad spectrum metalloprotease inhibitor, RS113456, have similar acute anti-inflammatory effects. *Laboratory Investigation,* Vol 81, No. 8, pp.1119-1131, ISSN 0023-6837

Cole-Strauss, A.; Gamper, H.; Holloman, W. K.; Muñoz, M.; Cheng, N. & Kmiec, E. B.(1999).Targeted gene repair directed by the chimeric RNA/DNA oligonucleotide in a mammalian cellfree extract. *Nucleic Acids Research,* Vol 27, No.5, pp.1323–1330, ISSN 0305-1048

Conlon, T. J.; Cossette, T.; Erger, K.; Choi ,Y. K.; Clarke, T.; Scott-Jorgensen, M.; Song, S.; Campbell-Thompson, M.; Cox, D. W.; Markovic ,V. D. & Teshima, I. E.(1982). Genes for immunoglobulin heavy chains and for α -1-antitrypsin are localized to specific regions of chromosome 14q. *Nature,* Vol 297, No. 5865, pp. 428–430. ISSN 0028-0836

Cox, D. W. (2001). In *The Metabolic Basis of Inherited Disease* , Scriver, C.; Beaudet, A.; Sly, W & Valle, D. (Eds), 5559-5586, ISBN-10: 0070607265, McGraw-Hill Inc, NewYork

Cruz, P. E.; Mueller, C.; Cossette, T. L.; Golant, A.; Tang, Q.; Beattie, S. G.; Brantly, M.; Campbell-Thompson, M.; Blomenkamp, K. S.; Teckman , J. H. & Flotte, T.R. (2007a). In vivo post-transcriptional gene silencing of alpha-1 antitrypsin by adeno-associated virus vectors expressing siRNA. *Laboratory Investigation* Vol 87, No.9, pp. 893-902, ISSN 0023-6837

Cruz, P. E.; Mueller, C. & Flotte, T.R. (2007 b).The promise of gene therapy for the treatment of alpha-1 antitrypsin deficiency. *Pharmacogenomics,* Vol 8, No. 9, pp.1191-1198, ISSN 1470-269X

Crystal , R. G.(1992). Gene therapy strategies for pulmonary diseases. *American Journal of Medicine,* Vol 92, No. 6A, pp.44S-52S, ISSN 1175-6365

Dabbagh, K.; Laurent, G. J.; Shock, A.; Leoni, P.; Papakrivopoulou, J. & Chambers, R. C. (2001). α-1-antitrypsin stimulates fibroblast proliferation and procollagen production and activates classical MAP kinase signalling pathways. *Journal of Cellular Physiology,* Vol 186, No.1, pp. 73-81, ISSN 0021-9541

Durai, S.; Mani, M.; Kandavelou, K.; Wu, J.; Porteus, M. H. & Chandrasegaran, S. (2005). Zinc finger nucleases: custom-designed molecular scissors for genome engineering of plant and mammalian cells. *Nucleic Acids Research,* Vol 33, No.18, pp. 5978-5990, ISSN 0305-1048

Dykes, D. D.; Miller, S. A. & Polesky, H. F. (1984). Distribution of α1-antitrypsin variants in a US white population. *Human Heredity* ,Vol *34,* No. 5, pp. 308-310, ISSN 0001-5652

Elliott, P. R.; Lomas, D. A.; Carrell, R.W. & Abrahams, J. P.(1996a). Inhibitory conformation of the reactive loop of α 1-antitrypsin. *Nature Structural Biology,* Vol *3,* No. 8, pp.676-681, ISSN 1072-8368

Elliott, P. R.; Stein, P. E.; Bilton, D.; Carrell, R.W. & Lomas, D.A. (1996b). Structural explanation for the deficiency of S α-1-antitrypsin. *Nature Structural Biology,* Vol 3, No.11, pp. 910–911, ISSN 1072-8368

Elliott, P. R.; Abrahams, J. P. & Lomas, D. A. (1998).Wild-type α 1- antitrypsin is in the canonical inhibitory conformation. *Journal of Molecular Biology,* Vol 275, No. 3, pp.419-425, ISSN 0022-2836

Elliott, P. R.; Pei, X.Y.; Dafforn, T. R. & Lomas, D. A. (2000). Topography of a 2.0 A° structure of α1-antitrypsin reveals targets for rational drug design to prevent conformational disease. *Protein Science,* Vol *9,* No. 7, pp.1274-1281, ISSN 0961-8368

Englehardt, J. F.; Ye, X.; Doranz, B. & Wilson, J. M. (1994a). Ablation of E2a in recombinant adenoviruses improves transgene persistence and decreases inflammatory response in mouse liver. *Proceeding of the National Academy of Science of the United State of America,* Vol 91, No. 13, pp. 6196-6200, ISSN 0027-8424

Englehardt, J. F.; Litzky , L. & Wilson, J. M.(1994b).Prolonged transgene expression in cotton rat lung with recombinant adenoviruses defective for E2a. *Human Gene Therapy,* Vol 5 , No. 10, pp.1217-1229, ISSN 1043-0342

Eriksson, S. (1965). Studies in α -1 antitrypsin deficiency. *Acta Medica Scandinavica* (suppl) Vol 432, pp.1–85, ISSN 0001-610116

Eriksson, S.; Alm, R. & Astedt, B. (1978). Organ cultures of human fetal hepatocytes in the study of extra-and intracellular α 1-antitrypsin. *Biochimica et Biophysica Acta,* Vol 542, No. 3, pp. 496-505. ISSN 0005-27369

Eriksson, S.; Carlson, J. & Velez, R. (1986). Risk of cirrhosis and primary liver cancer in α 1-antitrypsin deficiency. *The New England Journal of Medicine,*Vol 314, No. 12, pp.736-739, ISSN 0028-4793

Fallaux, F. J.; Kranenburg, O.; Cramer, S. J.; Houweling, A.; Van Ormondt, H.; Hoeben, R. C. & Van der Eb, A. J. (1996). Characterisation of 911: a new helper cell line for the titration and propagation of early region 1-deleted adenoviral vectors. *Human Gene Therapy* Vol 7, No.2, pp. 215-222, ISSN 1043-0342

Fields, B.N. and Knipe, D.M. (1986). In: *Fundamental Virology.* 1064 pp, ISBN 0-88167-683-7, Raven Press, New York

Fischer, D.; Bieber, T.; Li, Y.; Elsässer, H. P. & Kissel, T. (1999). A novel nonviral vector for DNA delivery based on low molecular weight, branched polyethylenimine: effect of molecular weight on transfection efficiency and cytotoxicity. *Pharmaceutical Research,* Vol 16, No.8, pp.1273–1279, ISSN 0724-8741

Flotte, T.R. (2002). Recombinant adeno-associated virus gene therapy for cystic fibrosis and α1-antitrypsin deficiency. *Chest,* Vol 121, No. 3, Supplement, pp.98S–102S, ISSN 0012-3692

Flotte, T. (March 2011).Alpha-1-antitrypsin Deficiency, In:*Project*, 20.3.2011, Available from http://www.gtc.ufl.edu/research/gtc-rppulm.htm#aa

Gao, G. P.; Alvira, M. R.; Wang, L.; Calcedo, R.; Johnston, J. & Wilson, J. M. (2002).Novel adeno-associated viruses from rhesus monkeys as vectors for human gene therapy. *Proceeding of the National Academy of Science of the United State of America*, Vol 99, No.18, pp.11854 -11859, ISSN 0027-8424

Garver, R. I.; Chytil, A.; Courtney, M. & Crystal. R. G. (1987). Clonal gene therapy: transplanted mouse fibroblast clones express human αl-antitrypsin gene *in vivo. Science*, Vol 237, No. 4816, pp. 762-764, ISSN 0036-8075

Geboes, K.; Ray, M. B.; Rutgeerts, P.; Callea, F.; Desmet, V. J. & Vantrappen, G. (1982). Morphological identification of α-1-antitrypsin in the human small intestine. *Histopathology*, Vol 6, No.1, pp.55-60, ISSN 0309-0167

Graham, F. L.; Smiley, J.; Russell, W. C. & Nairn, R.(1977). Characteristics of a human cell line transformed by DNA from human adenovirus type 5.*Journal of General Virology*, Vol 36, No.1, pp. 59-72, ISSN 0022-1317.

Hauck, B. & Xiao, W.(2003).Characterization of tissue tropism determinants of adeno-associated virus type 1. *The Journal of Virology,*Vol 77, No. 4, pp.2768-2774, ISSN 0022-538X

Heresi, G.A. & Stoller, J. K. (2008). Augmentation therapy in alpha-1 antitrypsin deficiency. *Expert Opinion on Biological Therapy* ,Vol 8, No. 4, pp.515–526, ISSN 1471-2598

Hubbard, R. C.; Brantly, M. I.; Sellers, S. E; Mitchell, M. E. & Crystal, R.G. (1989). Anti-neutrophil-elastase defenses of the lower respiratory tract in alpha 1-antitrypsin deficiency directly augmented with an aerosol of α1-antitrypsin. *Annals of Internal Medicine,* Vol 111, No.3, pp. 206–212, ISSN 0003-4819

Hubbard, R. C. & Crystal, R. G. (1990). Strategies for aerosol therapy of alpha l-antitrypsin deficiency by the aerosol route. *Lung*, Vol 168, Supplement , pp.565-578, ISSN 0341-2040

Huntington, J. A.; Read, R. J. & Carrell, R. W. (2000). Structure of a serpinprotease complex shows inhibition by deformation. *Nature,* Vol 407, No. 6806, pp. 923-926, ISSN 0028-0836

Ikari, Y.; Mulvihill, E. & Schwartz, S. M.(2001). α1-proteinase inhibitor, α1-antichymotrypsin, and α2-macroglobulin are the antiapoptotic factors of vascular smooth muscle cells *Journal of Biological Chemistry*, Vol *276,* No.15, pp. 11798-11803, ISSN 0021-9258

Jaffe, H. A.; Danel, C.; Longenecker, G.; Metzger, M.; Setoguchi ,Y.; Rosenfeld, M. A.; Gant, T.W.; Thorgeirsson, S. S.; Stratford-Perricaudet, L. D.; Perricaudet, M, et al. (1992). Adenovirus-mediated in vivo gene transfer and expression in normal rat liver. *Nature Genetics,* Vol 1, No.5, pp. 372–378, ISSN 1061-4036.

Janciauskiene, S. M.; Nita, I. M. & Stevens, T. (2007). α1-antitrypsin, old dog, new tricks. α1-antitrypsin exerts *in vitro* anti-inflammatory activity in human monocytes by elevating cAMP.*Journal of Biological Chemistry* ,Vol 282, No.12, pp. 8573-8582, ISSN 0021-9258

Jeannin, P.; Lecoanet-Henchoz, S.; Delneste, Y.; Gauchat, J. F. & Bonnefoy, J. Y. (1998). α-1 antitrypsin up-regulates human B cell differentiation selectively into IgE- and IgG4-secreting cells. *European Journal of Immunology,* Vol 28, No. 6, pp.1815-1822, ISSN 0014-2980

Jeppsson, J. O. (1976). Amino acid substitution Glu→Lys in α1-antitrypsin PiZ. *FEBS Letters,* Vol 65, No. 2, pp.195-197, ISSN 0014-5793

Jie, Z.; Cai, Y.; Yang, W.; Jin, M.; Zhu, W. & Zhu, C. (2003).Protective effects of α (1)-antitrypsin on acute lung injury in rabbits induced by endotoxin. *Chinese Medical Journal,* Vol 116, No.11, pp. 1678-1682, ISSN 0366-6999

Johnson, D. & Travis, J. (1978). Structural evidence for methionine at the reactive site of human α-1-proteinase inhibitor. *Journal of Biological Chemistry* , Vol 253, No. 20, pp. 7142-7144, ISSN 0021-9258

Kang, Y.; Stein, C. S.; Heth, J. A .; Sinn, P. L .; Penisten, A. K.; Staber, P. D.; Ratliff, K. L.; Shen, H.; Barker, C. K.; Martins, I.; Sharkey, C. M .; Sanders, D. A.; McCray, P. B. Jr. & Davidson, B.L. (2002). In vivo gene transfer using a nonprimate lentiviral vector pseudotyped with Ross River virus glycoproteins. *Journal of Virology,* Vol 76, No. 18, pp. 9378 - 9388, ISSN 0022-538X

Kay, M. A.; Baley, P.; Rothenberg, S.; Leland, F.; Fleming, L.; Ponder, K. P.; Liu, T.; Finegold, M.; Darlington, G.; Pokorny, W, et al. (1992). Expression of human α- 1-antitrypsin in dogs after autologous transplantation of retroviral transduced hepatocytes. *Proceeding of the National Academy of Science of the United State of America,* Vol 89, No. 1, pp. 89–93, ISSN 0027-8424

Kay, M. A.; Graham, F.; Leland, F. & Woo S. L.(1995).Therapeutic serum concentrations of human alpha-1-antitrypsin after adenoviral-mediated gene transfer into mouse hepatocytes. *Hepatology,* Vol 21, No.3, pp.815-819, ISSN 1665-2681

Kim, S. J.; Woo, J. R.; Seo, E. J.; Yu, M. H. & Ryu, S. E. (2001). A 2.1 A° resolution structure of an uncleaved α1-antitrypsin shows variability of the reactive center and other loops. *Journal of Molecular Biology* , Vol 306, No.1, pp. 109-119, ISSN 0022-2836

Kochanek, S.; Clemens, P. R.; Mitani, K.; Chen, H. H.; Chan, S. & Caskey, C. T. (1996).A new adenoviral vector : replacement of all viral coding sequences with 28 kb of DNA independently expressing both full-length dystrophin and betagalactosidase. *Proceeding of the National Academy of Science of the United State of America,* Vol 93, No.12, pp.5731-5736, ISSN 0027-8424

Koj, A.; Regoeczi, E.; Toews, C. J.; Leveille, R. & Gauldie, J. (1978). Synthesis of antithrombin. III and α-1-antitrypsin by the perfused rat liver. *Biochimica et Biophysica Acta,* Vol 539, No. 4, pp. 496-504. ISSN 0005-2736

Kotin, R. M. & Berns K. I.(1989).Organization of adeno-associated virus DNA in latency infected Detroit 6 cells. *Virology,* Vol 170, No.2, pp. 460-467, ISSN 0042-6822

Kueppers, F. & Christopherson, M. J. (1992). α1-antitrypsin: further genetic heterogeneity revealed by isoelectric focusing. *The American Journal of Human Genetics, Vol* 30, No.4, pp. 359-365, ISSN 0002-9297

Laurell C-B. & Eriksson S. (1963).The electrophoretic alpha-l-globulin pattern of serum in alpha-l-antitrypsin deficiency. *Scandivian Journal of Clinical Laboratory & Investigation,* Vol 15, No. 2, pp. 132-140, ISSN 0036-5513

Lemarchand, P.; Jaffe, H. A.; Danel, C.; Cid, M. C.; Kleinman, H. K.; Stratford-Perricaudet, L. D.; Perricaudet, M.; Pavirani, A.; Lecocq, J. P. & Crystal, R. G.(1992).Adenovirus-mediated transfer of a recombinant human alpha 1-antitrypsin cDNA to human endothelial cells. *Proceeding of the National Academy of Science of the United State of America,* Vol 89, No. 14, pp.6482-6486, ISSN 0027-8424

Libert, C.; Van Molle, W.; Brouckaert, P. & Fiers, W. (1996). α1-antitrypsin inhibits the lethal response to TNF in mice. *The Journal of Immunology,* Vol 157, No.11, pp.5126-5129, ISSN 0022-1767

Liqun Wang, R.; McLaughlin, T.; Cossette, T.; Tang, Q.; Foust, K.; Campbell-Thompson, M.; Martino, A.; Cruz , P.; Loiler , S.; Mueller, C. & Flotte, T. R.(2009). Recombinant AAV serotype and capsid mutant comparison for pulmonary gene transfer of alpha-1-antitrypsin using invasive and noninvasive delivery. *Molecular Therapy,* Vol 17, No.1, pp. 81-87, ISSN 1525-0016

Lomas, D. A.; Evans, D. L.; Finch, J. T. & Carrell, R. W.(1992). The mechanism of Z α1-antitrypsin accumulation in the liver. *Nature,* Vol 357, No. 6379, pp. 605-607, ISSN 0028-0836

Lomas, D. A.; Finch, J. T.; Seyama, K.; Nukiwa, T. & Carrell R.W. (1993). α-1-antitrypsin Siiyama (Ser53] Phe): further evidence for intracellular loop-sheet polymerization. *Journal of Biological Chemistry,* 268, No.21, pp.15333–15335, ISSN 0021-9258

Lu, Y.; Choi , Y. K.; Campbell-Thompson, M.; Li ,C.; Tang, Q.; Crawford, J. M.; Flotte, T. R. & Song, S.(2006). Therapeutic level of functional human α-1 antitrypsin (hAAT) secreted from murine muscle transduced by adeno-associated virus (rAAV1) vector. *The Journal of Gene Medicine,* Vol 8, No.6, pp. 730–735, ISSN 1099-498X

Mahadeva, R.; Chang, W. S.; Dafforn, T. R.; Oakley, D. J.; Foreman, R. C.; Calvin, J.; Wight, D. G. & Lomas, D. A.(1999). Heteropolymerization of S, I, and Z α-1-antitrypsin and liver cirrhosis. *The Journal of Clinical Investigation* , Vol 103, No.7, pp. 999–1006, ISSN 0021-9738

Manno, C. S.; Pierce, G. F.; Arruda , V. R.; Glader, B.; Ragni, M.; Rasko , J. J.; Ozelo, M. C.; Hoots, K.; Blatt , P.; Konkle, B.; Dake, M.; Kaye, R.; Razavi, M.; Zajko, A.; Zehnder, J.; Rustagi, P. K.; Nakai , H.; Chew, A.; Leonard, D.; Wright, J. F.; Lessard, R. R.; Sommer , J. M.; Tigges, M.; Sabatino, D.; Luk, A.; Jiang, H.; Mingozzi, F.; Couto, L.; Ertl, H. C.; High, K.A. & Kay, M.A.(2006).Successful transduction of liver in hemophilia by AAV-Factor IX and limitations imposed by the host immune response. *Nature Medicine,* Vol 12, No.3, pp. 342-347, ISSN 1078-8956

Manno, C. S.; Chew, A. J.; Hutchison, S.; Larson , P. J.; Herzog, R. W.; Arruda, V. R.; Tai, S. J.; Ragni , M. V.; Thompson, A.; Ozelo, M.; Couto, L. B.; Leonard, D. G.; Johnson, F. A.; McClelland, A.; Scallan, C.; Skarsgard, E.; Flake, A. W.; Kay, M. A.; High, K.A. & Glader, B. (2003).AAV-mediated factor IX gene transfer to skeletal muscle in patients with severe hemophilia B. *Blood* , Vol 101, No.8, pp. 2963-2972, ISSN 0006-4971

Matsunaga, E.; Shiokawa, S.; Nakamura, H.; Maruyama, T.; Tsuda, K. & Fukumaki Y.(1990). Molecular analysis of the gene of the α-1-antitrypsindeficiency variant, Mnichinan. *The American Journal of Human Genetics,* Vol 46, No. 3, pp. 602–612, ISSN 0002-9297

McLean, C.; Greene, C. M. & McElvaney, N. G.(2009).Gene targeted therapeutics for liver disease in alpha-1 antitrypsin deficiency. *Biologics,* Vol 3, pp. 63-75, ISSN 1177-5475.

McNab, G. L.; Ahmad, A.; Mistry, D. & Stockley, R. A.(2007). Modification of gene expression and increase in alpha1-antitrypsin secretion after homologous recombination in alpha1-antitrypsin defi cient monocytes. *Human Gene Therapy,* Vol 18, No.11, pp. 1171–1177, ISSN 1043-0342

Miller, A. D. (1992).Human gene therapy comes of age. *Nature,* Vol 357, No. 6378, pp. 455-460, ISSN 0028-0836

Moriya, K.; Yoshikawa, M.; Saito , K.; Ouji,Y.; Nishiofuku, M.; Hayashi, N.; Shizaka, S. & Fukui, H.(2007). Embryonic stem cells develop into hepatocytes after intrasplenic transplantation in CCl4-treated mice. *World Journal of Gastroenterology,* Vol 13, No.6, pp. 866–873, ISSN 1007-9327

Morral, N.; Parks, R. J.; Zhou, H.; Langston, C.; Schiedner, G.; Quinones, J.; Graham, F. L.; Kochanek, S. & Beaudet, A. L. (1998). High doses of a helper-dependent adenoviral vector yield supraphysiological levels of alpha1-antitrypsin with negligible toxicity. *Human Gene Therapy,* Vol 9, No.18, pp. 2709-2716, ISSN 1043-0342

Morsy, M. A.; Gu, M.; Motzel, S.; Zhao, J.; Lin, J.; Su, Q.; Allen, H.; Franlin, L.; Parks, R. J.; Graham, F. L.; Kochanek, S.; Bett, A. J. & Caskey, C. T.(1998).An adenoviral vector deleted for all viral coding sequences results in enhanced safety and extended expression of a leptin transgene. *Proceeding of the National Academy of Science of the United State of America,* Vol 95, No.14, pp. 7866-7877, ISSN 0027-8424

Mulligan, R. C. (1993). The basic science of gene therapy. *Science,* Vol 260, No. 5110, pp.926-932, ISSN 0036-8075

Nukiwa, T.; Brantly, M.; Ogushi, F.; Fells, G.; Satoh, K.; Stier, L.; Courtney, M. & Crystal, R. G. (1987a).Characterization of the M1(Ala213) type of α1-antitrypsin, a newly recognized, common "normal" α1- antitrypsin haplotype. *Biochemistry,* Vol 26, No.17, pp. 5259-5267, ISSN 0006-2960

Nukiwa, T.; Takahashi, H.; Brantly, M.; Courtney, M. & Crystal, R. G. (1987b). α-1-antitrypsin null Granite Falls , a nonexpressing α-1-antitrypsin gene associated with a frameshift to stop mutation in a coding exon. *Journal of Biological Chemistry,* Vol 262, No. 25, pp.11999–12004, ISSN 0021-9258

Ozaki, I.; Zern, M. A.; Liu, S.; Wei, D. L.; Pomerantz, R. J. & Duan, L.(1999). Ribozymemediated specific gene replacement of the alpha1-antitrypsin gene in human hepatoma cells. *Journal of hepatology,* Vol 31, No.1, pp.53–60, ISSN 0169-5185

Parks, R. J.; Chen, L.; Anton, M.; Sankar, U.; Rudnicki , M. A. & Graham, F. L.(1996).A helper-dependent adenovirus vector system: removal of helper virus by Cre-mediated excision of the viral packaging signal. *Proceeding of the National Academy of Science of the United State of America,* Vol 93, No.24, pp. 13565-13570, ISSN 0027-8424

Pellestor, F. & Paulasova, P. (2004).The peptide nucleic acids (PNAs), powerful tools for molecular genetics and cytogenetics. *European Journal of Human Genetics*, Vol 12, No.9, pp.694–700, ISSN 1018-4813

Perlmutter, D. H.; Cole, F. S.; Kilbridge, T. H.; Rossing, T. H. & Colten, H. R. (1985). Expression of the α 1-proteinase inhibitor gene in human monocytes and macrophages. *Proceedings of the National Academy of Sciences of the United States of America*, Vol *82*,No.3, pp. 795-799, ISSN 0027-8424

Plotnick, M. I.; Samakur, M.; Wang, Z. M.; Liu, X.; Rubin, H.; Schechter, N. M. & Selwood, T. (2002).Heterogeneity in serpin protease complexes as demonstrated by differences in the mechanism of complex breakdown. *Biochemistry* Vol 41, No.1, pp.334-342, ISSN 0006-2960

Qiu, P.; Ziegelhoffer, P. & Yang, N. S. (1996).Gene gun delivery of mRNA in situ results in efficient transgene expression and genetic immunization. *Gene Therapy*, Vol 3, No.3, pp. 262-268, ISSN 0969-7128

Rabinowitz, J. E.; Rolling, F.; Li, C.; Conrath, H.; Xiao, W.; Xiao, X. & Samulski, R. J. (2002).Cross-packaging of a single adeno-associated virus (AAV) type 2 vector genome into multiple AAV serotypes enables transduction with broad specificity. *The Journal of Virology*, Vol 76, No. 2, pp.791-801, ISSN 0022-538X

Ray, M. B.; Geboes, K.; Callea, F. & Desmer, V. J. (1977). α -1-antitrypsin immunoreactivity in islet cells of adult human pancreas. *Cell and Tissue Research,* Vol 185, No.1, pp.63-68, ISSN 0302-766X

Richard, J. (March 2011) . AAV Gene Terapy for AAT deficiency,In: *Summary*,20.3.2011, Available from http://www.labome.org/grant/r01/dk/aav/gene/aav-gene-therapy-for-aat-deficiency-7943012.html

Rizzuto, G.; Cappelletti, M.; Maione, D.; Savino, R.; Lazzaro, D.; Costa, P.; Mathiesen, I.; Cortese, R.; Ciliberto, G.; Laufer , R.; La Monica, N. & Fattori , E.(1999). Efficient and regulated erythropoietin production by naked DNA injection and muscle electroporation. *Proceeding of the National Academy of Science of the United State of America*, Vol 96, No. 11, pp. 6417-6422, ISSN 0027-8424

Roe, T. Y.; Reynolds, T. C.; Yu, G. & Brown, P. O.(1993).Integration of murine leukaemia virus DNA depends on mitosis. *The EMBO Journal*, Vol 12, No.5, pp. 2099-2108, ISSN 0261-4189

Rols, M. P.; Delteil, C.; Golzio, M.; Dumond, P.; Cros, S. & Teissie , J. (1998). In vivo electrically mediated protein and gene transfer in murine melanoma. *Nature Biotechnology*, Vol 16, No.2, pp. 168-171, ISSN 1087-0156

Rosenfeld, M. A.; Siegfried, W.; Yoshimura, K.; Yoneyama, K.; Fukayama, M.; Stier, L. E.; Paakko, P. K.; Gilardi, P.; Stratford-Perricaudet , L. D.; Perricaudet, M, et al.(1991).Adenovirus-mediated transfer of a recombinant α-1-antitrypsin gene to the lung epithelium in vivo. *Science*, Vol 252, No.5004, pp. 431–434.

Ryu, S. E.; Choi, H. J.; Kwon, K. S.; Lee, K. N. & Yu, M. H. (1996)The native strains in the hydrophobic core and flexible reactive loop of a serine protease inhibitor : crystal structure of an uncleaved α1- antitrypsin at 2.7 A°. *Structure*, Vol 4, No. 10, pp. 101181-1192, ISSN 0969-2126

Saito, K.; Yoshikawa, M.; Ouji, Y.; Moriya, K.; Nishiofuku, M.; Ueda, S.; Hayashi, N.; Ishizaka, S. & Fukui, H. (2006).Promoted differentiation of cynomolgus monkey ES cells into hepatocyte- like cells by co-culture with mouse fetal liver-derived cells. *World Journal of Gastroenterology*, Vol 12, No.42, pp. 6818–6827, ISSN 1007-9327

Salahuddin, P. (2010). Genetic variants of alpha1-antitrypsin. *Current Protein & Peptide Science,* Vol 11, No.2, pp.101-117, ISSN 1389-2037

Samulski, R. J.; Chang, L. S. & Shenk, T. (1989). Helper-free stocks of recombinant adeno-associated viruses:normal integration does not require viral gene expression. *The Journal of Virology*, Vol 63, No.9, pp.3822-3828, ISSN 0022-538X

Sandhaus, R. A. (2004). α1-Antitrypsin deficiency. 6: New and emerging treatments for α1-antitrypsin deficiency. *Thorax*, Vol 59, No.10, pp.904–909, ISSN 0040-6376

Schiedner, G.; Morral, N.; Parks, R. J.; Wu , Y.; Koopmans, S. C.; Langston, C.; Graham, F. L.; Beaudet, A. L. & Kochanek, S.(1998). Genomic DNA transfer with a high-capacity adenovirus vector results in improved *in vivo* gene expression and decreased toxicity. *Nature Genetics*, Vol 18, No.2, pp. 180-183, ISSN 1061-4036

Schroeder, W. T.; Miller, M. F.; Woo, S. L. & Saunders, G. F.(1985).Chromosomal localization of the human α-1-antitrypsin gene (PI) to 14q31–32. *The American Journal of Human Genetics,* Vol 37, No 5, pp. 868–872, ISSN 0002-9297

Scott, C. F.; Carrell, R. W.; Glaser, C. B.; Kueppers, F.; Lewis , J. H. & Colman, R. W. (1986). α-1-antitrypsin- Pittsburgh: a potent inhibitor of human plasma factor XIa, kallikrein, and factor XIIf. *The Journal of Clinical Investigation,* Vol 77, No.2, pp.631–634, ISSN 0021-9738

Seyama, K.; Nukiwa, T.; Souma, S.; Shimizu, K. & Kira, S. (1995). α-1 -antitrypsin-deficient variant Siiyama (Ser53 [TCC] to Phe53 [TTC]) is prevalent in Japan: status of α-1-antitrypsin deficiency in Japan. *American Journal of Respiratory and Critical Care Medicine,* Vol 152, No. 6, pp. 2119–2126, ISSN 1073-449X

Seyama, K.; Nukiwa, T.; Takabe, K.; Takahashi, H.; Miyake, K. & Kira, S. (1991). Siiyama (serine 53 (TCC) to phenylalanine 53 (TTC)): a new α- 1- antitrypsin-deficient variant with mutation on a predicted conserved residue of the serpin backbone. . *Journal of Biological Chemistry*, Vol 266, No.19, pp. 12627-12632, ISSN 0021-9258

Sharp, H. L.; Bridges, R. A.; Krivit, W. & Freier, E. F. (1969). Cirrhosis associated with α -1-antitrypsin deficiency: a previously unrecognized inherited disorder. *Journal of Laboratory and Clinical Medicine,* Vol 73, No.6, pp. 934-939, ISSN 0022-2143

Sifers, R. N.; Brashears-Macatee, S.; Kidd, V. J.; Muensch, H. & Woo, S.L. (1988). A frameshift mutation results in a truncated α-1-antitrypsin that is retained within the rough endoplasmic reticulum. *Journal of Biological Chemistry,* Vol 263, No.15, pp. 7330–7335, ISSN 0021-9258

Skinner, R.; Chang, W. S. W.; Jin, L.; Pei, X.; Huntington, J. A.; Abrahams, J. P.; Carrell, R. W. & Lomas, D. A. (1998). Implications for function and therapy of a 2.9 A° structure of binary-complexed antithrombin. *Journal of Molecular Biology*, Vol *283*, No.1, pp. 9-14, ISSN 0022-2836

Song, S.; Morgan, M.; Ellis, T.; Poirier, A.; Chesnut, K.; Wang, J.; Brantley, M.; Muzyczka, N.; Byrne, B. J.; Atkinson, M. & Flotte, T. R. (1998). Sustained secretion of human α -1-antitrypsin from murine muscle transduced with adeno-associated virus vectors. *Proceeding of the National Academy of Science of the United State of America*, Vol 95, No.24, pp.14384–14388, ISSN 0027-8424

Song, S.; Embury, J.; Laipis, P. J.; Berns, K. I.; Crawford, J. M. & Flotte T. R.(2001). Stable therapeutic serum levels of human α -1 antitrypsin (AAT) after portal vein injection of recombinant adeno-associated virus (rAAV) vectors. *Gene Therapy*, Vol 8, No.17, pp.1299–1306, ISSN 0969-7128

Song, S.; Scott-Jorgensen, M.; Wang, J.; Poirier, A.; Crawford, J.; Campbell-Thompson, M. & Flotte, T.R.(2002). Intramuscular administration of recombinant adenoassociated virus 2 alpha-1 antitrypsin (rAAV-SERPINA1) vectors in a nonhuman primatemodel: safety and immunologic aspects. *Molecular Therapy,* Vol 6, No. 3, pp. 329–335, ISSN 1525-0016

Stecenko, A. A. & Brigham, K. L. (2003). Gene therapy progress and prospects: alpha-1 antitrypsin. *Gene Therapy,* Vol 10, No.2, pp.95–99, ISSN 0969-7128

Stein, C. S.; Pemberton, J. L.; van Rooijen, N. & Davidson, B. L. (1998). Effects of macrophage depletion and anti-CD40 ligand on transgene expression and redosing with recombinant adenovirus. *Gene Therapy,* Vol 5, No.4, pp. 431-439, ISSN 0969-7128

Stein, C. S.; Martins, I. & Davidson, B. L. (2005). The lymphocytic choriomeningitis virus envelope glycoprotein targets lentiviral gene transfer vector to neural progenitors in the murine brain. *Molecular Therapy,* Vol 11, No.3, pp.382–389, ISSN 1525-0016

Stoll, S. M.; Sclimenti, C. R.; Baba, E. J.; Meuse, L.; Kay, M. A. & Calos, M. P. (2001).Epstein-Barr virus/human vector provides high-level, long-term expression of alpha1-antitrypsin in mice. *Molecular Therapy,* Vol 4, No.2, pp. 122-129, ISSN 1525-0016

Stratikos, E.; Gettins, P. G. W. (1997). Major proteinase movement upon stable serpin-proteinase complex formation. *Proceedings of the National Academy of Sciences of the United States of America*, Vol 94, No.2, pp .453-458, ISSN 0027-8424

Stratikos, E. & Gettins, P. G. W. (1998).Mapping the serpin-proteinase complex using single cysteine variants of α1-proteinase inhibitor Pittsburgh. *Journal of Biological Chemistry,* Vol 273, No. 25, pp.15582-15589, ISSN 0021-9258

Stratikos, E. & Gettins, P.G.W. (1997). Formation of the covalent serpinproteinase complex involves translocation of the proteinase by more than 70 A° and full insertion of the reactive center loop into beta-sheet A. *Proceedings of the National Academy of Sciences of the United States of America*, Vol 96, No.9, pp. 4808-4813, ISSN 0027-8424

Summerford, C. & Samulski, R. J. (1998).Membrane-associated heparin sulphate proteoglycan is a receptor for adeno-associated virus type 2 virions. *The Journal of Virology*, Vol 72, No.2, pp. 1438-1445, ISSN 0022-538X

Summerford, C.; Bartlett, J. S. & Samulski, R. J. (1999).AlphaVbeta5 integrin: a co-receptor for for adeno-associated virus type 2 infection. *Nature Medicine, Vol* 5, No.1, pp. 78-82, ISSN 1078-8956

Sveger, T. (1976). Liver disease in α 1-antitrypsin deficiency detected by screening of 200 000 infants. *The New England Journal of Medicine,* Vol 294, No.24, pp. 1316-1321, ISSN 0028-4793

Taylor, G. & Gumbleton, M. (2004). Aerosols for macromolecular delivery: design challenges and solutions. *American Journal of Drug Delivery,* Vol 2, No.3, pp.143–155, ISSN 1175-9038

Travis, J. (1988). Structure, function, and control of neutrophil proteinases. *American Journal of Medicine,* Vol 84, No. 6A, pp.37-42, ISSN 1175-6365

Turino, G. M.; Barker, A. F.; Brantly, M. L.; Cohen, A. B.; Connelly, R. P.; Crystal, R. G.; Eden, E.; Schluchter, M. D. & Stoller, J. K. (1996). Clinical features of individuals with PI * SZ phenotype of α-1- antitrypsin deficiency. α-1-Antitrypsin Deficiency

Registry Study Group. *American Journal of Respiratory and Critical Care Medicine*, Vol 154, No. 6, pp. 1718–1725, ISSN 1073-449X

Virella-Lowell, I.; Zusman, B.; Foust, K.; Loiler, S.; Conlon, T.; Song, S.; Chesnut, K. A.; Ferkol, T. & Flotte, T. R. (2005). Enhancing rAAV vector expression in the lung. *The Journal of Gene Medicine*, Vol 7, No.7, pp. 842-850, ISSN 1099-498X

Wang, D.; Haviland, D. L.; Burns , A. R.; Zsigmond, E. & Wetsel , R. A. (2007).A pure population of lung alveolar epithelial type II cells derived from human embryonic stem cells. *Proceeding of the National Academy of Science of the United State of America*, Vol 104, No.11, pp.4449–4454, ISSN 0027-8424

Wasungu, L. & Hoekstra, D. (2006). Cationic lipids, lipoplexes and intracellular delivery of genes. *Journal of Control Release*, Vol 116, No.2, pp. 255–264, ISSN 0168-3659.

Weiss, G.; Goossenn, B.; Doppler, W.; Fuchs, D.; Pantopoulos, K.; Werner-Felmayer, G.; Wachter, H. & Hentze, M. W. (1993). Translational regulation via iron-responsive elements by the nitric oxide/NOsynthase pathway. *The EMBO Journal*, Vol 12, No. 9, pp.3651-3657, ISSN 0261-4189

Wickham, T. J.; Mathias, P.; Cheresh, D. A. & Nemerow, G. R.(1993). Integrins alpha v beta 3 and alpha v beta 5 promote adenovirus internalization but not virus attachment. *Cell*, Vol 73, No.2, pp.309-319, ISSN 0092-8674

Wightman, L.; Kircheis, R.; Rössler, V.; Carotta, S.; Ruzicka, R.; Kursa, M. & Wagner, E. (2001). Different behavior of branched and linear polyethylenimine for gene delivery *in vitro* and *in vivo*. *The Journal of Gene Medicine*, Vol 3, No.4, pp. 362–372, ISSN 1099-498X

Wilczynska, M.; Fa, M.; Ohlsson, P. I. & Ny, T. (1995).The inhibition mechanism of serpins: evidence that the mobile reactive center loop is cleaved in the native protease-inhibitor complex. *Journal of Biological Chemistry*, Vol 270, No. 50, pp. 29652-29655, ISSN 0021-9258

Wilczynska, M.; Fa, M.; Karolin, J.; Ohlsson, P. I.; Johansson, L. B. A. & Ny, T. (1997). Structural insights into serpin-protease complexes reveal the inhibitory mechanism of serpins. *Nature Structural Biology*, Vol 4, No.5, pp. 354-357, ISSN 1072-8368

Wolff, J. A.; Malone, R. W.; Williams, P.; Chong, W.; Acsadi, G.; Jani, A. & Felgner, P. L. (1990). Direct gene transfer into mouse muscle *in vivo*. *Science*, Vol 247, No.4949, pp.1465–1468, ISSN 0036-8075

Wong, L. F.; Azzouz, M.; Walmsley, L. E.; Askham, Z.; Wilkes, F. J.; Mitrophanous, K. A.; Kingsman, S. M. & Mazarakis, N. D. (2004). Transduction patterns of pseudotyped lentiviral vectors in the nervous system. *Molecular Therapy*, Vol 9, No.1, pp.101 - 111.

Wood, A. M. & Stockley, R. A. (2007). Alpha one antitrypsin deficiency: from gene to treatment. *Respiration*, Vol 74, No.5, pp. 481-492, ISSN 0025-7931

Xiao, W.; Chirmule, N.; Berta, S. C.; McCullough, B.; Gao, G. & Wilson, J. M. (1999).Gene therapy vectors based on adeno-associated virus type 1. *The Journal of Virology*, Vol 73, No.5, pp. 3994-4003, ISSN 0022-538X

Yamashiro, D. J; Fluss, S. R. & Maxfield, F.R. (1983). Acidification of endocytic vesicles by an ATP-dependent proton pump. *The Journal of Cell Biology*, Vol 97, No.3, pp. 929–934, ISSN 0021-9525

Yang, N. S.; Burkholder, J.; Roberts, B.; Martinell, B. & McCabe, D. (1990). In vivo and in vitro gene transfer to mammalian somatic cells by particle bombardment.

Proceeding of the National Academy of Science of the United State of America, Vol 87, No.24, pp. 9568-9572, ISSN 0027-8424

Yang, Y.; Nunes, F.A.; Berensi, K.; Gonczol, E.; Englehardt, J. F. & Wilson, J. M. (1994). Inactivation of E2a in recombinant adenoviruses improves the prospect for gene therapy in cystic fibrosis. *Nature Genetics*, Vol 7, No.3, pp. 362-369, ISSN 1061-4036

Yang, Y.; Jooss, K. U.; Su, Q.; Ertl, H. C. & Wilson, J. M. (1996). Immune responses to viral antigens versus transgene product in the elimination of recombinant adenovirus-infected hepatocytes in vivo. *Gene Therapy*, Vol 3, No.2, pp.137-144, ISSN 0969-7128

Zhang, B.; Lu, Y.; Campbell-Thompson, M.; Spencer, T., Wasserfall, C., Atkinson, M. & Song, S. (2007). α1-antitrypsin protects β-cells from apoptosis. *Diabetes*, Vol 56, No. 5, pp.1316-1323, ISSN 0012-1797

Zhou, Q. J.; Xiang, L. X.; Shao, J. Z.; Hu, R. Z.; Lu, Y. L.; Yao, H. & Dai, L. C.(2007). In vitro differentiation of hepatic progenitor cells from mouse embryonic stem cells induced by sodium butyrate. *Journal of Cellular Biochemistry*, Vol 100, No.1, pp. 29–42, ISSN 0730-2312

22

Recent Developments in Gene Therapy Research Targeted to Cerebellar Disorders

Hirokazu Hirai and Akira Iizuka
Gunma University Graduate School of Medicine
Japan

1. Introduction

The cerebellum plays an important role in coordinated movement, motor learning and vestibular function. Cerebellar damage results in impaired body balance and disturbance in gait and posture. The cerebellum is impaired by various genetic diseases, such as spinocerebellar ataxia and mucopolysaccharidosis, and these diseases could be good candidates for gene therapy. There are at least two challenges that should be overcome before the clinical application of gene therapy is used to treat cerebellar disorders. The first challenge results from its large size, as the cerebellum is the second largest component of the central nervous system. The cerebellum can be subdivided into three main parts: the cerebrocerebellum, the vestibulocerebellum and the spinocerebellum (see Section 2 for details). Each subdivision in the cerebellum plays a distinct role and, to attain a satisfactory rescue of the cerebellar function by gene therapy, a therapeutic gene should be delivered efficiently and extensively into the large cerebellum.

The second challenge is to deliver a gene into specific target cell populations in the cerebellum. In Parkinson's disease, which is caused by degeneration of nigra-striatal dopaminergic neurons, cell type-specific delivery of a therapeutic gene is a secondary matter, as the supply of sufficient amounts of dopamine, irrespective of neurons or glia, in the striatum is most critical for the functional recovery of the basal ganglia. By contrast, specific cell populations within the cerebellum, such as cerebellar Purkinje cells, Bergman glia or neurons in the deep cerebellar nuclei, are selectively impaired in most cerebellar diseases, such as spinocerebellar ataxia. Thus, affected cell types differ depending on the disease type, and the selective delivery of a therapeutic gene to a subset of affected cell types could be a key advance for rescuing cells that are degenerating from progressive damage, restoring cerebellar function and, ultimately, helping patients to recover from cerebellar ataxia.

To this end, we have developed methods that allow for Purkinje cell-specific and Bergmann glia-specific gene expression in mice by modifying the culture conditions of lentiviral vector-producing human embryonic kidney (HEK) 293FT cells in combination with cell-type-specific promoters in lentiviral vectors. Moreover, a new injection technique for efficient and widespread gene delivery into the cerebellar cortex has been devised, which takes advantage of the anatomical location of the cerebellum. Using the newly developed gene transfer method for the cerebellum, we aimed to restore the abnormal phenotypes of two types of ataxic mice, both of which are affected in Purkinje cells by different pathologies. The results showed that the efficient and widespread delivery of therapeutic genes into Purkinje cells significantly restored ataxia and morphological and functional abnormalities of these cells in mutant mice. In this chapter, we describe our method that efficiently permits the selective gene delivery to cerebellar Purkinje cells or Bergmann glia and the rescue of two examples of ataxic mice. We also describe existing problems that should be resolved for the future clinical application of lentiviral vectors to cerebellar disorders.

2. Cerebellar organization and neural circuits in the cerebellum

The cerebellum can be subdivided into three main parts based on differences in their sources of input. The largest subdivision in humans is the cerebrocerebellum, which occupies most of the lateral hemisphere and is involved in the regulation of highly skilled movements, including speech. The vestibulocerebellum is the phylogenetically oldest part of the cerebellum; it comprises the caudal lobes of the cerebellum, including the flocculus and the nodulus, and is primarily engaged in the regulation of movements underlying posture and equilibrium. The last of the major subdivisions is the spinocerebellum, which occupies the median and paramedian zone of the cerebellar hemispheres. The spinocerebellum is the only part that receives input directly from the spinal cord. The lateral part and central part (vermis) of the spinocerebellum are involved in the movements of distal and proximal muscles, respectively. The vermis also regulates eye movements in response to vestibular inputs.

The cerebellar cortex contains 5 neurons, the granule cell, the Purkinje cell and three inhibitory interneurons (stellate cell, basket cell and Golgi cell) and is divided into three morphologically distinct parts: the granule cell layer, the Purkinje cell layer, and the molecular layer (Fig. 1a and b). The granule cell layer contains numerous granule cells, in which Golgi cells are scattered. The Purkinje cell layer is a monolayer that consists of the soma of Purkinje cells and Bergmann glia; the Purkinje cells extend their well-differentiated dendrites into the molecular layer (Fig. 1c), where stellate cells and basket cells are located. The Bergmann glia also extend their processes into the molecular layer (Fig. 1b).

A major input to the cerebellar cortex are the mossy fibers, axon bundles projecting from neurons in the thalamus, the brain stem and the spinal cord (Fig. 1b). The excitation of granule cells triggered by mossy fibers is transferred through the axons called parallel fiber to Purkinje cells. One Purkinje cell has more than one hundred thousand dendritic spines (Fig. 1d, arrows), on which parallel fiber terminals make excitatory synapses. Parallel fiber - Purkinje cell synapses are tightly wrapped by processes of Bergmann glia, so as to quickly take up the glutamate released from parallel fiber terminals. In this context, the Bergmann glia prevent the prolonged excitation of Purkinje cells and the spillover of glutamate that would activate the adjacent synapses.

Another excitatory input to the cerebellar cortex is the climbing fiber that originates from neurons in the inferior olivary nucleus of the medulla oblongata. The climbing fiber makes excitatory synapses directly on proximal dendrites of Purkinje cells and neurons in the deep cerebellar nuclei. Excitatory activity of granule cells and Purkinje cells is modulated by 3 types of inhibitory interneurons: Golgi cells, stellate cells, and basket cells. The Purkinje cells eventually integrate the information entered into the cerebellar cortex and send an inhibitory signal as the sole source of output from the cerebellar cortex to neurons in the deep cerebellar nuclei.

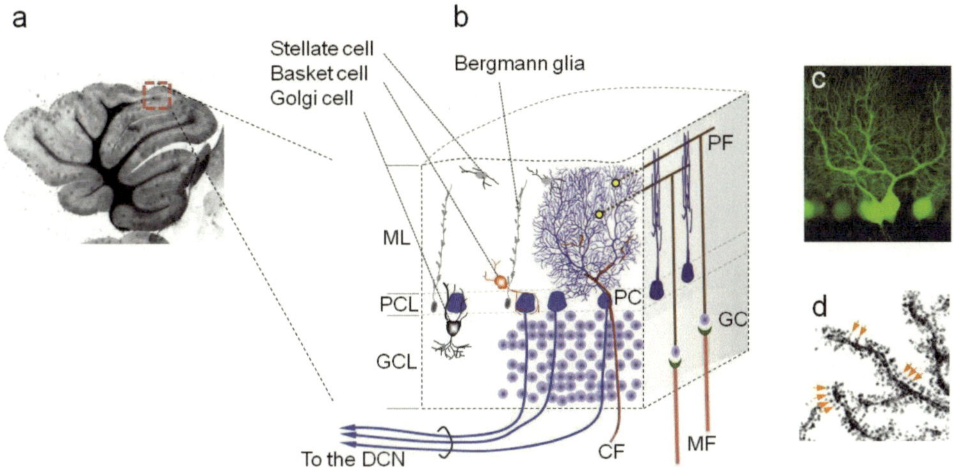

Fig. 1. Projections to and neural circuits in the cerebellar cortex. (a) A sagittal section of the vermis of a mouse cerebellum. (b) A schematic diagram of the cerebellar cortex that enlarges the square region in (a). ML, molecular layer; PCL, Purkinje cell layer; GCL, granule cell layer. A Purkinje cell (PC) receives excitatory inputs via parallel fibers (PF) and climbing fibers (CF) and sends inhibitory signals to neurons of the deep cerebellar nuclei (DCN). GC, granule cell, MF, Mossy fiber. (c) Well-differentiated dendrites of Purkinje cells are visualized by GFP expression. (d) Dendritic spines of Purkinje cells (arrows).

3. Disorders of the cerebellum

As cerebellar defects can be easily detected from overt ataxia, such as widespread gait and motor coordination deficits, numerous types of mutant mice with cerebellar degeneration have been isolated over the past 50 years. These mutant mice have contributed significantly to the elucidation of cerebellar physiology. At present, in parallel with advances in the development of viral vectors, we may be able to restore cerebellar defects of ataxic mice by a potential therapeutic gene delivery. Such rescue experiments have significant implications in terms of the future clinical application of gene therapy for patients suffering from cerebellar diseases. The following subsections summarize the cerebellar abnormalities and genetic defects identified in ataxic mice and humans.

3.1 Spontaneously occurring ataxic mice

Table 1 summarizes well-known murine mutants that cause cerebellar impairment. Recently, the genes responsible for those mutants have been identified and include missense mutations, nonsense mutations or frameshift mutations in the causative genes. The *hotfoot* mice are spontaneously occurring recessive mutants (Guastavino et al., 1990) that carry mutations in *Grid2*, which encodes the δ2 glutamate receptor (GluRδ2) (Wang et al., 2003). To date, more than 10 mutant alleles have been identified; among these, *hotfoot5J* mice have been shown to carry a point mutation in exon 12 of *Grid2*, which creates a stop codon in the region encoding transmembrane 3 of GluRδ2 protein (Wang et al., 2003). The aberrant GluRδ2 protein is easily degraded and is not detected in Purkinje cells of *hotfoot5J* mice; therefore, *hotfoot5J* mice are mutants lacking GluRδ2 function.

Mouse name	Chromosome	Gene	Major cell defect	Age of onset
Hotfoot (*Grid2^ho^*)	6	*Grid2* deletion (Loss of function)	Purkinje cell	3 weeks postnatal
Staggerer (*ROR^sg^*)	9	*Rora* deletion (Loss of function)	Purkinje cell	1 week postnatal
PCD (*Agtpbp1^pcd^*)	13	*Agtpbp* deletion (Loss of function)	Purkinje cell	3 weeks postnatal
Lurcher (*Grid2^Lc^*)	6	*Grid2* missense mutation (Gain of malfunction)	Purkinje cell	2 weeks potnatal

Table 1. Genetic abnormalities and affected cell types in spontaneously occurring ataxic mice.

Other loss-of-function mutants are *Staggerer* and Purkinje cell degeneration (pcd) mice. The *staggerer* mutation causes a functional impairment in a transcription factor, retinoid-related orphan receptor α (RORα), which belongs to the nuclear receptor superfamily (Boukhtouche et al., 2006; Gold et al., 2007). *Staggerer* mice have a 122-base pair deletion within the ligand binding domain (LBD) of the RORα gene (Hamilton et al., 1996). For PCD mice, 8 independent alleles have been identified, which carry genetic mutations in the *Nna1* gene, encoding a putative nuclear protein (Fernandez-Gonzalez et al., 2002; Wang & Morgan, 2007). Most of the *pcd* alleles represent complete loss-of-function mutations. Because it is reasonable to postulate that aberrant phenotypes in loss-of-function mutants may be restored by introducing the intact gene, and, as Purkinje cells are the main cell type impaired in the loss-of-function mutants discussed here (*hotfoot*, *staggerer* and *pcd*), the efficient delivery of the intact gene into the specific subset of cells (Purkinje) may be a promising therapy for the recovery of those mutant mice from cerebellar degeneration and, ultimately, ataxia.

There are two important points that should be addressed. First, gene delivery should be performed before Purkinje cells are substantially lost or irreversibly damaged. Purkinje cells of *pcd* mice die gradually from approximately 18 days of age and are virtually lost by 4 months of age. Similarly, the Purkinje cell number in *staggerer* mice begins to decrease in the first week after birth, and at least 75-90% of Purkinje cells are lost in adult mutants (Vogel et al., 2000). The degeneration of Purkinje cells causes secondary defects of granule cells and neurons in the inferior olivary nucleus. Therefore, later gene delivery results in less or no functional recovery in *staggerer* and *pcd* mutants.

Another important point is that gene delivery should be carried out before the Purkinje cell loses its plasticity. The compensation of a missing gene during an inappropriate time may result in the insufficient restoration of Purkinje cell abnormalities. By the second to third postnatal week, Purkinje cells extend dendrites and make a hundred thousand synapses with different counterparts. A series of developmental processes requires the strictly regulated expression of numerous genes, suggesting that the exogenous delivery of an intact gene after termination of this period may have little therapeutic impact. This period, in which the brain displays a heightened sensitivity to exogenous stimuli (and still maintains capacity to respond to gene therapy), is referred to as the "critical period". The critical period differs depending on the defects of the mutant animals; thus, a careful examination using animal models can provide clues to deduce the critical period for the human cerebellum.

The Lurcher (*Lc*) mouse is an autosomal semidominant mutant that displays the degeneration of virtually all of the cerebellar Purkinje cells (Vogel et al., 2007). In heterozygous mice (*Lc*/+), cerebellar Purkinje cells specifically start to degenerate in a cell-autonomous manner by postnatal day 8 (P8), and most die during the second postnatal week.; other cell types are eventually affected by secondary mechanisms (Wetts & Herrup, 1982). *Lc*/+ mice exhibit severe ataxia during the third postnatal week, when approximately 90% of the Purkinje cells have disappeared. *Lc* is caused by an alanine to threonine mutation in the highly conserved third hydrophobic segment of GluRδ2 (Zuo et al., 1997). As this region works as the gate of a cation channel (Kohda et al., 2000), the mutation converts the receptor into a constitutively leaky cation channel. Thus, lurcher is a gain-of-function mutation, suggesting that a simple delivery of the wild-type GluRα2 would not have a significant therapeutic impact on *Lc* Purkinje cells. A suppression of the mutant protein expression via, for example, RNA interference would be a promising gene therapy against disorders caused by a toxic-gain-of-function mutation.

3.2 Human cerebellar diseases potentially treatable with gene therapy

3.2.1 Spinocerebellar ataxia

The cerebellum is impaired by various diseases, including neurodegenerative and enzyme-deficient disorders. Spinocerebellar ataxia (SCA) is one of the representative diseases that affect the cerebellum. Approximately one third of the SCA in patients is hereditary. So far, at least 29 types of SCA result from chromosomal loci of the causal genes (Carlson et al., 2009), in which the major lesion of SCA type 1 (SCA1), SCA2, SCA6, SCA14, SCA17 and SCA31 affects Purkinje cells. Neurons in the deep cerebellar nuclei are impaired in SCA3, and cortical Bergmann glia are primarily degenerated in SCA7. The well-known cause of hereditary SCAs is the abnormal expansion of trinucleotide (CAG) repeats in the coding region of genes responsible for the diseases. This expansion produces mutant proteins having an abnormally expanded polyglutamine stretch, leading to the formation of nuclear aggregates with other proteins that are critical for cellular functions. This type of hereditary SCAs is called polyglutamine disease and includes SCA1, SCA2, SCA3, SCA6, SCA7 and SCA17. As these diseases are caused by the production of toxic polyglutamine proteins (polyQ), a potential therapeutic approach would be to reduce the mutant polyQ by, for example, RNA interference (Xia et al., 2004) or the facilitation of their degradation. The latter may include the enhancement of the ubiquitin-proteasome pathway (Al-Ramahi et al., 2006; Matsumoto et al., 2004; Torashima et al., 2008; Wang & Monteiro, 2007) and autophagy (Menzies et al., 2010; Menzies & Rubinsztein, 2010; Williams et al., 2006).

Autosomal dominant SCA14, characterized by severe cerebellar atrophy and ataxia, is caused by a missense mutation of the *PRKCG* gene, which encodes the protein kinase C (PKC) γ gene. γPKC-deficient mice show only mild ataxia and no gross morphological abnormalities in the cerebellum (Chen et al., 1995; Kano et al., 1995), suggesting that the gain-of-toxic function, rather than loss-of-function, of γPKC underlies the pathology of SCA14. Therefore, a decrease in the amount of mutant γPKC protein is thought to be an effective therapy for SCA14. Indeed, recent studies have shown the allele-specific inhibition of mutant gene expression (Alves et al., 2008; Hu et al., 2009), and such mutant allele-targeted RNA interference may result in better therapeutic efficacy.

3.2.2 Mucopolysaccharidosis

Lysosomal storage diseases (LSDs) are inherited metabolic disorders characterized by the accumulation of undigested macromolecules in the lysosomes due to a significant decrease or a complete absence in the activity of soluble lysosomal enzymes (Neufeld, 1991). As most lysosomal enzymes are ubiquitously expressed, a deficiency in a single enzyme affects peripheral organs, as well as various regions of the brain, including the cerebellum. There are approximately 50 forms of inherited LSDs in humans with incidences of 1 in 7,000 live births (Haskins, 2009). LSDs are usually grouped biochemically by the accumulated metabolite into 3 subgroups: mucopolysaccharidoses (MPS), sphingolipidoses, and mucolipidoses.

The potential treatments for LSDs include bone marrow or cord blood transplantation, enzyme replacement and gene therapy. Among the LSDs, those due to soluble lysosomal enzyme deficiencies are generally considered good candidates for gene therapy. These include MPS I, MPS IIIB and Niemann-Pick AB diseases (Sands & Davidson, 2006). To overcome the blood-brain barrier (BBB), viral vectors should be applied intrathecally (Watson et al., 2006) or directly into the brain parenchyma (Dodge et al., 2005), except in neonates having an incomplete BBB (Hartung et al., 2004; Kobayashi et al., 2005). Recent studies using knockout mouse models of MPS I and Niemann-Pick type A disease have shown a significant rescue of the phenotypic manifestations of the diseases upon intravenous and intrathecal application of adeno-associated virus (AAV) or lentiviral vectors expressing a deficient enzyme (Dodge et al., 2005; Hartung et al., 2004; Kobayashi et al., 2005; Watson et al., 2006). In addition, the injection of AAV vectors expressing the deficient gene, acid sphingomyelinase, into the deep cerebellar nuclei alleviated storage accumulation and corrected behavior deficits in the mouse model of Niemann-Pick type A disease (Dodge et al., 2005). These results suggest that viral vector-based gene transfer is promising for clinical gene therapy of patients with LSDs.

4. Viral vector-mediated gene delivery to the cerebellum

Vectors derived from retrovirus, Sindbis virus, adenovirus, lentivirus and AAV are widely used for gene transfer to mammalian cells; the properties of these vectors are summarized in Table 2. Retroviral vectors can express a foreign gene only in proliferating cells because they cannot pass through the nuclear membrane of host cells: the viral genome that enters into the cytoplasm of an infected cell can access the host chromosome only when the nuclear membrane disappears during mitosis. Exploiting this unique feature of retroviral vectors, they have been used to label neural stem cells (Kageyama et al., 2003; Levison et al., 2003; Namba et al., 2007).

Vectors	Gene expression	Insert size	Exchange of a promoter	Toxicity	Tropism	Period for gene expression	Inflammatory potential
Lenti	Stable	8 kb	○	(-)	broad	~7 days	Low
Retro	Stable	8 kb	○	(-)	Dividing cells only	~7 days	Low
AAV	Stable	<4.7 kb	○	(-)	broad	5~7 days	Low
Adeno	Transient (2months)	30 kb	○	(+)	Glia tropic	3~5 days	High
Sindbis	Cell death in 1-2 days	6 kb	×	(+++)	Neuro tropic	< 1 day	Very high

Table 2. Properties of different viral vectors.

Vectors based on Sindbis virus, a member of the Togaviridae family in the alphavirus subfamily, can infect non-dividing cells, including neurons, and replication occurs entirely in the cytoplasm of the infected cell as an RNA molecule (Griffin, 1998). Therefore, a high level of gene expression starts quickly after infection. One drawback of the Sindbis virus vector is high toxicity, as infected cells deteriorate within a couple of days.

Adenoviral vectors are widely used as gene transfer vectors. They can accommodate a large gene of ~30 kb and infect both neurons and glia, with a higher tropism for glia. Therefore, adenoviral vectors have been used to modify the function of Bergmann glia (Iino et al., 2001). Adenoviral vectors can exert toxicity to infected cells by triggering immune responses, and gene expression generally lasts only for ~2 months (Terashima et al., 1997). The features of adenoviral vectors, including their high infectivity in glial cells and immunogenicity, in combination with the introduction of an apoptosis-triggering gene are often applied to the gene therapy of malignant glioma (Horowitz, 1999; Jiang et al., 2009; Parker et al., 2009; Shinoura & Hamada, 2003).

Vectors derived from lentiviruses, a genus of slow viruses of the Retroviridae family, can replicate in non-dividing neurons with little toxicity to the infected cells (Escors & Breckpot). Moreover, stable gene expression lasts for more than several years. In the cerebellum, lentiviral vectors pseudotyped with vesicular stomatitis virus glycoprotein (VSVG) can infect various types of cortical cells that include Purkinje cells, stellate cells, basket cells, Golgi cells, Bergmann glia and astrocytes (Croci et al., 2006; Torashima et al., 2006a). The properties of lentiviral vectors are described in more detail in the next section (Subsection 4.1).

AAV is a non-pathogenic, small (20 nm), icosahedral and non-enveloped virus that belongs to the genus Dependovirus of the Parvoviridae family. Similar to lentiviral vectors, it infects both dividing and non-dividing cells with very little toxicity and a minimal immune response in the infected cells. To date, a number of AAV serotypes and over one hundred AAV variants have been isolated from adenovirus stocks or from human and non-human primate tissues (Gao et al., 2005; Wu et al., 2006). For gene transfer to cerebellar cells, AAV serotype 1, serotype 2 and serotype 5 (AAV1, AAV2 and AAV5) vectors have been used for the successful transduction of Purkinje cells (Alisky et al., 2000; Hirai, 2008; Kaemmerer et al., 2000; Xia et al., 2004). Thus, lentiviral vectors and AAV vectors, which have the potential to transduce Purkinje cells with almost no substantial toxicity, are promising as gene therapy vectors for cerebellar disorders that affect Purkinje cells. Because of the lack of pathogenicity, AAV vectors are increasingly becoming the vectors of choice for a wide range of gene therapy approaches. One major limitation of AAV vectors is the insert capacity, which is less than 4.7 kb, whereas lentiviral vectors have a higher capacity, up to 8 kb, for transgene accommodation (Table 2) (Hirai, 2008).

4.1 Factors that control the tropism of lentiviral vectors for cerebellar neurons and glia

As the VSVG binds to the phospholipids that constitute cellular membranes, VSVG-pseudotyped lentiviral vectors are thought to infect mammalian cells without cell-type preference. In the cerebellar cortex, lentiviral vectors have successfully transduced Purkinje cells, three types of interneurons, Bergmann glia and astrocytes, but not granule cells. The efficient transduction of Golgi cells and astrocytes present in the granule cell layer suggest that the injected viral solution is accessible to granule cells: however, no or few transduced granule cells, if any, were detected upon injection of lentiviral vectors to the adult cerebellum *in vivo* (Croci et al., 2006; Torashima et al., 2006a).

The observed lentiviral tropism for Purkinje cells is affected by the serum-lot quality and cultivation period of the HEK293FT cells used for lentiviral production (Torashima et al., 2006b). A three-day culture that causes the degeneration and death of HEK293FT cells results in the production of glia-tropic lentiviral vectors. Although the mechanism underlying this phenomenon has not been clarified, increases in the protease activity in the culture medium seems to be involved because the addition of a protease inhibitor in medium reversed the shift of lentiviral tropism from Purkinje cells to Bergmann glia (our unpublished observation). These results suggest that VSVG is modulated by a protease released from dead HEK293FT cells, leading to the alteration of lentiviral tropism.
The L7/PCP2 promoter is a Purkinje cell-specific promoter, and the Gfa2 promoter works as an astrocyte-specific promoter. Therefore, the combination of the cultivation period of HEK293 FT cells for lentiviral production and the accommodation of the L7 or Gfa2 promoter into lentiviral vectors permits us to specifically transduce Purkinje cells or Bergmann glia, respectively. However, these cell-type specific promoters generally have weak promoter strength. Therefore, the modification of these promoters, by the addition of an enhancer sequence and/or a significant increase in the viral titer by ultracentrifugation, is needed to attain sufficient levels of transgene expression.

4.2 A method that enables efficient and widespread gene delivery to the cerebellum

The cerebellum is a second largest organ in the mammalian CNS. Neurodegenerative diseases and congenital enzyme deficiency usually affect the entire cerebellar cortex, ranging from the vermis to the hemisphere, lobule 1 to lobule 10.
For effective gene therapy, a wide range of therapeutic gene delivery methods is indispensable. Figure 2a is a photo of our viral injection system for the rodent brain.
The injection of viral solutions to the brain parenchyma mechanically damages the tissue around an injection site, and ~1 μl is usually the limit for mouse brain regions, such as the striatum and hippocampus. However, we found that when injected at a speed of 0.2 - 0.3 μl/minute, it was possible to apply 10 μl of viral solution to the subarachnoidal space over lobule 6 of the cerebellar cortex (Fig. 2b) without substantial damage to the cortical tissue. Injected viral particles spread through subarachnoidal spaces and infect Purkinje cells via their well-differentiated dendrites, leading to markedly efficient transduction of the Purkinje cells (Fig. 3). We have also verified that this injection method is applicable to neonatal pups and mature mice (Fig. 2c) (Sawada et al., 2010; Torashima et al., 2006a; Torashima et al., 2006b).

5. Lentiviral vector-based rescue of mice with cerebellar ataxia

5.1 Hotfoot5J mice

Hotfoot mice are spontaneously occurring recessive mutants (Guastavino et al., 1990), and mice homozygous for the mutation showed severe ataxia with jerky tapping of the hindlimbs, which can be noted by two weeks after birth. The *Hotfoot5J* allele possesses a point mutation in exon 12 of the GluRδ2 gene, which creates a stop codon in the region encoding transmembrane 3 (Wang et al., 2003). Aberrant GluRδ2 protein is easily degraded and not detected in the Purkinje cells of *hotfoot5J* mice. Therefore, *hotfoot5J* mice are thought to exhibit a similar phenotype to that of GluRδ2 knock-out mice (Kashiwabuchi et al., 1995). Accordingly, we determined whether the ataxia of *hotfoot5J* mice could be reliably rescued by lentiviral-vector-based expression of the recombinant wild-type GluRδ2 gene (Iizuka et al., 2009).

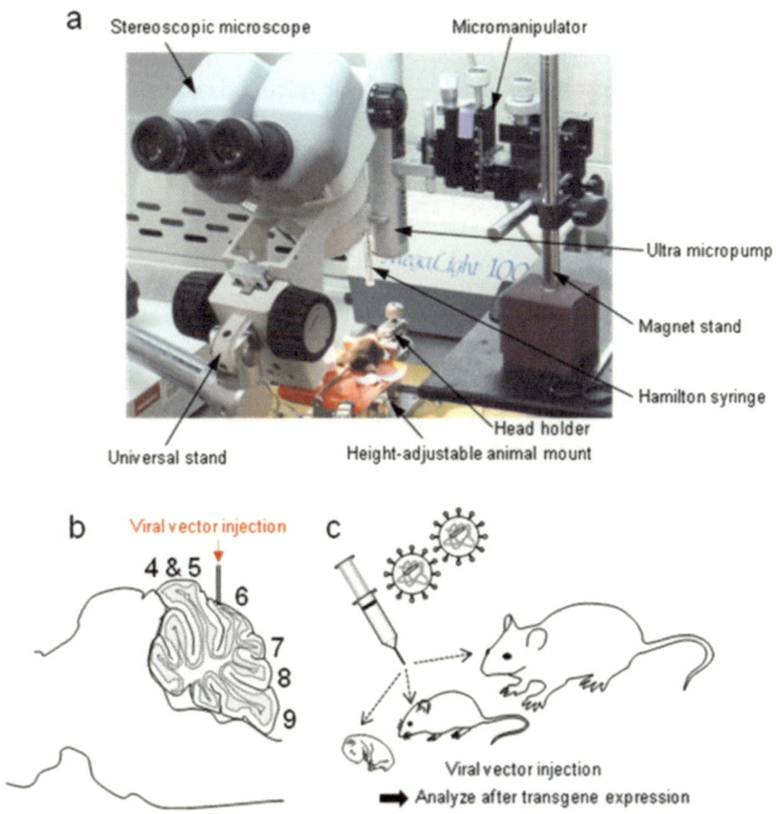

Fig. 2. Injection of viral vectors into the mouse cerebellum. (a) A viral vector injection setup. Viral vectors are injected very slowly with a speed of 0.2-0.3 μl/minute using an ultramicropump. (b) A schematic of the sagittal view of a mouse cerebellum depicting a viral injection site. (c) A schematic showing the availability of this injection method from a neonatal pup to a mature mouse.

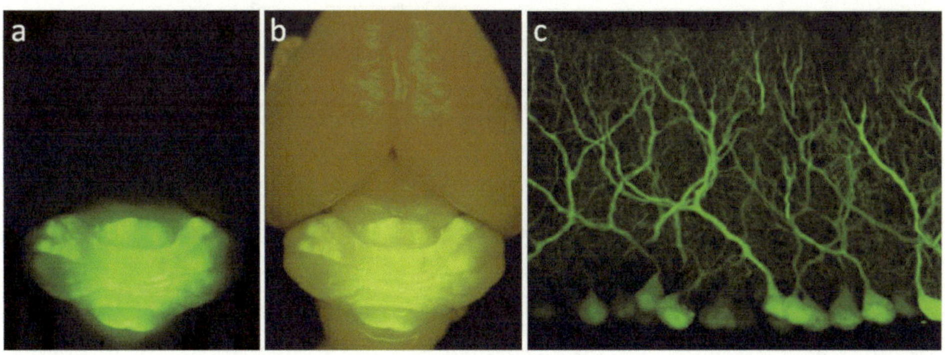

Fig. 3. Highly efficient transduction of Purkinje cells. Lentiviral vectors expressing GFP was injected as shown in Fig. 2. (a and b) Stereoscopic images of GFP fluorescence (a) and the superimposition with the whole brain (b) 7 days after the viral injection. (c) A GFP fluorescent image of Purkinje cells in the sagittal section.

Lentiviral vectors expressing GluRδ2 plus GFP or GFP alone were injected into lobule 6 of the *hotfoot5J* cerebella at P6, and the motor control ability was assessed at P30 by footprints and a rotarod test. The footprint pattern of mutant mice was markedly ameliorated by the expression of GluRδ2 plus GFP (Fig. 4).

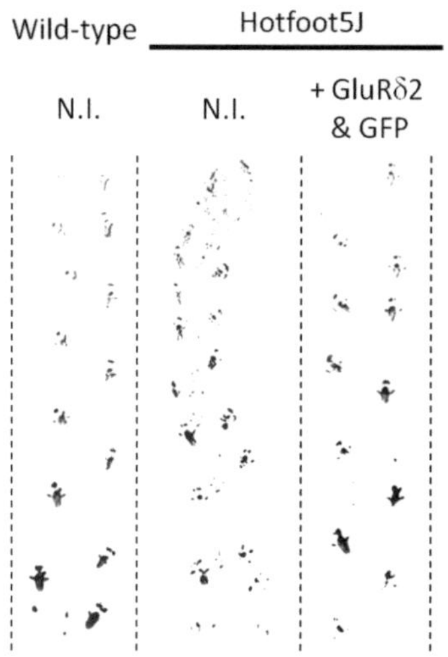

Fig. 4. Footprints of wild-type and *hotfoot5J* mice at P30. Ink was placed on the hindpaws of a non-injected wild-type mouse, a non-injected *hotfoot5J* mouse and *hotfoot5J* mice treated with GluRδ2 plus GFP (+ GluRδ2 & GFP); their footprints are shown. N.I., non-injected.

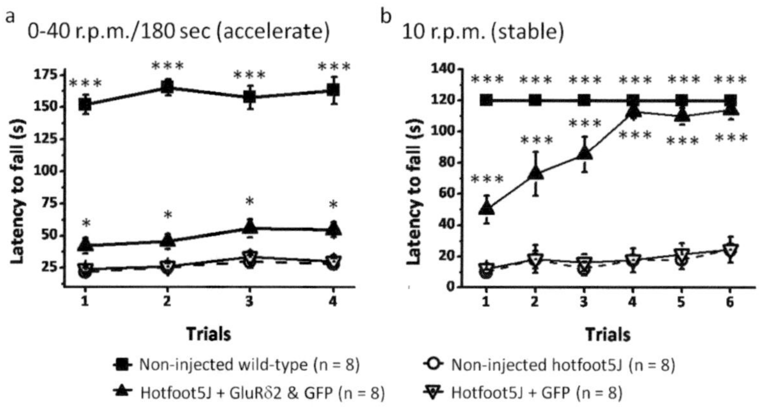

Fig. 5. Rescue of rotarod performance of *hotfoot5J* mice treated with GluRδ2 plus GFP. (a and b) Mice were assessed by two different tasks, an accelerating rod that reached 40 rpm from 0 rpm in 3 min (a) and a stably rotating rod with a speed of 10 rpm (b). The results of non-injected wild-type mice, non-injected *hotfoot5J* mice and *hotfoot5J* mice injected with lentiviral vectors expressing GluRδ2 plus GFP or GFP alone are presented. Asterisks indicate statistically significant differences compared with non-injected *hotfoot5J* mice: *$p < 0.05$, ***$p < 0.001$ (One-way ANOVA).

In the rotarod analysis, mice treated with GluRδ2 plus GFP showed significantly better performance at both acceleration and fixed-rod-speed tasks than non-injected mutant mice (Fig. 5), whereas neither the footprint pattern (not presented) nor the rotarod performance (Fig. 5) of *hotfoot5J* mice was altered by the injection of lentiviral vectors expressing only GFP. However, the rescue of ataxia by GluRδ2 expression was obviously incomplete; GluRδ2-treated *hotfoot5J* mice showed far poorer rotarod performance, particularly in the accelerating rod task (Fig. 5a), than wild-type mice. This was due partly to the expression of recombinant GluRδ2 in restricted lobules of *hotfoot5J* cerebellum.
Following the immunohistochemical examination, the GluRδ2 immunoreactivity was absent in the Purkinje cells from the non-injected *hotfoot5J* mice, whereas efficient GluRδ2 expression was detected in the dendritic spines of Purkinje cells from *hotfoot5J* mice treated with lentiviral vectors expressing GluRδ2 plus GFP.

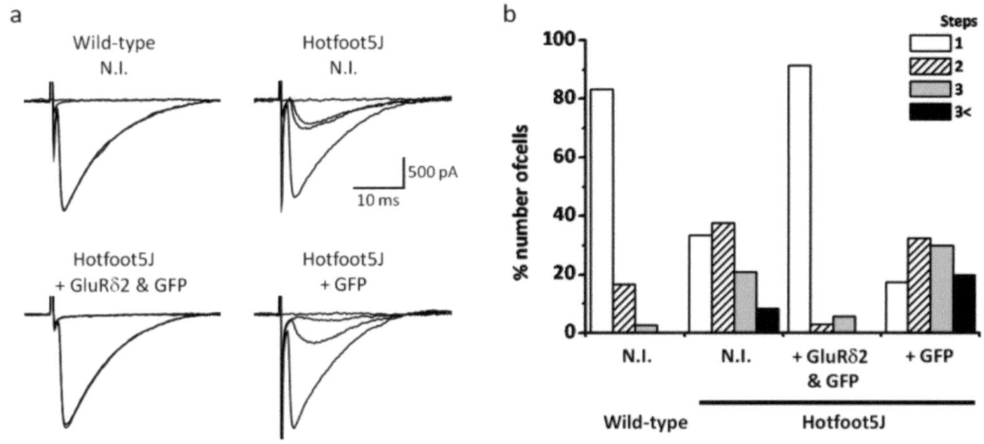

Fig. 6. Rescue from the persistent multiple CF innervation of *hotfoot5J* Purkinje cells by GluRδ2 expression. (a) Representative CF-EPSCs recorded from Purkinje cells clamped at −10 mV in non-injected wild-type, non-injected *hotfoot5J*, GluRδ2/GFP-treated *hotfoot5J*, and GFP-expressing *hotfoot5J* mice are shown. Scale bar, 500 pA, 10 ms. (B) Frequency histograms of Purkinje cells in terms of the number of discrete CF-EPSC steps in Purkinje cells from non-injected wild-type (42 cells, 3 animals), non-injected *hotfoot5J* (48 cells, 4 animals), GluRδ2/GFP-treated *hotfoot5J* (35 cells, 3 animals), and GFP-expressing *hotfoot5J* (40 cells, 3 animals) mice. N.I., non-injected.

Previous electrophysiological studies indicated that the multiple climbing fiber innervation of Purkinje cells continued even after maturation in the GluRδ2 knockout mice. GluRδ2$^{-/-}$ Purkinje cells were innervated persistently by multiple climbing fibers (Hashimoto et al., 2001; Ichikawa et al., 2002; Kashiwabuchi et al., 1995), and we examined whether the multiple innervations of *hotfoot5J* Purkinje cells were restored by the expression of recombinant GluRδ2 using a patch-clamp technique. Only 18% of the Purkinje cells in P31-P35 wild-type mice, and more than 60% of the Purkinje cells from age-matched GluRδ2-null mice, were innervated by multiple climbing fibers (Fig. 6). The failure of the developmental removal of surplus climbing fibers was completely rescued by the lentiviral vector-mediated expression of GluRδ2 plus GFP. However, no significant rescue was observed in *hotfoot5J* cerebella expressing GFP alone. These results suggest a therapeutic potential of lentiviral vector-based gene therapy for cerebellar disorders that result from a loss-of-function gene mutation.

5.2 The SCA model mice

Polyglutamine diseases, including several autosomal dominant types of SCA, are inherited neurodegenerative diseases caused by expanded polyQ accumulation in neurons (Koshy & Zoghbi, 1997). Recent studies have identified proteins that facilitate the degradation of polyQ aggregates through a ubiquitin-proteasome pathway in cultured cells. Previously, Yanagi and colleagues have identified a novel guanosine triphosphatase (GTPase), CRAG, as one of those proteins. Furthermore, these authors have shown that CRAG triggers the nuclear translocation of a CRAG-polyQ complex, leading to the degradation of polyQ in HeLa cells (Qin et al., 2006). Because the expression of CRAG decreases in the adult brain, it is plausible that a reduced level of CRAG could underlie the onset of polyglutamine diseases. Therefore, we examined the potential of CRAG expression for treating polyglutamine disease and tested our hypothesis by lentivirally introducing CRAG into the cerebellar neurons of mice overexpressing polyQ in the cerebellum.

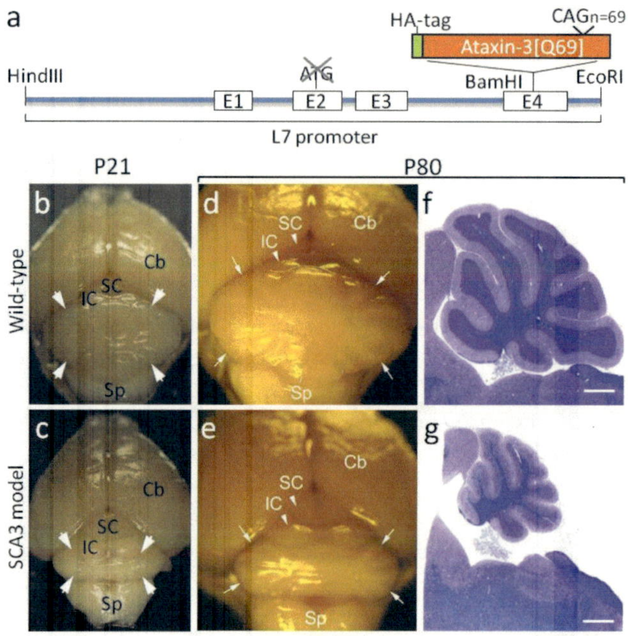

Fig. 7. Severe cerebellar atrophy in the PolyQ mouse at P21 and P80. (a) A schematic depicting the transgene that drives the mutant ataxin-3(Q69) under the control of the L7 promoter; an HA-tag was fused at the N-terminus of the truncated ataxin-3. Wild-type (b d, and f) and SCA3 model (c, e, and g) mice were fixed at P21 (b and c) or P80 (d-g). (b-e) A dorsal view of the whole brain; cerebella are indicated by arrows. Cb; cerebrum, IC; inferior colliculus, SC; superior colliculus, Sp; spinal cord. (f and g) Klüver–Barrera staining of sagittal sections of the cerebellum from a P80 SCA3 model mouse (g) and a wild-type littermate (f). Scale bars, 500 μm.

For this project, we generated transgenic mice (SCA model mice) expressing an expanded polyQ in cerebellar Purkinje cells using a truncated form of human ataxin-3, the gene responsible for Machado-Joseph disease (SCA3) with 69 CAG triplet repeats (ataxin-3[Q69]) (Kawaguchi et al., 1994; Yoshizawa et al., 2000) (Fig. 7a). The transgene expression was driven by a Purkinje cell-specific L7 promoter (Hirai et al., 2005). The SCA model mice started to show ataxic gait at approximately P10, which became more obvious as they developed further.

The cerebella of SCA model mice at P21 and P80 were substantially smaller than that of wild-type littermates (Fig. 7b-g). A low magnification of the sagittal sections of the SCA model mouse cerebellum showed that the overall structure of the cortex was not grossly affected (Fig. 7g). However, examination at a higher magnification revealed that the Purkinje cells were markedly disarranged, concomitant with a substantial impairment of dendritic differentiation (Fig. 8).

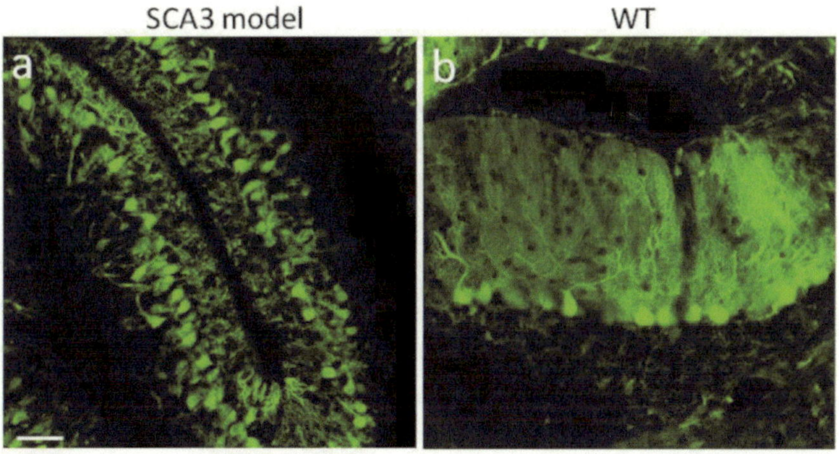

Fig. 8. Drastic morphological alteration in Purkinje cells of the SCA3 model mouse. Cerebellar sections from a P21 SCA3 model mouse (a) and a wild-type littermate (b) immunolabeled for calbindin. Note the markedly decreased thickness of the molecular layer and disarrangement of the Purkinje cell soma in the SCA3 model mouse cerebellum. Scale bar, 50 μm.

Immunostaining of the cerebellar sections for the hemagglutinin (HA)-tag at the N-terminus of polyQ revealed a weak and diffuse accumulation of polyQ mainly in the nucleus of Purkinje cells at P21. The polyQ was markedly increased and formed numerous inclusion bodies in or around the Purkinje cell bodies by P80. In addition to the immunoreactivity in the Purkinje cell layer, small inclusion bodies with strong immunoreactivity for polyglutamine and ubiquitin were detected in the axon terminals of the Purkinje cells in the deep cerebellar nuclei.

Lentiviral vectors expressing CRAG GTPase were injected into the midline cerebellar lobules of P21-P25 mice. The effect of CRAG or GFP expression was assessed by a rotarod test, in which mice were challenged with an accelerating rod paradigm just before or 4 or 8 weeks after the viral injection (Fig. 9a). The rotarod performance of the non-injected SCA3 model mice and the model mice expressing GFP alone deteriorated slightly at 8 weeks. In contrast, the performance of mice treated with CRAG was significantly improved at both 4 and 8 weeks after the injection, as compared with the results of non-injected mice. To examine the effect of CRAG expression on motor learning, mice were evaluated again by a rotarod test with a different paradigm, in which the rod speed was fixed at 5 rpm, and the trial was repeated 6 times. Non-injected SCA3 model mice and those treated with GFP showed almost no improvement in the performance even at the 6th trial (Fig. 9b). In contrast, mice treated with CRAG learned quickly how to stay on the rod, indicating the rescue of motor learning ability.

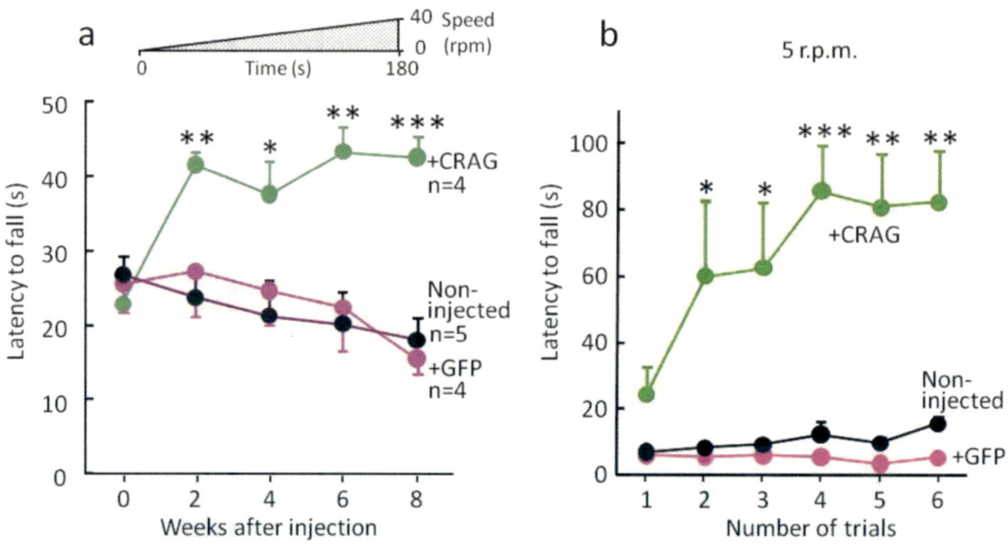

Fig. 9. Rescue of the ataxic phenotype in polyQ mice upon the lentivector-mediated expression of CRAG. (a and b) Results of the rotarod test. The rod was accelerated from 0 rpm and reached the maximum speed (40 rpm) in 3 min, as depicted above the graph (a). Mice treated with wild-type CRAG, but not those treated with GFP, exhibited significant improvement (a) (n = number of individual mice in each cohort). In the stable rod speed paradigm (5 rpm) administered 8 weeks after the injection, mice treated with CRAG learned quickly how to walk on the rod and showed a drastically better performance, compared with the non-injected and GFP-expressing mice (b). *$p<0.05$, **$p<0.01$, ***$p<0.001$, compared with results of non-injected mice.

We next examined the cerebellar sections from untreated mice or mice treated with the lentiviral vectors by immunohistochemistry. Whereas strong labeling with numerous polyQ inclusions was observed in the cerebellar slices from non-injected polyQ mice and those injected with virus expressing GFP, the overall labeling with an anti-HA antibody for polyQ was faint and diffusely distributed in the cytoplasm and nuclei of the Purkinje cells in CRAG-expressing slices (Fig. 10a-d). Notably, the arrangement and dendritic differentiation of the Purkinje cells was altered upon the expression of CRAG. Double immunolabeling for calbindin and Flag-tag fused with CRAG showed that only the CRAG-expressing Purkinje cells extended dendrites. Consistently, the molecular layer was significantly wider in the cerebella of polyQ mice treated with CRAG than in those of non-injected animals ($p<0.01$, Fig. 10e). These *in vivo* data substantiated previous cell-culture-based results and further extended the usefulness of the targeted delivery of genes facilitating the ubiquitin-proteasome pathway as a gene therapy against polyglutamine diseases and other neurodegenerative disorders.

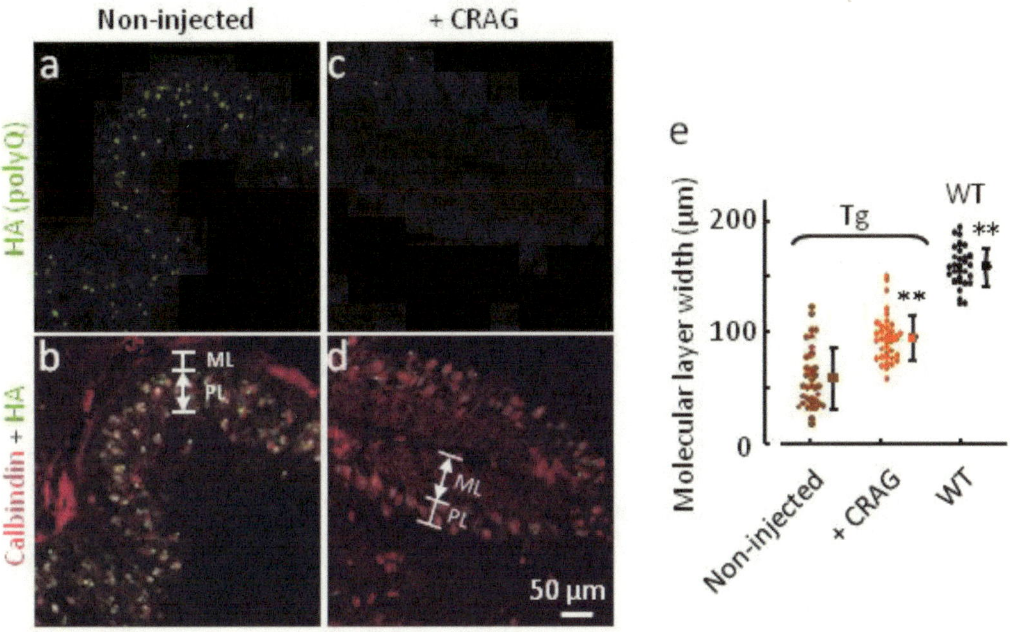

Fig. 10. Degradation of polyQ aggregates in Purkinje cells by lentiviral-vector-mediated expression of CRAG. (a-d) Cerebellar sections from mice receiving no injection (a and b) or treated with CRAG (c and d). Upper panels are fluorescent images of polyQ immunolabeled for HA (green), which were merged with those of Purkinje cells immunolabeled for calbindin (magenta, lower panels). ML; molecular layer, PL; Purkinje cell layer. (e) A graph of the thickness of the molecular layer. The thickness of the molecular layer in the cerebellum from SCA3 model mice (Tg) treated without (Non-injected) or with CRAG and their wild-type littermates (WT) was measured, and the data were plotted on the graph. The average ± SD is presented beside the each plot. Three animals in each experimental group and virus vectors obtained from at least two independent cultures were used for quantitative analysis. Asterisks indicate significant differences compared with results of non-injected mice, **$p<0.01$.

6. Underlying problems for the clinical application of lentiviral vectors to cerebellar diseases

6.1 The significantly larger size of human cerebellum compared with the mouse cerebellum

Figure 11 is a comparison of the mouse cerebellum with that of the cynomolgus monkey. Although our injection method allowed us to deliver a transgene very efficiently to mouse cerebellar cells, the human cerebellum is much larger than that of the cynomolgus monkey. Therefore, it is a tremendous challenge to attain the efficient transduction of Purkinje cells in the human cerebellum. To overcome this volume problem, we are exploring ways to increase the amount of the viral solution from 10 μl to 1,000 μl and the number of injection sites from one to, for example, three points.

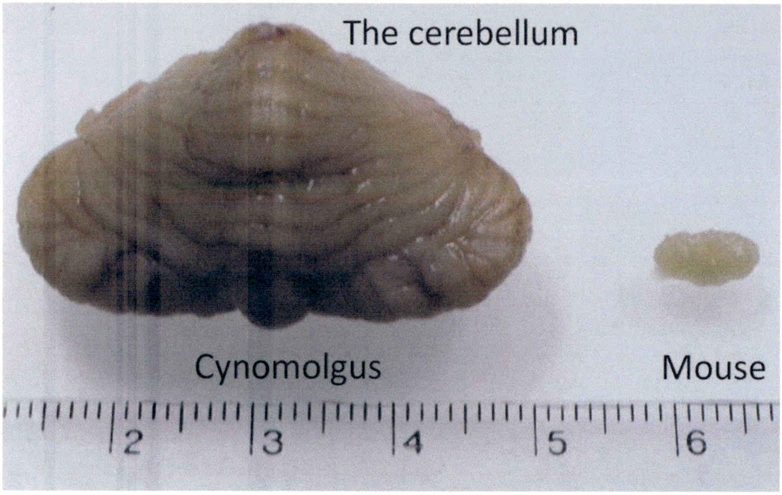

Fig. 11. Comparison of the mouse cerebellum (right) with that of the cynomolgus monkey (left).

6.2 Side effects that might be caused by the use of lentiviral vectors

6.2.1 Toxicity of lentiviral vector infection on Purkinje cells

Infection with Borna disease virus, an RNA virus tropic for cerebellar neurons, has been shown to cause developmental, neuroanatomical and behavioral abnormalities (Rubin et al., 1999). HIV infection has also been shown to cause a decreased expression of mRNA and protein of AMPA-type glutamate receptors in cerebellar Purkinje cells (Everall et al., 1995). Compared with adenoviral vectors that have immunogenicity, lentiviral vectors cause almost no immune responses to infected cells and are thought to exert little toxicity on host cells. However, it has not been fully clarified whether the infection of high-titer lentiviral vectors lacks an adverse influence on neurons *in vivo*. To clarify the influence of high-titer lentiviral vector infection and the subsequent expression of the transgene, we injected lentiviral vectors having a titer of 1.0 x 10^{10} transduction units (TUs) into the neonatal rat cerebellum. Neonates were used for examining lentiviral toxicity because the brain is extremely vulnerable to developmental damage following perinatal insult.

Lentiviral vectors expressing GFP under the control of the murine stem cell virus (MSCV) promoter were injected into the cerebellar cortex of neonatal rat pups. Three weeks after treatment, the GFP-expressing Purkinje cells were compared with control Purkinje cells from phosphate-buffered, saline-injected mice. An analysis of the dendritic tree showed that the total dendrite length in the GFP-expressing Purkinje cells was almost 80% of that in the control Purkinje cells. Furthermore, an electrophysiological examination showed that the short-term synaptic plasticity at the parallel fiber–Purkinje cell synapses and climbing fiber–Purkinje cell synapses was significantly altered in the GFP-expressing Purkinje cells. In contrast, the morphological and functional maldevelopment of infected Purkinje cells was attenuated substantially when lentiviral vectors with much weaker promoter activity were used. These results suggest that the maldevelopment of the Purkinje cells was caused mainly by the subsequent expression of a high amount of GFP driven by the strong MSCV promoter and that the toxic influence of lentiviral vector infection itself was minimal.

6.2.2 Insertional mutagenesis

Upon infection of a retrovirus into a cell, the viral RNA is inserted into the cytoplasm, where the RNA is reverse-transcribed into DNA by reverse transcriptase, which is then inserted into the host genome by an integrase. The viral genome sequence integrated into the host chromosome is called a "provirus". The provirus insertion may disrupt regions of the host genome that are critical for cellular functions, such as the control of the cell cycle or apoptosis; this process is called "insertional mutagenesis". In fact, *ex vivo* gene therapy using a murine leukemia virus (MLV) vector caused leukemia in 3 of the 11 children that were being treated for X-linked SCID (Hacein-Bey-Abina et al., 2003). However, lentiviral vectors are considered to be less likely to disturb the regulation and expression of host genes because of a difference of integration sites between the MLV vectors and lentiviral vectors: MLV vectors integrate primarily in promoter regions and CpG islands, whereas lentiviral vectors integrate into transcriptionally active genes (Mitchell et al., 2004; Schroder et al., 2002). Although it is not clear whether insertional mutagenesis can lead to the transformation of postmitotic neurons, lentiviral vectors do infect and cause insertional mutagenesis in glial cells with proliferative properties. Therefore, the risk of insertional mutagenesis should be considered when lentiviral vectors are used clinically to treat neurological diseases (Jakobsson & Lundberg, 2006).

7. Conclusion

The cerebellum develops significantly after birth (Goldowitz & Hamre, 1998), and, therefore, the expression of various genes is strictly regulated. Cerebellar granule cell precursors that proliferate vigorously in the external granule cell layer migrate along the processes of Bergmann glia to form the internal granule cell layer during the first postnatal two weeks in rodents. The migrating granule cells supply trophic factors, such as brain-derived neurotrophic factor (BDNF), which stimulates the Purkinje cells to form differentiated dendrites (Schwartz et al., 1997). During the migration process, parallel fibers, granule cell axons, (Granule cell axons are called "parallel fibers") make synapses with extending dendrites of Purkinje cells. Synaptic clefts between the parallel fibers and dendritic spines of a Purkinje cell are wrapped by processes of Bergmann glia that reuptake released glutamate, thereby modulate the synaptic transmission. Thus, 5 neurons and Bergmann glia in the cerebellar cortex concertedly elaborate the functional cerebellar neuronal circuit. One attractive therapy against diseases that impair Purkinje cells is the transplantation of Purkinje cells or their precursors engineered from stem cells into the damaged cerebellum. However, unless other cells surrounding Purkinje cells, such as the granule cells and interneurons, have sufficient plasticity, the transplanted Purkinje cells are not properly integrated to form a functional network, resulting in little therapeutic impact.

In contrast, gene therapy aims to salvage degenerating Purkinje cells by delivering a therapeutic gene. Accordingly, when Purkinje cells are not lost, this approach is theoretically more effective than stem cell-based cell replacement therapy for diseases that impair Purkinje cells; this is despite the fact that the surrounding cells have only limited plasticity. To attain sufficient therapeutic efficacy in gene therapy, the broad and efficient gene delivery to cerebellar neuronal or glial cells is indispensable, and this has been a significant challenge for decades. However, the problem is being solved by recent marked progress in both lentiviral and AAV vectors. The further accumulation of knowledge, including therapeutic genes and the critical period corresponding to distinct cerebellar defects, along with the development of animal models, would facilitate the clinical application of viral vector-based gene therapy for patients with various cerebellar disorders.

8. Acknowledgment

This work was supported by KAKENHI (19670003) and the Funding Program for Next Generation World-Leading Researchers (LS021).

9. References

Al-Ramahi, I., Lam, Y. C., Chen, H. K., de Gouyon, B., Zhang, M., Perez, A. M., et al. (2006). CHIP protects from the neurotoxicity of expanded and wild-type ataxin-1 and promotes their ubiquitination and degradation. *J Biol Chem,* Vol. 281, No. 36, pp. 26714-26724.

Alisky, J. M., Hughes, S. M., Sauter, S. L., Jolly, D., Dubensky, T. W., Jr., Staber, P. D., et al. (2000). Transduction of murine cerebellar neurons with recombinant FIV and AAV5 vectors. *Neuroreport,* Vol. 11, No. 12, pp. 2669-2673.

Alves, S., Nascimento-Ferreira, I., Auregan, G., Hassig, R., Dufour, N., Brouillet, E., et al. (2008). Allele-specific RNA silencing of mutant ataxin-3 mediates neuroprotection in a rat model of Machado-Joseph disease. *PLoS One,* Vol. 3, No. 10, pp. e3341.

Boukhtouche, F., Doulazmi, M., Frederic, F., Dusart, I., Brugg, B., & Mariani, J. (2006). RORalpha, a pivotal nuclear receptor for Purkinje neuron survival and differentiation: from development to ageing. *Cerebellum,* Vol. 5, No. 2, pp. 97-104.

Carlson, K. M., Andresen, J. M., & Orr, H. T. (2009). Emerging pathogenic pathways in the spinocerebellar ataxias. *Curr Opin Genet Dev,* Vol. 19, No. 3, pp. 247-253.

Chen, C., Kano, M., Abeliovich, A., Chen, L., Bao, S., Kim, J. J., et al. (1995). Impaired motor coordination correlates with persistent multiple climbing fiber innervation in PKC gamma mutant mice. *Cell,* Vol. 83, No. 7, pp. 1233-1242.

Croci, C., Fasano, S., Superchi, D., Perani, L., Martellosio, A., Brambilla, R., et al. (2006). Cerebellar neurons and glial cells are transducible by lentiviral vectors without decrease of cerebellar functions. *Dev Neurosci,* Vol. 28, No. 3, pp. 216-221.

Dodge, J. C., Clarke, J., Song, A., Bu, J., Yang, W., Taksir, T. V., et al. (2005). Gene transfer of human acid sphingomyelinase corrects neuropathology and motor deficits in a mouse model of Niemann-Pick type A disease. *Proc Natl Acad Sci U S A,* Vol. 102, No. 49, pp. 17822-17827.

Escors, D., & Breckpot, K. (2010). Lentiviral vectors in gene therapy: their current status and future potential. *Arch Immunol Ther Exp (Warsz),* Vol. 58, No. 2, pp. 107-119.

Everall, I. P., Hudson, L., al-Sarraj, S., Honavar, M., Lantos, P., & Kerwin, R. (1995). Decreased expression of AMPA receptor messenger RNA and protein in AIDS: a model for HIV-associated neurotoxicity. *Nat Med,* Vol. 1, No. 11, pp. 1174-1178.

Fernandez-Gonzalez, A., La Spada, A. R., Treadaway, J., Higdon, J. C., Harris, B. S., Sidman, R. L., et al. (2002). Purkinje cell degeneration (pcd) phenotypes caused by mutations in the axotomy-induced gene, Nna1. *Science,* Vol. 295, No. 5561, pp. 1904-1906.

Gao, G., Vandenberghe, L. H., & Wilson, J. M. (2005). New recombinant serotypes of AAV vectors. *Curr Gene Ther,* Vol. 5, No. 3, pp. 285-297.

Gold, D. A., Gent, P. M., & Hamilton, B. A. (2007). ROR alpha in genetic control of cerebellum development: 50 staggering years. *Brain Res,* Vol. 1140, No., pp. 19-25.

Goldowitz, D., & Hamre, K. (1998). The cells and molecules that make a cerebellum. *Trends Neurosci,* Vol. 21, No. 9, pp. 375-382.

Griffin, D. E. (1998). A review of alphavirus replication in neurons. *Neurosci Biobehav Rev,* Vol. 22, No. 6, pp. 721-723.

Guastavino, J. M., Sotelo, C., & Damez-Kinselle, I. (1990). Hot-foot murine mutation: behavioral effects and neuroanatomical alterations. *Brain Res,* Vol. 523, No. 2, pp. 199-210.

Hacein-Bey-Abina, S., Von Kalle, C., Schmidt, M., McCormack, M. P., Wulffraat, N., Leboulch, P., et al. (2003). LMO2-associated clonal T cell proliferation in two patients after gene therapy for SCID-X1. *Science,* Vol. 302, No. 5644, pp. 415-419.

Hamilton, B. A., Frankel, W. N., Kerrebrock, A. W., Hawkins, T. L., FitzHugh, W., Kusumi, K., et al. (1996). Disruption of the nuclear hormone receptor RORalpha in staggerer mice. *Nature,* Vol. 379, No. 6567, pp. 736-739.

Hartung, S. D., Frandsen, J. L., Pan, D., Koniar, B. L., Graupman, P., Gunther, R., et al. (2004). Correction of metabolic, craniofacial, and neurologic abnormalities in MPS I mice treated at birth with adeno-associated virus vector transducing the human alpha-L-iduronidase gene. *Mol Ther,* Vol. 9, No. 6, pp. 866-875.

Hashimoto, K., Ichikawa, R., Takechi, H., Inoue, Y., Aiba, A., Sakimura, K., et al. (2001). Roles of glutamate receptor delta 2 subunit (GluRdelta 2) and metabotropic glutamate receptor subtype 1 (mGluR1) in climbing fiber synapse elimination during postnatal cerebellar development. *J Neurosci,* Vol. 21, No. 24, pp. 9701-9712.

Haskins, M. (2009). Gene therapy for lysosomal storage diseases (LSDs) in large animal models. *ILAR J,* Vol. 50, No. 2, pp. 112-121.

Hirai, H. (2008). Progress in transduction of cerebellar Purkinje cells in vivo using viral vectors. *Cerebellum,* Vol. 7, No. 3, pp. 273-278.

Hirai, H., Miyazaki, T., Kakegawa, W., Matsuda, S., Mishina, M., Watanabe, M., et al. (2005). Rescue of abnormal phenotypes of the delta2 glutamate receptor-null mice by mutant delta2 transgenes. *EMBO Rep,* Vol. 6, No. 1, pp. 90-95.

Horowitz, J. (1999). Adenovirus-mediated p53 gene therapy: overview of preclinical studies and potential clinical applications. *Curr Opin Mol Ther,* Vol. 1, No. 4, pp. 500-509.

Hu, J., Matsui, M., Gagnon, K. T., Schwartz, J. C., Gabillet, S., Arar, K., et al. (2009). Allele-specific silencing of mutant huntingtin and ataxin-3 genes by targeting expanded CAG repeats in mRNAs. *Nat Biotechnol,* Vol. 27, No. 5, pp. 478-484.

Ichikawa, R., Miyazaki, T., Kano, M., Hashikawa, T., Tatsumi, H., Sakimura, K., et al. (2002). Distal extension of climbing fiber territory and multiple innervation caused by aberrant wiring to adjacent spiny branchlets in cerebellar Purkinje cells lacking glutamate receptor delta 2. *J Neurosci,* Vol. 22, No. 19, pp. 8487-8503.

Iino, M., Goto, K., Kakegawa, W., Okado, H., Sudo, M., Ishiuchi, S., et al. (2001). Glia-synapse interaction through Ca2+-permeable AMPA receptors in Bergmann glia. *Science,* Vol. 292, No. 5518, pp. 926-929.

Iizuka, A., Takayama, K., Torashima, T., Yamasaki, M., Koyama, C., Mitsumura, K., et al. (2009). Lentiviral vector-mediated rescue of motor behavior in spontaneously occurring hereditary ataxic mice. *Neurobiol Dis,* Vol. 35, No. 3, pp. 457-465.

Jakobsson, J., & Lundberg, C. (2006). Lentiviral vectors for use in the central nervous system. *Mol Ther,* Vol. 13, No. 3, pp. 484-493.

Jiang, H., Gomez-Manzano, C., Lang, F. F., Alemany, R., & Fueyo, J. (2009). Oncolytic adenovirus: preclinical and clinical studies in patients with human malignant gliomas. *Curr Gene Ther,* Vol. 9, No. 5, pp. 422-427.

Kaemmerer, W. F., Reddy, R. G., Warlick, C. A., Hartung, S. D., McIvor, R. S., & Low, W. C. (2000). In vivo transduction of cerebellar Purkinje cells using adeno-associated virus vectors. *Mol Ther,* Vol. 2, No. 5, pp. 446-457.

Kageyama, R., Hirata, H., & Hatakeyama, J. (2003). Retroviral vectors for gene delivery to neural precursor cells. *Int Rev Neurobiol,* Vol. 55, No., pp. 123-147.

Kano, M., Hashimoto, K., Chen, C., Abeliovich, A., Aiba, A., Kurihara, H., et al. (1995). Impaired synapse elimination during cerebellar development in PKC gamma mutant mice. *Cell,* Vol. 83, No. 7, pp. 1223-1231.

Kashiwabuchi, N., Ikeda, K., Araki, K., Hirano, T., Shibuki, K., Takayama, C., et al. (1995). Impairment of motor coordination, Purkinje cell synapse formation, and cerebellar long-term depression in GluR delta 2 mutant mice. *Cell,* Vol. 81, No. 2, pp. 245-252.

Kawaguchi, Y., Okamoto, T., Taniwaki, M., Aizawa, M., Inoue, M., Katayama, S., et al. (1994). CAG expansions in a novel gene for Machado-Joseph disease at chromosome 14q32.1. *Nat Genet,* Vol. 8, No. 3, pp. 221-228.

Kobayashi, H., Carbonaro, D., Pepper, K., Petersen, D., Ge, S., Jackson, H., et al. (2005). Neonatal gene therapy of MPS I mice by intravenous injection of a lentiviral vector. *Mol Ther,* Vol. 11, No. 5, pp. 776-789.

Kohda, K., Wang, Y., & Yuzaki, M. (2000). Mutation of a glutamate receptor motif reveals its role in gating and delta2 receptor channel properties. *Nat Neurosci,* Vol. 3, No. 4, pp. 315-322.

Koshy, B. T., & Zoghbi, H. Y. (1997). The CAG/polyglutamine tract diseases: gene products and molecular pathogenesis. *Brain Pathol,* Vol. 7, No. 3, pp. 927-942.

Levison, S. W., Druckman, S. K., Young, G. M., & Basu, A. (2003). Neural stem cells in the subventricular zone are a source of astrocytes and oligodendrocytes, but not microglia. *Dev Neurosci,* Vol. 25, No. 2-4, pp. 184-196.

Matsumoto, M., Yada, M., Hatakeyama, S., Ishimoto, H., Tanimura, T., Tsuji, S., et al. (2004). Molecular clearance of ataxin-3 is regulated by a mammalian E4. *Embo J,* Vol. 23, No. 3, pp. 659-669.

Menzies, F. M., Huebener, J., Renna, M., Bonin, M., Riess, O., & Rubinsztein, D. C. (2010). Autophagy induction reduces mutant ataxin-3 levels and toxicity in a mouse model of spinocerebellar ataxia type 3. *Brain,* Vol. 133, No. Pt 1, pp. 93-104.

Menzies, F. M., & Rubinsztein, D. C. (2010). Broadening the therapeutic scope for rapamycin treatment. *Autophagy,* Vol. 6, No. 2, pp. 286-287.

Mitchell, R. S., Beitzel, B. F., Schroder, A. R., Shinn, P., Chen, H., Berry, C. C., et al. (2004). Retroviral DNA integration: ASLV, HIV, and MLV show distinct target site preferences. *PLoS Biol,* Vol. 2, No. 8, pp. E234.

Namba, T., Mochizuki, H., Onodera, M., Namiki, H., & Seki, T. (2007). Postnatal neurogenesis in hippocampal slice cultures: early in vitro labeling of neural precursor cells leads to efficient neuronal production. *J Neurosci Res,* Vol. 85, No. 8, pp. 1704-1712.

Neufeld, E. F. (1991). Lysosomal storage diseases. *Annu Rev Biochem,* Vol. 60, No., pp. 257-280.

Parker, J. N., Bauer, D. F., Cody, J. J., & Markert, J. M. (2009). Oncolytic viral therapy of malignant glioma. *Neurotherapeutics,* Vol. 6, No. 3, pp. 558-569.

Qin, Q., Inatome, R., Hotta, A., Kojima, M., Yamamura, H., Hirai, H., et al. (2006). A novel GTPase, CRAG, mediates promyelocytic leukemia protein-associated nuclear body formation and degradation of expanded polyglutamine protein. *J Cell Biol,* Vol. 172, No. 4, pp. 497-504.

Rubin, S. A., Bautista, J. R., Moran, T. H., Schwartz, G. J., & Carbone, K. M. (1999). Viral teratogenesis: brain developmental damage associated with maturation state at time of infection. *Brain Res Dev Brain Res,* Vol. 112, No. 2, pp. 237-244.

Sands, M. S., & Davidson, B. L. (2006). Gene therapy for lysosomal storage diseases. *Mol Ther,* Vol. 13, No. 5, pp. 839-849.

Sawada, Y., Kajiwara, G., Iizuka, A., Takayama, K., Shuvaev, A. N., Koyama, C., et al. (2010). High transgene expression by lentiviral vectors causes maldevelopment of Purkinje cells in vivo. *Cerebellum,* Vol. 9, No. 3, pp. 291-302.

Schroder, A. R., Shinn, P., Chen, H., Berry, C., Ecker, J. R., & Bushman, F. (2002). HIV-1 integration in the human genome favors active genes and local hotspots. *Cell,* Vol. 110, No. 4, pp. 521-529.

Schwartz, P. M., Borghesani, P. R., Levy, R. L., Pomeroy, S. L., & Segal, R. A. (1997). Abnormal cerebellar development and foliation in BDNF-/- mice reveals a role for neurotrophins in CNS patterning. *Neuron,* Vol. 19, No. 2, pp. 269-281.

Shinoura, N., & Hamada, H. (2003). Gene therapy using an adenovirus vector for apoptosis-related genes is a highly effective therapeutic modality for killing glioma cells. *Curr Gene Ther,* Vol. 3, No. 2, pp. 147-153.

Terashima, T., Miwa, A., Kanegae, Y., Saito, I., & Okado, H. (1997). Retrograde and anterograde labeling of cerebellar afferent projection by the injection of recombinant adenoviral vectors into the mouse cerebellar cortex. *Anat Embryol (Berl),* Vol. 196, No. 5, pp. 363-382.

Torashima, T., Koyama, C., Iizuka, A., Mitsumura, K., Takayama, K., Yanagi, S., et al. (2008). Lentivector-mediated rescue from cerebellar ataxia in a mouse model of spinocerebellar ataxia. *EMBO Rep,* Vol. 9, No. 4, pp. 393-399.

Torashima, T., Okoyama, S., Nishizaki, T., & Hirai, H. (2006a). In vivo transduction of murine cerebellar Purkinje cells by HIV-derived lentiviral vectors. *Brain Res,* Vol. 1082, No. 1, pp. 11-22.

Torashima, T., Yamada, N., Itoh, M., Yamamoto, A., & Hirai, H. (2006b). Exposure of lentiviral vectors to subneutral pH shifts the tropism from Purkinje cell to Bergmann glia. *Eur J Neurosci,* Vol. 24, No. 2, pp. 371-380.

Vogel, M. W., Caston, J., Yuzaki, M., & Mariani, J. (2007). The Lurcher mouse: fresh insights from an old mutant. *Brain Res,* Vol. 1140, No., pp. 4-18.

Vogel, M. W., Sinclair, M., Qiu, D., & Fan, H. (2000). Purkinje cell fate in staggerer mutants: agenesis versus cell death. *J Neurobiol,* Vol. 42, No. 3, pp. 323-337.

Wang, H., & Monteiro, M. J. (2007). Ubiquilin interacts and enhances the degradation of expanded-polyglutamine proteins. *Biochem Biophys Res Commun,* Vol. 360, No. 2, pp. 423-427.

Wang, T., & Morgan, J. I. (2007). The Purkinje cell degeneration (pcd) mouse: an unexpected molecular link between neuronal degeneration and regeneration. *Brain Res,* Vol. 1140, No., pp. 26-40.

Wang, Y., Matsuda, S., Drews, V., Torashima, T., Meisler, M. H., & Yuzaki, M. (2003). A hot spot for hotfoot mutations in the gene encoding the delta2 glutamate receptor. *Eur J Neurosci,* Vol. 17, No. 8, pp. 1581-1590.

Watson, G., Bastacky, J., Belichenko, P., Buddhikot, M., Jungles, S., Vellard, M., et al. (2006). Intrathecal administration of AAV vectors for the treatment of lysosomal storage in the brains of MPS I mice. *Gene Ther,* Vol. 13, No. 11, pp. 917-925.

Wetts, R., & Herrup, K. (1982). Interaction of granule, Purkinje and inferior olivary neurons in lurcher chimeric mice. II. Granule cell death. *Brain Res,* Vol. 250, No. 2, pp. 358-362.

Williams, A., Jahreiss, L., Sarkar, S., Saiki, S., Menzies, F. M., Ravikumar, B., et al. (2006). Aggregate-prone proteins are cleared from the cytosol by autophagy: therapeutic implications. *Curr Top Dev Biol,* Vol. 76, No., pp. 89-101.

Wu, Z., Asokan, A., & Samulski, R. J. (2006). Adeno-associated virus serotypes: vector toolkit for human gene therapy. *Mol Ther,* Vol. 14, No. 3, pp. 316-327.

Xia, H., Mao, Q., Eliason, S. L., Harper, S. Q., Martins, I. H., Orr, H. T., et al. (2004). RNAi suppresses polyglutamine-induced neurodegeneration in a model of spinocerebellar ataxia. *Nat Med,* Vol. 10, No. 8, pp. 816-820.

Yoshizawa, T., Yamagishi, Y., Koseki, N., Goto, J., Yoshida, H., Shibasaki, F., et al. (2000). Cell cycle arrest enhances the in vitro cellular toxicity of the truncated Machado-Joseph disease gene product with an expanded polyglutamine stretch. *Hum Mol Genet,* Vol. 9, No. 1, pp. 69-78.

Zuo, J., De Jager, P. L., Takahashi, K. A., Jiang, W., Linden, D. J., & Heintz, N. (1997). Neurodegeneration in Lurcher mice caused by mutation in delta2 glutamate receptor gene. *Nature,* Vol. 388, No. 6644, pp. 769-773.

23

Role of Gene Therapy in the Management of Unilateral Vocal Fold Paralysis

Kevin Fung
Department of Otolaryngology – Head and Neck Surgery, University of Western Ontario, London, London Health Sciences Center – Victoria Hospital London, Ontario, Canada

1. Introduction

Vocal cord paralysis can occur as a result of injury to the recurrent laryngeal nerve (RLN). Possible causes include iatrogenic surgical injury (cardiac, thoracic, neck), neoplasm (e.g. thyroid, esophagus, lung) or neurological disease. Injury to the RLN results in vocal cord paresis or paralysis. Poor or absent movement of one or both vocal folds causes difficulties with voice, swallowing or breathing. This can have a substantial negative effect on quality of life due to poor vocal function, aspiration, and upper airway obstruction in the rare event of bilateral RLN injury.

2. Anatomy of the recurrent laryngeal nerve

Injury to the RLN can occur at any point along the course of the nerve, which spans the neck and thorax. The RLN is a branch of the vagus nerve, and has an extensive and complex anatomical course, beginning at the brainstem, coursing through the skull base, within the carotid sheath in the neck, into the thorax, looping around the aortic arch (left RLN), around the subclavian artery (right RLN), within the tracheoesophageal groove, posteromedial to the thyroid gland, and enters the larynx at the posteroinferior border of the cricoid cartilage. The RLN provides motor supply to the thyroarytenoid muscle, posterior cricoarytenoid muscle, lateral cricoarytenoid muscle, and interarytenoid muscles. It also provides sensory supply to the glottis and infraglottic larynx.

3. Current management options for unilateral vocal cord paralysis

Standard options for management of unilateral vocal cord paralysis include observation, voice and swallowing therapy, and surgery.

4. Observation

Patients sometimes exhibit variable clinical improvement with expectant management. This can be due to (i) spontaneous nerve regeneration, or (ii) natural compensation for glottic insufficiency by strengthening of the contralateral vocal cord.

5. Voice and swallowing therapy

A referral to an experienced speech language pathologist is commonly employed in cases of severe functional deficit where patients are reluctant or unfit to pursue surgery. Voice and swallowing rehabilitation has been shown to be effective, especially in motivated patients.

6. Surgery

Medialization of the paralyzed vocal cord aims to close the glottic gap, resulting in improvement in voice and aspiration. Specific procedures can be classified into endolaryngeal and extralaryngeal. Endolaryngeal procedures include injection laryngoplasty, whereby a 'filler' substance is injected into the paraglottic space, either percutaneously or endoscopically. Percutaneous approaches are performed in the clinic as an office-based procedure, and can be done safely under endoscopic guidance with local anaesthesia transorally, through the thyrohyoid membrane, through the thyroid cartilage, or most commonly, through the cricothyroid membrane. "Filler" substances commonly employed include calcium hydroxyapatite, collagen, and autologous fat. Extralaryngeal procedures include medialization laryngoplasty (thyroplasty), arytenoid adduction, and cricothyroid subluxation with adduction arytenopexy. The most commonly performed extralaryngeal procedure is the medialization thyroplasty. This is done in the operating room with IV sedation. The laryngeal framework is approached transcervically, and an alloplastic implant (such as Gortex™ or silastic) is inserted into the paraglottic space after drilling a window through the thyroid cartilage. This operation can be safely performed as an outpatient in selected patients (Zhao et al., 2010). Although implants can be hand-carved, contemporary thyroplasty systems include fully or partially pre-fabricated implants with gender-specific sizers and templates, for improved technical precision.

7. Pitfalls and shortcomings of current therapies

Although current therapies have been shown to be clinically effective, they represent static solutions to a dynamic problem. Physiologic vocal cord function is not actually restored. The ability to restore physiologic vocal cord movement depends upon developing strategies to maintain survival of injured or vulnerable neurons and to stimulate axonal regeneration to appropriate laryngeal muscles (Hogikyan et al. 2001, Rubin et al. 2003).

8. Nerve regeneration

Spontaneous natural nerve recovery can occur, but axon regrowth may fail to reach the laryngeal muscles, or fail to reinnervate the correct muscles (Crumley et al. 2000). Non-selective reinnervation of adductor and abductor laryngeal muscles results in synkinesis, which explains the variable clinical outcomes observed with expectant management.

It is known that neurotrophic and neuroprotective growth factors can prevent nerve degeneration following injury. Administration of these growth factors through the central nervous system (CNS) is an appealing strategy. However, technical access to these neurons is challenging, and direct injection is ineffective, since trophic factors diffuse poorly, and can cause injury to adjacent neuronal structures. A novel and innovative approach that is minimally invasive and avoids systemic side effects is remote delivery utilizing a viral vector, and forms the fundamental basis of the emerging evidence from investigations into the potential role of gene therapy for treatment of recurrent laryngeal nerve injury.

9. Gene therapy – a promising novel strategy for treatment of RLN injury

The remote delivery of genes encoding therapeutic growth factors to the CNS is an attractive management strategy, because it avoids the potential pitfalls of direct CNS injection (into the brainstem or spinal cord) and systemic administration. In this approach, viral vectors can be injected into the peripheral nervous system and be transported in a retrograde fashion to the CNS (Boulis et al. 1999, Rubin et al. 2001). Several viral vectors have been described for in vivo gene transfer in the nervous system, including herpes simplex virus, retroviruses, adenovirus, and adeno-associated virus (AAV). Contemporary bench techniques can impact virus attenuation, thereby preventing the negative consequences of local proliferation, and allow the addition of potentially therapeutic genes.

Previous research by our group has shown that an AAV vector, remotely injected into the RLN, travels in a retrograde fashion to the rat brainstem (Rubin et al. 2001) and that injection of an adenoviral vector into a crushed RLN added no additional injury compared with crush alone (Shiotani et al. 1999).

An experimental model of RLN injury for the study of viral gene therapy has been previously described (Fung et al., 2008, Figure 1). In this model, a standardized crush injury was induced to the RLN. Immediately following crush, there was a dramatic, measurable decrease in nerve–endplate contact percentage, and spontaneous recovery was observed by three weeks post-injury. Recovery was confirmed both endoscopically as well as histologically by determining a high nerve-endplate contact percentage. Nerve-endplate contact was quantified by a rigorous method of evaluation of immunohistochemically stained rat larynges for neurofilament and motor endplates. We showed that this method reliably quantified the anatomical integrity of neuromuscular connections in laryngeal muscle.

There are promising results from a study (Sabowski et al., 2009) investigating the effects of remote administration of an engineered zinc-finger protein transcription factor, Ad-32Ep65-Flag (Ad-p65). This factor has been found to induce expression of vascular endothelial growth factor (VEGF; also called VEGF-A). VEGF has well known neuroprotective effects. Subsequent work demonstrated that remote injection of Ad-p65 after RLN crush accelerated the return of vocal fold mobility and the percentage of nerve-endplate contacts in the thyroarytenoid muscle. Similar results have been described with adenoviral GDNF gene transfer (Araki et al., 2006). This study observed faster motor nerve conduction velocity of the RLN and quicker recovery rate of vocal fold movement following gene transfer.

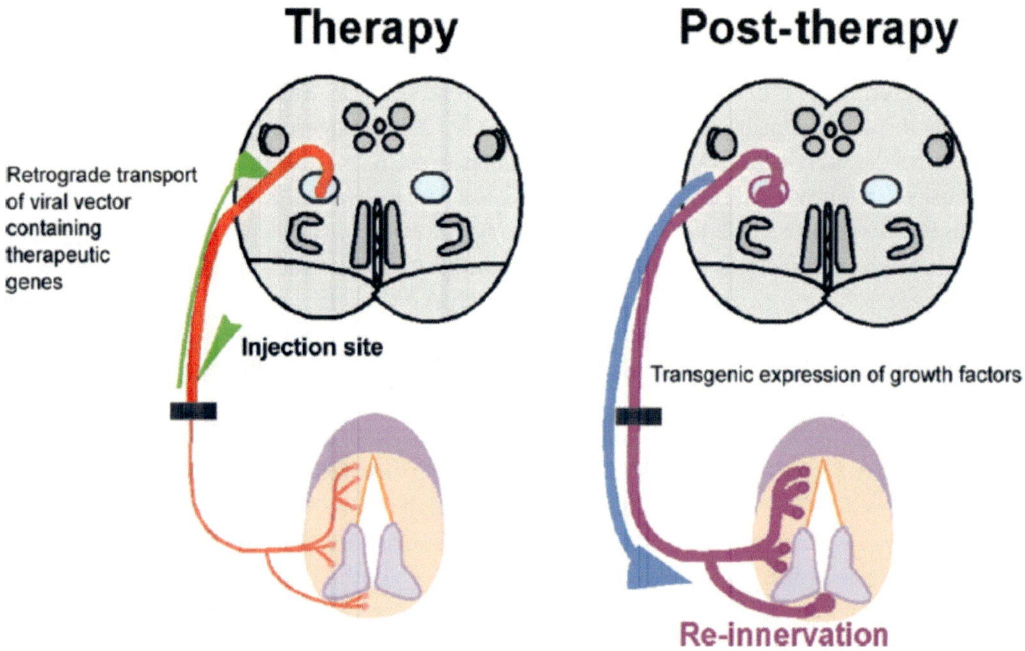

*reproduced from Fung et al. (2008)

Fig. 1.

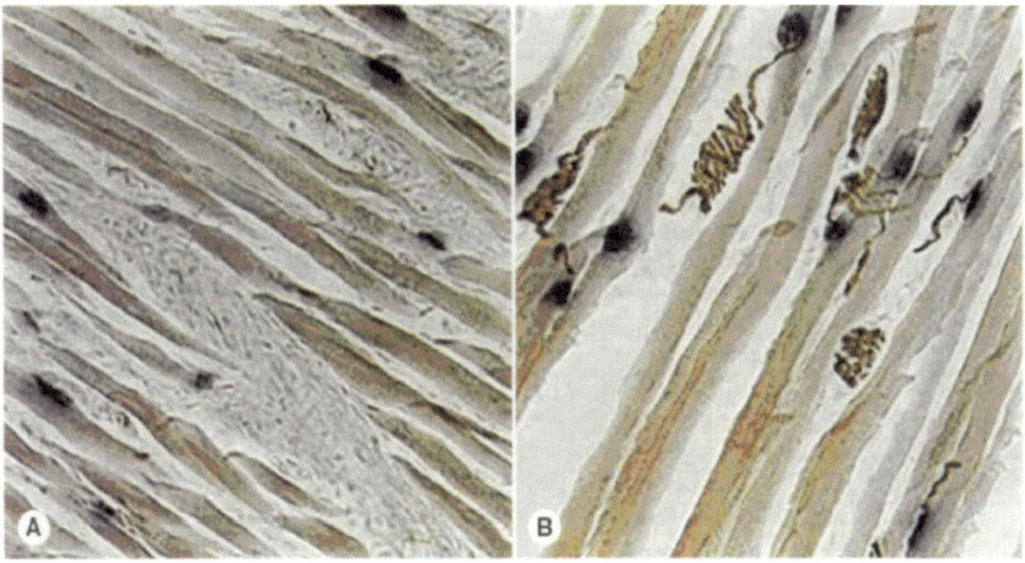

Reproduced from Fung et al. (2008)

Fig. 2. (A) Dennervation, as evidenced by low neuron-motor endplate contact percentage, following crush injury.
(B) Reinnervation, as evidence by high neuron-motor endplate contact percentage, following 3 weeks of recovery.

10. Conclusion

Gene therapy is a promising methodology that may enhance our ability to minimize nerve injury while maximizing functional outcome. Research using this model to investigate the potential therapeutic role of viral gene therapy for the treatment of recurrent laryngeal nerve injury is ongoing.

11. References

Zhao X, Roth K, Fung K. Type I thyroplasty: risk stratification approach to inpatient versus outpatient postoperative management. J Otolaryngol Head Neck Surg. 2010 Dec;39(6):757-61.

Hogikyan ND. Johns MM. Kileny PR. Urbanehek M. Carroll WR. Kuzon WM Jr. Motion-specific laryngeal reinnervation using muscle-nerve-muscie neurotization. Ann Otol Rhinol Laryngol 2001:110:801-10.

Rubin A. Mobley B. Hogikyan N, et al.. Delivery of an adenoviral vector to the crushed recurrent laryngeal nerve. Laryngoscope 2003;! 13:985-9.

Crumley RL. Laryngeal synkinesis revisited. Ann Otol Rhinol Laryngol 2000:109:365-71.

Boulis NM.Turner DE. Dice JA. Bhatia V. Peldman EL. Characterization of adenoviral gene expression in spinal cord after remote vector delivery. Neurosurgery 1999:45:131 -8.

Rubin AD. Hogikyan ND. Sullivan K. Boulis N. Feldman EL. Remote delivery of rAAV-GFP to the rat brainstem through the recurrent laryngea! nerve. Laryngoscope 2001:111:2041-5.

Shiotani A, O'Malley BW Jr, Coleman ME, Flint PW. Human insulin-like growth factor 1 gene transfer into paralyzed rat larynx: single vs multiple injection. Arch Otolaryngol Head Neck Surg 1999;125:555–60

Fung K, Hogikyan ND, Heavner SB, Ekbom D, Feldman EL. Development and characterisation of an experimental recurrent laryngeal nerve injury model for the study of viral gene therapy. Journal of Laryngology & Otology (2008), 122, 500–505.

Heavner SB, Rubin AD, Fung K, Old M, Hogikyan ND, Feldman EL. Dysfunction of the Recurrent Laryngeal Nerve and the Potential of Gene Therapy. Ann Otol Rhinol Laryngol 2007; 116(6): 441-448.

Sakowski SA, Heavner SB, Lunn JS, Fung K, Oh SS, Spratt SK, Hogikyan ND, Feldman EL. Neuroprotection using gene therapy to induce vascular endothelial growth factor-A expression. Gene Ther. 2009 Nov;16(11):1292-9.

Araki K, Shiotani A, Watabe K, Saito K, Moro K, Ogawa K. Adenoviral GDNF gene transfer enhances neurofunctional recovery after recurrent laryngeal nerve injury. Gene Ther. 2006 Feb;13(4):296-303.

Fluorescence Cross-Correlation Spectroscopy for Real-Time Monitoring of Exogenous DNA Behavior in Living Cells

Akira Sasaki and Masataka Kinjo
Graduate School of Advanced Life Science, Hokkaido University
Japan

1. Introduction

Many kind of DNA transfection techniques have been developed and widely used in the field of biochemical assay (Boussif et al., 1995, Chu et al., 1987, Felgner et al., 1987). Since recent development of fluorescent proteins such as green fluorescent protein (GFP), its variants and bio sensors, DNA transfection techniques play a greater role in the field of cell biology especially in bioimaging studies. DNA transfection is also used as a key technology to gene therapy (Selkirk, 2004, Schaffert et al., 2008). Thus the development of gene delivery vector with high efficiency is expected. Gene delivery systems with artificial nonviral vectors are widely used in the research field of cell biology and also in the clinical field as gene therapy to promote exogenous gene expression or inhibit production of a target protein. Nonviral vectors have advantages such as a low immune response and no risk of a disorder, which might be caused by native viral vector genome integration (Thomas et al., 2003). However, nonviral vectors need to overcome the disadvantage of low gene expression efficiency compared with native viral vectors (Luo et al., 2000). To increase the expression efficiency, it is needed to know gene delivery mechanisms. In general, complexes of exogenous DNAs and a cationic polymer or cationic lipid, commonly used as nonviral vectors, are internalized to target cells by endocytosis. Then a sequential process progresses spontaneously with escape from endosomes, dissociation of complexes, and diffusion of naked DNAs in the cytoplasm to the nucleus (Fig. 1) (Elouahabi et al., 2005).
However, such dynamic properties of transfected DNAs are not yet clearly distinguished because of the lack of suitable technique to observe intracellular DNA behavior. Fluorescence correlation spectroscopy (FCS) is a method based on observation of fluorescence intensity fluctuations that is the result of single fluorescent molecules diffuse in and out of small detection area (Fig. 2A, B) (Eigen et al., 1994). FCS technique can be applied for quantification of the absolute number of fluorescently labeled particles and measuring the molecular weight or size with extremely high sensitivity in a small sample volume, and a physical separation procedure is not needed. Therefore, FCS has currently employed to investigate molecular size or interactions *in vitro* and *in vivo* (Kinjo et al., 1995, Kitamura et al., 2006, Remaut et al., 2007, Kinjo et al., 2010). Dual color fluorescence cross-correlation spectroscopy (FCCS), an extended technique of FCS, can monitor molecular interactions directly in addition to parameters given from FCS measurements (Saito et al., 2004, Kogure et al., 2006, Bacia et al., 2007, Kim et al., 2007).

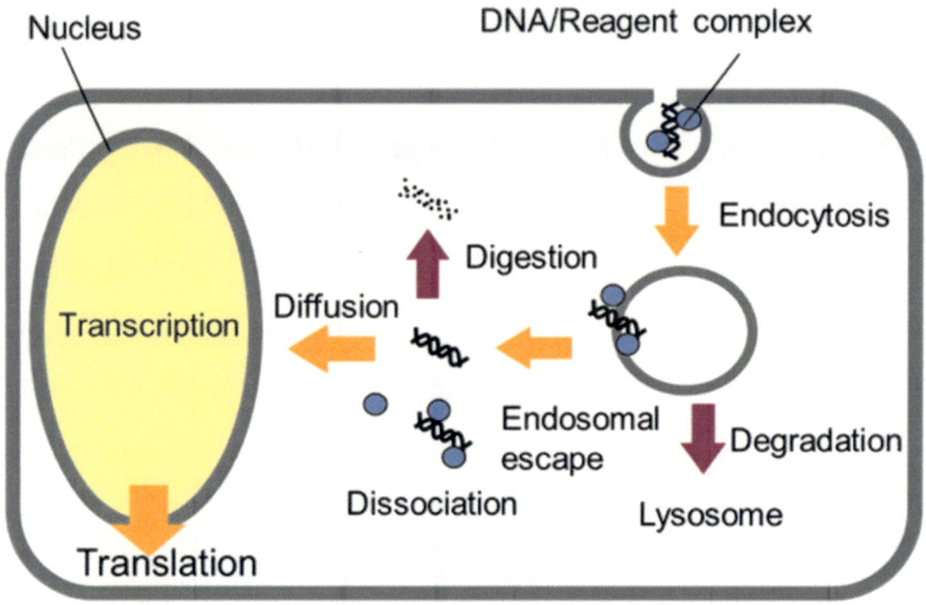

Fig. 1. Schematic diagram of intracellular gene delivery pathway.

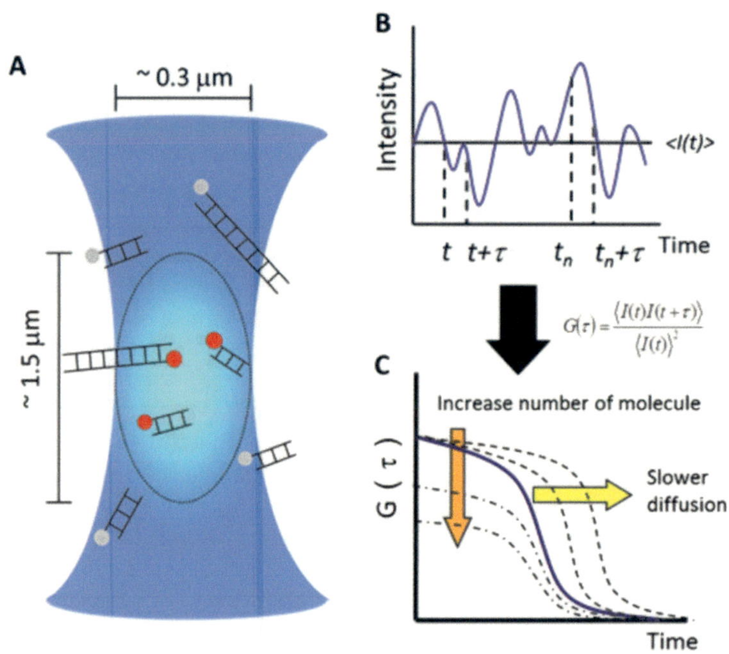

Fig. 2. Schematic diagram of FCS. (A) Schematic of observation area of FCS (confocal volume). (B) Obtained fluctuation of fluorescence intensity. (C) Autocorrelation functions (ACFs).

When the two target molecules are interacting, they will move together through the observation area and have synchronized fluorescence fluctuations in both two channels (Fig. 3A). On the other hand, the fluctuations are not correlated when these molecules move independently of one another (Fig. 3B). In this chapter, We describe the advantages of FCCS technique for the research field of gene therapy. In our research, FCCS technique was applied to study i) the behavior of exogenous DNA in living cells (Sasaki et al., 2010) and ii) the formation of DNA/carrier complex. In these cases, FCCS revealed the DNA degradation by nucleases and DNA-cationic polymer interactions to form DNA/carrier complex in real-time.

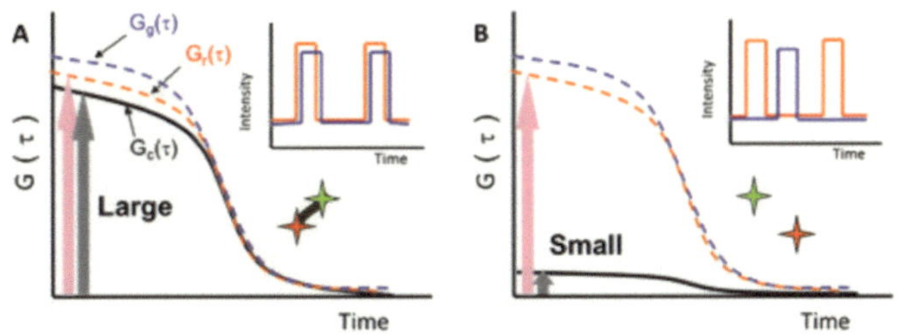

Fig. 3. Schematic diagram of FCCS. Auto and Cross-correlation functions (CCFs) of two fluorescent probes are connected (A) or separated (B).

2. Analysis of fluorescence cross-correlation spectroscopy

The FCCS setup consists of excitation, detection, and data processing systems similar to that of a typical laser-scanning confocal fluorescence microscope with high numerical-aperture (NA) objective.

Laser beams are focused on the coverslip via a confocal optic system to subfemto-liter size of observation area is generated. Emitted fluorescence signal is detected two avalanche photodiode (APD) through dichroic mirror (DM) and filter sets (barrier filter; BF) for each color channels (Fig. 4).

The FCS data are interpreted in terms of autocorrelation functions (G(τ)) (Fig. 2C), that give information on the diffusion time (DT) and the number of molecules (N) in observation area. Diffusion constant can be estimated from DT and size of observation area (Eigen et al., 1994).

The fluorescence autocorrelation functions of the red and green channels, $G_r(\tau)$ and $G_g(\tau)$, and the fluorescence cross-correlation function, $G_c(\tau)$, are calculated by

$$G_x(\tau)=\frac{\langle I_i(t)\cdot I_j(t+\tau)\rangle}{\langle I_i(t)\rangle\langle I_j(t)\rangle} \tag{1}$$

where τ denotes the time delay. I_i is the fluorescence intensity of the red channel (i = r) or green channel (i = g), $G_r(\tau)$ and $G_g(\tau)$ denote the autocorrelation functions of red (i = j = x = r), and green (i = j = x = g) respectively, or $G_c(\tau)$ denotes cross-correlation function (i = r, j = g, and x = c). Acquired G(τ) were generally fitted by a one- (i = 1) or two-component model (i = 2) as

$$G(\tau) = 1 + \frac{1 - f + f\exp(-\tau/\tau_t)}{N(1-f)} \sum_i F_i \left(1 + \frac{\tau}{\tau_i}\right)^{-1} \left(1 + \frac{\tau}{s^2\tau_i}\right)^{-1/2} \quad (2)$$

where F_i and τ_i are the fraction and diffusion time of component i, respectively. N is the average number of fluorescent particles in the observation area defined by radius ω and length 2z, and s is the structural parameter representing the ratio s = z/ω. The diffusion time (τ_i) corresponds to the average time for diffusion of fluorescent particles across the detection area, which reflects the size of particles. f is the average fraction of triplet state molecules and τ_t is triplet relaxation time (Widengren et al., 1995, Rigler et al., 1993). The distribution histogram of diffusion times was constructed using the CONTIN algorithm (Provencher, 1982, Björling et al., 1998).

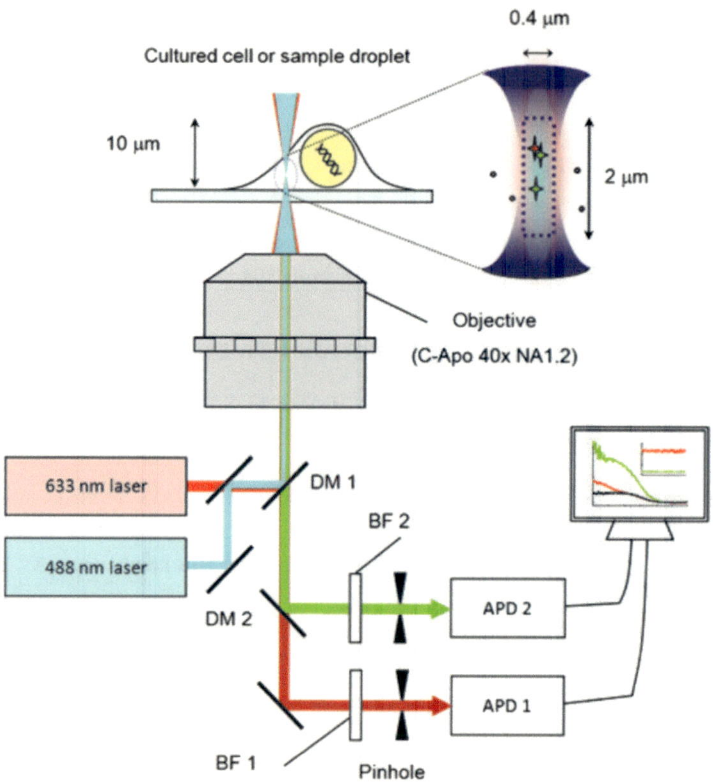

Fig. 4. Experimental setup for FCS and FCCS.

Instead of evaluating discrete diffusion processes with distinct species and their characteristic diffusion times, the dynamic motion of DNAs in the cell can be distributed with regard to their diffusion times using the distribution function $P(\tau D_i)$. The average numbers of red fluorescent particles (N_r), green fluorescent particles (N_g), and particles that have both red and green fluorescence (N_c) can be calculated by

$$N_r = \frac{1}{G_r(0) - 1}, \quad N_g = \frac{1}{G_g(0) - 1} \quad (3)$$

$$N_c = \frac{G_c(0) - 1}{[G_r(0) - 1] \cdot [G_g(0) - 1]} \tag{4}$$

respectively. When N_r and N_g are constant, ($G_c(0)$–1) is directly proportional to N_c. For quantitative evaluation of cross-correlations among various samples, the cross-correlation amplitude is normalized by autocorrelation amplitude (relative cross-correlation amplitude; RCA). RCA can be calculated by

$$RCA_g = \frac{G_c(0) - 1}{G_g(0) - 1} \tag{5}$$

$$RCA_r = \frac{G_c(0) - 1}{G_r(0) - 1} \tag{6}$$

respectively. The ratio of interacted molecule in red or green molecules can be obtained from equations 3 and 4 as

$$\frac{G_c(0) - 1}{G_g(0) - 1} = \frac{N_c}{N_r} \tag{7}$$

$$\frac{G_c(0) - 1}{G_r(0) - 1} = \frac{N_c}{N_g} \tag{8}$$

respectively. RCA_g shows the ratio of interacted molecules in the red molecules (N_c/N_r) (Eqs. 5 and 7) and RCA_r shows the ratio of interacted molecules in the green molecules (N_c/N_g) (Eqs. 6 and 8). FCCS measurement also gives the parameter of photon counts per molecule (CPM) of each fluorescent species. CPM is represented by count rate divided by number of particles.

3. Monitoring exogenous DNA degradation in living cells

Physical approaches such as microinjection (Zhang et al., 2008) and electroporation (Somiari et al., 2000) are performed to incorporate naked DNAs directly into cytoplasm and/or nucleus across the plasma membrane. On the other hand, DNAs are released into cytoplasm as naked shape and then the DNAs diffuse in the cytoplasm to the nucleus in the case of using gene carrier. The diffusion of exogenous DNAs in cytoplasm is relatively slow compared with that in solution (Dauty et al., 2005), and it is hard that large DNA goes cross the nuclear membrane in short time. Under such conditions in cytoplasm, the existence of nuclease degradation in cytoplasm is suggested (Pollard et al., 2001, Lechardeur et al., 1999, Fisher et al., 1993). It is presumed that the translocation and nuclear uptake of transfected DNA compete with digestion. Therefore, it is important to investigate behavior of naked exogenous DNAs in cytoplasm to achieve efficient gene delivery and expression. The cytoplasmic degradation for exogenous DNAs can work as a barrier against efficient gene delivery. However, little is known about the degradation mechanism because it is difficult to characterize the degradation process of exogenous DNA in living cells. The purpose of this section was to investigate the mechanism of exogenous DNA degradation in situ, in cytoplasm, by analyses of diffusion properties of DNAs and to determine the effects of cytoplasmic degradation on the gene expression rate. Thus we employed FCS to measure the diffusion properties of DNAs, and FCCS to monitor the degradation of DNAs by cytoplasmic nucleases at the single molecule level. Furthermore, we predicted that exonucleases would work as the main barrier in cytoplasm, so a capped or redundant structure was attached to the transfected DNA to enhance the expression of the protein EGFP.

3.1 Diffusion analysis of constructed DNAs in solution

A series of linear DNAs from 23 bp to 500 bp that were labeled with rhodamine green (RG) and Cy5 on both 5'ends (RG-DNA-Cy5) were synthesized by PCR. Autocorrelation curves of the green fluorescence channel ($G_g(\tau)$) and red fluorescence channel ($G_r(\tau)$), and a cross-correlation curve ($G_c(\tau)$) were obtained by FCCS measurements of RG-DNA-Cy5 in solution (Fig. 5A-D).

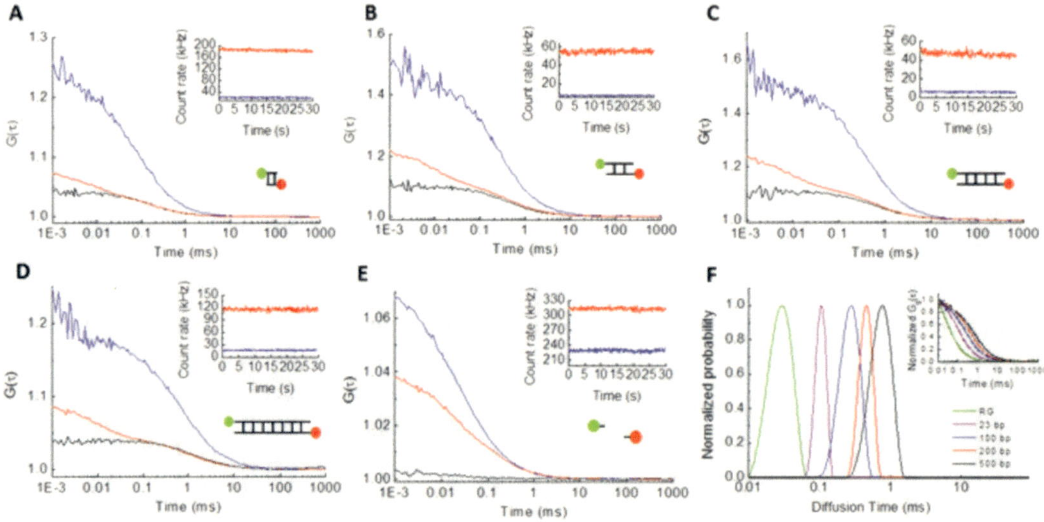

Fig. 5. Characterization of double-fluorescent-labeled DNAs in solution. Auto- and cross-correlation curves of (A) RG-23bp-Cy5 (B) RG-100bp-Cy5 (C) RG-200bp-Cy5 (D) RG-500bp-Cy5 DNA in 10 mM Tris-HCl (pH 7.4). (Insets) The fluorescence intensities in the red (red line) and green (blue line) channels during FCCS measurement. Blue, red and black lines represent $G_g(\tau)$, $G_r(\tau)$ and $G_c(\tau)$, respectively. (E) Auto- and cross-correlation curves of a mixture of RG-primer and Cy5-primer (23 mer each) as a negative control. (F) Distributions of diffusion times $P(\tau D_i)$ of various sizes of RG-DNA-Cy5 calculated from autocorrelation curves of the green channel by CONTIN algorithm. (Inset) Normalized autocorrelation curves $G_g(\tau)/G_g(0)$ (dot) with fitted curves (line) of DNAs in 10 mM Tris-HCl (pH 7.4) at room temperature.

To assess the degree of cross-correlation amplitude, relative cross-correlation amplitude (RCA) was calculated by dividing $G_c(0)-1$ by $G_r(0)-1$. The RCA value was 0.908±0.020 (mean ± S.D.) for the 500 bp DNA, which had double-fluorescent labels, and 0.104±0.023 for the mixture of fluorescent primers that were used in the PCR reactions (Fig. 5E). The RCA value represents the fraction of DNAs that have RG and Cy5 fluorophores at both DNA ends, thus intact DNAs. To extract information concerning the relative abundance and length of the

DNA from the autocorrelation curve, we used the CONTIN algorithm. The algorithm can determine the distribution of the correlation time with multiple peaks and its probability without any prior assumption about the number of peaks. Figure 5F shows the distributions of diffusion times that were calculated from the autocorrelation curve of the green channel (inset) by using the CONTIN algorithm. The spectra of diffusion times of RG-DNA-Cy5 were separated from each other. This result suggested that the length of the DNA could be estimated with sufficient resolution in this range and length.

3.2 Enzymatic degradation analysis in solution

To confirm whether FCS and FCCS could identify the degradation mechanisms of different kind of nucleases, we monitored the DNA degradation with DNase I (an endonuclease that acts randomly), exonuclease III (an exonuclease that acts in the 3′ to 5′ direction) and BAL31 nuclease (an exonuclease that acts in both 5′ to 3′ and 3′to 5′ directions) in solution. The nucleases were added to RG-500bp-Cy5 solution in a droplet (50 μl) on a coverslip and FCCS measurements were performed as a function of time (Fig. 6).

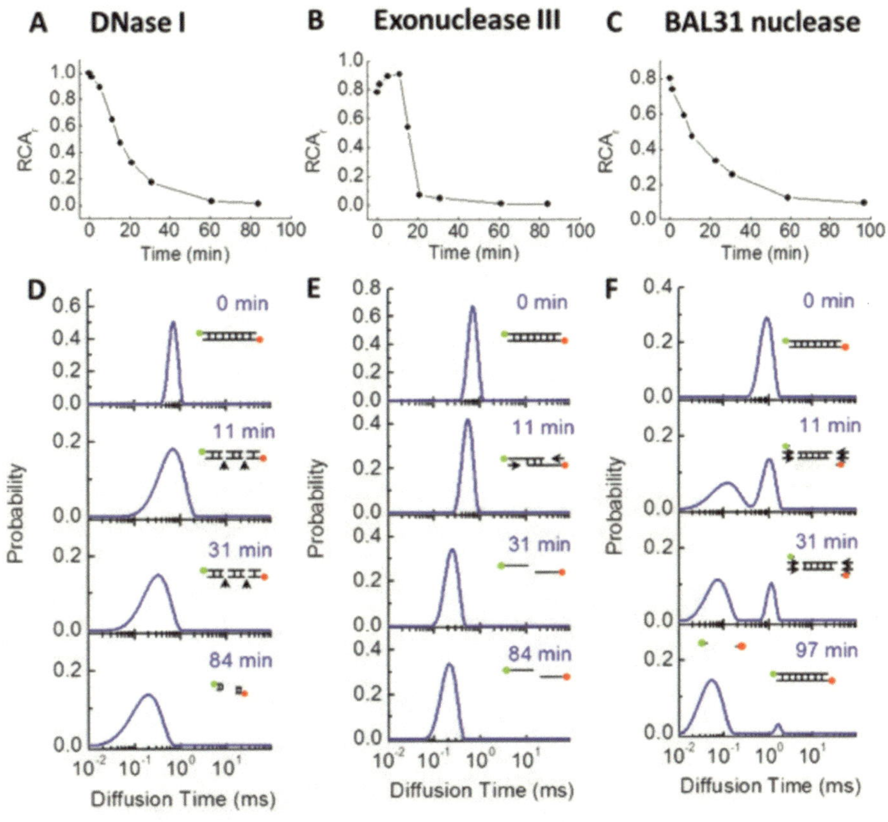

Fig. 6. Relative cross-correlation amplitudes, $(G_c(0)-1)/(G_r(0)-1)$ after addition of (A) 0.0001 U μl^{-1} DNase I, (B) 0.02 U μl^{-1} exonuclease III, and (C) 0.001 U μl^{-1} BAL31 nuclease. Distributions of diffusion times $P(\tau D_i)$ calculated by CONTIN algorithm from $G_g(\tau)$ at several time points after the addition of DNase I (D), exonuclease III (E) and BAL31 nuclease (F).

Figure 6A, B and C show the RCA changes of cross-correlation curves of RG-500bp-Cy5 with the three different type of nucleases. With DNase I and BAL31 nuclease, RCA values rapidly decreased after the nuclease addition. In contrast, with exonuclease III, the RCA value did not decrease until 11 min. This indicated that the fluorophores did not separate in the initial phase of degradation (Fig. 6E insets). The RCA value was not changed without addition of a nuclease in the measurement time (data not shown). We regarded 11 min as the initial phase, 31 min as the transient phase and 84–97 min as the stable phase of enzymatic reaction in Figure 6A, B and C. We performed CONTIN analysis and compared distributions of diffusion times in each phase (Fig. 6D–F). Changing of distribution of diffusion time and RCA show some kind of fingerprint of enzyme activity. The distribution peak became wider and shifted to the left with addition of DNase I (Fig. 6D). The peak width reflects the various lengths of DNA fragments generated by DNase I random degradation. In the case of exonuclease III, the enzyme generates two kinds of single-stranded DNA with the same sizes as the final products. The diffusion time shifted to the left at 31 min after nuclease addition without widening of the peak (Fig. 6E). Interestingly, two distribution peaks were detected with the BAL31 nuclease (Fig. 6F). A faster peak of diffusion times represents small fragments of DNA, with a level of diffusion time comparable to that of the RG fluorophore and a slower peak represents intact DNA. This result is reasonable since the BAL31 nuclease degrades the DNA from both the 5′ and 3′ends where the fluorophore is attached. Thus, we could identify the different enzymatic behaviors by using FCCS and distribution analysis of FCS without any separation method such as gel electrophoresis or gel filtration.

3.3 Detection of diffusion properties of exogenous DNAs in cytoplasm

To classify nuclease activity in the cytoplasm of living cells, fluorescent-labeled DNAs were directly introduced into the cytoplasm of living cells by the bead-loading method (Manders et al., 1999, Nagaya et al., 2002). RG-23bp-Cy5 localized largely in the nucleus (Figs. 7A, B, C) though, RG-100bp-Cy5 did not distribute into the nucleus (Figs. 7E, F, G, 8A and C).

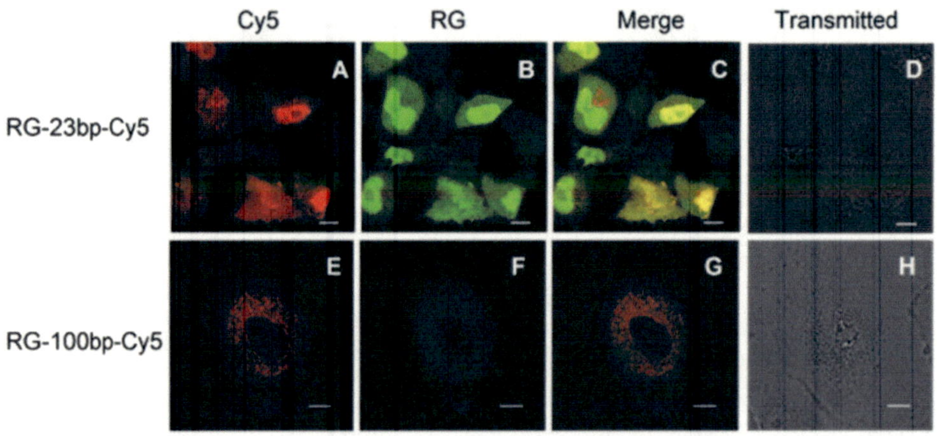

Fig. 7. LSM images of DNA loaded HeLa cells. LSM images of cells 30 min after loading of RG-23bp-Cy5 (A–D) or RG-100bp-Cy5 (E–H). Green (A, E), red (B, F), merged fluorescence images (C, G) and transmitted images (D, H), respectively. Scale bar represents 10 μm.

Auto- and cross-correlation curves of RG-100bp-Cy5 were obtained at the crosshair point in the image of laser scanning microscopy (LSM) of a living cell in which DNAs were incorporated into the cytoplasm (Fig. 8A, C). High cross-correlation amplitude was detected within 10 min after loading (Fig. 8B). However, cross-correlation amplitude was reduced after 45-min incubation at 37°C in the same cell (Fig. 8D). This reduction indicated that exogenous DNA was degraded in cytoplasm. DNA diffusion properties were also analyzed by distributions of diffusion times from autocorrelation curves using the CONTIN algorithm. At 45 min after loading of DNA, a faster peak (around 0.2 ms) appeared in distributions of diffusion times (Fig. 8D inset).

To determine the origin of each peak in the distributions of diffusion times, autocorrelation curves $G_g(\tau)$s of different DNA sizes that were obtained for the cytoplasm of HeLa cells, and were averaged (N = 4–8) and analyzed using the CONTIN algorithm (Fig. 9). Two peaks of diffusion times were detected in each measurement; faster peaks were of the same order of diffusion time as the free RG fluorophore.

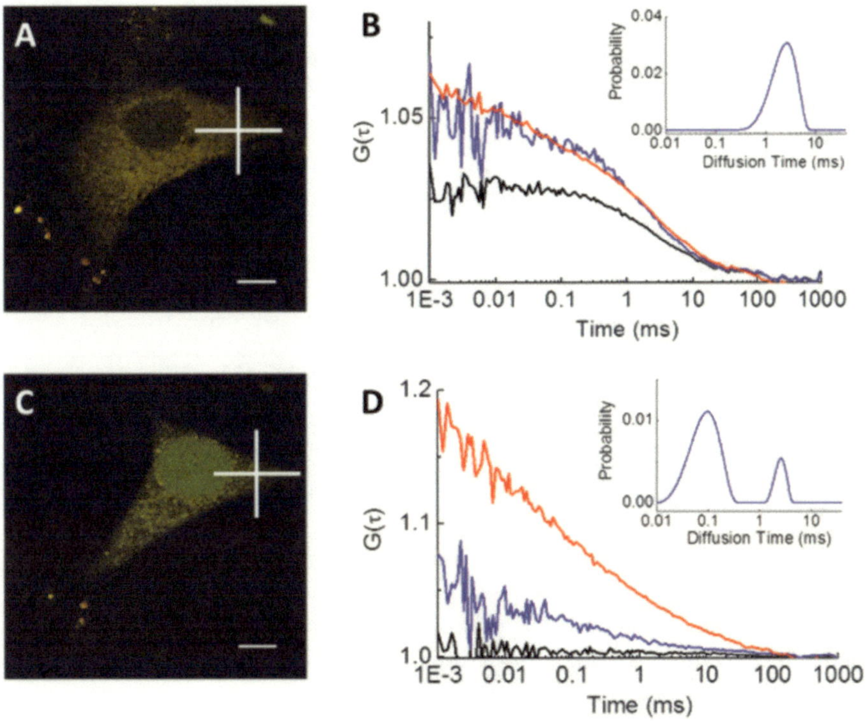

Fig. 8. Nuclease degradation of double-fluorescent-labeled DNAs in cytoplasm of a living COS7 cell. LSM images of (A) 10 min and (C) 45 min after loading of DNAs in the same cell. Auto- and cross-correlation curves of RG-100bp-Cy5 DNA at the crosshairs in the LSM image of (B) panel A (D) panel C. Scale bar represents 10 μm. RG, Cy5 and Cross represent $G_g(\tau)$, $G_r(\tau)$ and $G_c(\tau)$, respectively. Distributions of diffusion times $P(\tau D_i)$ of DNAs calculated by CONTIN algorithm (B, D insets).

On the other hand, the diffusion times of the slower peaks shifted to the right according to the increase in size of incorporated DNA (Fig. 9B). The diffusion times of DNAs in cytoplasm were 5–10 times slower than those in solution. This ratio was in good agreement with the previously reported value (Dauty et al., 2005) and this result agreed well with the 5′ to 3′ exonuclease degradation models in solution (Fig. 6F). Finally, the appearance of 5′ to 3′ exonuclease activity was expected as barrier activity in cytoplasm by comparison of incorporated exogenous DNAs using the distribution pattern of diffusion times. Distribution analysis of diffusion times using CONTIN algorithm clearly showed different peak patterns for different enzymatic activities. The distributions of diffusion times had two peaks in cytoplasm. The diffusion time of the faster peak was almost the same as that of fluorescent dye alone, whereas the other, slower peak depended on the size of the DNA that was incorporated. Moreover, moderately sized DNA fragments were not detected in the cytoplasm. Taken together, these findings helped us to determine that (i) how, (ii) when, and (iii) where incorporated DNAs were degraded in the living cell. (i) The main mechanism of exogenous DNA degradation in cytoplasm was 5′ to 3′ exonuclease activity rather than endonucleases. (ii) The time scale of degradation (<45 min) was determined by real-time measurement of optical method without invasive treatment. (iii) The location of DNA degradation was not in small compartments but in cytoplasm because the monitored DNAs were distributed homogenously and had free diffusion values.

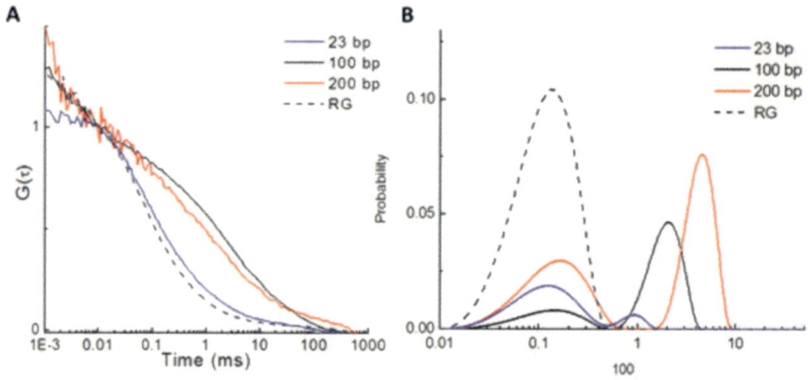

Fig. 9. Relationship between DNA size and diffusion time in living HeLa cells. (A) The average of $G_g(\tau)$ curves in HeLa cytoplasm at 30 min after RG-23bp-Cy5, RG-100bp-Cy5 and RG-200bp-Cy5 loading. (B) Distributions of diffusion times $P(\tau D_i)$ of DNAs calculated from the average of $G_g(\tau)$ curves using CONTIN algorithm. RG dye was also tested as a reference.

3.4 Effect of DNA end-capping on the EGFP expression efficiency

To confirm the enzymatic activity of the 5′ to 3′ exonuclease in cytoplasm, we carried out an inhibition experiment for the enzyme using end-capped or redundant DNAs and monitoring the expression rate of EGFP. If exonuclease degradation works as a barrier against DNA transfection, the use of longer DNA and/or end-capped-DNA that protects the coding regions from each terminal (Fig. 10) should increase the expression efficiency. We synthesized linear DNAs of various redundancy lengths and capped on both DNA ends by a hairpin-shape oligonucleotide (Zanta et al., 1999, van der Aa et al., 2005). The end-capped DNA remained intact after incubation with exonuclease III (data not shown). Fig. 11 shows

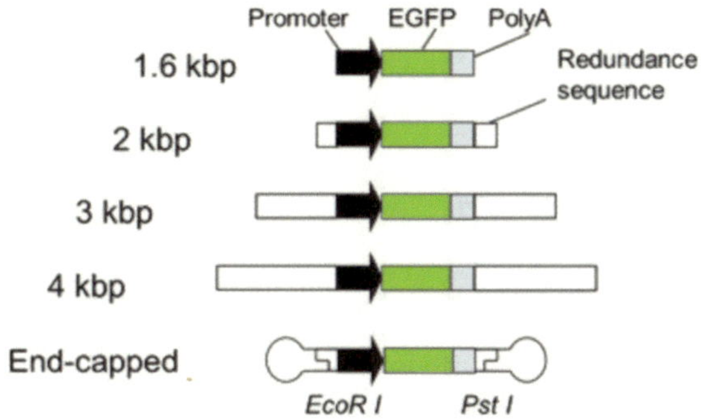

Fig. 10. Schematic diagram of various sizes of DNA expressing EGFP and end-capped DNA.

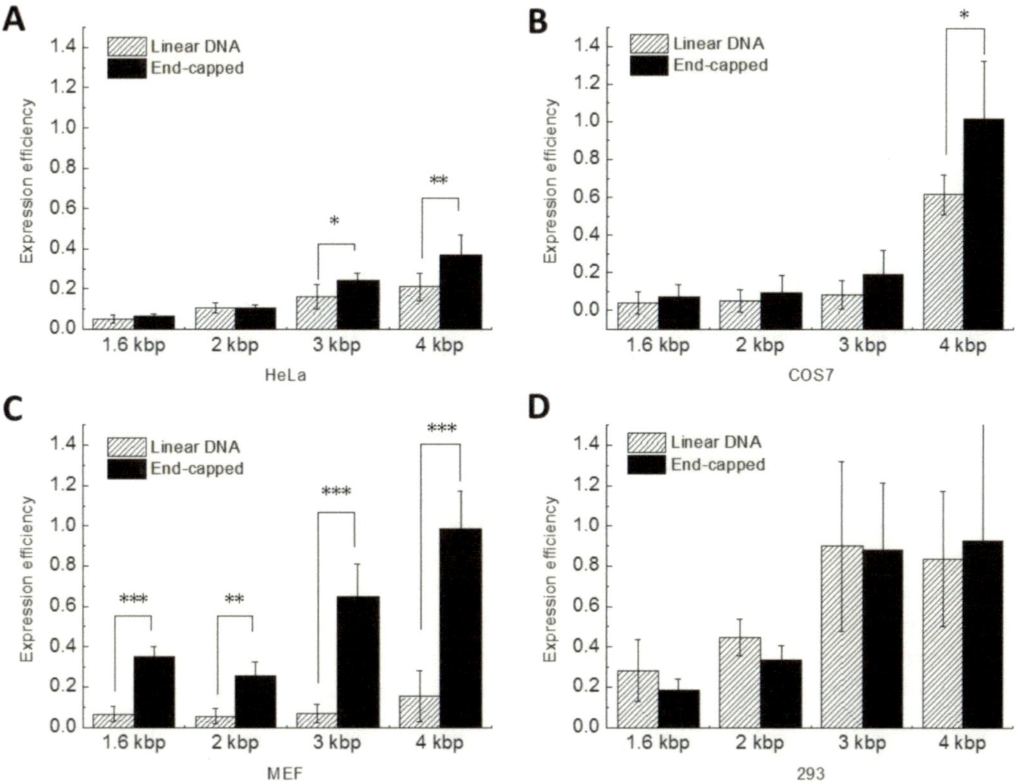

Fig. 11. Effect of DNA protection against exonucleases on expression efficiency with a cationic lipid. (A) HeLa, (B) COS7, (C) MEF and (D) 293 cells were transfected with 1 μg of uncapped or capped linear DNA per well. Complexes were formed with LipofectAmine 2000 reagent. Expression efficiency (E/Ep) is expressed as the mean ± S.D. of 4–5 different experiments. To normalize the values from each individual experiment, the expression rate of DNA was divided by the rate using the pEGFP-C1 plasmid. *, $P<0.05$; **, $P<0.01$; ***, $P<0.001$ (Student's t test). Striped bars, uncapped linear DNA; brack bars, end-capped DNA.

the expression efficiencies of DNAs in HeLa, COS7, MEF and 293 cells, respectively. The expression efficiency was based on the EGFP expression per copy of transfected DNA ($N \cdot M/W$), the value was divided by the expression of pEGFP-C1 plasmid for normalization ($N_p \cdot M_p/W_p$). The final expression efficiency was calculated by following equation,

$$Expression\ efficiency = \frac{N \cdot M/W}{N_p \cdot M_p/W_p} \quad (9)$$

where N, W, and M represent the number of EGFPs obtained from FCS measurement, the transfected DNA weight and molecular weight of transfected DNA, respectively. N_p, W_p and M_p represent the values with the pEGFP-C1 plasmid as a reference.

Expression efficiencies of short DNAs such as that with a 1.6 kbp length were lower than those of other lengths in each cell line. When the expression efficiencies of non-capped PCR products and capped DNAs were compared, it was clear that DNA capping significantly increased the expression efficiency of 4 kbp DNA in HeLa, COS7 and MEF cells. However, the end capping did not enhance the expression rate for short DNA lengths. In MEF cells, uncapped DNAs of all lengths were little expressed and capped DNAs exhibited ~10-fold greater gene expression than the uncapped DNAs. The effect of DNA capping was not observed in 293 cells. Although there were differences in the cell lines, the results obtained for HeLa, COS7 and MEF cells confirmed the effect of exonuclease degradation on DNA transfection. The nuclease activity was inhibited by capped structures on the 3′ and 5′ ends of the DNA. Interestingly, the end-capping effect on the expression rate was different in the cell lines. In MEF cells, which are generally said to be hard to transfect (Ewert et al., 2006), the end-capping effect was significant (Fig. 11C). On the other hand, in 293 cells, which are generally used in transfection assays because of their high expression efficiency, no end-capping effect was observed (Fig. 11D). These results agreed with previous reports that the transfected plasmids were more stable in 293 cells than in COS, NIH-3T3, HeLa cells (Alwine, 1985). In summary, our results show that exonuclease activity is related to transfection efficiency, though the level of exonuclease activitity in cytoplasm might be different depending on the cell line.

Here we propose new concept of nuclease characterization by monitoring the degradation patterns of oligonucleotides based on the fragment size and direction of degradation in living cells. The concept is similar to conventional ones such as an analysis by using radioisotope-labeled oligonucleotides and a size determination by gel electrophoresis. The relationship between the exogenous DNA expression level and DNA stability by extension of DNA fragments was studied using the luciferase assay in vitro and in vivo (Hirata et al., 2007); however, this assay in a cell homogenate only provides information on bulk DNA stability, not on the individual DNA degradation mechanism. Our approach is, therefore, replacement of the conventional concept by diffusion measurement using a fluorescent tag and coincident analysis using FCS and FCCS so that sensitivity is enhanced to the single molecule level and a physical separation procedure is not needed. Therefore, our method can be employed for measurements in single living cells.

4. Monitoring complex formation between gene carriers and nucleic acids

The association and dissociation between DNA and gene carriers are important *in vitro* and *in vivo*. The efficiency of DNA internalization depends on the properties of DNA/carrier complexes such as their sizes. The size is determined by affinity between DNAs and carriers and the ratio of DNAs to carrier molecules. The FCCS method has the advantage that it does not need physical separation procedures, so the association and dissociation of DNA and carriers can be directly monitored not only in solution but also in living cells.

4.1 Quantum dot based gene carrier

Quantum dots (QDs) are nanometer-sized semiconductor crystals that emit visible to infrared fluorescence depending on their composition and diameter. QDs have several advantages such as high resistance to photobleaching, high brightness and narrow emission wavelengths with broad excitation spectra. QDs are comprised of an inorganic core, inorganic shell and an organic coating to solubilize them to the water phase. Since the surface to volume ratio of a QD is relatively high, QDs can be used as scaffold particles for carrying ligands, therapeutic agents and gene delivery carriers.
Cationic polymers can condense with DNA by electrostatic interaction to form complexes that promote internalization of exogenous DNA into cells. Polyethyleneimine (PEI) is an efficient gene carrier, that has a proton-sponge effect (Boussif et al., 1995). PEI solubilizes QDs to water so it is also useful for surface coating of QDs (Duan et al., 2007, Zhu et al., 2005).

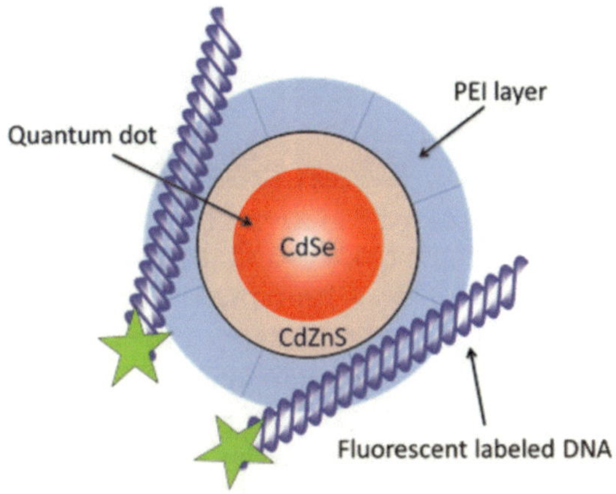

Fig. 12. Diagram of PEI-QD. PEI-coated QD forms a complex with DNA.

CdSe/CdZnS QD cores that emit 605 nm fluorescence were synthesized (Jin et al., 2010) and PEI (average molecular weight about 10000) was added and heated to 60°C in tetrahydrofuran. The resulting precipitates of PEI-coated QDs were dissolved in water (PEI-QDs). The PEI-QD solution was then mixed with a plasmid that coded red fluorescent protein, mKate2 (pmKate2-N). To visualize the localization of the plasmid, a sample plasmid was stained with YOYO-1 iodide. Then the plasmid/PEI-QD complex was added to cultured HeLa cells. After 24-hour incubation, fluorescence emission of expressed mKate2 was detected (Fig. 13). The result showed that PEI-QD had the potential to introduce plasmid vectors into cells. Fluorescence of QDs and YOYO-1 colocalized at large complexes, though free molecules or small complexes were not visible by the conventional microscopy, so methods that can detect their diffusion at the single molecule level, such as FCS and FCCS, are needed.

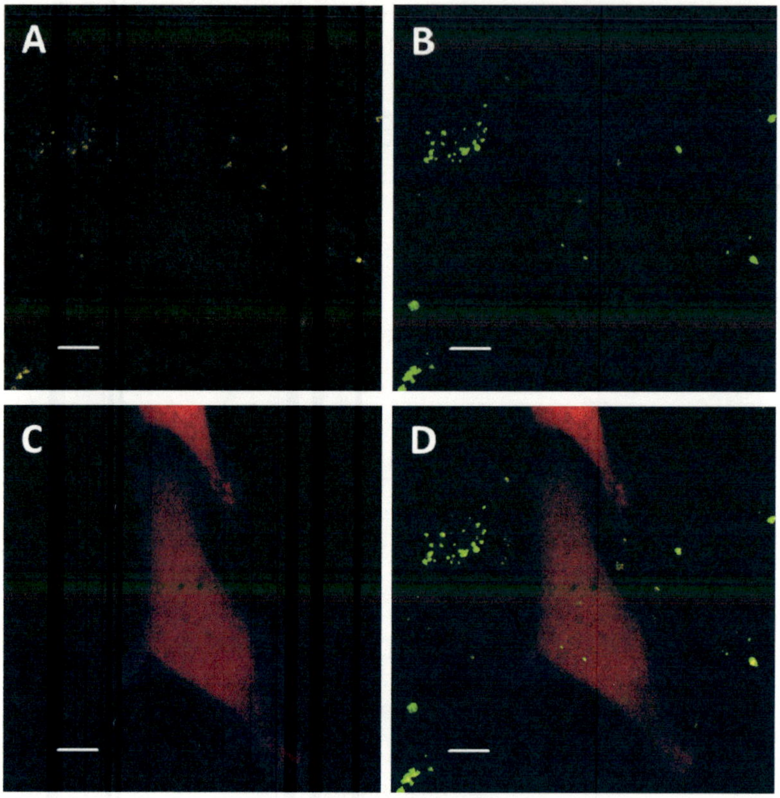

Fig. 13. LSM images of DNA transfected HeLa cells. LSM images of cells 24 hours after addition of PEI-QD/pmKate2-N. QDs (A), YOYO-1 (B), mKate2 (C) and merged fluorescence images (D) respectively. Scale bar represents 10 μm.

4.2 Monitoring of DNA/PEI complex formation in vitro

The efficiency of gene delivery by DNA/carrier complexes depends on the size of the complex and the dissociation kinetics in cells.

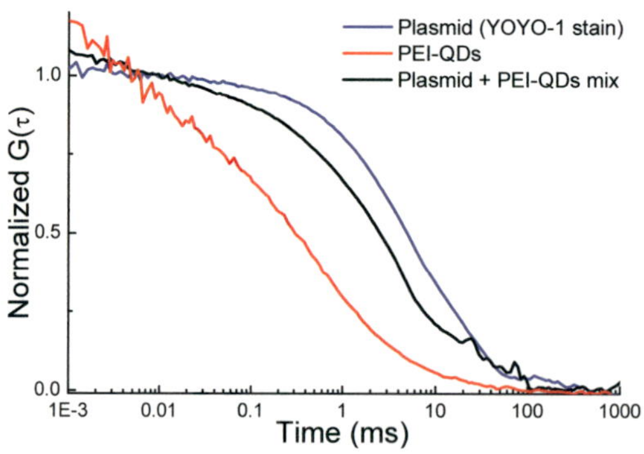

Fig. 14. Normalized autocorrelation curves of plasmid DNA (blue line), PEI-QDs (red line) and a mixture of the plasmid and PEI-QD (black line) in solution.

To develop an efficient gene carrier, it is necessary to characterize the properties of the DNA/carrier complexes. Previously the characterization of complexes was carried out by gel electrophoresis (Eastman et al., 1997).

Currently, there are several FCS studies of DNA/carrier association and dissociation (Van Rompaey et al., 2001, Braeckmans et al., 2010). By using FCS, the size and the ratio of the DNA to the gene carrier are evaluated in solution from the values of the diffusion time and CPM, which are obtained by FCS measurements (see section 2). A 4 kbp circular-shaped plasmid was mixed the PEI-QDs and FCS measurements were carried out. The diffusion time of the plasmid decreased due to the compaction of DNA by the interaction with the cationic gene carrier (Fig. 14).

On the other hand, FCCS can monitor the interaction of DNA with a gene carrier directly. FCS monitors the change of the diffusion time (or molecular size) though the interaction cannot be distinguished if the diffusion time is decreased or not changed due to the change of the molecular shape. For demonstration, PEI-QDs and rhodamine green-labeled 500 bp linear DNA (RG-500bp) were mixed at various ratios, and then FCCS measurements were carried out with single-laser excitation at 488 nm (Fujii et al., 2007). Fluorescence emissions were collected from two channels for rhodamine green and QD. The increase of autocorrelation amplitude of the green channel (RG-500bp) made observation of the DNA complex possible (Fig. 15). The cross-correlation amplitude was also increased (Fig. 15). This high cross-correlation amplitude directly shows the incorporation of RG-500bp and the PEI-QDs.

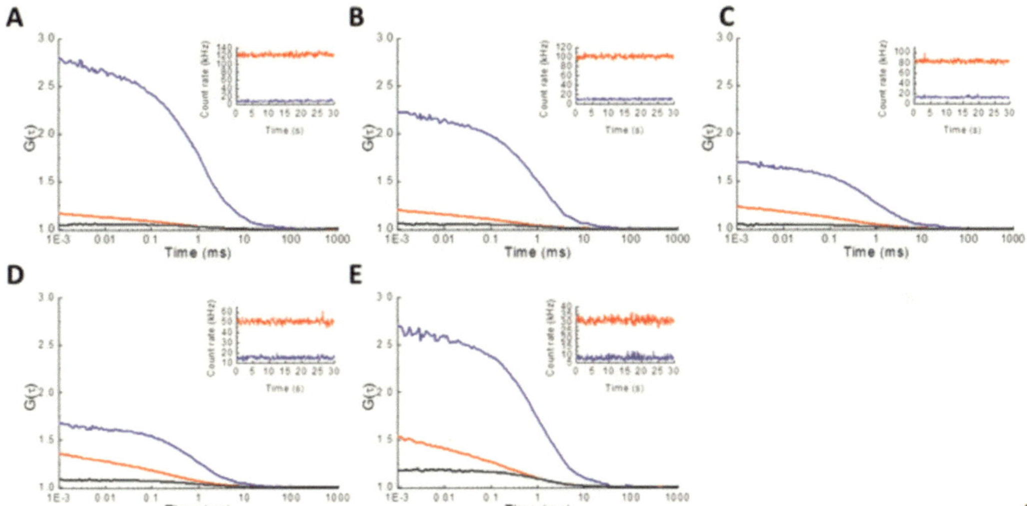

Fig. 15. Cross-correlation analysis of RG-500bp and PEI-QDs. The correlation curves of various RG-500bp/PEI-QD ratios (A; 0.5, B; 1, C; 2, D; 4, E; 8). Blue, red and black lines represent $G_g(\tau)$, $G_r(\tau)$ and $G_c(\tau)$, respectively.

The RCA_r value was increased according to the increase of the PEI-QD concentration (Fig. 16A). At a low DNA/QD ratio, the number of PEI-QDs in solution was larger than the number of RG-500bp so there were many QDs that did not interact with DNA. On the other hand, RCA_g was decreased at once by the decrease of PEI-QD because of the relative decrease of interacting partners (Fig. 16C). The numbers of RG-500bp and PEI-QDs contained in the complexes could be estimated from the value of CPM. The CPMs of the green channel were 4 to 8 times larger than the value of a single RG-500bp and the CPMs of the red channel were comparable to the value of a single PEI-QD (Fig. 16B). These results indicated that 4 to 8 RG-500bp molecules and a single PEI-QD particle were contained in the complexes under the tested conditions. At high ratios of DNA/QDs, DNA and QDs may aggregate so that RCA_r and CPM_g are increased. The FCCS technique has strong advantages to investigate the properties of DNA carriers such as the strength of binding between DNA and the carrier, the size of the complex and the amount of DNA and number of carriers contained in the complex.

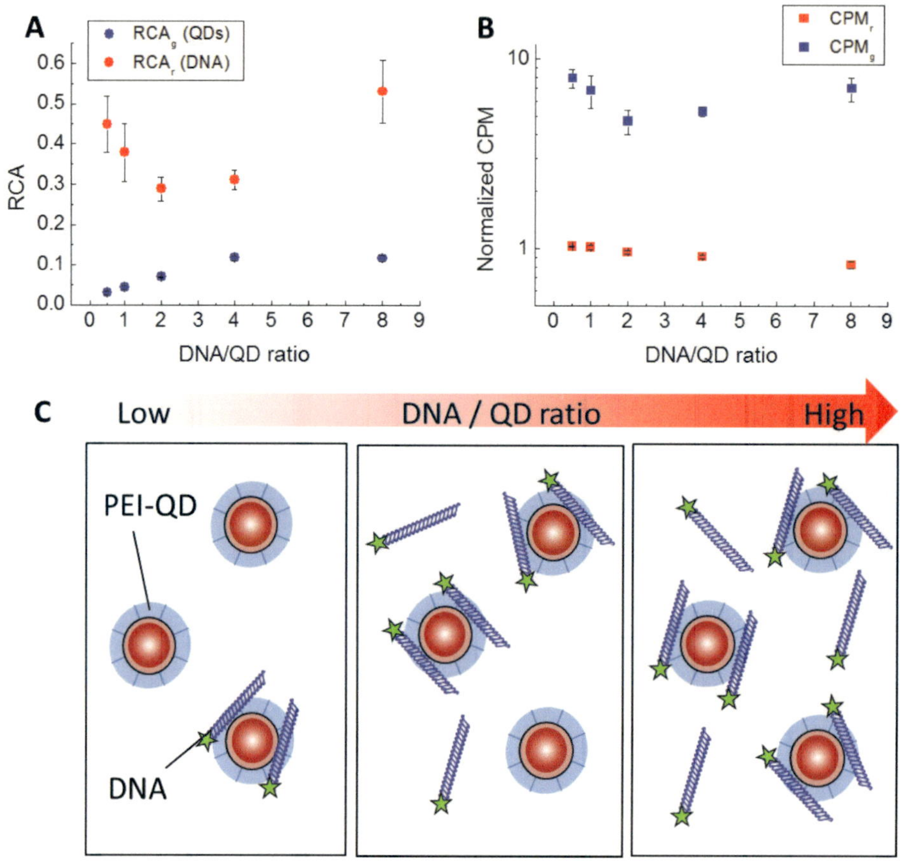

Fig. 16. RCA values (A) and normalized CPM (B) of RG-500bp/PEI-QD complexes. CPM values were normalized by the CPM of a single RG-500bp or PEI-QD. Note that RCA_g shows the ratio of interacting molecules among the red molecules (N_c/N_r). RCA_r shows the ratio of interacting molecules among the green molecules (N_c/N_g) (see Eq. 7 and 8). (C) Schematic diagrams of DNA/QD interactions at various ratios.

5. Conclusion

It is necessary to ascertain the fate of exogenous DNA for the development of nonviral gene therapy. FCS and FCCS, which provide spatiotemporal information on diffusion properties and interactions of biomolecules, were employed for analyses in living cells. FCCS experiments revealed rapid DNA degradation in cytoplasm. In addition, the DNA degradation mechanism in cytoplasm due to 5′ to 3′ exonuclease was estimated by measuring DNA diffusion properties at the single molecule level. The methods using noninvasive monitoring of the diffusion properties of DNA provide information on the fate of intracellular exogenous DNA and the efficiency of DNA integration in living cells. Understanding of these intracellular events should help with the development of novel efficient gene delivery methods.

FCS and FCCS are rapidly becoming widely used to detect movements and interactions of biomolecules in living cells (Chenette, 2009, Lidke et al., 2009), and various related applications such as two-focus FCS (Yu et al., 2009), raster image correlation spectroscopy (RICS) (Digman et al., 2009) and multi-point total internal reflection-fluorescence correlation spectroscopy (TIR-FCS) (Ohsugi et al., 2006, 2009) have been developed. FCS, FCCS and these techniques will shed new light on cell biology and gene therapy.

6. Acknowledgements

The authors thank Professor Takashi Jin (Osaka University) for providing various types of quantum dot cores. Our research was partly supported by Grants-in-Aid for Scientific Research (A) 18207010 and (S)21221006, by Grants-in-Aid for Exploratory Research (20657035) from the JSPS, and No. 19058001 in Priority Area "Protein Community."

7. References

Alwine, J., (1985). Transient gene expression control: effects of transfected DNA stability and trans-activation by viral early proteins. *Mol Cell Biol*, 5 (5), 1034-42.

Bacia, K. & Schwille, P., (2007). Practical guidelines for dual-color fluorescence cross-correlation spectroscopy. *Nat Protoc*, 2842-2856.

Björling, S.; Kinjo, M.; Földes-Papp, Z.; Hagman, E.; Thyberg, P. & Rigler, R., (1998). Fluorescence correlation spectroscopy of enzymatic DNA polymerization. *Biochemistry*, 37 (37), 12971-8.

Boussif, O.; Lezoualc'h, F.; Zanta, M.; Mergny, M.; Scherman, D.; Demeneix, B. & Behr, J., (1995). A versatile vector for gene and oligonucleotide transfer into cells in culture and in vivo: polyethylenimine. *Proc Natl Acad Sci U S A*, 92 (16), 7297-301.

Braeckmans, K.; Buyens, K.; Naeye, B.; Vercauteren, D.; Deschout, H.; Raemdonck, K.; Remaut, K.; Sanders, N. N.; Demeester, J. & De Smedt, S. C., (2010). Advanced fluorescence microscopy methods illuminate the transfection pathway of nucleic acid nanoparticles. *J Control Release*, 148 (1), 69-74.

Chenette, EJ.; (2009). Milestone 10 FCS and FRAP: illuminating cellular processes. *Nat Milestones*, S13-S14

Chu, G.; Hayakawa, H. & Berg, P., (1987). Electroporation for the efficient transfection of mammalian cells with DNA. *Nucleic Acids Res*, 15 (3), 1311-26.

Dauty, E. & Verkman, A., (2005). Actin cytoskeleton as the principal determinant of size-dependent DNA mobility in cytoplasm: a new barrier for non-viral gene delivery. *J Biol Chem*, 280 (9), 7823-8.

Digman, M.; Wiseman, P.; Horwitz, A. & Gratton, E., (2009). Detecting protein complexes in living cells from laser scanning confocal image sequences by the cross correlation raster image spectroscopy method. *Biophys J*, 96 (2), 707-16.

Duan, H. & Nie, S., (2007). Cell-penetrating quantum dots based on multivalent and endosome-disrupting surface coatings. *J Am Chem Soc*, 129 (11), 3333-8.

Eastman, S. J.; Siegel, C.; Tousignant, J.; Smith, A. E.; Cheng, S. H. & Scheule, R. K., (1997). Biophysical characterization of cationic lipid: DNA complexes. *Biochim Biophys Acta*, 1325 (1), 41-62.

Eigen, M. & Rigler, R., (1994). Sorting single molecules: application to diagnostics and evolutionary biotechnology. *Proc Natl Acad Sci U S A*, 91 (13), 5740-7.

Elouahabi, A. & Ruysschaert, J., (2005). Formation and intracellular trafficking of lipoplexes and polyplexes. *Mol Ther*, 11 (3), 336-47.

Ewert, K.; Evans, H.; Zidovska, A.; Bouxsein, N.; Ahmad, A. & Safinya, C., (2006). A columnar phase of dendritic lipid-based cationic liposome-DNA complexes for gene delivery: hexagonally ordered cylindrical micelles embedded in a DNA honeycomb lattice. *J Am Chem Soc*, 128 (12), 3998-4006.

Felgner, P.; Gadek, T.; Holm, M.; Roman, R.; Chan, H.; Wenz, M.; Northrop, J.; Ringold, G. & Danielsen, M., (1987). Lipofection: a highly efficient, lipid-mediated DNA-transfection procedure. *Proc Natl Acad Sci U S A*, 84 (21), 7413-7.

Fisher, T.; Terhorst, T.; Cao, X. & Wagner, R., (1993). Intracellular disposition and metabolism of fluorescently-labeled unmodified and modified oligonucleotides microinjected into mammalian cells. *Nucleic Acids Res*, 21 (16), 3857-65.

Fujii, F. & Kinjo, M., (2007). Detection of antigen protein by using fluorescence cross-correlation spectroscopy and quantum-dot-labeled antibodies. *Chembiochem*, 8 (18), 2199-203.

Hirata, K.; Nishikawa, M.; Kobayashi, N.; Takahashi, Y. & Takakura, Y., (2007). Design of PCR-amplified DNA fragments for in vivo gene delivery: size-dependency on stability and transgene expression. *J Pharm Sci*, 96 (9), 2251-61.

Jin, T.; Sasaki, A.; Kinjo, M. & Miyazaki, J., (2010). A quantum dot-based ratiometric pH sensor. *Chem Commun (Camb)*, 46 (14), 2408-10.

Kim, S.; Heinze, K. & Schwille, P., (2007). Fluorescence correlation spectroscopy in living cells. *Nat Methods*, 963-973.

Kinjo, M.; Sakata, H. & Mikuni, S., (2010). First steps for fluorescence correlation spectroscopy of living cells. *Live Cell Imaging – A Laboratory Manual - second edition*, pp. 229-238, ISBN 978-0-87969-892-8.

Kinjo, M. & Rigler, R., (1995). Ultrasensitive hybridization analysis using fluorescence correlation spectroscopy. *Nucleic Acids Res*, 23 (10), 1795-9.

Kitamura, A.; Kubota, H.; Pack, C.; Matsumoto, G.; Hirayama, S.; Takahashi, Y.; Kimura, H.; Kinjo, M.; Morimoto, R. & Nagata, K., (2006). Cytosolic chaperonin prevents polyglutamine toxicity with altering the aggregation state. *Nat Cell Biol*, 8 (10), 1163-70.

Kogure, T.; Karasawa, S.; Araki, T.; Saito, K.; Kinjo, M. & Miyawaki, A., (2006). A fluorescent variant of a protein from the stony coral Montipora facilitates dual-color single-laser fluorescence cross-correlation spectroscopy. *Nat Biotechnol*, 24 (5), 577-81.

Lechardeur, D.; Sohn, K.; Haardt, M.; Joshi, P.; Monck, M.; Graham, R.; Beatty, B.; Squire, J.; O'Brodovich, H. & Lukacs, G., (1999). Metabolic instability of plasmid DNA in the cytosol: a potential barrier to gene transfer. *Gene Ther*, 6 (4), 482-97.

Lidke, D. & Wilson, B., (2009). Caught in the act: quantifying protein behaviour in living cells. *Trends Cell Biol*, 19 (11), 566-74.

Luo, D. & Saltzman, W., (2000). Synthetic DNA delivery systems. *Nat Biotechnol*, 18 (1), 33-7.

Manders, E.; Kimura, H. & Cook, P., (1999). Direct imaging of DNA in living cells reveals the dynamics of chromosome formation. *J Cell Biol*, 144 (5), 813-21.

Nagaya, H.; Wada, I.; Jia, Y. & Kanoh, H., (2002). Diacylglycerol kinase delta suppresses ER-to-Golgi traffic via its SAM and PH domains. *Mol Biol Cell*, 13 (1), 302-16.

Ohsugi, Y.; Saito, K.; Tamura, M. & Kinjo, M., (2006). Lateral mobility of membrane-binding proteins in living cells measured by total internal reflection fluorescence correlation spectroscopy. *Biophys J*, 91 (9), 3456-64.

Ohsugi, Y. & Kinjo, M., (2009). Multipoint fluorescence correlation spectroscopy with total internal reflection fluorescence microscope. *J Biomed Opt*, 14 (1), 014030.

Pollard, H.; Toumaniantz, G.; Amos, J.; Avet-Loiseau, H.; Guihard, G.; Behr, J. & Escande, D., (2001). Ca2+-sensitive cytosolic nucleases prevent efficient delivery to the nucleus of injected plasmids. *J Gene Med*, 3 (2), 153-64.

Provencher, S., (1982). A constrained regularization method for inverting data represented by linear algebraic or integral-equations. *Comput Phys Commun*, 27 (3), 213-227.

Provencher, S., (1982). CONTIN - A general-purpose constrained regularization program for inverting noisy linear algebraic and integral-equations. *Comput Phys Commun*, 27 (3), 229-242.

Remaut, K.; Lucas, B.; Raemdonck, K.; Braeckmans, K.; Demeester, J. & De Smedt, S., (2007). Can we better understand the intracellular behavior of DNA nanoparticles by fluorescence correlation spectroscopy? *J Control Release*, 121 (1-2), 49-63.

Rigler, R.; Mets, U.; Widengren, J. & Kask, P., (1993). Fluorescence correlation spectroscopy with high count rate and low-background - analysis of translational diffusion. *Euro Biophys J Biophys Let*, 169-175.

Sasaki, A. & Kinjo, M.; (2010). Monitoring intracellular degradation of exogenous DNA using diffusion properties. *J Control Release*, 143(1), 104-11.

Saito, K.; Wada, I.; Tamura, M. & Kinjo, M., (2004). Direct detection of caspase-3 activation in single live cells by cross-correlation analysis. *Biochem Biophys Res Commun*, 324 (2), 849-54.

Schaffert, D. & Wagner, E., (2008). Gene therapy progress and prospects: synthetic polymer-based systems. *Gene Ther*, 15 (16), 1131-8.

Selkirk, S., (2004). Gene therapy in clinical medicine. *Postgrad Med J*, 80 (948), 560-70.

Somiari, S.; Glasspool-Malone, J.; Drabick, J.; Gilbert, R.; Heller, R.; Jaroszeski, M. & Malone, R., (2000). Theory and in vivo application of electroporative gene delivery. *Mol Ther*, 2 (3), 178-87.

Thomas, C.; Ehrhardt, A. & Kay, M., (2003). Progress and problems with the use of viral vectors for gene therapy. *Nat Rev Genet*, 4 (5), 346-58.

van der Aa, M.; Koning, G.; van der Gugten, J.; d'Oliveira, C.; Oosting, R.; Hennink, W. & Crommelin, D., (2005). Covalent attachment of an NLS-peptide to linear DNA does not enhance transfection efficiency of cationic polymer based gene delivery systems. *J Control Release*, 101 (1-3), 395-7.

Van Rompaey, E.; Engelborghs, Y.; Sanders, N.; De Smedt, S. C. & Demeester, J., (2001). Interactions between oligonucleotides and cationic polymers investigated by fluorescence correlation spectroscopy. *Pharm Res*, 18 (7), 928-36.

Widengren, J.; Mets, U. & Rigler, R., (1995). Fluorescence correlation spectroscopy of triplet-states in solution - a theoretical and experimental-study. *J Physical Chem*, 13368-13379.

Yu, S.; Burkhardt, M.; Nowak, M.; Ries, J.; Petrásek, Z.; Scholpp, S.; Schwille, P. & Brand, M., (2009). Fgf8 morphogen gradient forms by a source-sink mechanism with freely diffusing molecules. *Nature*, 461 (7263), 533-6.

Zanta, M.; Belguise-Valladier, P. & Behr, J., (1999). Gene delivery: a single nuclear localization signal peptide is sufficient to carry DNA to the cell nucleus. *Proc Natl Acad Sci U S A*, 96 (1), 91-6.

Zhang, Y. & Yu, L., (2008). Microinjection as a tool of mechanical delivery. *Curr Opin Biotechnol*, 19 (5), 506-10.

Zhu, J.; Tang, A.; Law, L. P.; Feng, M.; Ho, K. M.; Lee, D. K.; Harris, F. W. & Li, P., (2005). Amphiphilic core-shell nanoparticles with poly(ethylenimine) shells as potential gene delivery carriers. *Bioconjug Chem*, 16 (1), 139-46.

Alpha-1 Antitrypsin Deficiency: Recent Developments in Gene Therapy Research

Catherine M. Greene and Noel G. McElvaney
Royal College of Surgeons in Ireland, Education and Research Centre, Beaumont Hospital, Dublin 9. Ireland

1. Introduction

Alpha-1 antitrypsin (AAT) deficiency is a hereditary disorder associated with mutations in the *SERPINA1* gene (Kelly et al., 2008; Greene et al., 2008). Over 100 different alleles have been identified however the most common disease-causing mutation, termed Z, encodes a glutamic acid to lysine substitution at position 342 of the mature AAT protein. As a member of the serine proteinase inhibitor family, the role of AAT is to inhibit serine proteases throughout the body but principally in the lung. The ZAAT protein fails to adopt the correct protein conformation and polymerises and accumulates intracellularly in AAT-producing cells. The liver is the major source of the body's pool of AAT. The major consequences of ZAAT accumulation in hepatocytes are toxic gain of function events leading to endoplasmic reticulum (ER) expansion and dilation and activation of multiple ER stress signalling pathways (Lomas et al., 1992; Teckman & Perlmutter, 2000; Lawless et al., 2004; Hidvegi et al., 2005; Hidvegi et al., 2007; Miller et al., 2007). These predispose to liver failure. The second major clinical consequence of ZAAT deficiency is a lower than normal antiprotease protective screen throughout the body, but most importantly in the lung (Lomas et al., 1993). ZAAT deficient individuals can develop emphysematous lung disease as early as in their 4th decade.

Gene therapies to treat both aspects of the disease are currently at various stages of development. For the liver disease approaches that can be considered include ribozymes, antisense, peptide nucleic acids and small-interfering RNAs; all designed to inhibit expression of the mutant gene (recently reviewed in McLean et al., 2009). For the lung disease gene therapies using non-viral, lentiviral and adeno-associated viral approaches to express the normal gene either locally or intramuscularly have been reported (Chulay et al., 2011; Brantly et al., 2006; Flotte et al., 2007; Argyros et al., 2008; Brantly et al., 2009; Liqun Wang et al., 2009); all aim to increase AAT levels in the circulation above the deficiency threshold of 11 μM. New approaches are focused on coupling haematopoietic stem cell therapy with AAT-lentiviral gene therapy (Ghaedi et al., 2010; Argyros et al., 2008). This chapter will review the history and current state-of-the-art in these areas.

2. Gene therapies targeting ZAAT-related liver disease

There are currently no available treatments for AAT deficiency-related liver disease other than transplantation. The 5-year survival is 83% for adults and 90% for children post transplant (Kemmer et al., 2008). As an alternative to transplantation gene therapy approaches aimed at inhibiting ZAAT expression in the liver can potentially be used to stop the production of the mutant Z protein, hence prohibiting the accumulation of the protein in the liver and providing protection against liver disease. Such approaches include the use of ribozymes, small interfering RNA (siRNA) and small DNA fragments (SDF), and a number of these genetic approaches designed to downregulate ZAAT expression have been tested in animals as therapies for liver disease in AAT deficiency. To date there have been no reports on the use of zinc-finger nucleases (ZFN) or peptide nucleic acids (PNA) to treat ZAAT-related liver disease (Figure 1). ZFNs are artificial restriction enzymes that can be engineered to target specific DNA sequences and exploit a cell's DNA repair machinery to precisely alter the genome; PNAs are synthetic DNA analogues that hybridize to complementary DNA or RNA to facilitate anti-gene or antisense inhibition, respectively (Jensen et al., 1997; Pellestor & Paulasova, 2004). It has been suggested that if ZAAT levels can be decreased to those similar or lower than MZ AAT heterozygotes there may be clinical benefit (Cruz et al., 2007) as heterozygous individuals rarely develop severe liver disease, particularly in childhood.

2.1 Ribozymes

Ribozymes are catalytic RNA molecules capable of cleaving RNA with high specificity. Their catalytic properties were discovered almost 30 years ago (Kruger et al., 1982) and they are now known to contain both a catalytic RNA domain that cleaves a target mRNA and a substrate-binding domain that contains an antisense sequence to the target mRNA sequence that enables them to bind to their target mRNA sequence through Watson–Crick base pairing (Trang et al., 2004). The best characterised ribozymes have hammerhead or hairpin shaped active centres; both are promising gene-targeting reagents.

Hammerhead ribozymes capable of cleaving AAT mRNA have been constructed and were shown to be effective at inhibiting ZAAT expression in a human hepatoma cell line (Zern et al., 1999). In this study the hepatoma cells were also stably transduced with a modified AAT cDNA capable of producing wildtype AAT protein, but resistant to cleavage by the ZAAT-targetted ribozyme. Later a bi-functional vector was constructed, which contained both the ribozyme and the ribozyme-resistant AAT gene. Once transduced into hepatoma cells, the cells showed effective expression of the transduced AAT under conditions where the endogenous AAT gene was inhibited (Ozaki et al., 1999). Effective gene therapy for ZAAT deficiency requires stable transduction of resting hepatocytes, ideally to deliver both wild-type AAT and to inhibit production of ZAAT. Duan *et al.* treated transgenic mice expressing the human ZAAT allele with a simian virus 40 (SV40)-derived vector carrying a ribozyme designed to target the human transcript. The mice showed a marked decrease of human AAT mRNA and protein in the liver, and serum levels of human AAT were decreased by up to 50% 3-16 weeks after transduction (Duan et al., 2004).

Together these data show promise for the use of ribozymes for ZAAT-related liver disease. Importantly ribozymes bind to their targets with high specificity however there can be problems with their use to knockdown gene expression *in vivo* as their activity *in vivo* is not usually sufficient to achieve the desired effects.

2.2 Small interfering RNA

RNA interference (RNAi) is the process of sequence-specific, post-transcriptional gene silencing. It is initiated by short double-stranded RNA (dsRNA) sequences called small

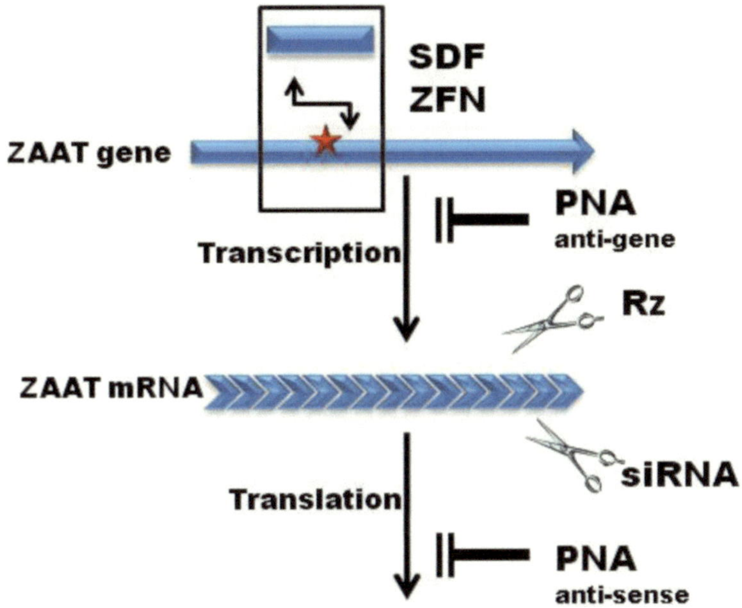

Fig. 1. Gene therapies for ZAAT-related liver disease. The Z mutation (shown by the red star) can be repaired using small DNA fragments (SDF) or zinc finger nucleases. Peptide nucleic acids (PNA) can inhibit the processes of transcription or translation whilst ribozymes (Rz) and siRNA target the mRNA and inhibit translation.

interfering RNA (siRNA) that are generated from longer transcripts by the enzyme Dicer. Each siRNA has specificity for a target RNA via its homology to sequences within the target gene (Elbashir et al., 2001). siRNAs form part of the RNA-induced silencing complex (RISC), a multi-component nuclease containing RNAse III, that enables the destruction of target mRNAs (Hammond et al., 2000). The argonaute protein within RISC incorporates one strand of an siRNA, known as the guide strand, and uses this as a template for recognizing complementary mRNA. Once found the target mRNA is cleaved by activation of the RNAse activity within RISC.

The delivery *in vivo* of siRNAs by liposomes or cationic lipids has been described. Other strategies for local or systemic administration of siRNA include electropulsation, delivery by viral vector, chemical modifications of siRNA molecules or polyamine or other encapsulation technologies. Targetting siRNAs directly to the liver can be achieved by local administration via injection through the hepatic portal vein and can prevent unwanted effects on normal host tissues. In 2007 studies describing the use of siRNAs designed to downregulate endogenous AAT within hepatocytes were reported. Using an adeno-associated virus (AAV) backbone three separate siRNA sequences were transduced singly or as a trifunctional construct into cell culture models. Whilst each siRNA had activity independently, the levels of AAT expression showed the greatest decrease, up to five-fold lower than controls, with the trifunctional construct. Following packaging of this construct into an AAV serotype 8 capsid, and transduction into the livers of transgenic mice overexpressing human ZAAT, a decrease in total and monomer ZAAT levels coupled with reversal of ZAAT accumulation was evident within the liver up to 3 weeks after vector injection (Cruz et al., 2007).

2.3 Small DNA fragments

The use of small DNA fragments (SDF) for homologous replacement of mutant genes allows targets to be directly altered by insertion, deletion or replacement. Theoretically direct conversion of the mutant sequence to a wild-type genotype ensues, thereby restoring the normal phenotype. The basis of this technology involves the introduction of small DNA fragments into cells that recombine with the genomic DNA at a targeted site, thereby producing a specific change in the sequence. The feasibility of using SDF targeting the AAT gene has been reported. SDFs encoding the normal AAT sequence were generated and transfected *ex vivo* into peripheral blood monocytes from control and ZAAT deficient individuals. The SDFs corrected the defective gene in ZAAT monocytes and treatment was associated with an increase in AAT secretion. A similar methodology to repair the ZAAT gene defect in hepatocytes should have beneficial effects on secretion, and could ultimately lead to protection of both the lung and liver in ZAAT deficient individuals (McNab et al., 2007).

3. Gene therapies to target ZAAT-related lung disease

There have been a number of gene therapy trials for the treatment of AAT deficiency-related lung disease. The first used cationic liposomes encapsulating a plasmid carrying the human AAT cDNA (Brigham et al., 2000). In this open-label study the liposomes were administered intranasally to 5 ZAAT deficient individuals. The results showed that AAT levels were increased at day 5 following administration and returned to baseline by day 14. Subsequent studies have improved on this by using non-pathogenic human parvovirus recombinant AAV vectors that are more efficient at transgene delivery and are more capable of extended transgene expression.

3.1 Intramuscular adeno-associated viral gene delivery

In 2006 Brantly *et al.* reported their results from a phase I trial of intramuscular injection of a recombinant adeno-associated virus serotype 2 vector (rAAV2) carrying the human AAT gene into 12 AAT deficient adults (Brantly et al., 2006). Subjects were divided into groups of three and allocated to one of four dose cohorts ranging from 2.1×10^{12} to 6.9×10^{13} vector genomes. Each was injected into the deltoid muscle of their non-dominant arm sequentially in a dose-escalating fashion. No vector-related adverse events occurred in any of the participants although anti-rAAV2 capsid antibodies were present and rose after vector injection. In this study just one subject exhibited low-level expression of wild-type AAT in their serum (82 nM) up to 30 days after receiving an injection of 2.1×10^{13} vector genomes. Residual AAT levels from previous AAT protein replacement therapy was blamed for interfering with the detection of any possible vector expression in most of the other individuals.

Later in another phase 1, open-label, dose-escalation clinical trial sustained AAT expression was achieved using a rAAV serotype 1 vector (Brantly et al., 2009). rAAV1 is substantially more efficient than rAAV2 in transducing skeletal muscle (Cruz et al., 2007). Once again subjects were dosed via intramuscular (i.m.) injection and those subjects who had been

receiving protein therapy discontinued its use for 28 or 56 days prior to vector administration. In those who received 2.2 x 10^{13} and 6.0 x 10^{13} vector genome particles normal AAT was expressed above background in all subjects. AAT expression was sustained at levels 0.1% of normal for at least 1 year in the highest dosage level cohort. Vector administration was well tolerated and there were no changes in hematology or clinical chemistry parameters however neutralizing antibody and IFN-gamma enzyme-linked immunospot responses to rAAV1 capsid were evident in all subjects at day 14.
The most recent report on this gene therapy approach describes the results of a preclinical evaluation of a rAAV1 vector expressing human AAT made using a recombinant herpes simplex virus production method that can achieve much higher yields enabling a substantial increase in dosage in clinical studies (Chulay et al., 2011). The toxicology study in mice treated i.m. with this vector showed that the HSV-produced vector had favorable characteristics in terms of purity, efficiency of transduction, and human AAT expression.

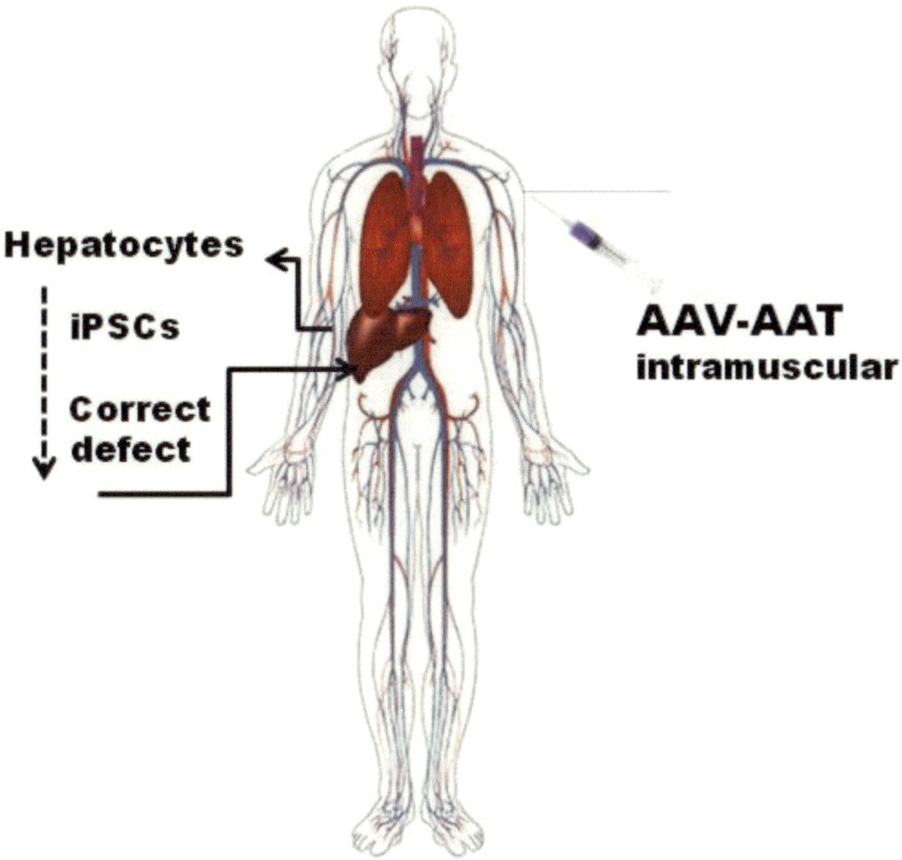

Fig. 2. Gene therapy strategies for ZAAT-related lung disease. The normal AAT gene can be introduced via intramuscular injection of an AAT-expressing adeno-associated virus (AAV) leading to production of normal AAT protein. Alternatively a patient's own cells can be harvested, induced to pluripotency (iPSCs) and the defect corrected *ex vivo* prior to autologous cell therapy.

Administration with this vector led to no significant differences in clinical findings or hematology and no gross changes in pathology although there were mild changes in skeletal muscle at the injection site. These consisted of focal chronic interstitial inflammation and muscle degeneration, regeneration and vacuolization in vector-injected animals. Vectors were detectable in blood 24 hours after dosing and declined thereafter, with no copies detectable 90 days after dosing. Antibodies to human AAT were detected in almost all treated animals, with antibodies to HSV detectable in most animals that received the highest vector dose. With higher doses of HSV-produced vector, the increase in serum human AAT levels was dose-dependent in females and, interestingly, greater than dose-proportional in males. Together all of these studies support continued development of rAAV1-AAT vectors for i.m. gene delivery for the treatment of AAT deficiency (Figure 2).

3.2 Viral gene delivery to the lung

Transduction of cells within the lung is an attractive approach for AAT gene therapy. Since somatic tissues are comprised of heterogeneous, differentiated cell lineages that can be difficult to specifically transfect (although this may have been largely overcome by the work of Flotte using i.m. injection (section 3.1)), methods have been tested to deliver gene therapies directly to cells within the lung. These include AAV and other viral methods to deliver the AAT gene directly to cells within the lung for local expression of AAT at the site where it is most needed to provide an antiprotease protective screen. Both integrating lentiviral systems and non-integrating AAV vectors are capable of gene transfer and expression *in vivo* in non-dividing cells and approaches using both viruses have been undertaken. Using recombinant AAV vectors Liqun Wang *et al.* evaluated the transduction and expression efficiencies of several rAAV serotypes and rAAV2 capsid mutants with specific pulmonary targeting ligands (Liqun Wang et al., 2009). Noninvasive intranasal delivery was compared with intratracheal lung delivery into the mouse lung. Of all the vectors tested they found that recombinant rAAV8 was the most efficient serotype at expressing AAT in the lung. Intratracheal administration was superior to intranasal delivery for most vectors. Limberis *et al.* also characterized a wide range of vectors and nine different serotypes of rAAV for their ability to transduce mouse and human ciliated airway epithelium (Limberis et al., 2009). In their studies rAAV5 and rAAV6 were found to be the most efficient at transducing mouse epithelium whilst only rAAV6 was as effective in human cells. Variants of AAV6 with targeted mutations were also tested. One of these, rAAV6.2, was more efficient than all the other rAAV vectors tested and shows promise for development and preclinical testing. In a separate AAT-rAAV6 study involving delivery to the lungs of mice and dogs, administrations led to increased and extended intrapulmonary AAT levels, however the animals developed immune responses including a lymphoproliferative response to the AAV capsid (Halbert et al., 2010). Another approach using intratracheal instillation of an AAT lentiviral system led to successful selective delivery of the AAT transgene to alveolar macrophages in the mouse lung (Wilson et al., 2010). These cells persisted in the alveoli and expressed AAT for the lifetime of the adult mouse and achieved localized secretion of therapeutic levels of AAT protein into the airway epithelial lining fluid. Using a mouse model of emphysema this approach ameliorated the progression of emphysema without inducing humoral or cellular immune responses.

3.3 Stem cell therapy and other approaches to gene delivery

An ideal gene therapy approach should enable persistent transgene expression without limitations of safety and reproducibility. Using an individual's own cells, cultured *in vitro* as the delivery platform for gene therapy is a new approach that can potentially circumvent these problems. The use of stem cells, either the induced pluripotent form or hematopoietic/mesencymal derived, has been considered for AAT gene therapy. For example, lentivirally transduced murine hematopoietic stem cells (HSCs) expressing a human AAT transgene have been developed (Wilson et al., 2008). Once transplanted into irradiated mouse recipients these HSCs maintained their multipotency, self-renewal potential, and could reconstitute the hematopoietic systems of both primary and secondary recipients. Furthermore these lentivirally-modified cells generated sustained and systemic expression of AAT *in vivo* for over 30 weeks. Other genetically modified mesenchymal stem cells (MSCs) have been used that, once differentiated into hepatocyte-like cells, offer a potentially unlimited source of cells for autologous transplant procedures (Ghaedi et al., 2010). These human MSCs were transduced with a lentiviral AAT expression vector and were shown to express major hepatocyte marker genes and AAT. This technology has potential as an *in vitro* source of cells for transplantation therapy of liver diseases in AAT-deficient patients. Another angle on this approach is being developed by Li *et al.* (Li et al., 2010). They assessed the feasibility of bone marrow (BM) cell-based liver gene delivery of human AAT. Their *in vitro* studies showed that both lentiviral and rAAV vectors expressing AAT can be transduced into these cells and transplanted into the liver where they differentiate into hepatocytes and express AAT, resulting in sustained levels of circulating AAT in the recipient mice. In another study they used adipose tissue as an abundant, accessible and replenishable source of adult stem cells (Li et al., 2011). Adipose tissue-derived mesenchymal stem cells (AT-MSCs) resemble bone marrow-derived mesenchymal stem cells (BM-MSCs). Having investigated the feasibility of AT-MSC-based liver gene delivery for the treatment of AAT deficiency by transducing mouse AT-MSCs with an rAAV1 vector carrying the human AAT gene, it was shown that when the cells were then transplanted into the mouse liver that they expressed human AAT. Importantly, no anti-human AAT antibodies were detected.

Human induced pluripotent stem cells (iPSC) also hold great promise for cell-based therapy and in cell studies of genetic diseases. A strategy using dermal fibroblasts from AAT-deficient individuals has generated a library of patient-specific human iPSC cell lines (Rashid et al., 2010). Once differentiated into hepatocytes the resulting cells exhibit properties of mature hepatocytes and recapitulate key pathological features of AAT deficiency including accumulation of misfolded AAT in the endoplasmic reticulum. Using an approach such as this it may be possible to generate iPSC hepatocytes from an AAT-deficient individual, repair the defect *in vitro* with for example SDFs, ribozymes or zinc finger nucleases and transplant these 'corrected' cells back into the original donor (Figure 2). The next step in advancing this technology will be to achieve this without the worry of endogenous effects mediated by reprogramming transgenes. A number of methods already exist for generating murine or neonatal iPSCs free of reprogramming transgenes however, until recently this was not the case for disease-specific iPSC from humans with inherited or degenerative diseases. Now a humanized version of a single lentiviral "stem cell cassette" vector to accomplish efficient reprogramming of normal or diseased skin fibroblasts obtained from humans has been developed (Somers et al., 2010). The human iPSCs generated using this vector contain a single viral integration that can excise to generate human iPSCs free of integrated transgenes. As a proof of principle, this strategy has been used to generate lung disease-specific iPSC lines from individuals with AAT deficiency-related emphysema. These cells have the ability to differentiate into developmental precursor tissue of lung epithelia and will prove invaluable for AAT-deficiency related investigations. However the most exciting aspect of this technology is its potential to generate safer autologous 'corrected' cell therapies similar to those described above.

It is sometimes suggested that non-viral episomal plasmid DNA (pDNA) vectors may offer some advantages over viral vectors in that they can be produced cheaply and in large quantities. Argyros *et al.* developed such a vector using the human AAT promoter to drive expression of a luciferase gene and achieve long-term expression in murine liver (Argyros et al., 2008). Over the course of the study the vector was maintained as an episome and did not replicate. Luciferase expression was detectable up to 6 months and this is believed to be by means of a unique scaffold/matrix attachment region (S/MAR) element that inhibits methylation of the AAT promoter.

4. Conclusion

Since the first human gene therapy trials using lymphocytes for the cellular delivery of the adenosine deaminase gene to patients with severe combined immune deficiency (SCID) and as tumour-infiltrating vehicles there has been a remarkable expansion in the development of gene therapy strategies (Culver et al., 1991a; 1991b; 1991c). The most promising data have come from therapies targeting monogenic disorders. With respect to ZAAT deficiency, rAAV2 vectors, and more recently rAAV1 due to its higher tropism for muscle cells, have shown great promise for delivery of the AAT gene. The advantages of AAV vectors include not only their lack of acute pathology but also their episomal nature. Occasional problems with adaptive immune responses to its capsid proteins have been encountered in some contexts (Manno et al., 2006), however newer generation vectors with greater safety and efficiency of gene transfer are constantly under development. Non-AAV gene therapy strategies for AAT-related lung disease, although less advanced, also show potential. Genetic therapies designed to down-regulate expression of ZAAT in hepatocytes to reverse the toxic gain of function in the liver are also less well developed, however the next decade is likely to see huge progress in this area. Finally the recent advent of various stem cell technologies can only enhance efforts in ZAAT deficiency and gene therapy research.

5. Acknowledgments

Funding for alpha-1 antitrypsin deficiency research in this department is gratefully acknowledged from the US. Alpha One Foundation, the Medical Research Charities Group and the Health Research Board of Ireland, Programmes for Research in Third Level Institutes administered by the Higher Education Authority, the Children's Medical and Research Centre, Crumlin Hospital and the Department of Health and Children.

6. References

Argyros, O., Wong, S.P., Niceta, M., Waddington, S.N., Howe, S.J., Coutelle, C., Miller, A.D. & Harbottle R.P. (2008). Persistent episomal transgene expression in liver following delivery of a scaffold/matrix attachment region containing non-viral vector. *Gene Ther* 15, 24, pp 1593-1605.

Brantly, M.L., Chulay, J.D., Wang, L., Mueller, C., Humphries, M., Spencer, L.T., Rouhani, F., Conlon, T.J., Calcedo, R., Betts, M.R., Spencer, C., Byrne, B.J., Wilson, J.M. & Flotte, T.R. (2009). Sustained transgene expression despite T lymphocyte responses in a clinical trial of rAAV1-AAT gene therapy. *Proc Natl Acad Sci U S A* 106, 38, pp 16363-16368.

Brantly, M.L., Spencer, L.T., Humphries, M., Conlon, T.J., Spencer, C.T., Poirier, A., Garlington, W., Baker, D., Song, S., Berns, K.I., Muzyczka, N., Snyder, R.O., Byrne, B.J. & Flotte, T.R. (2006). Phase I trial of intramuscular injection of a recombinant adeno-associated virus serotype 2 alpha l-antitrypsin (AAT) vector in AAT-deficient adults. *Hum Gene Ther* 17, 12, pp 1177-1186.

Brigham, K.L., Lane, K.B., Meyrick, B., Stecenko, A.A., Strack, S., Cannon, D.R., Caudill, M. & Canonico, A.E. (2000). Transfection of nasal mucosa with a normal alpha1-antitrypsin gene in alpha1-antitrypsin-deficient subjects: comparison with protein therapy."*Hum Gene Ther* 11, 7, pp 1023-1032.

Chulay JD, Ye GJ, Thomas DL, Knop DR, Benson JM, Hutt JA, Wang G, Humphries M, Flotte TR (2011). Preclinical Evaluation of a Recombinant Adeno-associated Virus Vector Expressing Human Alpha-1 Antitrypsin Made Using a Recombinant Herpes Simplex Virus Production Method. *Hum Gene Ther* 22, 2,155-165.

Cruz, P.E., Mueller, C., Cossette, T.L., Golant, A., Tang, Q., Beattie, S.G., Brantly, M., Campbell-Thompson ,M., Blomenkamp, K.S., Teckman, J.H. & Flotte TR. (2007). In vivo post-transcriptional gene silencing of alpha-1 antitrypsin by adeno-associated virus vectors expressing siRNA. *Lab Invest* 87, 9, pp. 893-902.

Culver, K., Cornetta, K., Morgan, R., Morecki, S., Aebersold, P., Kasid, A., Lotze, M., Rosenberg, S.A., Anderson, W.F., & Blaese, R.M. (1991a). Lymphocytes as cellular vehicles for gene therapy in mouse and man. *Proc Natl Acad Sci U S A* 88, 8, pp. 3155-3159.

Culver, K.W., Anderson, W.F. & Blaese, R.M. (1991b). Lymphocyte gene therapy. *Hum Gene Ther* 2, 2, 107-109.Culver, K.W., Osborne, W.R., Miller, A.D., Fleisher, T.A., Berger, M., Anderson, W.F. &

Blaese, R.M. (1991c). Correction of ADA deficiency in human T lymphocytes using retroviral-mediated gene transfer. *Transplant Proc* 23, 1 Pt 1, 170-171.

Duan, Y.Y., Wu, J., Zhu, J.L., Liu, S.L., Ozaki, I., Strayer, D.S. & Zern, M.A. (2004). Gene therapy for human alpha1-antitrypsin deficiency in an animal model using SV40-derived vectors. *Gastroenterology* 127, 4, pp.1222-12232.

Elbashir, S.M., Martinez, J., Patkaniowska, A., Lendeckel ,W. & Tuschl, T. (2001). Functional anatomy of siRNAs for mediating efficient RNAi in *Drosophila melanogaster* embryo lysate. *EMBO J* 20, 23, pp. 6877-6888.

Flotte, T.R., Conlon, T.J., Poirier, A., Campbell-Thompson, M. & Byrne, B.J. (2007). Preclinical characterization of a recombinant adeno-associated virus type 1-pseudotyped vector demonstrates dose-dependent injection site inflammation and dissemination of vector genomes to distant sites. *Hum Gene Ther* 18, 3, 245-256.

Ghaedi, M., Lotfi, A.S. & Soleimani, M. (2010). Establishment of lentiviral-vector-mediated model of human alpha-1 antitrypsin delivery into hepatocyte-like cells differentiated from mesenchymal stem cells. *Tissue Cell* 42, 3, pp. 181-189.

Greene, C.M., Miller, S.D., Carroll, T., McLean, C., O'Mahony, M., Lawless, M.W., O'Neill, S.J., Taggart, C.C. & McElvaney NG (2008). Alpha-1 antitrypsin deficiency: a conformational disease associated with lung and liver manifestations. *J Inherit Metab Dis* 31, 1, pp. 21-34.

Halbert, C.L., Madtes, D.K., Vaughan, A.E., Wang, Z., Storb, R., Tapscott, S.J. & Miller, A.D.(2010). Expression of human alpha1-antitrypsin in mice and dogs following AAV6 vector-mediated gene transfer to the lungs. *Mol Ther* 18, 6, pp. 1165-1172.

Hammond, S.M., Bernstein, E., Beach, D. & Hannon GJ.. (2000). An RNA-directed nuclease mediates post-transcriptional gene silencing in *Drosophila* cells. *Nature* 404, 6775, pp. 293-296.

Hidvegi, T., Mirnics, K., Hale, P., Ewing, M., Beckett, C. & Perlmutter DH. (2007). Regulator of G Signaling 16 is a marker for the distinct endoplasmic reticulum stress state associated with aggregated mutant alpha1-antitrypsin Z in the classical form of alpha1-antitrypsin deficiency. *J Biol Chem* 282, 38, pp. 27769-27780.

Hidvegi, T., Schmidt, B.Z., Hale, P. & Perlmutter, D.H. (2005). Accumulation of mutant alpha1-antitrypsin Z in the endoplasmic reticulum activates caspases-4 and -12, NFkappaB, and BAP31 but not the unfolded protein response. *J Biol Chem* 280, 47, 39002-39015.

Jensen, K.K., Orum, H., Nielsen, P.E. & Nordén, B. (1997). Kinetics for hybridization of peptide nucleic acids (PNA) with DNA and RNA studied with the BIAcore technique. *Biochemistry* 36, 16, pp. 5072-5077.

Kelly, E., Greene, C.M., Carroll, T.P., McElvaney, N.G. & O'Neill SJ. (2010) Alpha-1 antitrypsin deficiency. *Respir Med* 104, 6, pp. 763-772.

Kemmer, N., Kaiser, T., Zacharias, V. & Neff, G,W. (2008). Alpha-1-antitrypsin deficiency: outcomes after liver transplantation. *Transplant Proc* 40, 5, 1492-1494.

Kruger, K., Grabowski, P.J., Zaug, A.J., Sands, J., Gottschling, D.E. & Cech TR.(1982). Self-splicing RNA: autoexcision and autocyclization of the ribosomal RNA intervening sequence of Tetrahymena. *Cell* 31, 1, pp. 147-157.

Lawless, M.W., Greene, C.M., Mulgrew, A., Taggart, C.C., O'Neill, S.J.& McElvaney, N.G.(2004). Activation of endoplasmic reticulum-specific stress responses associated with the conformational disease Z alpha 1-antitrypsin deficiency. *J Immunol* 172, 9, pp. 5722-5726.

Li, H., Lu, Y., Witek, R.P., Chang, L.J., Campbell-Thompson, M., Jorgensen, M., Petersen, B. & Song, S. (2010). *Ex vivo* transduction and transplantation of bone marrow cells for liver gene delivery of alpha1-antitrypsin. *Mol Ther* 18, 8, pp. 1553-1558.

Li, H., Zhang, B., Lu, Y., Jorgensen, M., Petersen, B. & Song, S. (2011) Adipose tissue-derived mesenchymal stem cell-based liver gene delivery. *J Hepatol.* In Press.

Limberis, M.P., Vandenberghe, L.H., Zhang, L., Pickles, R.J. & Wilson, J.M. (2009).Transduction efficiencies of novel AAV vectors in mouse airway epithelium in vivo and human ciliated airway epithelium in vitro. *Mol Ther* 17, 2, pp. 294-301.

Liqun Wang, R., McLaughlin, T., Cossette, T., Tang, Q., Foust, K., Campbell-Thompson, M., Martino, A., Cruz, P., Loiler, S., Mueller, C. & Flotte TR.(2009). "Recombinant AAV serotype and capsid mutant comparison for pulmonary gene transfer of alpha-1-antitrypsin using invasive and noninvasive delivery." *Mol Ther* 17, 1, pp. 81-87.

Lomas, D.A., Evans, D.L., Finch, J.T. & Carrell, R.W. (1992). The mechanism of Z alpha 1-antitrypsin accumulation in the liver. *Nature* 357, 6379, pp. 605-607.

Lomas, D.A., Evans, D.L., Stone, S.R., Chang, W.S. & Carrell, R.W (1993). Effect of the Z mutation on the physical and inhibitory properties of alpha 1-antitrypsin. *Biochemistry* 32, 2, 500-508.

Manno, C,S., Pierce, G.F., Arruda, V.R., Glader, B., Ragni, M., Rasko, J.J., Ozelo, M.C., Hoots, K., Blatt, P., Konkle, B., Dake, M., Kaye, R., Razavi, M., Zajko, A., Zehnder, J., Rustagi, P.K., Nakai, H., Chew, A., Leonard, D., Wright, J.F., Lessard, R.R., Sommer, J.M., Tigges, M., Sabatino, D., Luk, A., Jiang, H., Mingozzi, F., Couto, L., Ertl, H.C., High, K.A. & Kay, M.A. (2006). Successful transduction of liver in hemophilia by AAV-Factor IX and limitations imposed by the host immune response. *Nat Med* 12, 3, pp. 342-347.

McLean, C., Greene, C.M. & McElvaney N.G. (2009). Gene targeted therapeutics for liver disease in alpha-1 antitrypsin deficiency. *Biologics* 3, pp.63-75.

McNab, G.L., Ahmad, A., Mistry, D. & Stockley, R.A. (2007). Modification of gene expression and increase in alpha1-antitrypsin (alpha1-AT) secretion afterhomologous recombination in alpha1-AT-deficient monocytes. *Hum Gene Ther* 18, 11, pp. 1171-1177.

Miller, S.D., Greene, C.M., McLean, C., Lawless, M.W., Taggart, C.C., O'Neill, S.J., & McElvaney, N.G. (2007). Tauroursodeoxycholic acid inhibits apoptosis induced by Z alpha-1 antitrypsin via inhibition of Bad. *Hepatology* 46, 2, pp. 496-503.

Ozaki, I., Zern, M.A., Liu, S., Wei, D.L., Pomerantz, R.J. & Duan L. (1999). Ribozyme-mediated specific gene replacement of the alpha1-antitrypsin gene in human hepatoma cells. *J Hepatol* 31, 1, pp. 53-60.

Pellestor, F. & P. Paulasova (2004). The peptide nucleic acids (PNAs), powerful tools for molecular genetics and cytogenetics. *Eur J Hum Genet* 12, 9, pp. 694-700.

Rashid, S.T., Corbineau, S., Hannan, N., Marciniak, S.J., Miranda, E., Alexander, G., Huang-Doran, I., Griffin, J., Ahrlund-Richter, L., Skepper, J., Semple, R., Weber, A., Lomas, D.A. & Vallier, L. (2010). Modeling inherited metabolic disorders of the liver using human induced pluripotent stem cells. *J Clin Invest* 120, 9, pp. 3127-3136.

Somers, A., Jean, J.C., Sommer, C.A., Omari, A., Ford, C.C., Mills, J.A., Ying, L., Sommer, A.G., Jean, J.M., Smith, B.W., Lafyatis, R., Demierre, M.F., Weiss, D.J., French, D.L., Gadue, P., Murphy, G.J., Mostoslavsky, G. & Kotton, D.N. (2010) Generation of transgene-free lung disease-specific human induced pluripotent stem cells using a single excisable lentiviral stem cell cassette. *Stem Cells* 28, 10, 1728-1740.

Teckman, J. H. & D. H. Perlmutter (2000). Retention of mutant alpha(1)-antitrypsin Z in endoplasmic reticulum is associated with an autophagic response. *Am J Physiol Gastrointest Liver Physiol* 279, 5, pp. G961-974.

Trang, P., Kim, K. & Liu, F. (2004). Developing RNase P ribozymes for gene-targeting and antiviral therapy. *Cell Microbiol* 6, 6, pp. 499-508.

Wilson, A.A., Kwok, L.W., Hovav, A.H., Ohle, S.J., Little, F.F., Fine, A. & Kotton,D.N. (2008). Sustained expression of alpha1-antitrypsin after transplantation of manipulated hematopoietic stem cells. *Am J Respir Cell Mol Biol* 39, 20, pp. 133-141.

Wilson, A.A., Murphy, G.J., Hamakawa, H., Kwok, L.W., Srinivasan, S., Hovav, A.H., Mulligan, R.C., Amar, S., Suki, B. & Kotton, D.N. (2010). Amelioration of emphysema in mice through lentiviral transduction of long-lived pulmonary alveolar macrophages. *J Clin Invest* 120, 1, pp. 379-389.

Zern, M.A., Ozaki, I., Duan, L., Pomerantz, R., Liu, S.L. & Strayer, D.S. (1999). A novel SV40-based vector successfully transduces and expresses an alpha 1-antitrypsin ribozyme in a human hepatoma-derived cell line. *Gene Ther* 6, 1, pp. 114-120.

26

Critical Stages in the Development of the First Targeted, Injectable Molecular-Genetic Medicine for Cancer

Erlinda M. Gordon and Frederick L. Hall
Magnahelix Inc. & Box Five Biomedical Consultants L.L.C.
U.S.A.

1. Introduction

Quietly, cautiously, and steadily, the field of modern medicine recently progressed across a new threshold with the development of Rexin-G, the first and so far, only, targeted injectable molecular genetic medicine to be validated in the clinic. Designed to function within the context and complexities of the human circulatory system, the "smart," "stealth," "highly-selective" nanoparticles embodied in Rexin-G travel beyond the reach of the most gifted surgeons, beyond the horizons of the finest catheters, to seek out the biochemical hallmarks of invasive cancers, and to deliver a lethal genetic payload where it is needed most—i.e., targeting the histopathology of the tumor microenvironment. In this invited review, we elaborate upon the critical stages of scientific discovery, molecular-genetic target validation, preclinical studies, pathotropic (disease-seeking) platform development, clinical trial design, molecular pharmacology, regulatory considerations, and GMP production & bioprocessing that, taken together, define the advancement of this tumor-targeted genetic medicine for cancer. In the course of delineating the developmental trajectory of Rexin-G into a series of logical and discrete stages, the authors have endeavored to extract, abstract, and represent a host of molecular biotechnological innovations in an accessible manner, providing (i) a useful overview of the converging fields of applied genetics, nanotechnology, and molecular biotechnology, and (ii) a conceptual basis for advancing new *pipeline* products in the emerging field of pathotropic medicine.

2. Setting the stage – targeting metastasis, one of the gravest medical needs

The problem of managing metastatic cancer, with its accompanying progression to evermore aggressive forms of the primary tumor cell (Bacac and Stamenkovic, 2008; Wong et al., 2009), remains one of the most daunting problems of modern medicine, thereby defining an unmet medical need. While many primary tumors can be eradicated by surgery if detected early in the course of disease progression, the appearance of metastatic disease is associated with a poor prognosis that worsens with the development of resistance to conventional chemotherapies (O'Day and Gorlick, 2009; Box et al., 2010; Verma et al., 2011). In the past ten years, there has been a frustrating lack of clinical advancements in the treatment of metastatic cancers (Di Marco et al., 2010, Stathis and Moore, 2010, Nieto et al., 2008). Once metastatic disease develops in pediatric sarcomas or in breast cancer, for example, the possibility of a cure is very limited or practically nonexistent (Krishnan et al., 2005; Gonzalez-Angulo et al., 2007). Moreover, this decade-long frustration has resulted in regulators, clinical investigators, and practicing oncologists effectively lowering their standards and expectations with regard to clinical trials and patient outcomes (Nieto et al., 2008; Allen et al., 2010; Verma et al., 2011). It is in this context that the call for innovative molecular targeted therapies emerged (Cappetta et al., 2011); it is in this context that the theoretical capability of tumor-targeted nanotechnology advanced (Gordon and Hall, 2005; Zolnick et al., 2010; Shapira et al., 2011); and it is in this context that the promise and potential of genetic medicine became apparent (Gordon et al., 2008; Sreeramoju and Libutti, 2010; Gordon and Hall, 2010).

At the turn of the 21st century, the advent of targeted genetic medicine faced three major challenges: (i) ***undeveloped biotechnology***—specifically, the problem of inefficient gene delivery *in vivo*; (ii) ***institutional incredulity***—regarding the feasibility of achieving tumor-targeting under physiological conditions; and (iii) ***scientific skepticism***—concerning the seemingly overwhelming bio-mathematics of the applied nanotechnologies required for effective tumor control. The first challenge was elucidated by the pharmaceutical industry, as it systematically withdrew from the field of genetic medicine, stating: "*From the beginning, the therapy's main difficulty has been a logistical one: how to deliver enough healthy genes to the appropriate site and get them to stay there long enough to cure or alleviate a disease....*" the consensus opinion being, "*improved gene delivery methods are needed in order to give human trials a better chance of success*" (Langreth and Moore, 1999). The second challenge was exemplified by a National Cancer Institute grant reviewer, circa 2000 (privileged communication), who stated that "*One couldn't possibly imagine that the systemic delivery of an extracellular matrix (ECM)-targeted gene delivery vector would accumulate appreciably inside a tumor nodule; more likely, the gene delivery would be restricted to the superficial 'stromal' layers, much like the peeling of an onion skin.*" The third challenge, that of insurmountable biomathematics, was addressed in a scholarly debate following a keynote presentation by the authors at the Cold Spring Harbor Laboratory 2001 meeting on "*Vector Targeting Strategies for Gene Therapy.*" In view of the first preclinical demonstrations of efficient, tumor-targeted gene delivery achieved under physiological conditions *in vivo*, there still remained considerable doubt concerning the feasibility of overcoming the rigors of physiology—dilution, filtration, immunological inactivation, fluid dynamics, and shear forces—to the extent needed to deliver a sufficient number of vector particles via the systemic circulation without utilizing infectious (self-replicating) viral components. Taken together, these formal challenges that prevailed at the cusp of the 21st century represented a formidable technological *barrier to entry* into the field of targeted genetic medicine, in general, and to the advancement of cancer gene therapy, in particular.

One by one, these imposing biopharmaceutical challenges were addressed and overcome during the course of a decade of scientific discovery, biotechnological innovation, translational research, and clinical development: a decade which may, in retrospect, be appropriately regarded as the *decennium mirabilis* of targeted genetic medicine—that "remarkable decade" wherein the clinical promise and potential of cancer gene therapy was ushered across the threshold of history. In technical scope, these challenges ranged from basic and applied molecular-genetics and virology, to medical nanotechnology, to the biophysics of tumor targeting and the constructs of therapeutic gene-delivery, to the advent of pathotropic (disease-seeking) medicine and the advancement of precision-targeted retrovectors, through a series of "proof-of-concept"preclinical studies and rigorous clinical trials, leading ultimately to the GMP bio-production and scale-up of the first fully-validated tumor-targeted gene delivery vector (i.e., Rexin-G) in accordance with the most exacting (U.S. FDA) demands of a Phase III/commercial oncology product. For the purposes of this invited review, these individual technological steps in the origination and development of Rexin-G for metastatic cancer are subdivided into discrete steps or *critical stages of development* that constitute the definitive biopharmacological foundations of a new field of medicine.

3. The pioneering stage – basic molecular-genetic research and discovery

"To heal him, we must touch something other than the coverlet of his bed!" exclaimed Ambroise Paré in 1569, extolling those physicians and surgeons in attendance that M. le Marquis de Auret was not yet beyond hope, but they would have to dig somewhat deeper into the fabric of nature to uncover a cure. This paternal challenge from one of the great pioneers of experimental medicine still echoes through the ages, compelling would-be healers to look beyond the superficiality and the plasticity of cellular signal transduction unto the final common pathways that function as prime *executive regulatory mechanisms* governing cell growth and viability. Indeed, after years of disappointing studies of experimental treatments for vascular proliferative disorders based on the disruption of cell receptor-mediated events, there emerged the appeal to look deeper—through an epoch of molecular-genetic research and discovery—for the executive enzymatic components of cellular growth control and those final common, highly-conserved biochemical pathways that physically execute the orderly progression of the mammalian cell division cycle (Siriam and Patterson, 2001; Ferguson and Patterson, 2003). It is in this deeper mechanistic understanding of the executive 'enzymatic engines' of the mammalian cell division cycle (Schwartz and Shah, 2005; Marretta and Ales, 2010), that the drug targets of a more effectual apothecary for both vascular proliferative disorders (Charron et al., 2006) and otherwise intractable cancers can be found (Johnson and Shapiro, 2010; Krystof and Uldrijan, 2010).

Located at the headwaters of oncogenesis, where growth-promoting proto-oncogenes meet and physically inactivate the predominant endogenous tumor suppressor proteins (Sherr and McCormick, 2002), a class of inducible regulatory proteins called "Cyclins" reside—along with their Cyclin-dependent, proline-directed protein kinase (CDK) partners (Hall and Vulliet, 1991; Pines, 1995) and their respective polypeptide CDK inhibitors, which themselves represent a potent form of physiological growth inhibition/tumor suppression (Viallard, et al., 2001; Wesierska-Gadek et al., 2011). In the course of the mammalian cell division cycle, the Cyclins appear in a sequential manner, in accordance with the progressive stages of the cell cycle [*note, the alphabetical designation Cyclins A through G denotes the order of scientific discovery/cloning, rather than the temporal induction of the gene product per se*], participating directly in the enzymatic activation of one or more cognate CDKs (Gerard and Goldbetter, 2009) while physically guiding the activated protein kinase complexes to specific substrates (first demonstrated by Peeper et al., 1993) and subcellular locations (Morgan, 1997). The operational result of progressive Cyclin expression and resulting CDK activation can be viewed conceptually as "feed-forward" regulatory control, overriding endogenous growth/tumor suppressor proteins and advancing the cell cycle beyond the limiting biochemical checkpoint(s). The reported incidence of specific Cyclin over-expression, gene amplification, and/or viral subversion of these Cyclin-dependent pathways, in association with the molecular mechanisms of carcinogenesis, are sufficient to warrant the formal designation of proto-oncogene to describe the growth-promoting role of these executive regulatory elements.

4. The mechanistic stage – molecular-genetic target validation

Among the so-called Cyclins, the *CYCG1* gene encoding human Cyclin G1 (Wu et al., 1994) is of particular bio-pharmaceutical importance; for it represents the molecular target of Rexin-G, the first targeted, injectable genetic medicine developed for diverse cancer indications. Indeed, recent clinical demonstrations of the broad-spectrum, single-agent, anti-tumor activity of Rexin-G have generated intense medical and scientific interest in the regulatory biology of Cyclin G1, as well as the molecular mechanisms-of-action of Rexin-G. In the course of its pharmaceutical development, it should be noted that the advanced molecular-genetic "knockout" construct embodied in Rexin-G is not dependent on the mechanisms of antisense-mediated gene suppression—which could possibly be overcome by the plasticity and the redundancy inherent in the Cyclin/CDK control elements as structurally- and functionally-related families of genes (Malumbres, 2005; Santamaria and Ortega, 2006; Satyanarayana and Kaldis, 2009)—but rather Rexin-G enforces the expression of a dominant-negative construct, i.e., a mutant form of the Cyclin-G1 protein, which effectively "blocks" the *executive biochemical pathways* governed by Cyclin G1, in the presence of a veritable "sea" of wild-type protein expression (see Xu et al., 2001). It is the blockade of these *executive biochemical pathways* (shown diagrammatically in Figure 1) that is invariably cytocidal to cancer cells and their associated proliferative neovasculature (Gordon et al., 2000, 2001; Gordon and Hall, 2010).
Mechanistically, the Cyclin G1 proto-oncogene is appreciably over-expressed in numerous cancers; its enforced expression promotes cell growth and effectively shortens the cell cycle (Smith et al., 1997), while its blockade by either antisense oligonucleotides or dominant-negative mutant constructs is decidedly lethal—via the active mechanisms of apoptosis—to both proliferative vascular cells (Zhu et al., 1997; Xu et al., 2001) and to a broad spectrum of cancer cells derived from all three germ layers (Skotzko et al., 1995; Chen et al., 1997; Hung et al., 1997; Gordon et al., 2001; Gordon et al., 2007; Gordon and Hall, 2010). Notably, in Cyclin G1-deficient mice, there is a significant reduction in the observed incidence of chemically-induced tumorigenesis (Jensen et al., 2003), which is consistent with a loss of antagonistic Cyclin G1-mediated effects on the levels and activities of the p53 tumor suppressor protein. As shown in Figure 1 (below), there is an intimate "negative-feedback" relationship between Cyclin G1 and at least two of the most prominent tumor suppressor proteins characterized to date: that is, the Retinoblastoma (Rb) tumor suppressor protein, which is genetically dysfunctional in many types of cancer, and the p53 tumor suppressor, which governs both apoptosis and senescence, in addition to regulating pivotal biochemical checkpoints involving DNA damage and enzymatic repair. In the first case, it appears that Cyclin G1, which is capable of forming complexes with multiple CDK partners (Piscopo and Hinds, 2008), participates in the inactivation of the Rb protein by directing site-specific protein phosphorylation events that ultimately enable cell cycle progression. In the second case, it appears that Cyclin G1 inactivates p53 (Ohtsuka et al., 2003, 2004), at least in part, by activating the MDM2 oncoprotein, which initiates the ubiquitin-mediated protein degradation of the p53 protein (Kimura and Nojima, 2002; Feng et al., 2011). In this case, it is important to note that both the Cyclin G1 effector and the MDM2 oncoprotein are transcriptionally activated (induced) by p53-dependent mechanisms (Okamoto and Beach,

1994; Moll and Petrenko, 2003), yet both of these regulatory proteins clearly function through additional biochemical pathways that are entirely independent of p53 (Zhang et al., 2005; Rayburn et al., 2009), which is genetically altered and/or inactivated in a large number of cancers.

Perhaps the most important aspect of target validation that can be discerned for Cyclin G1 as a drug target—and thus Rexin-G as an anti-cancer agent—is the recent finding that nature itself has seen fit to target this executive regulatory locus through endogenous microRNAs (Feng et al., 2011; Huang and He, 2011) that exert stringent control of Cyclin G1 expression. A series of high-throughput screens investigating the role of microRNAs in the pathogenesis of human hepatocellular carcinoma (HCC) identified miR-122 as the preeminent species of microRNA that is either missing or severely down-regulated in approximately 70% of HCC cancers and in all of the HCC-derived cancer cell lines (Gramantieri et al., 2007). Importantly, these studies identified Cyclin G1 as a gene target of miR-122, further validating the inverse correlation between miR-122 and Cyclin G1 expression that exists in primary liver carcinomas. Assuredly, the biochemical mechanism by which miR-122 expression decreased the viability of liver cancer cells was determined to be via apoptosis (Wu et al,. 2009); and enforced expression of miR-122 by adenoviral vectors has been shown to induce both cell cycle arrest and apoptosis in a number of different cancer cell lines (Ma et al., 2010) .

It was further determined that the pathological loss of miR-122 expression in liver cancer was not only correlated with an increased proliferative potential of the cancer cells, but with the extent of disease progression and metastasis (Coulouarn et al, 2009); while the re-expression of miR-122 was demonstrated to inhibit both the tumorigenic properties (Bai et al., 2009) and the metastatic potential (Tsai et al., 2009). In terms of molecular-genetic mechanisms of action, it was confirmed that, by modulating Cyclin G1 expression, miR-122 influences the stability and the transcriptional activity of p53, as it reduces the metastatic *invasiveness* of HCC-derived cell lines (Fornari et al., 2009). Moreover, the inhibitory effect of experimentally-restored miR-122 expression on Cyclin G1 levels serves to increase the sensitivity of HCC cells to doxorubicin-induced apoptosis, thereby establishing a mechanistic basis for the future development of combined chemotherapy and RNA-based cancer therapies. Taken together with the emerging molecular biology of Cyclin G1 (see Figure 1), it now appears that the biopharmaceutical agent, Rexin-G (a RNA-based genetic medicine), essentially restores a natural *tumor suppressor function* that is inherent in a normally-abundant species of microRNA—a species of microRNA that is lost with the pathogenesis of cancer, particularly that of invasive metastatic cancer.

Fig. 1 legend: As a mitotically-activated (or transformed) cell becomes 'competent' to proliferate and passes through the sequential phases of cell growth and DNA synthesis on to cell division, Cyclin G1 plays a pivotal role in governing the executive enzymatic activities of key regulatory components, including the checkpoints sensing DNA damage and repair. Normally held tightly in check (by microRNA-122), the growth-associated Cyclin G1 stands at the headwaters of cell cycle progression: advancing the cell cycle (arrows) through a myriad of enzymatic complexes, (i) by regulating site-directed protein phosphorylation by cyclin-dependent protein kinases (CDKs), which phosphorylate and inactivate the Rb tumor suppressor protein (blunted arrows), and (ii) by activating the cellular oncoprotein MDM2, which in turn inactivates the p53 tumor suppressor protein (blunted arrows) by initiating its destruction. Cyclin G1 governs the enzymatic activities of such key regulatory enzymes by transcriptional control of downstream elements, enzymatic activation/inactivation of the executive enzymes, and by directing the regulatory complexes to specific substrates and/or specific subcellular locations.

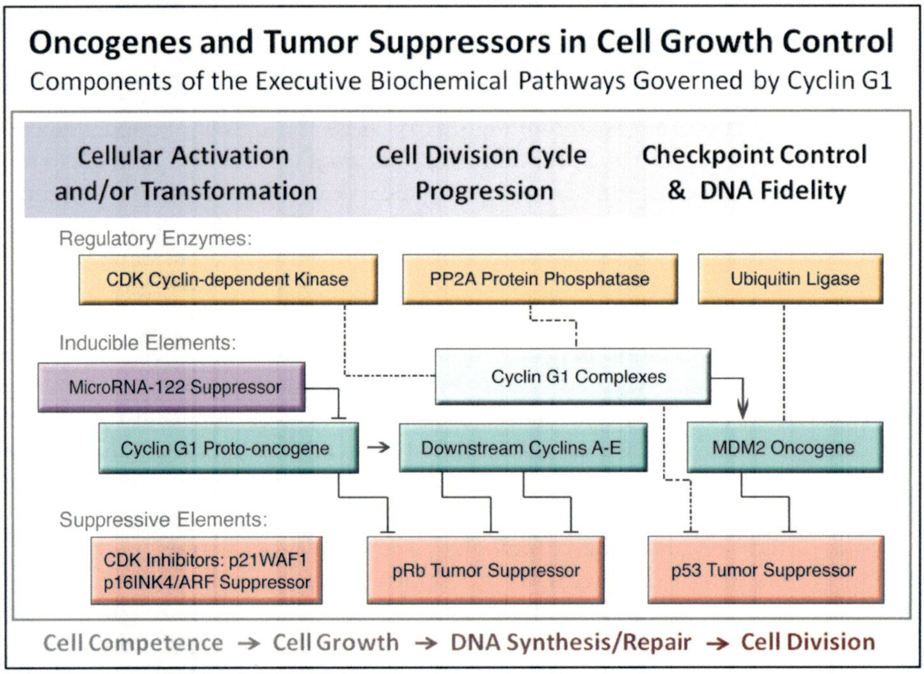

Fig. 1. Diagram depicting the major enzymatic activities, proto-oncogenes, and tumor suppressor proteins operating in the executive biochemical pathways governed by Cyclin G1.

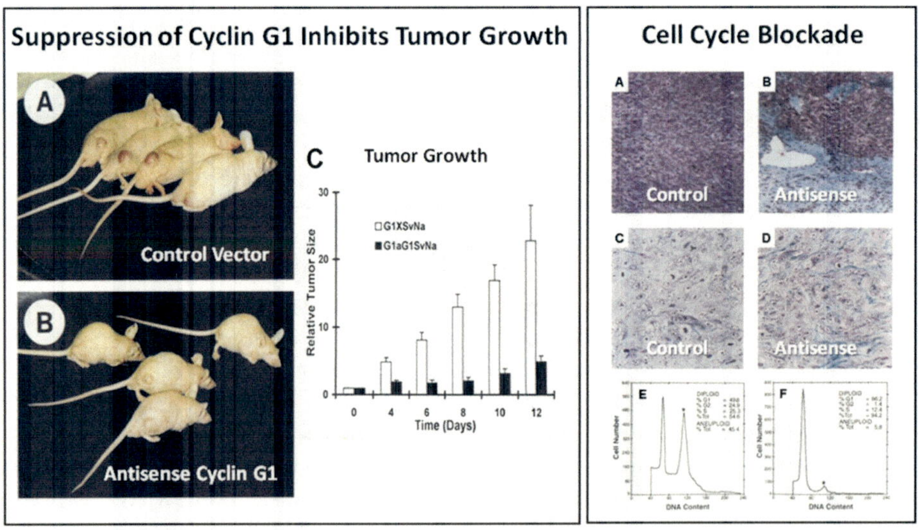

Fig. 2. Retroviral vector-mediated gene transfer of an antisense Cyclin G1 construct inhibits osteosarcoma growth in nude mice.

Following the identification of Cyclin G1 as a strategic therapeutic locus, a series of preclinical studies provided the initial *proofs-of-concept* (Skotzko et al., 1995; Chen et al., 1997; Gordon and Hall, 2010), thereby validating the therapeutic potential of cyclin G1 "knockout" constructs as anti-cancer agents by direct injection of therapeutic gene-delivery vehicles, or *vectors*, into tumor xenografts in experimental animals. As shown in Figure 2, both the reduction of tumor growth and the accompanying blockade of cell cycle progression are readily apparent. However, the more pressing technological challenge to reach beyond the obvious accessibility of localized primary tumors, and to address the fundamental problem of metastatic disease—i.e., to deliver the therapeutic potential of Cyclin-G1 knockout constructs where they are needed most—remained to be accomplished by a separate and distinct stage of scientific innovation.

Fig. 2 legend: Down-regulation of Cyclin G1 expression inhibits the proliferation of human osteosarcoma cells, as shown in rapidly growing subcutaneous tumors in athymic nude mice (Left Panel) treated by direct injection of either a Control (A) or Antisense Cyclin G1 vector (B); comparative tumor growth over time is shown in C. Histological analysis of tumor nodules (Right Panel) from Control (A,C,E) versus Antisense Cyclin G1 treated animals (B,D,F) demonstrates a significant reduction in the mitotic index in Antisense Cyclin G1-treated animals, which is confirmed by FACS analysis (E vs F), revealing a decrease in the number of cells in S and G2/M phases of the cell cycle (Chen et al., 1997). Cytocidal activity is confirmed by an increased incidence of apoptotic nuclei in the Antisense Cyclin G1-treated osteosarcoma cells (Skotzko et al., 1995).

5. The advent of pathotropic targeting – an enabling therapeutic gene delivery platform

In the course of scientific research and development it is often "The Road Not Taken," that is, the conscious decision to take the *road less traveled by*, that turns out to make the most significant difference in terms of historical outcome. In the case of targeted gene delivery, it was the conscious decision to target a *common* histopathological property of the metastatic process, rather than the unique and ever-changing surface features (ligands, receptors, etc) of the individual cancer cells, that made all the difference in terms of enhancing the efficiency of tumor-targeting under the most demanding of physiological conditions. Indeed, in the process of metastasis and metastatic tumor formation, both nascent and underlying extracellular matrix (ECM) proteins are characteristically exposed; and it is this characteristic exposure of one particular class of ECM proteins, the ubiquitous and determinative collagens (i.e., *collagen patefacio,* from Gordon and Hall, 2009), that now forms the basis for *disease-seeking* (or Pathotropic) tumor targeting. By conceptually grasping the *physiological surveillance function* that is inherent in the von Willebrand blood coagulation factor (vWF), which normally guides platelets to the sites of vascular injuries, and then physicochemically transposing a synthetic derivative of this *physiological surveillance function*, via genetic engineering, onto the surface of a nanoparticle-sized gene delivery vector (Hall et al., 2000; Gordon et al., 2000, 2002), the fields of molecular biotechnology and nanotechnology converged to enable the medical oncologist to reach beyond the mere coverlets of the proverbial bedside and to expose the very fabric of the nature of the metastatic disease process (Gordon and Hall, 2005, 2007). It is the advent of pathotropic targeting which would ultimately serve as the enabling biotechnological platform for therapeutic gene delivery *in vivo,* enabling the development of tumor-targeted gene therapy vectors that could be administered systemically, which would then seek-out sites of cancerous histopathology and accumulate to high levels in primary tumors and in the remote, occult, and otherwise inaccessible lesions of cancer metastasis.

6. The definitive proofs of principle - targeting metastasis *in vivo* in pertinent models of cancer

Comprised of (i) a structural multi-lamellar capsule (or retrovector core), (ii) a genetic payload of various designs, and (iii) a pathotropic envelope protein, the first tumor-targeted gene delivery vectors were initially designed to carry unique "marker genes," in the place of a therapeutic RNA construct, in order to study the kinetics and biodistribution of the circulating nanoparticles under well-defined experimental conditions, as well as the overall efficiency of the resulting gene transfer events. As shown in Figure 3 (below), which depicts a classic subcutaneous tumor xenograft model in which human tumor cells are flagrantly grafted into the flanks of athymic mice, the tumor-targeted vector is subsequently introduced into the systemic circulation through the tiny tail vein of the sleeping animal. The tumor-targeted nanoparticle must not only withstand the intense turbulence and dilution of the general circulation in this model, it must transit the heart, pass through the extensive filtering networks of the lungs, and transit the heart once again, before it is pumped through the aortic arch and a mere fraction of the blood flow is distributed to the flanks on the first pass. Nevertheless, the targeted nanoparticles are demonstrably partitioned into the tumor xenografts within a matter of minutes with intense avidity, where they can be seen to leave the fenestrated circulation within the tumors and begin to spread throughout the tumor nodules, much like a particulate dye accumulates from solution (by high affinity) into a natural sponge. With this constant pathotropic partitioning and resulting accumulation of vector particles in high local concentrations within the tumor nodules, it is clear that the targeted nanoparticles are highly active in terms of effectuating marker gene delivery to the proliferative cancer cells, as evidenced by the quantitative efficiency of the resulting transgene expression.

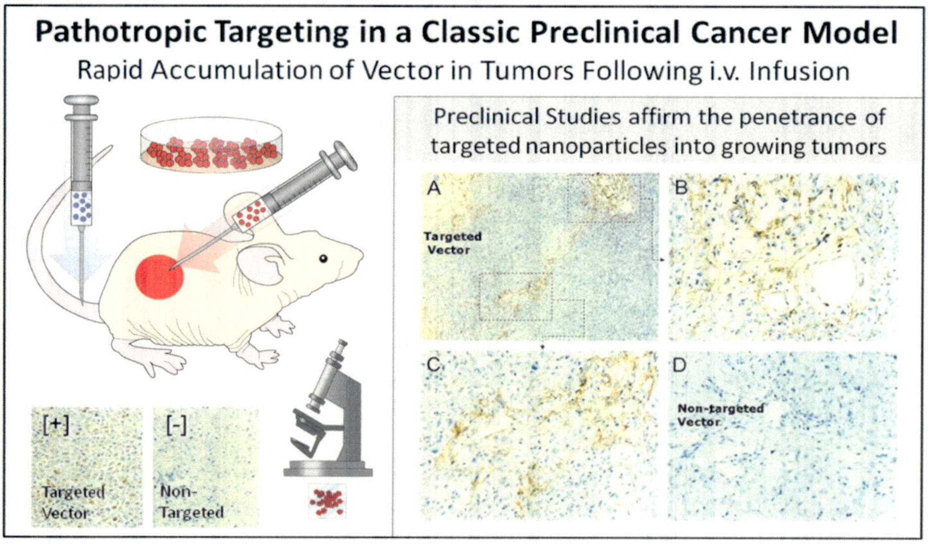

Fig. 3. Redistribution and gene transfer activity of a tumor-targeted retrovector bearing a marker gene into subcutaneously-implanted tumor xenografts in athymic mice.

Fig. 3 legend: Human pancreatic cancer cells were implanted in this classic cancer model (Left Diagram) followed by intravenous infusions of a tumor-targeted gene transfer vector (+) or non-targeted control vector (-). Immunohistochemical staining for the retrovector envelope protein (Right Panel) demonstrated appreciable accumulation of the targeted vector within 60 minutes of infusion (brown stain, A), which can be seen spreading out from the vasculature into the interstitial matrices of the tumor nodule (higher magnification, B, and C), in comparison with the non-targeted control vector where little if any accumulation can be found. Immunohistochemical staining for the β-galactosidase marker gene (Lower Left) confirmed high levels of transgene expression with the targeted vector.

Moving on to a somewhat more pertinent model of metastatic pancreatic cancer, where metastasis to the liver is all too common, additional characterization of the *physiological surveillance function* of these tumor-targeted nanoparticles was revealed, along with a striking demonstration of the high degree of selectivity of this targeted gene delivery platform for tumor cells and their associated neovasculature, while sparing normal liver cells in the immediate vicinity. In the model of metastatic pancreatic cancer shown in Figure 4 (below), the tumor-targeted retrovector bearing the designated marker gene was instilled at certain stages following the development of the liver metastasis. In the earliest stages of metastasis, where small groups and clusters of cancers cells invade the liver—before a distinctive tumor nodule is apparent - the vector demonstrates a striking ability to follow the submicroscopic biochemistries of tumor cell invasion, tracking the path of the invasive cancer cells, and delivering its transgene payload (marker gene) selectively to the invasive tumor cells while sparing the normal liver parenchyma. With the onset of neoangiogenesis, it becomes clear that, in addition to delivering the marker gene to the proliferative tumor cells, the pathotropically-targeted vector efficiently targets the vasculature of these aggressive tumors as well; thus the major focus of the transgene gene delivery is restricted to metastatic cancer cells and their attendant blood supply. These findings further indicate that an appropriate therapeutic (i.e., cytocidal) payload would exhibit significant anti-angiogenic properties, as well as anti-tumor activities.

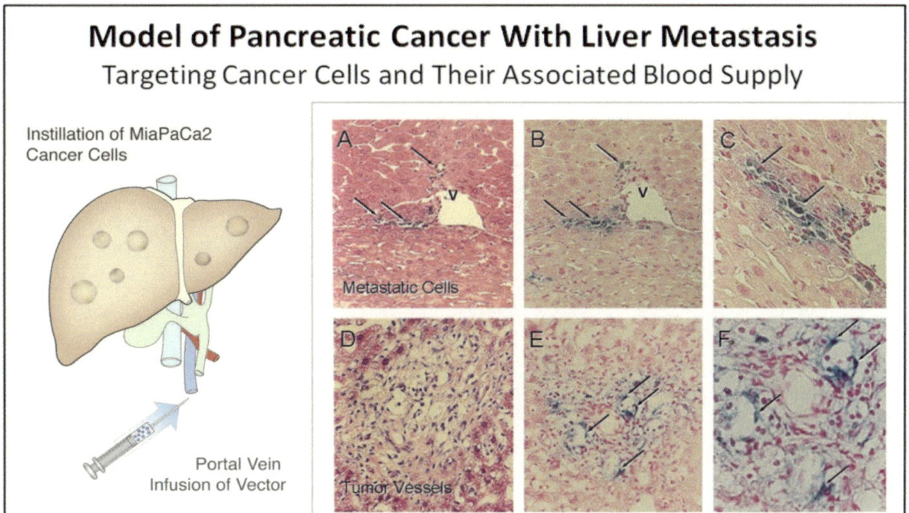

Fig. 4. Pathotropic vector bearing a marker gene identifies cellular targets for gene transfer in a murine model of pancreatic cancer metastatic to the liver.

Fig. 4 legend: Human pancreatic cancer cells were infused via the portal vein into the liver (Left Panel) followed, three days later, by portal vein infusions of a tumor-targeted gene transfer vector bearing a β-galactosidase marker gene at various stages of tumor formation (Right Panel). H&E staining of the earliest stage of metastasis (A) shows a small group of pancreatic cancer cells exiting a hepatic vein and migrating into the liver parenchyma. Histochemical staining for the marker gene expression (blue-green stain in B, enlarged in C) demonstrates efficient and selective gene delivery to the cancer cells. Following the establishment of the liver tumors with onset of neoangiogenesis (H&E stain of vessels shown in D), transfer of the β-galactosidase marker gene is seen in the proliferative endothelial cells of the tumor vessels (E and F).

Replacing the marker gene cassette with a cytocidal dominant-negative Cyclin G1 construct resulted in the development of the therapeutic anti-cancer agent designated Rexin-G, an acronym that conveys its molecular engineering roots: *Retroviral expression vector bearing an inhibitory construct of the Cyclin G1 gene*. Pioneering studies in the aforementioned preclinical cancer models with this *killer gene* as the genetic payload, resulted in the first demonstrations of clinical efficacy for targeted gene delivery *in vivo*: (i) corroborating the high-efficiency of tumor-targeted gene delivery with evidence of clinical efficacy, (ii) establishing the initial dose-response curves of an emergent pharmacology, (iii) confirming the fundamental biochemical mechanisms-of-action as enforced apoptosis, and (iv) revealing the characteristic hallmarks of tumor destruction and regression under the onslaught of this targeted cytocidal genetic medicine. As shown in Figure 5, repeated intravenous infusions of Rexin-G administered in a tumor xenograft model induced significant inhibition of tumor growth while altering the entire histology of the residual tumor nodules: as areas of focal vascular destruction (anti-angiogenesis) and massive tumor necrosis are observed among distinctive zones of overt cellular degeneration and reparative fibrosis.

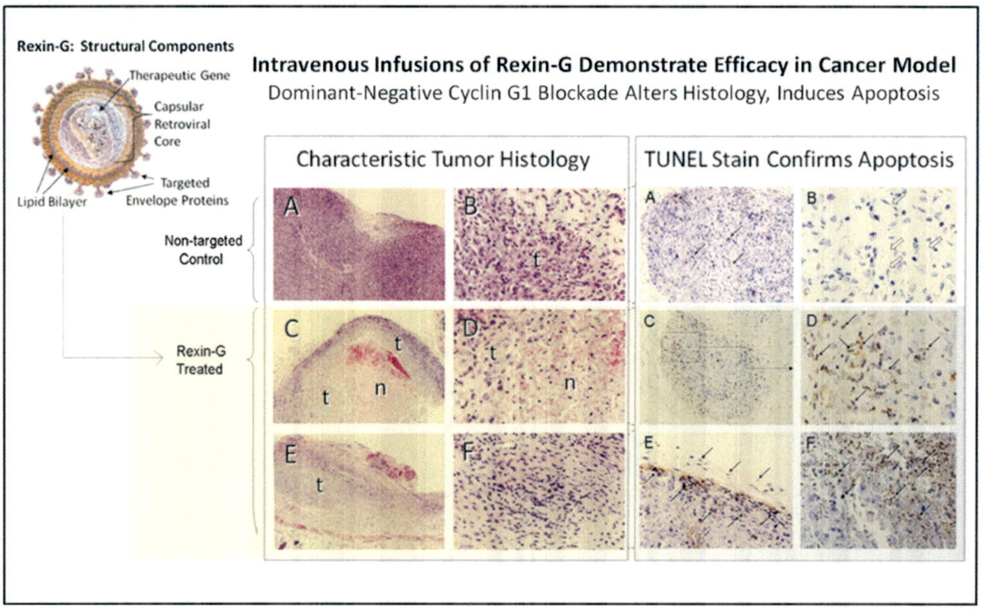

Fig. 5. Repeated intravenous infusions of Rexin-G abate the growth and alter the histology of pancreatic cancer xenografts in athymic mice.

Further histological analysis confirms that the major mechanism-of-action responsible for the observed tumor destruction is the induction of apoptosis by Rexin-G, which is evident in both the cancer cells and the endothelial cells of the associated tumor neovasculature. In addition to these histological indications of tumor destruction attributed to Rexin-G (Gordon et al., 2000, 2001) is the recruitment of tumor infiltrating lymphocytes to clean up the resultant tumor debris (see Figure 6).

Fig. 5 legend: Human pancreatic cancer cells were established as subcutaneous xenografts in the flanks of the experimental animals, followed one week later, by tail vein infusions of a tumor-targeted Rexin-G or a non-targeted vector (as indicated). Histological analysis of tumors from control vector- (A,B) versus Rexin-G vector-(C-F) treated animals (Left Panel) showed massive and focal necrosis (n) of tumor cells (t), along with zones of vascular disruption (C), and fibrosis (F). TUNEL staining for the detection of DNA fragmentation (Right Panel) confirmed the primary mechanism-of-action to be apoptosis (brown stain, arrows), which is rare in control tumors (A) with their robust vascular beds (B), but is readily evident in the disrupted vasculature (C,D) and in the dying tumor cells (E,F) of the Rexin-G treated animals.

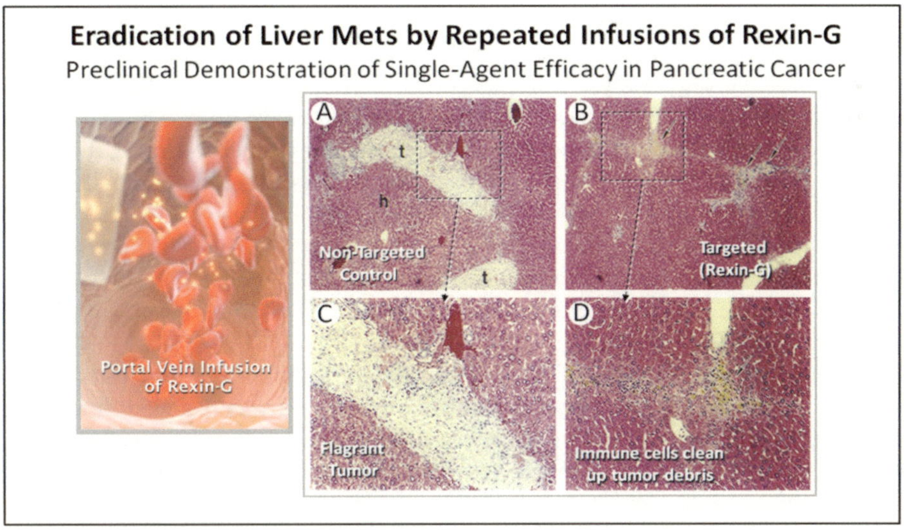

Fig. 6. Complete eradication of liver metastases by repeated infusions of Rexin-G retrovector in a murine model of metastatic pancreatic cancer.

Fig. 6 legend: Flagrant tumors are shown in control animals (A, enlarged in C) vs no evidence of active tumor cells in Rexin-G -treated mice (B, enlarged in D). Note: Resident Kupffer cells (macrophages in the liver) are observed to be engorged with hemosiderin indicative of phagocytosis of tumor debris. Analysis of dose-response (Gordon et al., 2000), in relation to inhibition of tumor growth, formed the basis of a more-predictive clinical pharmacology.

7. The 1st clinical stage – phase I studies establish clinical feasibility and overall safety

The definitive demonstrations of selective tumor targeting, predictable mechanisms-of-action, and single-agent efficacy in preclinical cancer models provided compelling impetus for expedient clinical development, which necessitated further evaluations of general safety, dose-response relationships, bio-distribution, pharmacokinetics, and monitoring of gene transfer in a series of scientific studies that ranged from mice, to rats, to rabbits, to larger animals (pigs). Taken as a whole, the resulting compilation of scientific evidence served to provide the *requisite documentation of general safety* and the *reasonable expectation of clinical benefit* that was critically analyzed by the NIH Recombinant DNA Advisory Committee (RAC), which was formed in 1974 in response to public concerns regarding the safety of manipulating genetic material through the use of recombinant DNA techniques. In accordance with its role as a federal advisory committee, the RAC forwarded its recommendations to the Director of the Office of Biotechnology Activities, in line with the General NIH Guidelines for basic and clinical research involving recombinant DNA molecules and human gene transfer trials, respectively. Critical review and analysis of scientific, safety, and ethical considerations by the RAC pertaining to the clinical utility and administration of Rexin-G in humans, was conducted in 2000 (Lenz et al., 2002) at which time, the appointed reviewers stated that the platform targeting biotechnologies embodied in Rexin-G were both elegant and important (Russell, RAC Transcript, 2000).

While it was initially envisioned that Rexin-G would be administered to human cancer patients regionally at first, via hepatic arterial infusions (Lenz et al., 2002), it so happened that a series of formal requests for Compassionate Use applications of Rexin-G in Stage IV metastatic pancreas cancer took precedent—in compliance with both U.S. FDA permissions and Philippine BFAD/FDA regulations—which served to propel the clinical advancement of Rexin-G. In terms of time, it served to validate the tumor-targeted gene delivery platform as a systemically administered agent. With federal allowances for such commendable international collaboration in place, Rexin-G was first deployed in the clinic in the Philippines in 2002, with the tacit acknowledgement that Epeius Biotechnologies would advance its clinical development program in the USA "as soon as practicable" (U.S. FDA Communications, 2002).

These pioneering clinical studies of Rexin-G in chemotherapy-resistant pancreatic cancer (Gordon et al., 2004) stand as the seminal foundations of targeted genetic medicine by (i) demonstrating the safety and single-agent anti-tumor activity of repeated intravenous infusions, (ii) affirming predicted dose-response relationships astutely extrapolated from pertinent preclinical data, and (iii) validating the tumoricidal mechanisms-of-action of Rexin-G, along with the now-classical hallmarks of tumor destruction (see Figure 7).

Fig. 7 legend: Combined PET-CT scan (Left Plate) shows central necrosis in 5 out of 6 visible lesions in one patient with chemo-resistant pancreatic cancer. An opportunistic surgical biopsy of a liver lesion after Rexin-G treatment (Right Plate) in another patient with chemo-resistant metastatic pancreatic cancer reveals characteristic zones of anti-angiogenesis (A), along with focal necrosis of tumor cells (A,B), overt apoptosis, verified by TUNEL stain (D,E), reparative fibrosis (A-f, Mason's Trichrome in C), and recruitment of tumor-infiltrating lymphocytes (F), including CD4+ helper (stained in F) and CD8+ killer T-cells (not shown).

The authors' report of unprecedented single-agent anti-tumor activity of Rexin-G observed in 3 out of 3 pancreatic cancer patients who were treated in the Philippines with increasing weekly doses of Rexin-G in an innovative *intra-patient dose-escalation regimen*—where careful analysis of drug safety was verified before escalating to progressively higher doses—gained Orphan Drug Designation for pancreatic cancer by the U.S. FDA in 2003, and federal funding from the FDA Orphan Products Development program in 2006. The first U.S.-based Phase I study established the overall safety of repeated infusions of Rexin-G and the lower rungs of the pharmacological dose-response curve for Stage IV pancreatic cancer (Galanis et al., 2008) compared to the higher, more-effective doses shown in succeeding advanced Phase I/II studies (shown in Figure 11; Chawla et al., 2010). Meanwhile, clinical development of Rexin-G advanced in the Philippines through a series of Phase I/II studies and an Expanded Access program, which extended the scope of clinical applications to a wider variety of cancers, including breast cancer, melanoma, and laryngeal CA (Gordon et al., 2006, 2007).

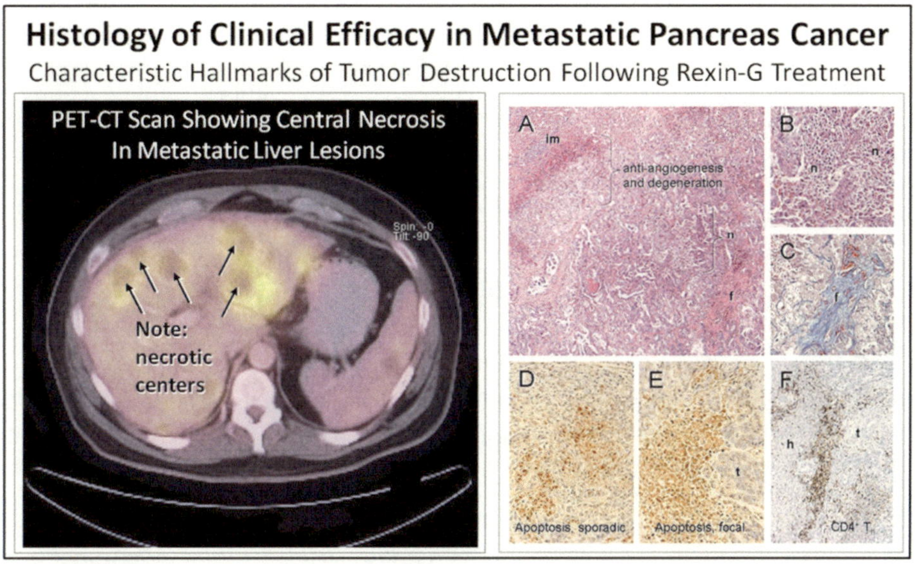

Fig. 7. Radiological and histological evidence of anti-tumor activity of Rexin-G.

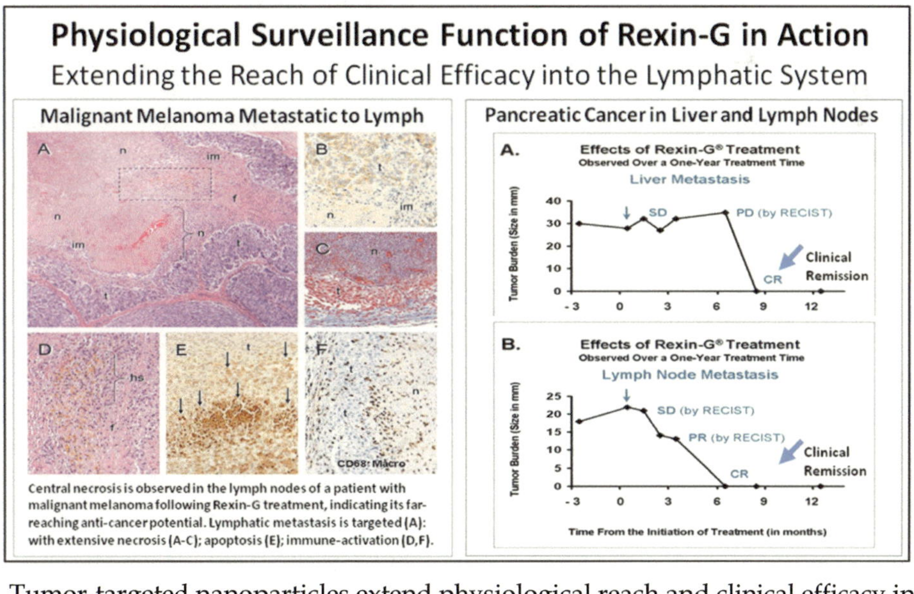

Fig. 8. Tumor-targeted nanoparticles extend physiological reach and clinical efficacy into the lymphatic system.

Among the most important insights gained from these pioneering clinical studies—insights which were not immediately apparent from the preclinical models—was the finding that the physiological surveillance function inherent in the Rexin-G nanoparticles was not only capable of targeting tumors by successive excursions through the general circulation, but was also capable of penetrating and eliminating cancer metastases in the lymphatic system (see Figure 8).

Fig. 8 legend: Biopsy of a surgically excised lymph node (Left Plate) in a patient with metastatic malignant melanoma exhibits the characteristic hallmarks of Rexin-G mediated tumor destruction along with its apoptotic mechanisms-of-action (legend). Monitoring stabilization of disease (SD), along with the observed decrease in the size and extent of lymph node metastasis (B) in a Stage IVb pancreatic cancer patient (Right Plate) encouraged clinical oncologists to "hold the course" of Rexin-G treatment, even in the face of slight progressive disease (PD) seen in the liver (A); an astute clinical decision that resulted in a clinical remission, initially observed after 9 months of Rexin-G treatment. Note: remission/survival ongoing > 2 yrs.

8. The 2nd clinical stage – phase II studies establish the molecular pharmacology

With the clinical feasibility and general safety of the Rexin-G retrovector formally established in the clinical setting, the U.S. FDA approved the stepwise escalation of Rexin-G dosage in a series of three *adaptive* and *advanced* Phase I/II studies for metastatic chemotherapy-resistant pancreas cancer, sarcoma, and breast cancer. The *adaptive* study designs were intended to further refine the analysis of Rexin-G bioactivity, in terms of pertinent tumor response criteria, while these inter-patient dose escalation studies were *advanced*, in as much as a Phase II evaluation of clinical efficacy was incorporated in each of the study designs. These studies demonstrated that Rexin-G was well tolerated, with no evidence of dose-limiting toxicities (DLT), and that Rexin-G exhibited dose-dependent anti-tumor activity when administered as a stand-alone therapy for pancreatic cancer and sarcoma (Chawla et al., 2009, 2010). Of particular importance was the availability of surgical specimens obtained during the course of Rexin-G treatment, where Rexin-G was permitted by study design to serve as both neoadjuvant therapy, to bring the cancer under control, and as post-surgical adjuvant therapy, to help prevent recurrence. The availability of such germane and opportune histology served to validate the predictable molecular and histological mechanisms of Rexin-G action (Hall et al., 2010; see Figure 9 below).

Fig. 9 legend: Immunostaining for the vector nanoparticles (Left Plate) demonstrates the generalized accumulation of vector particles within the tumor (light brown staining material A, versus Control, with no primary antibody B); moreover, the natural propensity/targeting of the retrovector envelope for the phosphate transporters that are abundant on proliferative cells results in targeting of tumor cells and associated vasculature (C-E). Right Plate: Immunostaining for Keratin identifies the islands tumor cells (A, insert) amidst extensive fibrosis (B, Trichrome stain), while TUNEL stain verifies active cancer cell death by apoptosis (C, D versus Control E). It is relevant to note that this patient with metastatic pancreatic cancer has enjoyed a sustained *surgical remission* with adjuvant Rexin-G therapy for over 2 years.

In the course of these advanced, adaptive Phase I/II studies, the clinical responses to Rexin-G were examined in a comprehensive manner, which included an analysis of tumor size (RECIST criteria), metabolic activity (International PET criteria), and changes in tumor density (CHOI criteria). From this, it was possible (i) to discern early tumor responses to Rexin-G treatment (recall Figure 7) in relation to its tumor-targeted mechanisms-of-action, and (ii) to refine the evaluation of clinical efficacy (previously established as RECIST for cytotoxic chemotherapy) and to apply more pertinent evaluation criteria to the emerging field of targeted biologics. In the case of an osteosarcoma patient, for example, the use of

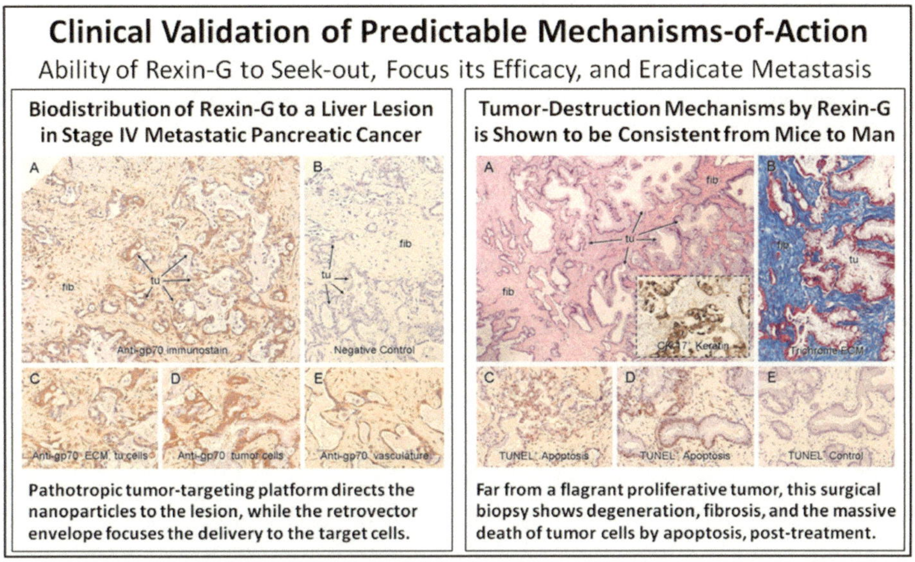

Fig. 9. Immunohistochemical staining of sections of a biopsied liver nodule obtained during Rexin-G treatment, revealing tumor-targeting and tumor-destroying mechanisms-of-action.

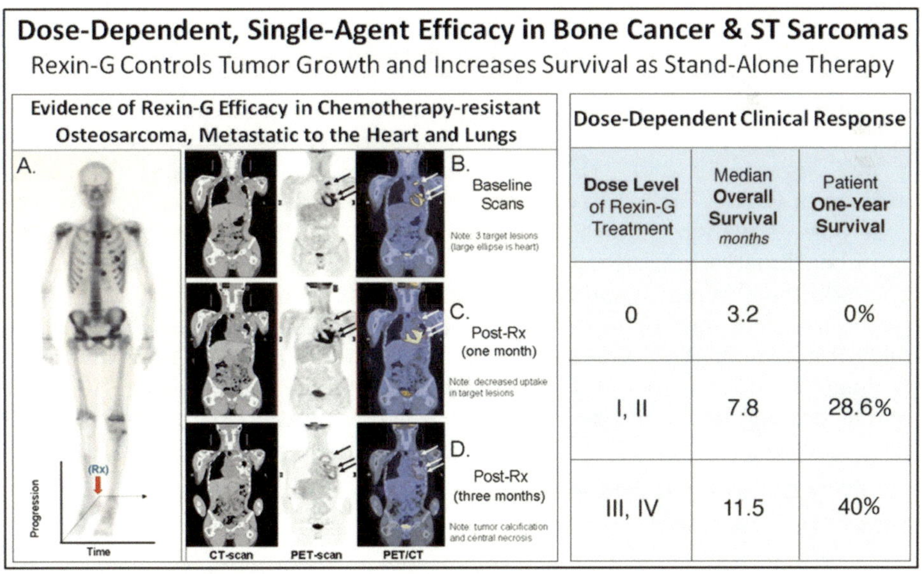

Dose Level of Rexin-G Treatment	Median Overall Survival *months*	Patient One-Year Survival
0	3.2	0%
I, II	7.8	28.6%
III, IV	11.5	40%

Fig. 10. Demonstration of dramatic anti-tumor activity of Rexin-G as monotherapy for osteosarcoma (by PET/CT scans) and dose-dependent overall survival time by analysis of a Phase I/II clinical study of Rexin-G in bone and soft tissue sarcomas.

RECIST criteria for evaluating tumor response was not reliable, since clinical efficacy was characterized more appropriately by the reduction in tumor metabolic activity (by PET scan), accompanied by extensive calcification of tumor nodules (see Figure 10).
Based on these findings, the U.S. FDA approved a Phase II study for osteosarcoma to be conducted concomitantly with the ongoing Phase I/II study for bone and soft tissue sarcomas (STS) that used the PET scan as the primary imaging tool for the evaluation of clinical efficacy. Aggregate analysis of these study results confirmed the overall safety of Rexin-G (with no DLT), its anti-tumor activity, and the positive dose-dependent impact on patient survival parameters (Figure 10) which, after all, represents a "gold standard" for the evaluation of clinical responses for a prospective anti-cancer agent.
Fig. 10 legend: Left Panel: Radiological examination of a 17-year old male patient after primary tumor excision and limb salvage surgery (A) reveals rapidly progressing metastases (insert) to lung and adrenal gland. Rexin-G infusions halted tumor progression, as evidenced by no new lesions, a significant (48%) reduction in tumor metabolic activity and overt calcification of the target lesions shown in follow-up PET-CT scans during Rexin-G treatment (baseline B, versus C and D). Right Panel: Analysis of the Phase I/II study data demonstrates a dose-dependent increase in patient survival parameters.
In these Phase I/II and Phase II studies of clinical safety and efficacy, it became increasingly evident that the observed dose-response phenomenology, as well as the predicted Calculus of Parity (Gordon et al., 2006; Gordon and Hall, 2007), had served to establish the basic foundations of an emerging clinical pharmacology for Rexin-G, providing estimates of optimal weekly doses, by determining the quantitative *threshold for bioactivity* for both pancreas cancer and sarcomas; and providing a practical estimate of the actual numbers of nanoparticles needed on a weekly basis to match an aggressive, chemotherapy-resistant tumor burden and, thus, to impact the fatal course of metastatic disease. This emergent clinical pharmacology has several important implications: First, it serves to address and to resolve the problem of exponential tumor cell growth, with the conclusion that it is indeed difficult, but not impossible, to provide sufficient numbers of targeted nanoparticles needed to meet and match a given tumor burden. Second, it affirms that chemo-resistant cancer patients do indeed die, as predicted, in the absence of sufficient quantitative intervention, in accordance with the results of the Rexin-G low-dose safety studies and the historical controls (see Figures 10 and 11). Most importantly, by establishing the quantitative pharmacology of Rexin-G action in end- or late-stage chemo-resistant cancer, these seminal Phase I/II dose-escalation studies serve to establish critical analytical parameters and meaningful benchmarks for further clinical studies—studies that will extend the utility of Rexin-G to additional types of solid tumors, to surgical oncologists who will employ it as neoadjuvant/adjuvant therapy to effectuate a curative surgery, to clinical oncologists who will deploy it in combination with other useful anticancer agents, and eventually to many cancer patients at much earlier stages of the disease, where the respective tumor burden could be matched and can no longer be considered either unreachable or insurmountable.

9. Regulatory considerations – efficacy & safety as the basis of pharmacology / toxicology

The conduct and the progression of clinical trials for an investigational new drug (IND) are carried out under stringent oversight by the clinical investigators, the medical and scientific authorities of the corporate sponsor, and the local and federal regulatory agencies, the latter of which provide an additional level of critical analysis and assurance that adequate safety considerations have been achieved prior to granting approval for a given cadre of patients to be treated at the next higher dose level, as specified in the clinical study design. In this regard, it is important to note that Rexin-G exhibited an exemplary safety profile in the adaptive Phase I/II studies sufficient to warrant an expedited dose escalation. As represented graphically in Figure 11, the enrollment of chemotherapy-resistant sarcoma patients in the Phase I/II study happened to outpace the enrollment of patients in the Phase I/II study for pancreatic cancer; and, as such, the scheduled dose-escalations proceeded to higher, more-effective doses in a shorter period of time. However, in view of (i) the documented safety of each preceding dose level, (ii) the evidence of dose-dependent tumor control, and (iii) the survival benefits achieved in the sarcoma study, the U.S. FDA granted permission for an *"across-the-board"* dose escalation for all three ongoing Phase I/II trials in an effort to improve cancer control and patient outcome. An examination of the resulting Kaplan-Meier survival curves (see Figure 11, below) affirms the astuteness of this regulatory approval, whereby the critical analysis of the bone and soft tissue sarcoma patients served, in effect, to extend the lives of the pancreatic cancer patients. In this context, the constructive philosophical adage, first introduced in the FDA Centennial Book chapter "A Primer on Pathotropic Medicine"(Gordon and Hall, 2007), is all the more compelling: *"When the pathotropic medication is of broad spectrum utility, as in the case of Rexin-G, it behooves the clinical investigator to expand the scope of the clinical applications to include a broad spectrum of different intractable metastatic cancers, with the realization that—given the appropriate interim analysis—each new patient's experience may benefit the next, and that additional penetrating insights can be gained upon extensive critical analysis performed in aggregate."* Hence, it is important to consider that the *safety* and *efficacy* data obtained from a relatively small number of patients in clinical trials of this investigational new drug are, in actuality, the prime scientific building blocks upon which the *toxicology*, the *pharmacology*, and ultimately the *praxis* of targeted genetic medicine will be constructed.

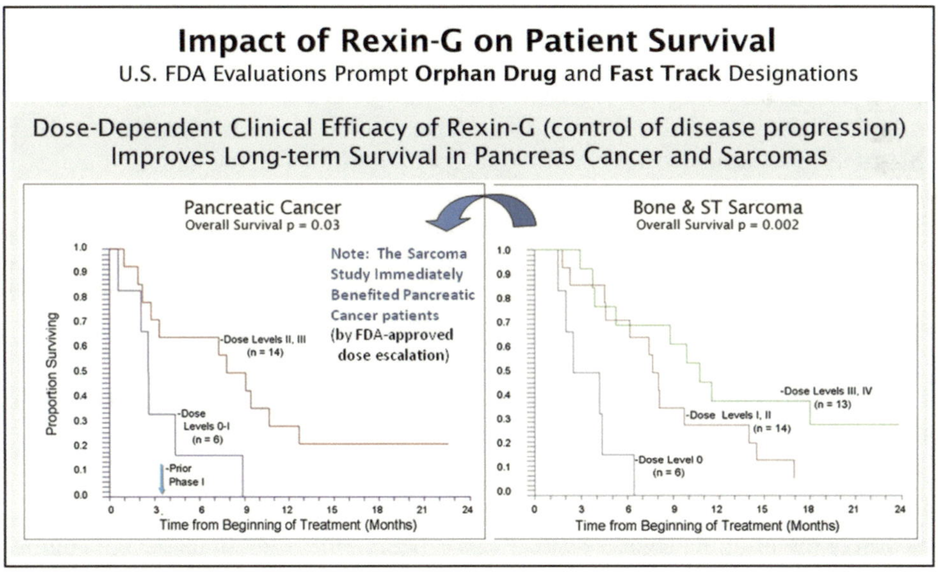

Fig. 11. Kaplan-Meier survival curves for two concomitant Phase I/II studies of Rexin-G administered as monotherapy to metastatic cancer patients who had previously failed standard chemotherapies.

Fig. 11 legend: Left Panel: Overall survival of pancreatic cancer patients is increased significantly from the previous Phase I safety studies (arrow) by successive dose escalation, which was expedited by critical analysis of an ongoing Phase I/II study of bone and soft tissue sarcoma (Right Panel) and subsequent allowance of an *across-the-board* dose escalation to effective clinical doses. Note, the dismal survival times observed in the lowest dose groups is in agreement with historical control data for each of these respective chemo-resistant cancers; while dose-dependent gains in overall survival are clinically, statistically significant.

In the Philippines, where the clinical development of Rexin-G proceeded to advance with similar regulatory oversight, data analysis, and guidance, the clinical studies were facilitated by the federal approval of an Expanded Access Program, wherein a larger and more diverse set of metastatic cancers - cancers originating from all three germ layers - were determined to be responsive to the anti-cancer bioactivity of Rexin-G. At this point, it became exceedingly important to standardize the GMP bio-manufacturing of Rexin-G to an even greater extent, and to undertake a program of research and development aimed at characterizing the *stability* of the drug product under conditions of long-term storage, which is measured in years. Following extensive analysis of product safety, efficacy, composition, purity, and long-term stability, Rexin-G was granted Accelerated Approval in 2007, receiving a Certificate of Product Registration from the Philippine Bureau of Food and Drugs (BFAD/Philippine FDA) enabling its commercialization for the treatment of all solid tumors that are determined to be resistant to standard chemotherapies. Thus, it is reasonable to expect that Rexin-G will follow a similar course of clinical development in the United States and worldwide, where clinical studies and regulatory oversight are comparable.

Following the registration of Rexin-G for all solid chemo-resistant tumors in the Philippines, and the attainment of its first Orphan Drug Designation for pancreatic cancer in the U.S, the clinical development of Rexin-G advanced steadily in the USA with the successful completion of three adaptive Phase I/II studies for sarcoma, breast cancer and pancreatic cancer, and a Phase II study for osteosarcoma (Chawla et al., 2009, 2010); in each of these studies, both primary and secondary endpoints were achieved. Formal critical evaluation of the U.S. safety and efficacy data, with due consideration for the unmet medical need, resulted in the granting of two additional *Orphan Drug Designations* for Rexin-G - with its implicit market protections and clinical development priorities for soft tissue sarcoma and osteosarcoma. In mid-2009, Rexin-G gained *Fast Track Product* designation from the U.S. FDA as 2nd-line treatment for pancreatic cancer, to expedite the development and validation of the tumor-targeted gene delivery platform and its therapeutic "payload."

10. The commercial product – GMP production, bio-processing, QA testing, and scale-up

As Rexin-G approaches the cusp of Phase III clinical trials in the USA for both pancreatic cancer and sarcomas, it is important to note that the clinical development of Rexin-G to date is a function of the multiple levels of safety and efficacy embodied in its design engineering, as is the observed broad-spectrum anti-cancer activity. Indeed, the molecular-genetic components of the Rexin-G retrovector are enhanced by the set of virtues and limitations inherent in the biotechnology platform, which work together to provide *four distinctive levels of safety* in coordination with *three distinctive levels of efficacy* (see Gordon and Hall, 2010). In terms of Safety: (i) the stealth vector platform allows repeated infusions without untoward immunologic reactions; (ii) the limitations of the retroviral core becomes a virtue, as the vector is capable of enforcing gene expression in proliferative / dividing cells only; (iii) the growth-associated designer gene is active against cancer cells and proliferative vasculature but not against normal non-dividing cells; and (iv) the pathotropic accumulation in cancerous tissues sequesters the vector away from non-target organs. In terms of Efficacy: (i) the cell cycle gene knockout provides for broad-spectrum anti-cancer activity, while (ii) the anti-angiogenic activity destroys tumor-associated vasculature, and (iii) the pathotropic targeting leads to effective drug accumulation where it is needed most, i.e., in cancerous lesions in the vicinity of target cancer cells. In terms of the therapeutic "designer gene" it bears reiteration that recent studies of functional genomics using high-throughput screening methodologies have served to validate the Cyclin G1 locus as a critical gene target for the key tumor-suppressive microRNA, miR-122 (Gramanteri et al., 2007; Fornari et al., 2009), thereby linking the loss of this natural endogenous molecular regulation (of the Cyclin G1 locus) to both the mechanisms of carcinogenesis (Bai et al., 2009) and the cytological progression of metastatic disease (Coulouarn et al., 2009). In light of such scientific validation of the drug target, it is increasingly apparent that, by inhibiting the executive oncogenic Cyclin G1 pathway in a highly selective manner, the molecular-genetic construct delivered by Rexin-G serves to restore a natural *tumor-suppressive function* that is lost or disabled with the onset of many cancers. In anticipation of the calculated need for higher-potency Rexin-G formulations, along with the need to produce much larger quantities of the Phase III clinical grade product—which essentially becomes the commercial product—coordinated research and development activities have focused on the large-scale biopharmaceutical manufacturing of Rexin-G under stringent GMP conditions, where an uncompromising effort was made to preserve the integrity of each and all of the structural and enzymatic components that constitute the functionality of the tumor-targeted nanoparticle, and to preserve the fidelity of the therapeutic transgene.

Physicochemically, the Rexin-G nanoparticle is assembled from a certified bank of *producer cells* under the instructive directions of three separate gene cassettes (called plasmids): 1. Gag (structural), 2. Pol (enzymatic), and 3. Envelope (cell recognition and entry), which come together in a process called transfection to determine the unique properties of the synthetic retrovector particles. Namely, the nano-sized particles are *replication incompetent*, packaging only the therapeutic gene of interest; they are *stealth* in terms of their low immunogenicity, enabling repeated intravenous infusions; they are *selective*, capable of delivering the therapeutic transgene to dividing cells only; and they are *pathotropically-targeted*, physically capable of seeking-out and accumulating in diseased tissues under physiological conditions. The use of the 'Split Genome' elements in biopharmaceutical manufacturing—i.e., the partitioning of the retrovector elements into three separate and distinct plasmids—renders the synthetic nanoparticles certifiably replication incompetent, while successive generations of R&D and improvements in plasmid structure and performance elevated the industry to a new *state-of-the-art* (see Gordon et al., 2008 for a review). The strategic utilization of a transient co-transfection system for the bioproduction of each large-scale batch of Rexin-G—as opposed to stable packaging or producer cell lines, which are susceptible and prone to genetic drift—is purposeful, in that it maintains all the refinements in retrovector design engineering in the final clinical product.

While the myriad details of biopharmaceutical GMP protocols, optimizations of cell factories, post-production bio-processing procedures, qualification of bioassays, product identity assessments, product purity testing, and sterility certification, along with the multitude of quality control and quality assurance issues and documentation that accompany these highly-standardized procedures is beyond the scope of this review, it should be emphasized nonetheless that these are among the most meticulously-prepared and thoroughly-documented records that are subjected to critical analysis by the FDA, under the auspices of Process Analytical Technology (PAT) and Chemistry, Manufacturing and Control (CMC) reviews. Suffice it to say that the developers of Rexin-G are in complete accord with the U.S. FDA's current perspective on modern drug quality systems, which states, *"...quality cannot be tested into products; it should be built-in or should be by design."*

By addressing and resolving a number of serious GMP and CMC issues that had previously plagued the biopharmaceutical industry, in terms of the consistency, variability, and industrial scale-up of complex biologics to the point of commercial feasibility, the developers of Rexin-G demonstrated the practical utility of applied research: improving the overall safety, efficiency, productivity, purity, scalability, economy-of-scale, and ultimately the affordability of the clinical grade biologic product for the benefit of cancer patients, the biopharmaceutical industry, and society.

In the context of this communication, it bears mention that the relative purity of Rexin-G, over that which was originally approved for use in humans and employed in years of clinical trials, has been increased more than 400X. In other words, the clinical product (now at 1 x 10e10 cfu/ml) is well over 99.7% more pure in terms of allowable excipients per dose. For example, a 500ml dose of Rexin-G at 2.5 x 10e7cfu/ml is now administered as 1.25 ml.

In January 2011, the U.S. FDA granted Phase 3 status for Rexin-G. What this means, in terms of clinical development, is that the Rexin-G product, with its advanced GMP manufacturing, bio-processing, and final formulation, meets rigorous FDA standards for obtaining a marketing license in the future; and that the developers can now proceed with its strategic, diversified Phase 3 drug development programs for osteosarcoma, soft tissue sarcoma, and pancreatic cancer where it has received Fast Track Designation and Orphan drug priorities.

11. The 3rd clinical stage – multiple phase III studies for U.S. product registration

Despite the enlightened intentions of the U.S. FDA Accelerated Approval program to shorten the development times of promising new drugs for serious medical illness - that is, to grant accelerated approval for new molecular entities on the basis of compelling Phase II trial data, followed by confirmatory post-approval trials - there has been a discernable reversion, in recent years, for the U.S. FDA to restrict Phase II efficacy endpoints and to encourage sponsors to design accelerated approval applications on the basis of interim analyses of protracted Phase III trials (Richey et al., 2009). Moreover, a number of adverse instances in the drug approval process have raised legitimate concerns by the FDA Oncology Drugs Advisory Committee (ODAC), which has essentially created new hurdles, for both clinically effective and ineffective agents alike, and has increased the focus on post-marketing studies (Goozner, 2010, 2011). Therefore, it cannot be considered either expedient or logical to undertake a program of clinical development for a new and potentially important oncology agent based solely on acceleration of its marketing approval. Rather, the heightened and politically-charged regulatory climate encourages the responsible sponsor to undertake a robust and long-term program of clinical development, which (i) strengthens and improves clinical validation of safety and efficacy, (ii) mitigates the risk that is inherent in the conduct of a single clinical trial, (iii) broadens clinical utility (and potential market share) by expanding clinical indications, and (iv) serves to inspire confidence and lasting support from regulatory bodies in the fullness of time.

Commensurate with the fundamental principles of basic science—the step-wise demonstrations of physiological tumor-targeting, predictable mechanisms-of-action, pharmacological safety, and single-agent anti-tumor activity, including dose-dependent survival benefits—is the strident recommendation of the primary inventors that the high-value biotechnology platform embodied in Rexin-G merits the implementation of a comprehensive, progressive, and diversified program of clinical development: a program of clinical development that not only meets but far exceeds the minimal requisites for federal regulatory approval. After all, the cancer genetics, the molecular biotechnologies, the functional genomics, and the medicinal nanotechnologies embodied within Rexin-G represent a *nano-architectural* triumph of modern medicine. It is within the most stringent guidelines and guidance of the U.S. FDA that Phase II and Phase III pivotal studies of Rexin-G are currently being designed: as first-line therapy in combination with anti-metabolites, as stand-alone therapy for second-line indications, and as neoadjuvant/adjuvant therapy in combination with surgical procedures.

With the clinical validation of the tumor-targeted gene delivery platform accomplished, and the biopharmaceutical evaluation of Rexin-G as a Phase 3 (i.e., commercial) product achieved, the end of one particular *Product Development Stage* (that of Rexin-G) signals the beginning of the next (introducing Reximmune-C). In light of the potential "pipeline" of pathotropically targeted anti-cancer agents, it was first reasoned, and then proven in preclinical studies, that the same bio-technological platform developed for the targeted delivery of the cytocidal *designer gene* could just as readily deliver an immune-stimulating cytokine gene directly to the same cancerous lesions, which would provide a highly-localized and personalized form of cancer vaccination (Gordon et al., 2007, 2008; Zolnik et al., 2010). This two-tier complementary approach—termed the *GeneVieve (Genes for Life) Protocol*—aimed at both tumor eradication and cancer vaccination, was evaluated in a limited number of patients who benefited from previous Rexin-G therapy (see Figure 12 below). The sequential delivery of Rexin-G followed by Reximmune-C, which bears a controllable construct of the granulocyte-macrophage colony-stimulating factor (GM-CSF) transgene, induced substantial tumor necrosis and recruitment of tumor-infiltrating lymphocytes in cancerous lesions without raising the baseline levels of the powerful cytokine in the patient's blood; thereby affirming both general safety and an effective Reximmune-C dose range (Cornelio et al., 2010). In the subsequent follow-up of the first 9 patients receiving the tumor-targeted cancer vaccination in a Phase I/II study of the GeneVieve Protocol, a large percentage (> 70%) of these otherwise poor prognosis patients exhibited an overall survival beyond one year (Ignacio et al., 2010). By meeting both primary and secondary study endpoints—defining a safe and effective dose range—these findings indicate that this strategic combination of two pathotropic medicines (Rexin-G plus Reximmune-C) is safe and well-tolerated, and may help control tumor growth and prolong survival, thus advancing the protocol and the molecular biotechnologies of personalized cancer vaccination as a feasible and promising approach.

Fig. 12 legend: Rationale: "Pathotropic" targeting of therapeutic gene delivery enables personalized cancer vaccinations *in situ* by means of simple intravenous infusions. Rexin-G and Reximmune-C are tumor-targeted retrovectors bearing a cytocidal cyclin G1 'knockout'

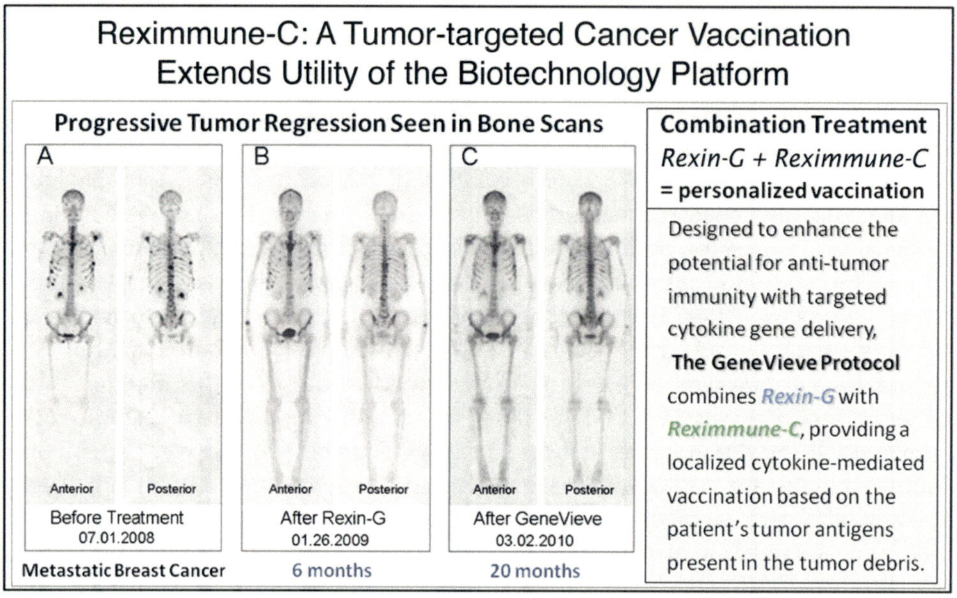

Fig. 12. Bone scans of a patient with metastatic breast cancer obtained at intervals following treatment with Rexin-G followed by a two-tier cancer vaccination with Rexin-G plus Reximmune-C (The GeneVieve Protocol).

construct and a controllable GM-CSF expression construct, respectively. The working hypothesis for this bipartite tumor-targeted cancer vaccination strategy is that the personalized vaccination of a patient against his/her own specific cancer type can be achieved by combining (1) a targeted vector bearing a tumoricidal payload, i.e. Rexin-G with (2) a targeted vector bearing a potent immuno-stimulatory gene, i.e. Reximmune-C. First, Rexin-G is administered to control tumor growth and to expose neoantigens within the tumor microenvironment, followed by defined pulses of Reximmune-C, which recruits the patient's immune cells into the lesions, thereby prompting immunologic activation, recognition of tumor neoantigens, and induction of an antitumor immunity. Baseline (A); post Rexin-G (B); post Rexin-G plus Reximmune C (C).

12. Looking back and then forward – reflections on proper values and valuations

Looking back over the past decade of scientific and medical achievement in the emerging field of targeted genetic medicine, the term *decennium mirabilis* seems all the more appropriate. The technological challenges that once stymied and precluded therapeutic gene delivery *in vivo* have all been overcome. The triad of forbidding challenges of *undeveloped biotechnology*, *institutional incredulity*, and *scientific skepticism* have been confronted and allayed by a significant amount of scientific and clinical data that heralded the advent of pathotropic targeting as an enabling biotechnological platform with a series of sound conclusions: (i) it is no longer impossible to reach the fabric of the nature of malignant disease itself (i.e., *collagen patefacio,* from Gordon and Hall, 2009); (ii) it is no longer impossible to deliver a sufficient number of therapeutic genes to the appropriate site and get them to stay there long enough to impact and reverse the course of metastatic disease

(Gordon and Hall, 2010; Hall et al., 2010); (iii) it is no longer appropriate to deny the mathematical potentiality of a targeted genetic medicine, in light of the quantitative demonstrations of single agent dose-dependent anti-tumor activity, along with the recent advances in biopharmaceutical vector production that have raised the potency of the clinical-grade vectors more than two orders of magnitude (Gordon and Hall, 2009). Indeed, as the development and validation of the world's first (Waehler et al., 2007; Gordon and Hall, 2010), but no longer only (see Reximmune-C; Gordon et al., 2007, 2008), tumor-targeted genetic medicine is recognized, the promise and potential of the platform have begun to percolate into the general medical literature, impacting the practice of clinical oncology (Hughes, 2009), medical imaging (Bjojani et al, 2010), medicinal nanotechnology (Peach et al., 2009), and gene therapy (Sverdlov, 2009), as well as the discussions of bedside bioethics (Toh, 2011) and the practical applications of tumor immunology (Zolnik et al., 2010).

Looking forward into the future, it is only a matter of *time* (see Gordon and Hall, 2009) when the progression of metastatic disease is no longer considered to be intractable, and the poor prognosis of chemotherapy-resistant cancer is summarily improved. It is also only a matter of *time*, when the potentially "disruptive" biotechnology is eventually viewed as enabling platform for further research and development, and the potential of the resulting "pipeline" becomes a value-added resource for the biopharmaceutical industry. As the Development Stage of this leading genetic medicine comes to a close, and the resources of the academic institutions and the idealistic enterprises that initially supported its advancement are expended in the process of serving such unmet medical needs, it would be expected that the pioneering inventors and the visionary business builders are eventually replaced by professional financial institutions and pharmaceutical conglomerates that are capable of supporting vast expenditures required for the progressive, diversified programs of late-stage clinical studies that will expand the clinical applications, optimize the protocols for a multitude of new treatment combinations, and ultimately extend the reach of pathotropically-targeted gene delivery into the evolving praxis of modern and post-modern medicine. One can only hope that the abiding values of inspiration and compassion that once fueled the hearts and minds of the physicians and scientists who carried this platform thus far for the benefit of the cancer patient, will not be lost entirely in the valuations to come.

13. Acknowledgements

The authors are grateful to Heather C. Gordon for astute medical and scientific illustrations and for assistance in the writing of the manuscript.

14. References

Ahmed, F., Steele, J.C., Herbert, J.M., et al. (2008). Tumor stroma as a target in cancer. *Curr Cancer Drug Targets,* Vol.8,No.6,447-53.

Allen. C., Paraskevakou, G., Liu, C., et al. (2008). Oncolytic measles virus strains in the treatment of gliomas. *Expert Opin Biol Ther,* Vol. 8,No. 2,213-320.

Andrews, B.K., & Berndt, M.C. (2004). Platelet physiology and thrombosis. *Thromb Res* Vol. 114,No. 5-6,447-53.

Bacac, M., & Stamenkovic, J. (2008). Metastatic cancer cell. *Annu Rev Pathol,* Vol. 3,221-47.Andrews, B.K., & Berndt, M.C. (2004). Platelet physiology and thrombosis. *Thromb Res* Vol. 114,No. 5-6,447-53.

Baek, W.K., Kim, D., Jung, N., et al. (2003). Increased expression of cyclin G1 in leiomyoma compared with normal myometrium. *Am J Obstet Gynecol,* Vol. 188, No. 3,634-39.

Bai, S., Nasser, M.W., Wang, B., et al. (2009). MicroRNA-122 inhibits tumorigenic properties of hepatocellular carcinoma cells and sensitizes these cells to sorafenib. *J Biol Chem,* Vol. 284,No. 46, 32015-27.

Berkhout, B., Verhoef, K., van Wamel, J.L.B., & Back, N.K.T. (1999). Genetic instability of live, attenuated human immunodeficiency virus Type 1 vaccine strains. *J Virol,* Vol. 73,No. 2,1138-45.

Bjojani, M.S., Van Dort, M., Rehemtulla, A., & Ross, B.D. (2010). Targeted Imaging and Therapy of Brain Cancer Using Theranostic Nanoparticles. Mol. Pharmaceutics, Vol. 7,No. 6,1921-9.

Blechacz, B., & Russell, S.J. (2008). Measles virus as an oncolytic vector platform. *Curr Gene Ther,* Vol. 8,No. 3,162-75.

Box, C., Rogers, S.J., Mendiola, M., & Eccles, S.A. (2010). Tumour microenvironments interactions: paths to progression and targets for treatment. *Semin Cancer Biol,* Vol. 20,No. 3,128-38.

Braun-Dullaeus, R.C., Mann, M.J., & Dzau, V.J. (1998). Cell cycle progression: new therapeutic target for vascular proliferative disease. *Circulation,* Vol. 98,82-89.

Braybrooks, J.P., Slade, A., Deplanque, G., et al. (2005). Phase I study of MetXia-P450 gene therapy and oral cyclophosphamide for patients with advanced breast cancer or melanoma. *Clin Cancer Res,* V.11,N.4,1512-20.

Burris, H. III, & Rocha-Lima, C. (2008). New therapeutic directions for advanced pancreatic cancer: Targeting the epidermal growth factor and vascular endothelial growth factor pathways. *The Oncologist,* Vol. 3,289-98.

Capetta, A., Lonardi, S., Pastorelli, D., et al. (2011). Advanced gastric cancer (GC) and cancer of the gastro-oesophageal junction (GEJ): focus on targeted therapies. *Crit Rev Oncol Hematol.* (Epub ahead of print January 2011).

Chawla, S.P., Chua, V.S., Kalra, A., et al. (2008). Phase II study of pathotropic nanoparticles bearing a cytocidal cyclin G1 construct (Rexin-G) reveals significant anti-tumor activity with no toxicity in chemo-resistant metastatic osteosarcoma. *The Cardiothoracic Surgery Network and CTOS 14th Annual Meeting,* London, U.K.Chawla, S.P., Chua, V.S., Mohan, V., et al. (2008). Phase I/II study of targeted gene delivery in vivo - intravenous infusions of Rexin-G - demonstrates significant biologic activity by FDG-PET-CT without toxicity in patients with progressive chemo-resistant sarcoma, breast cancer and pancreatic cancer. *J Clin Oncol,* Vol. 26,(May 20 suppl: abstract # 14509).

Chawla, S.P., Chua, V.S., Fernandez, L., et al. (2009). Phase I/II and Phase II studies of targeted gene delivery in vivo: intravenous Rexin-G for chemotherapy-resistant sarcoma and osteosarcoma. *Mol Ther.* Vol. 17,1651-7.

Chawla, S.P., Chua, V.S., Fernandez, L. (2010). Advanced Phase I/II studies of targeted gene delivery in vivo: Intravenous Rexin-G for gemcitabine-resistant metastatic pancreatic cancer. *Mol Ther.* Vol. 18,No. 2,435-41.

Chen, D.S., Zhu, N.L., Hung, G., et al. (1997). Retroviral vector-mediated transfer of an antisense cyclin G1 construct inhibits osteosarcoma tumor growth in nude mice. *Hum Gene Ther,* Vol. 8,1679-86.

Chen, H.H., Cawood, R., & Seymour, L.W. (2008). Toward more effective gene delivery. *Genome Biol,* Vol. 9,1-301.

Chua, V.S., Chawla, S.P., Kalra, A., et al. (2008). Phase I/II study of targeted gene delivery in vivo - intravenous infusion of pathotropic nanoparticles bearing a cytocidal cyclin G1 gene (Rexin-G) - demonsrtrates anti-tumor activity in chemo-resistant metastatic bone and soft tissue sarcoma. *The Cardiothoracic Surgery Network and CTOS 14 Annual Meeting,*London, U.K.

Coulouarn, C., Factor, V.M., Andersen, J.B., et al. (2009). Loss of miR-122 expression in liver cancer correlates with suppression of the hepatic phenotype and gain of metastatic properties. *Oncogene,* Vol. 28,No. 40,3526-36.

Cornelio, G.H., Lorenzo, C.C., Lopez, F.F., et al. (1997). Phase I study of sequential targeted gene delivery: Intravenous infusions of Rexin-G followed by Reximmune-C induce tumor necrosis and recruitment of tumor infiltrating lymphocytes in cancerous lesions. *J Clin Oncol,* Vol. 26,(May 20 suppl: abstract # 3077).

Cornelio, G.H., Lorenzo, C.C., Lopez, F.F., et al. (2008). Phase I study of sequential targeted gene delivery: Intravenous infusions of Rexin-G followed by Reximmune-C induce tumor necrosis and recruitment of tumor infiltrating lymphocytes in cancerous lesions. *J Clin Oncol,* Vol. 26 (May 20 suppl; abstr 3077).

Csikasz-Nagy, A., Novak, B., & Tyson, J.J. (2008) Reverse engineering models of cell cycle regulation. *Adv Exp Med Biol,* Vol. 641,88-97.

Dalba, C., Bellier, B., Kasahara, N., & Klatzmann, D. (2007). Replication-competent vectors and empty virus-like particles: new retroviral vector designs for cancer gene therapy or vaccines. *Mol Ther,*Vol.15,No.3,457-66.

Davis, J.J., & Fang, B. (2005). Oncolytic virotherapy for cancer treatment: challenges and solutions. *J Gene Med,* Vol. 7,No. 11, 1380-9.

Di Marco, M., Di Cicilia, R,. Macchini, M.,et al. (2010). Metastatic pancreatic cancer: is gemcitabine still the best standard treatment? (Review). *Oncol Rep,* Vol. 23,No. 5,1183-92.

Ding, L., Getz, G., Wheeler, D.A., et al. (2008). Somatic mutations affect key pathways in lung adenocarcinoma. *Nature,* Vol. 455,No. 7216,1069-75.

Dingli, D., & Russell, S.J. (2002). Genetic targeting of retroviral vectors, In: *Vector Targeting for Therapeutic Gene Delivery.* Curiel, D.T., & Douglas, J.T., 267-291, John Wiley & Sons, Inc., New Jersey, U.S.A.

Feng, Z., Zhang, C., Wu, R., & Hu, W. (2011). Tumor suppressor p53 meets microRNAs. *J Mol Cell Biol,* Vol. 3,No. 1,44-50. Ferguson, J.E. III., & Patterson, C. (2003). Break the cycle: the role of cell-cycle modulation in the prevention of vasculoproliferative diseases. *Cell,* Vol. 2,No. 3,211-19.

Fornari, F., Gramantieri, L., Giovannini, C., et al. (2009). MiR-122/cyclin G1 interaction modulates p53 activity and affects doxorubicin sensitivity of human hepatocarcinoma cells. *Cancer Res,* Vol. 69,No. 14,5761-7.

Fressinaud, E., Mazurier, C., & Meyer, D. (2002). Molecular genetics of type 2 von Willebrand disease. *Int J Hematol,* Vol. 75,No. 1,9-18.

Galanis, E., Carlson, S.K., Foster, N.R., et al. (2008). Phase I trial of a pathotropic retroviral vector expressing a cytocidal cyclin G1 construct (Rexin-G) in patients with advanced pancreatic cancer. *Mol Ther,* Vol. 16,No. 5,979-84.

Gerard, C., & Goldbeter, A. (2009). Temporal self-organization of the cyclin/Cdk network driving the mammalian cell cycle. *Proc Natl Acad Sci U S A,* Vol. 106,No. 51,21643-8.

Gonzalez-Angulo, A.M., Morales-Vasquez, F., & Hortobagyi, G.N. (2007). Overview of resistance to systemic therapy in patients with breast cancer. *Adv Exp Med Biol,* Vol. 608,1-22.

Goozner, M. (2010). FDA increases focus on postmarketing studies. *J Natl Cancer Inst,* Vol. 102,No.17,1302-4.

Goozner, M. (2011). Accelerated drug approval: FDA may get tougher; companies cite hurdles. *J Natl Cancer Inst,* Vol. 103;No. 6,455-7.

Gordon, E.M., Liu, P.X., Zhen, S.H., et al. (2000). Inhibition of metastatic tumor growth in nude mice by portal vein infusions of matrix-targeted retroviral vectors bearing a cytocidal cyclin G1 construct. *Cancer Res,* Vol. 60,3343-7.

Gordon, E.M., Liu, P.X., Chen, Z.H., et al. (2001). Systemic administration of a matrix-targeted retroviral vector is efficacious for cancer gene therapy in mice. *Hum Gene Ther,* Vol. 12,193-204.

Gordon, E.M., Zhu, N.L., Prescott, M.F., et al. (2001). Lesion-targeted injectable vectors for vascular restenosis. *Hum Gene Ther,* Vol. 12,1277-87.

Gordon, E.M., Hall, F.L., Beart, R.W. Jr., & Anderson, W.F. (2002). Genetic Engineering of Targeted Retroviral Vectors, In: *Vector Targeting for Therapeutic Gene Delivery,* Curiel, D.T., & Douglas, J.T., 293-320, Wiley-Liss, Inc.,New Jersey,USA.

Gordon, E.M., Cornelio, G.H., Lorenzo, C.C., et al. (2004). First clinical experience using a 'pathotropic' injectable retroviral vector (Rexin-G) as intervention for Stage IV pancreatic cancer. *Int J Oncol,* Vol. 24,177-85.

Gordon, E.M., & Hall, F.L. (2005). Nanotechnology blooms, at last (Review). *Oncol Reports,* Vol. 13,1003-7.

Gordon, E.M., Lopez, F.F., Cornelio, et al. (2006). Pathotropic nanoparticles for cancer gene therapy. Rexin-G™: Three-year clinical experience. *Int J Oncol,* Vol. 29,1053-64.

Gordon, E.M., & Hall, F.L. (2007). A Primer on Pathotropic Medicine, In: *Celebrating One Hundred Years of the Food and Drug Administration. A Special Centennial Edition,* 80-83, Brooklands New Media L.T.D., Oswestry, Shropshire, U.K.

Gordon, E.M., Chan, M.T., Geraldino, N., et al. (2007). Le morte du tumour: Histological features of tumor destruction in chemo-resistant cancers following intravenous infusions of pathotropic nanoparticles bearing therapeutic genes. *Int J Oncol,* Vol. 30,1297-307.

Gordon, E.M., Levy, J.P., Reed, R.A., et al. (2008). Targeting metastatic cancer from the inside: A new generation of targeted gene delivery vectors enables personalized cancer vaccination in situ. *Int J Oncol,*Vol.33,665-75.

Gordon, E.M., & Hall, F.L. (2009). The 'timely' development of Rexin-G: First targeted injectable gene vector (Review). Int J Oncol Vol. 35,229-38.

Gordon, E.M., & Hall, F.L. (2010). Rexin-G, a targeted genetic medicine for cancer. *Expert Opin Biol Ther,* Vol. 10,No. 5,819-32.

Gramantieri, L., Ferracin, M., Fornari, F., et al. (2007). Cyclin G1 is a Target of miR-122a, a MicroRNA Frequently Down-regulated in Human Hepatocellular Carcinoma. *Cancer Res,* Vol.67,No. 13,6092-9.

Greenman, C., Stephens, P., Smith, R., et al. (2007). Patterns of somatic mutation in human cancer genomes. *Nature,* Vol. 446,No. 7132,153-8.

Hall, F.L., & Vulliet, P.R. (1991). Proline-directed protein phosphorylation and cell cycle regulation. *Curr Opin Cell Biol,* Vol. 3,No. 2,176-84.

Hall, F.L., Liu, L., Zhu, N.L., et al. (2000). Molecular engineering of matrix-targeted retroviral vectors incorporating a surveillance function inherent in von Willebrand factor. *Hum Gene Ther,* Vol. 11,983-93.

Hall, F.L., Levy, J.P., Reed, R.A., et al. (2010). Pathotropic targeting advances clinical oncology: tumor-tartgeted localization of therapeutic gene delivery. *Oncol Rep.* Vol. 24,No. 4,829-33.

Han, X., Kasahara, N., & Kan, Y.W. (1995). Ligand-directed retroviral targeting of human breast cancer cells. *Proc Natl Acad Sci USA,*Vol. 92,No. 21,9747-51.

Harrop, R., Drury, N., Shingler, W., et al. (2007). Vaccination of colorectal cancer patients with modified vaccinia ankara encoding the tumor antigen 5T4 (Trovax) given alongside chemotherapy induces potent immune responses. *Clin Cancer Res,* Vol. 13,No. 15,4487-94.

Harrop, R., Drury, N., Shingler, W., et al. (2008). Vaccination of colorectal cancer patients with Trovax alongside chemotherapy (5-fluorouracil, leukovorin and irinotecan) is safe and induces potent immune responses. *Cancer Immunol Immunother,* Vol. 57,No. 7,977-86.

Hendrie, P.C., & Russell, D.W. (2005). Gene targeting with viral vectors. *Mol Ther,* Vol. 12,No. 1,9-17.

Huang, S., & He, X. The role of microRNAs in liver cancer progression. (2011). *Br J Cancer,* Vol. 104,No. 2,235-40.

Hughes, D.P.M. (2009). Strategies for the targeted delivery of therapeutics for osteosarcoma. *Expert Opinion on Drug Delivery,* Vol. 6,No. 12,1311-21.

Ignacio, J.G., Chawla, S.P., Manalo, R.E., et al. (2010). A Phase I/II Study of Intravenous Rexin-G and Reximmune-C for Cancer Immunotherapy: The GeneVieve Protocol. *J Clin Oncol,* Vol. 28 (May suppl; abstr 2546).

Jensen, M.R., Factor, V.M., Fantozzi, A., et al. (2003). Reduced hepatic tumor incidence in cyclin G1-deficient mice. *Hepatology,* Vol. 37,No. 4,862-70.

Johnson, N., & Shapiro, G.I. (2010). Cyclin-dependent kinases (cdks) and the DNA damage response: rationale for cdk inhibitor-chemotherapy combinations as an anticancer strategy for solid tumors. *Expert Opin Ther Targets,* Vol. 14, No. 11,1199-212.

Kan, O., Griffiths, L., Baban, D., et al. (2001). Direct retroviral delivery of human cytochrome P450 2B6 for gene-directed enzyme prodrug therapy of cancer. *Cancer Gene Ther,* Vol. 8,No. 7,473-82.

Karapetis, C.S., Khambata-Ford, S., Jonker, D.J., et al. (2008). K-ras mutations and benefit from cetuximab in advanced colorectal cancer. *N Engl J Med,* Vol. 359, No. 17,1757-65.

Kasahara, N., Dozy, A.M., & Kan, Y.W. (1994). Tissue-specific targeting of retroviral vectors through ligand-receptor interactions. *Science,* Vol. 266,No. 5189,1373-6.

Kimura, S.H., Ikawa, M., Ito, A., et al. (2001). Cyclin G1 is involved in G1/M arrest in response to DNA damage and in growth control after damage recovery. *Oncogene*, Vol. 20,No. 25,3290-300.

Kimura, S.H., & Nojima, H. (2002). Cyclin G1 associates with MDM2 and regulates accumulation and degradation of p53 protein. *Genes to Cells*, Vol. 7,869-80.

Krishnan, K., Khanna, C., & Helman,L.J. (2005). The biology of metastases in pediatric sarcomas. *Cancer J*, Vol.11,No.4,306-13.

Krystof, V., & Uldrijan, S. (2010). Cyclin-dependent kinase inhibitors as anticancer drugs. *Curr Drug Targets*, Vol. 1,No. 3,291-302.

Kwon, S.H., Park, J.C., Ramachandran, S., et al. (2008). Loss of cyclin g1 expression in human uterine leiomyoma induces apoptosis. *Reprod Sci*, Vol. 15,No. 4,400-10.

Lavillette, D., Russell, S.J., & Cosset, F.L. (2001). Retargeting gene delivery using surface-engineered retroviral vector particles. *Curr Opin Biotechnol*, Vol. 12,No. 5, 461-6.

Ley, T.J., Mardis, E.R., Ding, L., et al. (2008). DNA sequencing of a cytogenetically normal acute myeloid leukaemia genome. *Nature*, Vol.456,No.7218,66-72.

Lenz, H.J., Anderson, W.F., Hall, F.L., & Gordon, E.M. (2002). Clinical Protocol: Tumor site specific Phase I evaluation of safety and efficacy of hepatic arterial infusion of a matrix-targeted retroviral vector bearing a dominant negative cyclin G1 construct as intervention for colorectal carcinoma metastatic to liver. *Hum Gene Ther*, Vol. 13,1515-37.

Liu, T., Kirn, D. (2007). Systemic efficacy with oncolytic virus therapeutics: Clinical proof-of-concept and future directions. *Cancer Res*, Vol. 67,No. 2,429-32.

Ma, L., Liu, J., Shen, J., et al. (2010). Expression of miR-122 mediated by adenoviral vector induces apoptosis and cell cycle arrest of cancer cells. *Cancer Biol Ther*, Vol. 9,No. 7,554-61.

Maeda, M., Ampo, K., Kiryu-Seo, S., et al. (2005). The p53-independent nuclear translocation of cyclin G1 in degenerating neurons by ischemic and traumatic insults. *Exp Neurol*, Vol. 193,No. 2,350-60.

Malumbres, M. (2005). Revisiting the "Cdk-centric" view of the mammalian cell cycle. *Cell Cycle*, Vol. 4,No. 2,206-10.

Maretta, R.M., & Ales, F. (2010). Cancer cell(s) cycle sequencing reveals universal mechanisms of apoptosis. *Mol Cell Biomech*, Vol. 7,No. 4,225-66.

McDonald, E.R. III, & El-Deiry, W.S. (2000). Cell cycle control as a basis for cancer drug development (Review). *Int J Oncol*, Vol. 16,No. 5,871-86.

Moll, U.M., & Petrenko, O. (2003). The MDM2-p53 Interaction. *Mol Cancer Res*, Vol. 1,1001-8.

Morgan, D.O. (1997). Cyclin-dependent kinases: engines, clocks, and microprocessors. *Annu Rev Cell Dev Biol*, Vol. 13,261-91.

Morita, N., Kiryu, S., & Kiyama, H. (1996). p53-independent cyclin G expression in a group of mature neurons and its enhanced expression during nerve regeneration. *J Neurosci*, Vol. 16,No. 19,5961-5966.

Morse, M. (2005).Technology evaluation: Rexin-G, Epeius Biotechnologies. *Curr Opin Mol Ther*, Vol. 7,No. 2,164-9.

Nalluri, S.R., Chu, D., Keresztes, R., Zhu, X., & Wu, S. (2008). Risk of venous thromboembolism with the angiogenesis inhibitor bevacizumab in cancer patients: A meta-analysis. *JAMA*, Vol. 300,No. 19,2277-85.

Nieto, J., Grossbard, M.L., & Kozuch, P. (2008). Metastatic pancreatic cancer 2008: Is the glass less empty? *The Oncologist*, Vol. 13,562-76.

Noureddini, S.C., & Curiel, D.T. (2005). Genetic targeting strategies for adenovirus. *Mol Pharm*, Vol. 2,No. 5,341-7.

O'Day, K., & Gorlick, R. (2009). Novel therapeutic agents for osteosarcoma. *Expert Rev Anticancer Ther*, Vol. 9,No. 4,511-23.

Ohtsuka, T., Ryu, H., Minamishima, Y.A., et al. (2003). Modulation of p53 and p73 levels by Cyclin G: implications of a negative feedback regulation. *Oncogene*, Vol. 22,No. 11,1678-88.

Ohtsuka, T., Jensen, M.R., Kim, H.G., et al. (2004). The negative role of cyclin G in ATM-dependent p53 activation. *Oncogene*, Vol. 23,5405-8.

Okamoto, K., & Beach, D. (1994). Cyclin G is a transcriptional target of the p53 tumor suppressor protein. *EMBO J*, Vol. 13,No. 20,4816-22.

Peach, M.S., Kumbar, S.G., Brown, J.L., & Laurencin, C.T. (2009) *Current Bioactive Compounds*, Vol. 5, No. 3,170-184.

Peeper, D.S., Parker, L.L., Ewen, M.E., et al. (1993). A- and B-type cyclins differentially modulate substrate specificity of cyclin-cdk complexes. *EMBO J*, Vol. 12,No. 5, 1947-54.

Perez, R., Wu, N., Klipfel, A.A., & Beart, R.W, Jr. (2003). A better cell cycle target for gene therapy for colorectabl cancer: cyclin G. *Gastrointest Surg*, Vol. 7,No. 7,884-9.

Pines, J. (1995). Cyclins, CDKs and cancer. *Semin Cancer Biol*, Vol. 6,No. 2,63-72.

Piscopo, D.M., & Hinds, P.W. (2008). A Role for the Cyclin Box in the Ubiquitin-Mediated Degradation of Cyclin-G1. *Cancer Res*, Vol. 68,No. 14,5581-90.

Prestwich, R.J., Harrington, K.J., Pandha, H.S., et al. (2008). Oncolytic viruses: a novel form of immunotherapy. *Expert Rev Anticancer Ther*, Vol. 8,No. 10,1581-8.

Raponi, M., Winkler, Dracopoli, N.C. (2008). KRAS mutations predict response to EGFR inhibitors. *Curr Opin Pharmacol*, Vol. 8,No. 4,413-8.

Rayburn, E.R., Ezell, S.J., & Zhang, R. (2009). Recent advances in validating MDM2 as a cancer target. *Anticancer Agents Med Chem*, Vol. 9,No. 8,882-903.

Reimer, C.L., Borras, A.M., Kurdistani, S.K., et al. (1999). Altered regulation of cyclin G in human breast cancer and its specific localization at replication foci in response to DNA damage in p53+/+ cells. *J Biol Chem*, Vol. 274,No. 16,11022-9.

Richey, E.A., Lyons, E.A., Nebeker, J.R., et al. (2009). Accelerated approval of cancer drugs: improved access to therapeutic breakthroughs or early release of unsafe and ineffective drugs? *J Clin Oncol*, Vol. 27,No. 26,4398-405.

Roodhart, J.M., Langenberg, M.H., Witteveen, E., & Voest, E.E. (2008). The molecular basis of class side effects due to treatment with inhibitors of the VEGF/FEGFR pathway. *Curr Clin Pharmacol*, Vol. 3,No. 2,132-43.

Ryu, B.Y., Zavorotinskaya, T., Trentin, B., & Albritton, L.M. (2008). The block to membrane fusion differs with the site of ligand insertion in modified retroviral envelope proteins. *J Gen Virol*, Vol. 89,No. 4,1049-1058.

Sandrin, V., Russell, S.J., & Cosset, F.L. (2003). Targeting retroviral and lentiviral vectors. *Curr Top Microbiol Immunol*, Vol. 281,137-78.

Santamaria, D., & Ortega, S. (2006). Cyclins and CDKs in development and cancer: lessons from genetically modified mice. *Front Biosci*,V.11,1164-88.

Satyanarayana, A., & Kaldis, P. (2009). Mammalian cell-cycle regulation: several Cdks, numerous cyclins and diverse compensatory mechanisms. *Oncogene*, Vol. 28,No. 33,2925-39.

Scappaticci, F.A., Skillings, J.R., Holden, S.N., et al. (2007). Arterial thromboembolic events in patients with metastatic carcinoma treated with chemotherapy and bevacizumab. J *Natl Cancer Inst*, Vol. 99,No. 16,1232-9.

Schaffer, D.V., Koerber, J.T., & Lim, K.I. (2008). Molecular engineering of viral gene delivery vehicles. *Annu Rev Biomed Eng*, Vol. 10,169-94.

Schneider, B.P., Wang, M., Radovich, M., et al. (2008). Association of vascular endothelial growth factor and vascular endothelial growth factor receptor-2 genetic polymorphisms with outcome in a trial of paclitaxel compared with paclitaxel and bevacizumab in advanced breast cancer. *J Clin Oncol*, Vol. 26,No. 28,4672-8.

Schwartz, G.K., & Shah, M.A. (2005). Targeting the cell cycle: a new approach to cancer therapy. *J Clin Oncol*, Vol. 20,No. 36,9408-21.

Seo, H.R., Lee, D.H., Lee, H.J., et al. (2006). Cyclin G1 overcomes radiation-induced G2 arrest and increases cell death through transcriptional activation of cyclin G1. *Cell Death Differ*, Vol. 13,No. 9,1475-84.

Shapira, A., Livney, Y.D., Broxterman, H.J., & Assaraf, Y.G. (2011). Nanomedicine for targeted cancer therapy: Towards the overcoming of drug resistance. *Drug Resist Updat*, Feb 15 (Epub ahead of print).

Sherr, C.J., & McCormick, F. (2002). The RB and p53 pathways in cancer. *Cancer Cell*, Vol. 2,No. 2,103-12.

Siriam, V., & Patterson, C. (2001). Cell cycle in vasculoproliferative diseases: potential interventions and routes of delivery. *Circulation*, Vol. 103.No. 19,2414-19.

Skotzko, M., Wu, L., Anderson, W.F., et al. (1995). Retroviral Vector-mediated Gene Transfer of Antisense Cyclin G1 (CYCG1) Inhibits Proliferation of Human Osteogenic Sarcoma Cells. *Cancer Res*, Vol. 55,5493-8.

Smith, M.L., Knotny, H.U., Bortnick, R., & Fornace, A.J. Jr. (1997). The p53-regulated cyclin G promotes cell growth: p53 downstream effectors cyclin G and Gadd45 exert different effects on cisplatin chemosensitivity. *Exp Cell Res*, Vol. 230,No. 1,61-68.

Sreeramoju, P., & Libutti, S.K. (2010). Strategies for targeting tumors and tumor vasculature for cancer therapy. *Adv Genet*, Vol. 69,135-52.

Stathis, A., & Moore, M.J. (2010). Advanced pancreatic carcinoma: current treatment and future challenges. *Nat Rev Clin Oncol*, Vol. 7,No. 3,163-72.

Sugimoto, M., & Miyata, S. (2002). Functional property of von Willebrand factor under flowing blood. *Int J Hematol*, Vol. 75,No. 1,19-24.

Sverdlov, E.D. (2009). Not gene therapy, but genetic surgery - the right strategy to attack cancer. *Molecular Genetics*, Microbiology and Virology, Vol. 24,No. 3,93-113.

Tai,C.K., & Kasahara,N. (2008). Replication-competent retrovirus vectors for cancer gene therapy. *Front Biosci*, Vol.13,3083-95.

Taylor, R.A., & Risbridger, G.P. (2008). Prostatic tumor stroma: a key player in cancer progression. *Curr Cancer Drug Targets*, Vol. 8,No. 6,490-7.

Thorne, S.H. (2008). Oncolytic vaccinia virus: from bedside to benchtop and back. *Curr Opin Mol Ther*, Vol. 10,No. 4,387-92.

Toh, H.C. (2011). Providing Hope in Terminal Cancer: When is it Appropriate and When is it Not? *Ann Acad Med Singapore*, Vol. 40,50-55.

Tsai, W.C., Shu, P.W., Lai, T.C., et al. (2009). MicroRNA-122, a tumor suppressor microRNA that regulates intrahepatic metastasis of hepatocellular carcinoma. *Hepatology*, Vol. 49,No. 5, 1571-82.

Valsamakis, A., Auwaerter, P.G., Rima, B.K., et al. (1999). Altered virulence of vaccine strains of measles virus after prolonged replication in human tissue. *J Virol*, Vol. 73,No. 10,8791-7.

Verma, N., & Swain, S.M. (2011). Bevacizumab and heart failure risk in patients with breast cancer: a thorn in the side? *J Clin Oncol*, Vol. 29,No. 6,603-6.

Viallard, J.F., Lacombe, F., Belloc, F., et al. (2001). [Molecular mechanisms controlling the cell cycle: fundamental aspects and implications for oncology]. [Article in French]. *Cancer Radiother*, Vol. 5,No. 2,109-29.

Vile, R., Ando, D., & Kirn, D. (2002). The oncolytic virotherapy treatment platform for cancer: Unique biological and biosafety points to consider. *Cancer Gene Ther*, Vol. 9,1062-7.

Waehler, R., Russel, S.J., & Curiel, D.T. (2007). Engineering targeted viral vectors for gene therapy. *Nat Rev Genet*, Vol. 8,No. 8,573-87.

Wesierska-Gadek, J., Maurer, M., Zulehner, N., & Komina, O. (2011). Whether to target single or multiple CDKs for therapy? That is the question. *J Cell Physiol*, Vol. 226,No. 2,341-9.

Witlox, M.A., Lamfers, M.L., Wuisman, P.I., et al. (2007). Evolving gene therapy approaches for osteosarcoma using viral vectors: review. *Bone*, Vol. 40,No. 4,797-812.

Wong, D., Hwang, J., Venook, A.P., et al. (2008). Serum CA19-9 decline compared to radiographic response as a surrogate for clinical outcomes in patients with metastatic pancreatic cancer receiving chemotherapy. *Pancreas*, Vol. 37,269-74.

Wood, L.D., Parsons, W., Jones, S., Lin, J., Sjoblom, T., Leary, R.J., Shen, D., Boca, S.M., Barber, T., Ptak, J., & Silliman, N., et al. (2007). The genomic landscapes of human breast and colorectal cancers. *Science*, Vol. 318,No. 5853,1108-13.

Wu, L., Liu, L., Yee, A., et al. (1994). Molecular Cloning of the human CYCG1 gene encoding a G-type cyclin: overexpression in osteosarcoma cells. *Oncol Rep*, Vol. 1,705-11.

Wu, X., Wu, S., Tong, L., et al. (2009). miR-122 affects the viability and apoptosis of hepatocellular carcinoma cells. *Gastroenterol*, Vol. 44,No. 11,1332-9.

Xu, F., Prescott, M.F., Liu, P.X., et al. (2001). Long term inhibition of neointima formation in balloon-injured rat arteries by intraluminal instillation of a matrix-targeted retroviral vector bearing a cytocidal mutant cyclin G1 construct. *Int J Mol Med*, Vol. 8,No. 1,19-30.

Zhang, Z., Wang, H., Li, M., et al. (2005). Novel MDM2 p53-independent functions identified through RNA silencing technologies. *Ann N Y Acad Sci*, Vol. 1058,205-14.

Zhang, Y., & Chatterjee, D.K. (2006). Liposomes, Dendrimers and other Polymeric Nanoparticles for Targeted Delivery of Anticancer Agents - a Comparative Study, In: *Nanomaterials for Cancer Therapy*, Chalia, S., Kumar, S.R., 338-70, Wiley-VCH Verlag GmbH & Company, KGaA, Weinheim.

Zhao, L., Samuels, T., Winckler, S., et al. (2003). Cyclin G1 has growth inhibitory activity linked to the ARF-Mdm2-p53 and pRb tumor suppressor pathways. *Mol Cancer Res*, Vol. 1,No. 3,195-206.

Zhu, N.L., Wu, L., Liu, P.X., et al. (1997). Downregulation of cyclin G1 expression by retrovirus-mediated antisense gene transfer inhibits vascular smooth muscle cell proliferation and neointima formation. *Circulation,* Vol. 96,No. 2,628-35.

Zolnick, B.S., Gonzales-Fernandez, A., Sadriah, N., & Dobrovolskaia, M.A. (2010). *Endocrinology,* Vol. 151,458-65.